Best of Incredibly Easy!®

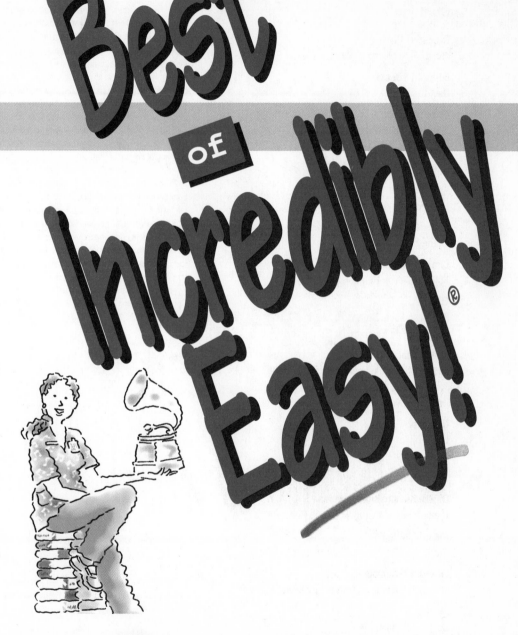

LIPPINCOTT WILLIAMS & WILKINS
A **Wolters Kluwer** Company

Philadelphia • Baltimore • New York • London
Buenos Aires • Hong Kong • Sydney • Tokyo

Staff

Executive Publisher
Judith A. Schilling McCann, RN, MSN

Editorial Director
David Moreau

Clinical Director
Joan M. Robinson, RN, MSN

Senior Art Director
Arlene Putterman

Art Director
Mary Ludwicki

Editorial Project Manager
Jaime Stockslager Buss

Clinical Project Manager
Collette Bishop Hendler, RN, BS, CCRN

Editors
Rita Breedlove, Brenna H. Mayer,
Julia VanTine Reichert, Liz Schaeffer

Copy Editors
Kimberly Bilotta (supervisor), Scotti Cohn,
Tom DeZego, Amy Furman, Shana Harrington,
Kelly Pavlovsky, Pamela Wingrod

Designer
Lynn Foulk

Illustrator
Bot Roda

Digital Composition Services
Diane Paluba (manager), Joyce Rossi Biletz

Manufacturing
Patricia K. Dorshaw (director), Beth J. Welsh

Editorial Assistants
Megan L. Aldinger, Karen J. Kirk, Linda K. Ruhf

Indexer
Barbara Hodgson

BESTIE010905 — D N O S
07 06 05   10 9 8 7 6 5 4 3 2 1

Library of Congress Cataloging-in-Publication Data
Best of incredibly easy.
    p. ; cm.
    Includes bibliographical references and index.
    1. Nursing — Handbooks, manuals, etc. I. Lippincott Williams
        & Wilkins.
    [DNLM: 1. Nursing Care — methods — Handbooks. WY 49
    B561 2006]
RT51.B42 2006
610.73 — dc22
ISBN 1-58255-446-3 (alk. paper)   2005015697

Contents

Contributors and consultants

Joanne M. Bartelmo, RN, MSN
Independent Consultant
Pottstown, Pa.

Betsy Baumgartner, RN, BA, BSN
Staff Nurse
Massachusetts General Hospital
Boston

Kim Cooper, RN, MSN
Nursing Department Chair
Ivy Tech State College
Terre Haute, Ind.

Lisa Cozier, RN
Staff Nurse
Cambria Heights, N.Y.

James Davis IV, RN, BSN
Clinical Leader ICU
Abington (Pa.) Memorial Hospital

Pamela Kovach, RN, BSN
Independent Consultant
Perkiomenville, Pa.

Monica Narvaez Ramirez, RN, MSN
Faculty
University of the Incarnate Word
School of Nursing and Health Professions
San Antonio, Tex.

Susan Riley, RN,C
Clinical Nurse IV
North Bay Medical Center
Fairfield, Calif.

Tracey J. Siegel, RN, MSN, APN,BC, CWOCN
Faculty
Charles E. Gregory School of Nursing
Perth Amboy, N.J.

INCREDIBLY EASY'S
GREATEST HITS

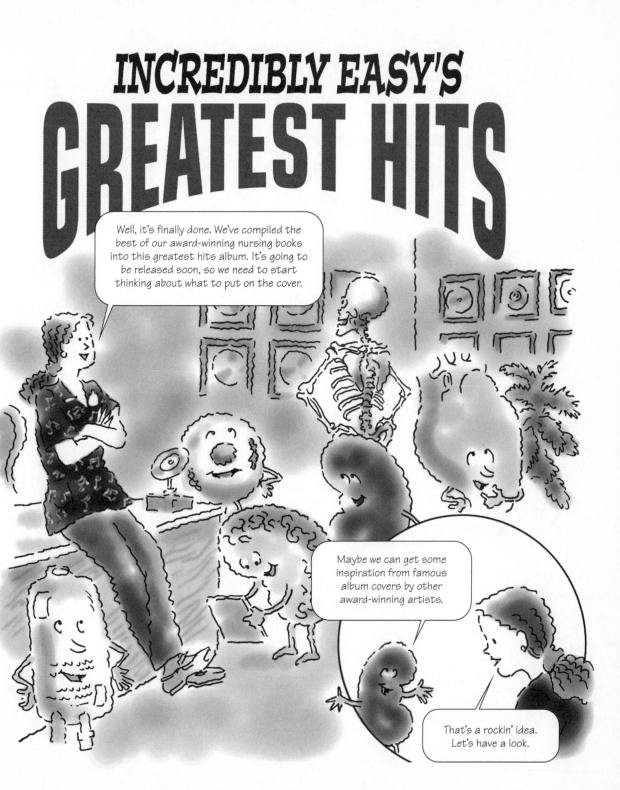

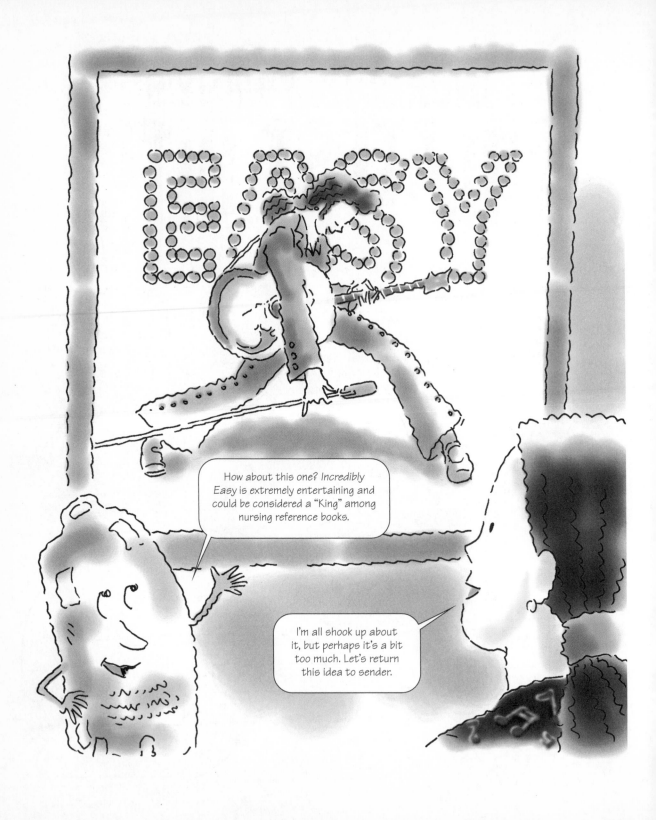

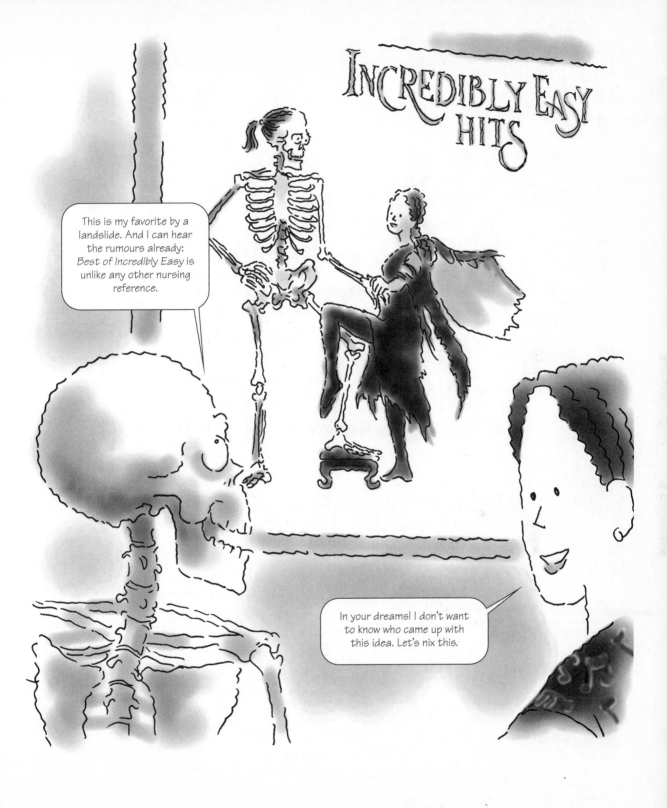

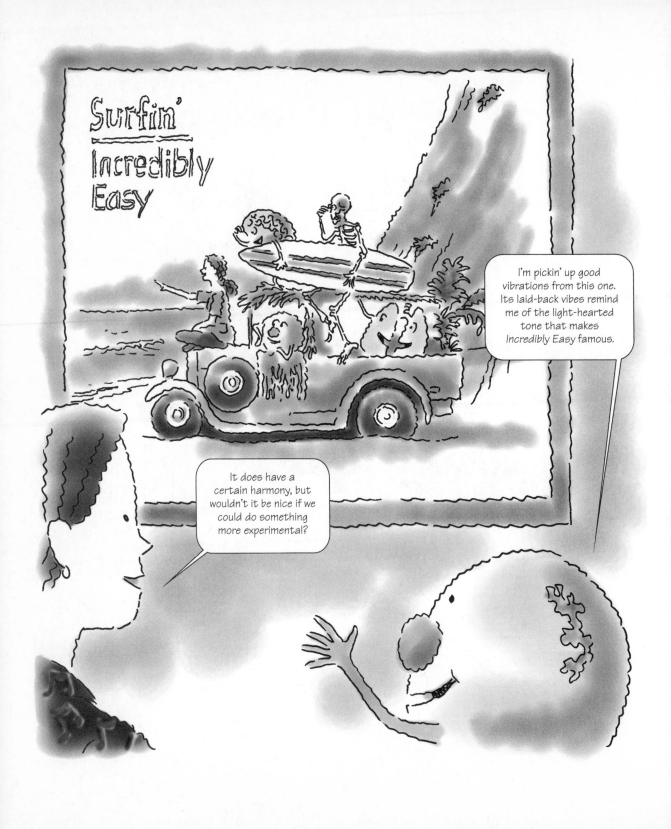

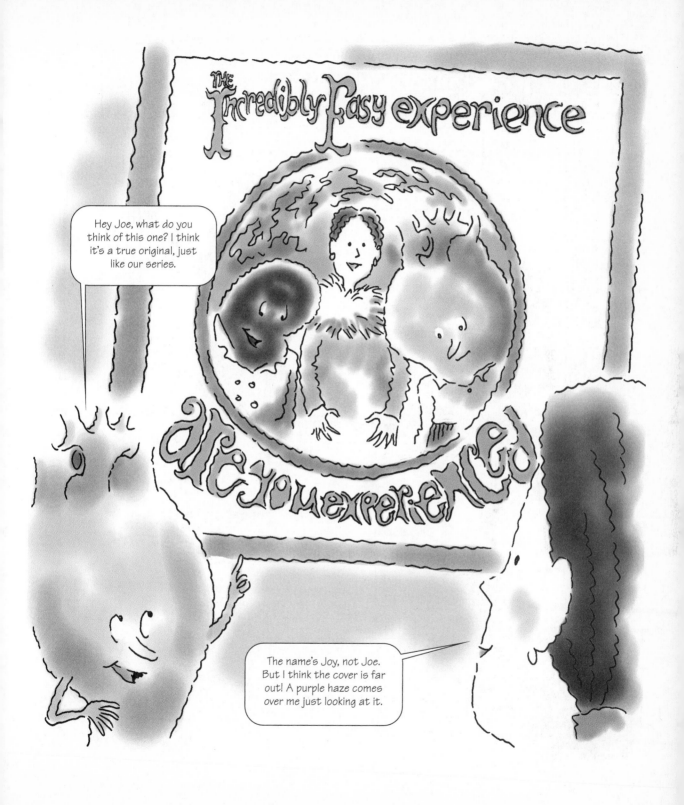

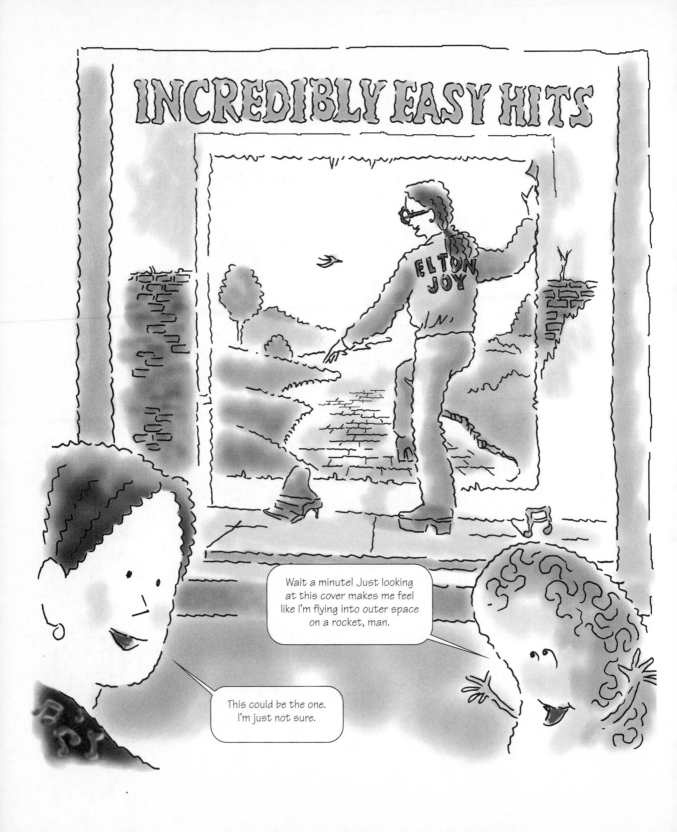

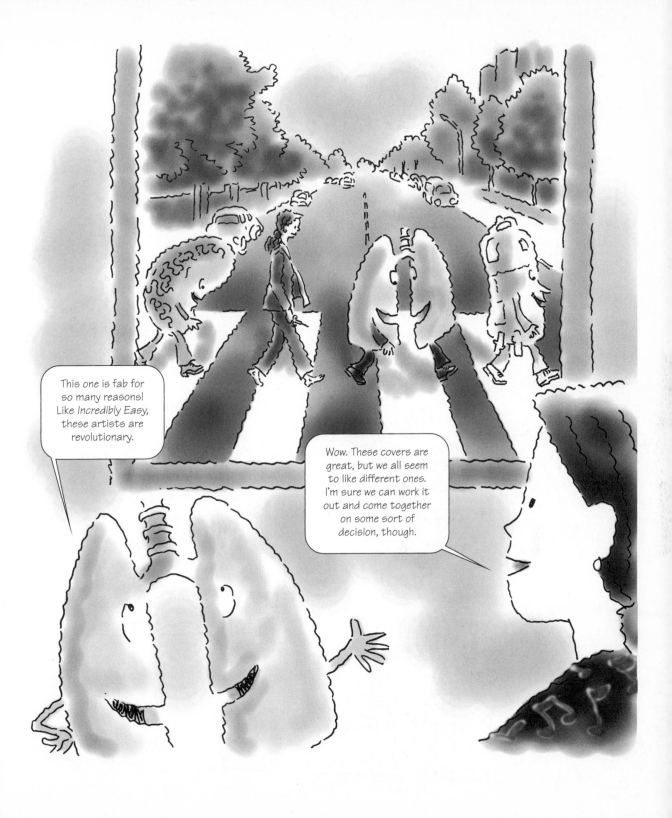

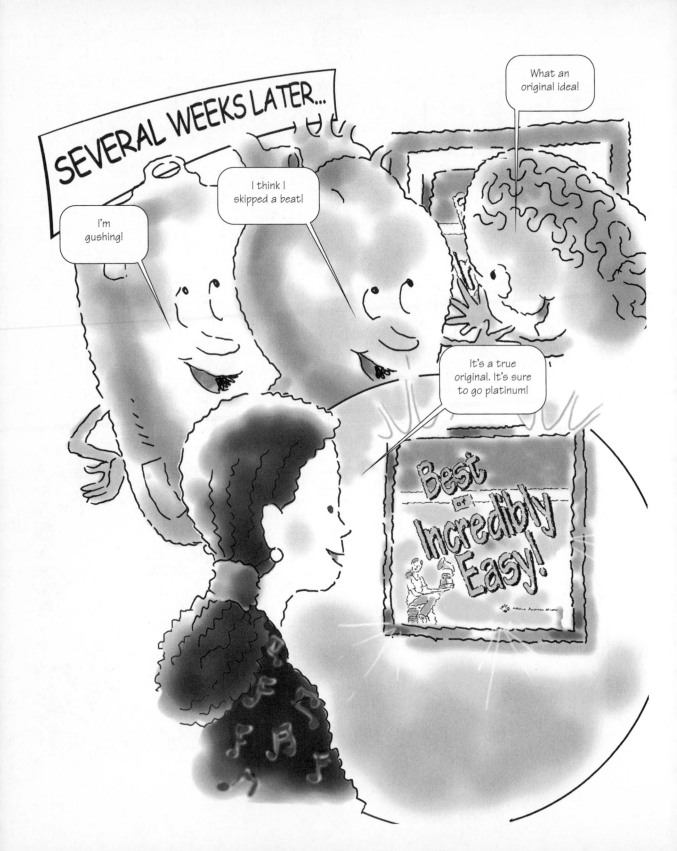

Health assessment

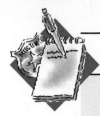

Just the facts

In this chapter, you'll learn:

♦ strategies to aid you in interviewing and obtaining a detailed health history from a patient

♦ questions to ask that pertain to each body system

♦ assessment techniques, including inspection, palpation, percussion, and auscultation.

Obtaining a health history

Any health assessment involves collecting a health history, including objective and subjective data:

• *Objective data* are obtained through observation and are verifiable. For example, if the patient seeks care for a rash, you can verify this complaint by looking at the rash. Therefore, the rash is objective data.

• *Subjective data* are obtained solely from the patient and can't be verified by anyone else. For example, if the patient tells you he has back pain, that information is subjective data because it's something that only he can verify.

> Take a moment to set the stage before taking the health history. A supportive, encouraging approach will make your patient feel much more at ease.

Beginning the interview

The way you conduct the interview can help set the patient at ease, which in turn can help you get the information you need. Here's how to make the most of an interview:

• Choose a quiet, private, well-lit area to help the patient feel more at ease.

• Make sure that the patient is comfortable. Sit facing him, 3′ to 4′ (1 to 1.5 m) away.

• Introduce yourself and then explain that the purpose of the health history and assessment is to identify key problems and gather information to help plan his care.
• Reassure the patient that everything he says will be kept confidential.
• Use touch sparingly. Many people aren't comfortable when strangers hug, pat, or touch them.

Watch what you say

• Assess the patient to see whether language barriers exist. Can he hear you? (See *Overcoming interviewing obstacles.*)
• Speak slowly and clearly, and use language that's easy to understand. Avoid medical terms and jargon.
• Address the patient formally—for example, "Mr. Jones." Don't use his first name unless he asks you to.

Communication strategies

You'll also want to use various strategies to make sure you communicate effectively.

Nonverbal communication strategies

Keep in mind that you and the patient communicate nonverbally as well as verbally. These tips can help you make effective use of nonverbal communication:

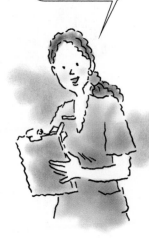

Reassure the patient that what he tells you will be kept confidential.

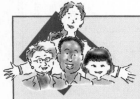

Bridging the gap

Overcoming interviewing obstacles

With a little ingenuity, you can conquer barriers to interviewing. For example, if a patient doesn't speak English, your facility may have a bank of interpreters you can call on for help. A trained medical interpreter—who's familiar with medical terminology, knows interpreting techniques, and understands the patient's rights—would be ideal. Be sure to tell the interpreter to translate the patient's speech verbatim.

Avoid using one of the patient's family members or friends as an interpreter. Doing so would violate the patient's right to confidentiality.

Breaking the sound barrier
Is your patient hearing impaired? You can overcome this barrier, too. First, make sure the light is bright enough for him to see your lips move. Then face him and speak slowly and clearly. If necessary, have the patient use an assistive device, such as a hearing aid or an amplifier. If the patient uses sign language, see whether your facility has a sign-language interpreter.

• Listen attentively and make eye contact frequently. (See *Overcoming cultural barriers*.)
• To encourage the patient to keep talking, nod your head or use other reassuring gestures, such as motioning with your hands for him to continue and maintaining eye contact.
• Watch for nonverbal clues, such as wringing of the hands, restlessness, and inability to maintain eye contact, that indicate the patient is uncomfortable or unsure about how to answer a question.
• Be aware of your own nonverbal behaviors, such as watching the clock, folding your arms, and making facial expressions, that might cause the patient to stop talking or become defensive.
• Observe the patient closely to see whether he understands each question. If he doesn't appear to understand, repeat the question using different words or familiar examples.

Verbal communication strategies

Verbal communication strategies include using open-ended and closed questions as well as such techniques as silence, facilitation, confirmation, reflection, clarification, summary, and conclusion:
• Asking *open-ended questions* lets the patient respond more freely. An example of an open-ended question is, "Why did you come to the emergency department today?" Questioning in this manner allows the patient to answer however he wishes.
• You may also choose to ask *closed-ended questions*. They may encourage the patient to give clear, concise feedback. An example of a closed question is, "Do you ever get headaches?" This question encourages the patient to give a one- or two-word response so you can quickly focus on a specific point.
• Allow moments of *silence* during the interview. Besides encouraging the patient to continue talking, this strategy also gives you a chance to assess his ability to organize thoughts.
• Using such phrases as "please continue" or "go on" encourages the patient to continue with his story. This technique is known as *facilitation*.
• *Confirmation* helps ensure that you and the patient are on the same track. Repeat the information the patient gives to help clear up misconceptions that you or he might have.
• Try using *reflection* — repeating something the patient has just said — to help you obtain more specific information. For example, a patient with a stomachache might say, "I know I have an ulcer." If so, you can repeat, "You know you have an ulcer?" Then the patient might say, "Yes. I had one before, and the pain is the same."
• When the patient gives vague or confusing information, use the technique of *clarification*. For example, if the patient says, "I can't stand this," your response might be, "What can't you stand?" Doing so gives the patient an opportunity to explain his statement.

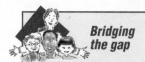

Bridging the gap

Overcoming cultural barriers

To maintain a good relationship with your patient, remember that his cultural behaviors and beliefs may differ from your own. For example, most people in the United States make eye contact when they talk with others. However, people in several other cultures—including Native Americans, Asians, and people from Arabic-speaking countries—may find eye contact disrespectful or aggressive.

• Restating the information the patient gave you, known as *summarization*, ensures that the data you've collected is accurate and complete. Doing so also signals that the interview is about to end.
• Indicate to the patient when you're ready to conclude the interview (*conclusion*). You can do this by saying, "I believe I have all of the information I need right now. Is there anything you want to add before I leave?" Doing so gives him the opportunity to gather his thoughts and make any pertinent final statements.

Questions to ask

A complete health history requires information from each of the following categories, obtained in this order:

 biographic data

 chief complaint

 medical history

 family history

 psychosocial history

 activities of daily living (ADLs).

Biographic data

Ask the patient for his name, address, telephone number, birth date, age, marital status, religion, and nationality. Find out with whom he lives, and get the name and telephone number of a person to contact in case of an emergency.

Also ask the patient about his health care, including the name of his primary doctor. Ask whether he has ever been treated for his current problem. Finally, ask whether he has prepared advance directives — documents that state his wishes about his health in the event of his physical or mental incapacitation. (See *Advance directives.*) If he can't furnish accurate information, ask him for the name of a friend or relative who can. Document the source of the information as well as whether an interpreter was needed.

Chief complaint

Ask the patient his primary health concern, also known as the *chief complaint.* Document this information in the patient's exact words to avoid misinterpretation. Ask how and when the symptoms developed, what led the patient to seek medical attention, and how the problem has affected his life and ability to function.

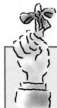

Memory jogger

To remember the categories you should cover in your health history, think, "Being Complete Makes For Proper Assessment:"

Biographic data

Chief complaint

Medical history

Family history

Psychosocial history

Activities of daily living.

Advance directives

The Patient Self-Determination Act allows patients to prepare advance directives, which are written documents that state their wishes regarding health care in the event they become incapacitated or unable to make decisions. Elderly patients in particular may have interest in advance directives because they tend to be concerned with end-of-life issues.

Direction for directives

If a patient doesn't have an advance directive in place, the health care facility must provide him with information about it, including how to establish one.

An advance directive may include:
• the name of the person authorized by the patient to make medical decisions if the patient can no longer do so
• specific medical treatment the patient wants or doesn't want
• instructions regarding pain medication and comfort—specifically, whether the patient wishes to receive certain treatment even if the treatment may hasten his death
• information the patient wants to relay to his loved ones
• the name of the patient's primary health care provider
• any other wishes.

Medical history

Ask the patient about past and current medical problems. Typical questions include:
• Have you ever been hospitalized? If so, when and why?
• What childhood illnesses did you have?
• Are you being treated for any problem? If so, what's the problem? What's your doctor's name?
• Have you ever had surgery? If so, when and why?
• Are you allergic to any drugs, foods, or anything in the environment? If so, what kind of allergic reaction do you have?
• Do you take any medications, including over-the-counter preparations? If so, how much do you take and how often do you take it? Do you use home remedies, herbal preparations, or dietary supplements?
• Do you use other alternative or complementary therapies?

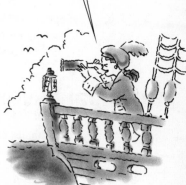

The health history explores the patient's past and present problems.

Family history

The patient's family history can provide information about his risk for certain illnesses. Typical questions include:

• Are your mother, father, and siblings living? If not, how old were they when they died? What were the causes of their deaths?
• If they're living, do they have diabetes, high blood pressure, heart disease, asthma, cancer, sickle cell anemia, hemophilia, cataracts, glaucoma, or other illnesses?

Psychosocial history

For the psychosocial history, ask the patient about his occupation (past and current), education, economic status, and responsibilities. Also ask these questions:
• How have you coped with medical or emotional crises in the past?
• Has your life changed recently? What changes in your personality or behavior have you noticed?
• How adequate is the emotional support you receive from family and friends?
• How close do you live to health care facilities? Can you get to them easily?
• Do you have health insurance?
• Are you on a fixed income?

Activities of daily living

Assess ADLs by asking the patient to describe his typical day. Make sure you ask about:
• appetite, special diets, and food allergies
• exercise habits
• sleep habits, including the number of hours he sleeps at night, what his sleep pattern is like, and whether he feels rested after sleep
• leisure activities and hobbies
• smoking habits (how many cigarettes or cigars per day)
• alcohol intake (amount per day)
• use of illicit drugs, such as marijuana and cocaine, and if so, frequency of use
• religious beliefs that could affect diet, dress, or health practices.

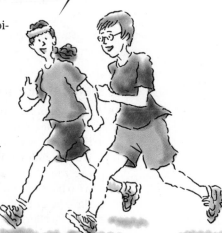

Your patient's daily activities, such as exercise habits, can reveal important information about her health.

Physical assessment

During the physical assessment, you'll use all of your senses and a systematic approach to collect information about the patient's health. An initial assessment guides your entire care plan.

Collecting the tools

Before you start a physical assessment, collect the necessary tools, including cotton balls, gloves, an ophthalmoscope, an otoscope, a penlight, a percussion hammer, safety pins, and a stethoscope.

Two heads are better than one

Use a stethoscope with a diaphragm and a bell. The diaphragm has a flat, thin, plastic surface that picks up high-pitched sounds such as breath sounds. The bell has a smaller, open end that picks up low-pitched sounds, such as third and fourth heart sounds.

All the better to see you with...

You'll need a penlight to illuminate the inside of the patient's nose and mouth, cast tangential light on lesions, and evaluate pupillary reactions. An ophthalmoscope enables you to examine the internal structures of the eye; an otoscope, the external auditory canal and tympanic membrane.

Other tools include cotton balls and safety pins to test sensation and pain differentiation, a percussion hammer to evaluate deep tendon reflexes, and gloves to protect the patient and you.

Preparing the patient

Before you start the assessment, briefly explain what you plan to do and why, how long it will take, what position changes it will require, and what equipment you'll use. As you perform the assessment, explain each step in detail. Document your findings up to this point in a concise paragraph.

Factor in his feelings

Keep in mind that the patient may be worried that you'll find a problem. He may also consider the assessment an invasion of his privacy because you're observing and touching sensitive, private and, perhaps, painful body areas.

Obtaining vital signs

Accurate measurements of the patient's vital signs provide critical information about body functions. The first time you assess a patient, record his baseline vital signs and statistics.

Body temperature

Body temperature is measured in degrees Fahrenheit (F) or degrees Celsius (C). Normal body temperature ranges from 96.7° to 100.5° F (35.9° to 38.1° C), depending on the route used for measurement.

Hyperthermia describes an oral temperature above 106° F (41.1° C); hypothermia, a rectal temperature below 95° F (35° C). (See *How temperature readings compare*.)

Pulse

To assess the pulse, palpate one of the patient's arterial pulse points and note its rate, rhythm, and amplitude. A normal pulse for an adult is between 60 and 100 beats/minute. The radial pulse is the most accessible. However, in cardiovascular emergencies, you may palpate for the femoral or carotid pulses. Normal pulse rate ranges between 100 and 190 beats/minute in infants and between 80 and 125 beats/minute in children. (See *Pinpointing pulse sites*.)

Feeling the beat

To palpate for a pulse, use the pads of your index and middle fingers. Press the area over the artery until you feel pulsations. If the rhythm is regular, count the beats for 30 seconds and then multiply by 2 to get the number of beats per minute. If the rhythm is irregular or the patient has a pacemaker, count the beats for 1 minute. When you take the pulse for the first time (or when you obtain baseline data), count the beats for 1 minute.

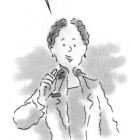

A normal pulse for an adult is between 60 and 100 beats/minute.

How temperature readings compare

You can take your patient's temperature in four ways. The chart below describes each method.

Method	Normal temperature	Used with
Oral	97.7° to 99.5° F (36.5° to 37.5° C)	Adults and older children who are awake, alert, oriented, and cooperative
Axillary (armpit)	96.7° to 98.5° F (35.9° to 36.9° C)	Infants, young children, and patients with impaired immune systems when infection is a concern
Rectal	98.7° to 100.5° F (37.1° to 38.1° C)	Infants, young children, and confused or unconscious patients
Tympanic (ear)	98.2° to 100° F (36.8° to 37.8° C)	Adults and children, conscious and cooperative patients, and confused or unconscious patients

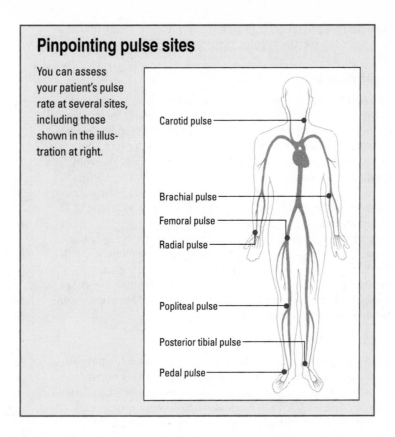

Pinpointing pulse sites

You can assess your patient's pulse rate at several sites, including those shown in the illustration at right.

Carotid pulse

Brachial pulse

Femoral pulse

Radial pulse

Popliteal pulse

Posterior tibial pulse

Pedal pulse

Off beat

When you note an irregular pulse:
• Evaluate whether the irregularity follows a pattern.
• Auscultate the apical pulse while palpating the radial pulse. You should feel the pulse every time you hear a heartbeat.
• Measure the difference between the apical pulse rate and radial pulse rate. This measurement, called the *pulse deficit,* indirectly evaluates the ability of each cardiac contraction to eject sufficient blood into the peripheral circulation.

Leaps and bounds

You must also assess the pulse amplitude. To do so, use a numerical scale or descriptive term to rate or characterize the strength. The following scale is commonly used:
• *absent pulse* — not palpable, measured as 0
• *weak* or *thready pulse* — hard to feel, easily obliterated by slight finger pressure, measured as +1
• *normal pulse* — easily palpable, obliterated by strong finger pressure, measured as +2

• *bounding pulse* — readily palpable, forceful, not easily obliterated by pressure from the fingers, measured as +3.

Respirations

As you count respirations, be aware of the depth and rhythm of each breath. To determine the respiratory rate, count the number of respirations for 60 seconds. A rate of 16 to 20 breaths/minute is normal for an adult. If the patient knows you're counting how often he breathes, he may unintentionally alter the rate. To avoid this, take his respirations while you take his pulse. The normal respiratory rate for an infant ranges between 30 and 80 breaths/minute depending on the age of the infant; for a child, a rate of 15 to 30 breaths/minute is considered normal.

Pay attention as well to the depth of the patient's respirations by watching his chest rise and fall. Is his breathing shallow, moderate, or deep? Observe the symmetry of his chest wall as it expands during inspiration and relaxes during expiration. Be aware that skeletal deformity, broken ribs, and collapsed lung tissue can cause unequal chest expansion.

Accessory to the act...of breathing

Watch for accessory muscle use, which can enhance lung expansion when oxygenation drops. Patient position during normal breathing may also suggest such problems as chronic obstructive pulmonary disease (COPD). Normal respirations are quiet and easy, so note any abnormal sounds, such as wheezing and stridor.

Blood pressure

Blood pressure measurements consist of systolic and diastolic readings. The systolic reading reflects the maximum pressure exerted on the arterial wall at the peak of left ventricular contraction. Normal systolic pressure ranges from 100 to 119 mm Hg. The diastolic reading reflects the minimum pressure exerted on the arterial wall during left ventricular relaxation. Normal diastolic pressure ranges from 60 to 79 mm Hg. Generally speaking, this reading is more significant than the systolic reading because it evaluates arterial pressure when the heart is at rest. (See *Blood pressure variations*.)

Unpronounceable and indispensable

The *sphygmomanometer*, a device used to measure blood pressure, consists of an inflatable cuff, a pressure manometer, and a bulb with a valve. To record a blood pressure, the cuff is centered over an artery, inflated, and deflated. As the cuff deflates, listen with a stethoscope for Korotkoff's sounds, which indicate the systolic and diastolic pressures. Blood pressure can be measured

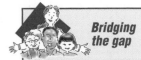

Bridging the gap

Blood pressure variations

Blood pressure may vary depending on the patient's race or sex. For example, black women tend to have higher systolic blood pressures than white women, regardless of age. Furthermore, after age 45, the average blood pressure of black women is almost 16 mm Hg higher than that of white women in the same age-group.

With this statistic in mind, carefully monitor the blood pressures of your black female patients, being alert for signs of hypertension. Early detection and treatment — combined with lifestyle changes — can help prevent such complications as stroke and kidney disease.

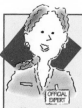

Advice from the experts

Tips for hearing Korotkoff's sounds

If you have difficulty hearing Korotkoff's sounds, try to intensify them by increasing vascular pressure below the cuff. Here are two techniques.

Raise an arm

Palpate the brachial pulse and mark its location with a pen to avoid losing the pulse spot. Apply the cuff and have the patient raise his arm above his head. Then inflate the cuff about 30 mm Hg above the patient's systolic pressure. Have him lower his arm until the cuff reaches heart level. Then deflate the cuff and take a reading.

Make a fist

Position the patient's arm at heart level. Inflate the cuff to 30 mm Hg above the patient's systolic pressure and ask him to make a fist. Have him rapidly open and close his hand approximately 10 times. Then deflate the cuff and take a reading.

from most extremity pulse points. The brachial artery is used for most patients because of its accessibility. (See *Tips for hearing Korotkoff's sounds*.)

Physical assessment techniques

No matter where you start your physical assessment, you'll use four techniques:

 inspection

 palpation

 percussion

 auscultation.

Abdominal exception

Use these techniques in sequence except when you perform an abdominal assessment. Because palpation and percussion can alter bowel sounds, the sequence for assessing the abdomen is inspection, auscultation, percussion, and palpation.

Inspection

Inspect the patient using vision, smell, and hearing to observe normal conditions and deviations. Performed correctly, inspection

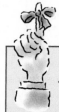

Memory jogger

To remember the order in which you should perform assessment of most systems, think, "I'll **P**roperly **P**erform **A**ssessment":

Inspection

Palpation

Percussion

Auscultation.

can reveal more than other techniques. As you assess each body system, observe for color, size, location, movement, texture, symmetry, odors, and sounds.

Palpation

Palpation requires you to touch the patient with different parts of your hands, using varying degrees of pressure. To do so, you need short fingernails and warm hands. Always palpate tender areas last. Tell the patient the purpose of your touch and what you're feeling. (See *Types of palpation*.)

Check out these features

As you palpate each body system, evaluate the following features:
- *texture* — rough or smooth?
- *temperature* — warm, hot, or cold?
- *moisture* — dry, wet, or moist?
- *motion* — still or vibrating?
- *consistency of structures* — solid or fluid-filled?
- *patient response* — any pain or tenderness?

Types of palpation

The two types of palpation, light and deep, provide different types of assessment information.

Light palpation
Perform light palpation to feel for surface abnormalities. Depress the skin ½" to ¾" (1 to 2 cm) with your finger pads, using the lightest touch possible. Assess for texture, tenderness, temperature, moisture, elasticity, pulsations, superficial organs, and masses.

Deep palpation
Deep palpation is used to feel internal organs and masses for size, shape, tenderness, symmetry, and mobility. Depress the skin 1½" to 2" (4 to 5 cm) with firm, deep pressure. If necessary, use one hand on top of the other to exert firmer pressure.

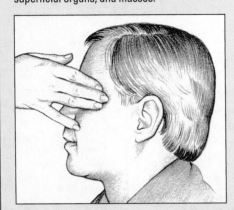
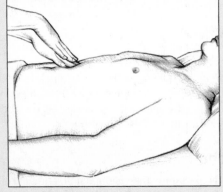

Percussion

Percussion involves tapping your fingers or hands quickly and sharply against parts of the patient's body, usually the chest or abdomen. The technique helps you locate organ borders, identify organ shape and position, and determine whether an organ is solid or filled with fluid or gas. (See *Types of percussion.*)

As you percuss, move gradually from areas of resonance to those of dullness and then compare sounds. Also, compare sounds on one side of the body with those on the other side.

Auscultation

Auscultation, usually the last step, involves listening for various breath, heart, and bowel sounds with a stethoscope. To prevent the spread of infection among patients, clean the heads and end pieces of the stethoscope with alcohol or a disinfectant before each use.

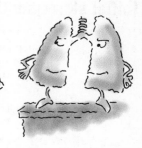

Go ahead and percuss me. I think you'll find that I'm rarely dull and I really resonate!

Types of percussion

You can perform percussion using the direct or indirect method.

Direct percussion

Direct percussion reveals tenderness. Using one or two fingers, tap directly on the body part. Ask the patient to tell you which areas are painful, and watch his face for signs of discomfort. This technique is commonly used to assess an adult patient's sinuses for tenderness.

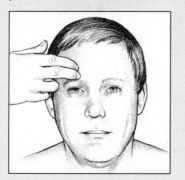

Indirect percussion

Indirect percussion elicits sounds that give clues to the makeup of the underlying tissue. Press the distal part of the middle finger of your nondominant hand firmly on the body part. Keep the rest of your hand off the body surface. Flex the wrist of your dominant hand. Using the middle finger of your dominant hand, tap quickly and directly over the point where your other middle finger touches the patient's skin. Listen to the sounds produced.

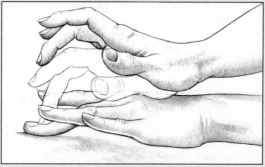

Assessing the skin

The skin covers the internal structures of the body and protects them from the external world. You might think of the skin as a "window" through which you can view changes taking place inside the body.

Initial skin questions

Most complaints about the skin involve itching, rashes, lesions, pigmentation abnormalities, or changes in existing lesions. Typical questions to ask about changes in a patient's skin include:
• How and when did your skin changes occur?
• Are the changes in the form of a skin rash or lesion?
• Is the change confined to one area, or has the condition spread?
• Does the area bleed or have drainage?
• Does the area itch?
• How much time do you spend in the sun, and how do you protect your skin from ultraviolet rays?
• Do you have allergies?
• Do you have a family history of skin cancer or other significant diseases?
• Do you have a fever or joint pain, or have you lost weight?
• Have you had a recent insect bite?
• Do you take any over-the-counter or prescription medications or herbal preparations? If so, which ones?
• What changes in your skin have you observed in the past few years?

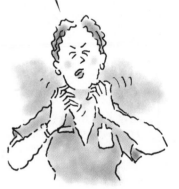

I'm itching to ask my patients about skin conditions.

Inspecting and palpating the skin

To assess the skin, you'll use the techniques of inspection and palpation, focusing on color, texture, turgor, moisture, and temperature. Gather the necessary equipment, including a clear ruler with centimeter and millimeter markings, tongue blade, penlight or flashlight, and magnifying glass. Wear gloves during your examination.

Color

Look for localized areas of bruising, cyanosis, pallor, and erythema. Check for uniformity of color and hypopigmented or hyperpigmented areas. Color changes may vary depending on skin pigmentation. (See *Detecting color variations in dark-skinned people.*)

Texture and turgor

Inspect and palpate the skin's texture, noting its thickness and mobility. It should look smooth and be intact. Skin that isn't intact may indicate local irritation or trauma.

Palpation also helps you evaluate the patient's hydration status. Dehydration and edema cause poor skin turgor. However, aging may also cause poor skin turgor, so turgor may not be a reliable indicator of an elderly patient's hydration status.

Moisture

Observe the skin's moisture content. The skin should be relatively dry, with a minimal amount of perspiration. Skin-fold areas should also be fairly dry.

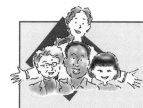

Bridging the gap

Detecting color variations in dark-skinned people

Listed below are ways to detect color variations in dark-skinned people to assess for cyanosis, edema, erythema, jaundice, pallor, petechiae, and rashes.

Cyanosis
Examine the conjunctivae, palms, soles, buccal mucosa, and tongue. Look for dull, dark color.

Edema
Examine the area for decreased color, and palpate for tightness.

Erythema
Palpate the area for warmth.

Jaundice
Examine the sclerae and hard palate in natural—not fluorescent—light, if possible. Look for a yellow color.

Pallor
Examine the sclerae, conjunctivae, buccal mucosa, tongue, lips, nail beds, palms, and soles. Look for an ashen color.

Petechiae
Examine areas of lighter pigmentation such as the abdomen. Look for tiny, purplish red dots.

Rashes
Palpate the area for skin texture changes.

Temperature

Palpate the skin bilaterally for temperature. Warm skin suggests normal circulation; cool skin, a possible underlying disorder. Distinguish between generalized and localized coolness and warmth.

Lesions

During your inspection, you may see normal variations in the skin's texture and pigmentation. Red lesions caused by vascular changes include hemangiomas, telangiectases, petechiae, purpura, and ecchymoses and may indicate disease. Normal variations include birthmarks, freckles, and nevi, or moles. Freckles are small, flat macules located primarily on the face, arms, and back. They're usually red brown to brown. Nevi are either flat or raised and may be pink, tan, or dark brown. Like birthmarks, they can be found on all areas of the body.

New or not?

When investigating a lesion, start by classifying it as primary or secondary. A primary lesion is new. Changes in a primary lesion constitute a secondary lesion. Examples of secondary lesions include fissures, scales, crusts, scars, and excoriations. (See *Identifying primary lesions*.)

It's what's inside that counts

Use a flashlight or penlight to determine whether a lesion is solid or fluid-filled. Macules, papules, nodules, wheals, and hives are solid lesions. Vesicles, bullae, pustules, and cysts are fluid-filled lesions.

Lesion lowdown

After you've identified the type of lesion, describe its characteristics, pattern, location, and distribution. A detailed description can help you determine whether the lesion is a normal or pathologic skin change.

Sizing up the situation

Measure the diameter of the lesion using a millimeter-centimeter ruler. If you estimate the diameter, you may not be able to determine subtle changes in size. If you note drainage, document the type, color, and amount. Also note whether the lesion has a foul odor, which can indicate a superimposed infection.

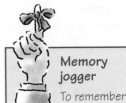

Memory jogger

To remember what to assess when evaluating a lesion, think of the letters **ABCDE:**

Asymmetry

Border

Color and configuration

Diameter and drainage

Evolution, or progression, of the lesion.

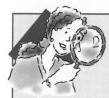

A closer look

Identifying primary lesions

Are you having trouble identifying your patient's lesion? Here's a quick look at three common lesions. Remember to keep a centimeter ruler handy to accurately measure the size of the lesion.

Macule
Flat, circumscribed area of altered skin color that is generally less than 1 cm; examples: freckle, flat nevus

Papule
Raised, circumscribed, solid area that's generally less than 1 cm; examples: elevated nevus, wart

Vesicle
Circumscribed, elevated lesion containing serous fluid that's less than 1 cm; example: early chickenpox

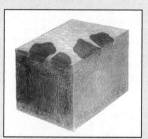 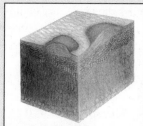 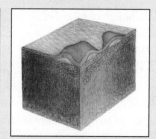

Assessing the eye

A thorough assessment of the patient's eyes and vision can help you identify problems that can affect the patient's health and quality of life.

Initial eye questions

To obtain an accurate history, first ask the patient these specific eye-related questions:
- Do you wear corrective lenses for distance or for reading?
- Are you experiencing blurred vision, blind spots, floaters, double vision, pain, discharge, or unusual sensitivity to light? Are you having trouble seeing at night?
- Have you ever had an eye injury or eye surgery?
- Have you ever had a lazy eye?
- Do you have allergies?
- When was your last eye examination?

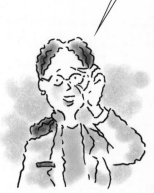

The eyes have it. An eye assessment can help you identify problems that can affect the patient's health and quality of life.

• Do you have a history of hypertension, diabetes, stroke, multiple sclerosis, syphilis, or human immunodeficiency virus (HIV)? Does anyone in your family have glaucoma, cataracts, vision loss, or retinitis?

• What medications do you take, including over-the-counter drugs, herbal preparations, eyedrops, and eyewashes?

• What do you do for a living and for recreation? Are you exposed to chemicals, fumes, flying debris, or infectious agents? If so, do you wear eye protection?

• How well are you managing your everyday activities? (if the patient is visually impaired or elderly)

Inspecting the eyes

Before you start your examination, gather the necessary equipment, including a good light source, a penlight, one or two opaque cards, an ophthalmoscope, vision-test cards, gloves, tissues, and cotton-tipped applicators.

Eyelid

Ask the patient to open and close his eyes to see whether they close completely. If the downward movement of the upper eyelid when gazing downward is delayed, it's called *lid lag*, which is a common sign of hyperthyroidism. Assess the lids for redness, edema, inflammation, or lesions. Observe whether the lower eyelids turn inward toward the eyeball, called *entropion*, or outward, called *ectropion*. Protrusion of the eyeball, called *exophthalmos* or *proptosis*, is also common in patients who have hyperthyroidism.

Crying or drying?

Inspect the eyes for excessive tearing or dryness. Excessive tearing is associated with such conditions as conjunctival or corneal foreign bodies, conjunctivitis, and thyrotoxicosis. Dryness or decreased tearing is associated with such conditions as sarcoidosis, Turner's syndrome, and Stevens-Johnson syndrome.

Conjunctiva

To inspect the bulbar conjunctiva, ask the patient to look upward. Gently pull down the lower eyelid. The bulbar conjunctiva should be clear and shiny. Note excessive redness, exudate, foreign bodies, and edema. Also, observe the sclera's color, which should be white to buff. In black patients, you may see flecks of tan. A bluish discoloration may indicate scleral thinning.

Getting an eye lift

To examine the palpebral conjunctiva, have the patient look down. Then lift the upper lid, holding the upper lashes against the eyebrow with your finger. The palpebral conjunctiva should be uniformly pink. In patients with a history of allergies, the palpebral conjunctiva may have a cobblestone appearance.

Cornea

To examine the cornea, shine a penlight first from both sides and then from straight ahead. The cornea should be clear and without lesions. To test corneal sensitivity, lightly touch the cornea with a wisp of cotton. (See *Assessing corneal sensitivity.*)

Iris

The iris should appear flat, and the cornea should appear convex. Excess pressure in the eye—such as that caused by acute angle-closure glaucoma—may push the iris forward, making the anterior chamber appear very small. The irises should be the same size, color, and shape.

Pupil

Pupils should be equal in size, round, and about one-fourth the size of the iris in normal room light. Unequal pupils generally indicate neurologic damage, iritis, glaucoma, or therapy with certain drugs. A fixed pupil that doesn't react to light can be an ominous neurologic sign.

In perfect agreement

Test the pupils for direct and consensual response. In a slightly darkened room, hold a penlight about 20″ (50.8 cm) from the patient's eyes, and direct the light at the eye from the side. Note the reaction of the pupil you're testing (direct response) and of the opposite pupil (consensual response). Both should react the same way. Also note sluggishness or inequality in the response. Repeat the test with the other pupil. *Note:* If you shine the light in a blind eye, neither pupil will respond. If you shine the light in a seeing eye, the pupils will respond consensually.

Willing to accommodate

To test the pupils for accommodation, place your finger approximately 4″ (10.2 cm) from the bridge of the patient's nose. Ask the patient to look at a fixed object in the distance and then at your finger. His pupils should constrict and his eyes converge as he focuses on your finger.

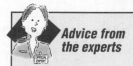

Advice from the experts

Assessing corneal sensitivity

To test corneal sensitivity, touch a wisp of cotton from a cotton ball to the cornea, as shown.

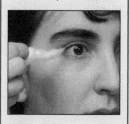

The patient should blink. If he doesn't, he may have suffered damage to the sensory fibers of cranial nerve V or to the motor fibers controlled by cranial nerve VI.

Keep in mind that people who wear contact lenses may have reduced sensitivity because they're accustomed to having foreign objects in their eyes.

Just a wisp
Remember that a wisp of cotton is the only safe object to use for this test. Even though a gauze pad or tissue is soft, it can cause corneal abrasions and irritation.

Testing visual acuity

To test the patient's far and near vision, use a Snellen chart and a near-vision chart. To test his peripheral vision, use confrontation. Before each test, ask the patient to remove corrective lenses if he wears them.

Snellen chart

Have the patient sit or stand 20' (6.1 m) from the chart, and then cover his left eye with an opaque object. Ask him to read the letters on one line of the chart and then move downward to increasingly smaller lines until he can no longer discern all of the letters. Have him cover his right eye and repeat the test. Finally, to test his binocular vision, have him read the smallest line he can read with both eyes uncovered. If the patient wears corrective lenses, have him repeat the test wearing them. Record his vision with and without correction.

The Big E

Use the Snellen E chart to test visual acuity in young children and other patients who can't read. Cover the patient's left eye to check the right eye, point to an E on the chart, and ask the patient to point which way the letter faces. Repeat the test with the left eye. If the test values between the two eyes differ by two lines, such as 20/30 in one eye and 20/50 in the other, suspect an abnormality such as amblyopia (reduced vision in an eye that appears normal during ophthalmoscopic examination).

Near-vision chart

To test near vision, cover one of the patient's eyes with an opaque object and hold a Rosenbaum near-vision card 14″ (35.6 cm) from his eyes. Have him read the line with the smallest letters he can distinguish. Repeat the test with the other eye. If the patient wears corrective lenses, have him repeat the test while wearing them. Record the visual accommodation with and without lenses.

Assessing eye muscle function

To evaluate extraocular muscles, you'll need to assess the corneal light reflex and the cardinal positions of gaze.

(Text continues on page 21.)

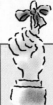

Memory jogger

To make sure that your pupil assessment is complete, think of the acronym PERRLA:

Pupils

Equal

Round

Reactive

Light-reacting

Accommodation.

If your patient can't read, use the Snellen E!

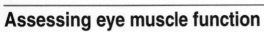

Sites for heart sounds

Normal heart sounds indicate events in the cardiac cycle, such as the closing of heart valves, and are reflected to specific areas of the chest wall. Auscultation sites are identified by the names of heart valves but aren't located directly over the valves. Rather, these sites are located along the pathway blood takes as it flows through the heart's chambers and valves.

When auscultating for heart sounds, place the stethoscope over the four sites illustrated below.

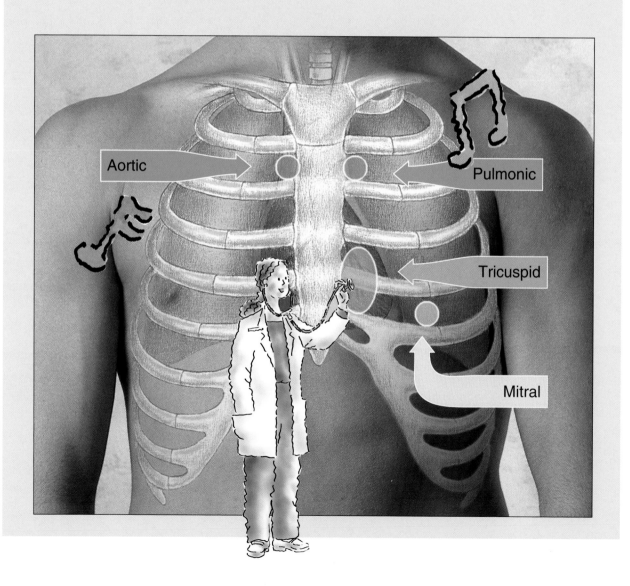

Cycle of heart sounds

When you auscultate a patient's chest and hear that familiar "lub-dub," you're hearing the first and second heart sounds, S_1 and S_2. At times, two other sounds may occur: S_3 and S_4.

Heart sounds are generated by events in the cardiac cycle. When valves close or blood fills the ventricles, vibrations of the heart muscle can be heard through the chest wall.

Varying sound patterns

The phonogram at right shows how heart sounds vary in duration and intensity. For instance, S_2 (which occurs when the semilunar valves snap shut) is a shorter-lasting sound than S_1 because the semilunar valves take less time to close than the atrioventricular valves, which cause S_1.

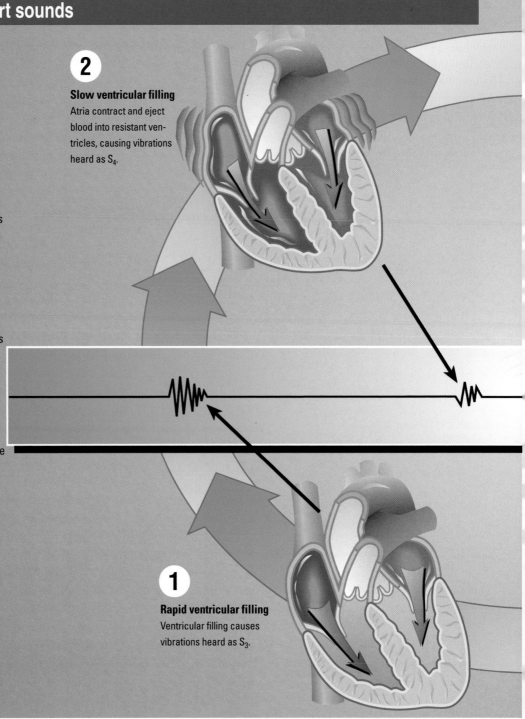

2

Slow ventricular filling
Atria contract and eject blood into resistant ventricles, causing vibrations heard as S_4.

1

Rapid ventricular filling
Ventricular filling causes vibrations heard as S_3.

Diastole

Systole

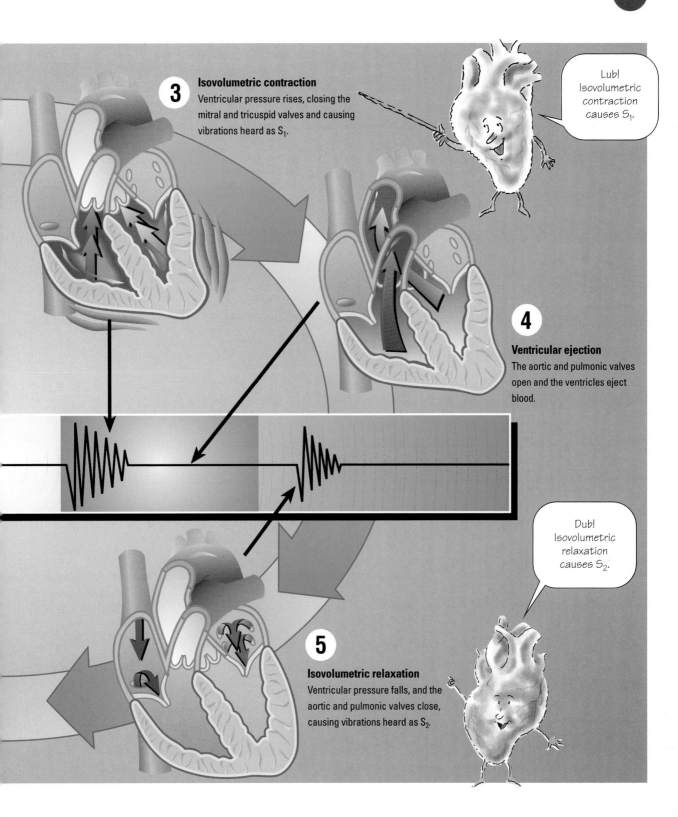

Understanding murmurs

Normally, heart valves close tightly and then open completely to let blood flow through. However, various conditions may alter blood flow through the valves, causing murmurs and, in many cases, increasing the workload of the heart.

The first two illustrations show a normal valve open and closed. The other illustrations portray three common reasons for the development of murmurs.

> Valve closure is normally an open-and-shut case.

Normal valve open

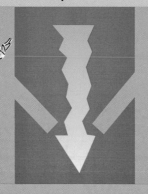

Normal valve closed

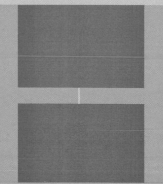

High blood flow

High blood flow through a normal valve may cause a murmur. Examples include an aortic systolic murmur, which can be caused by anemia and a subsequent compensatory increase in cardiac output.

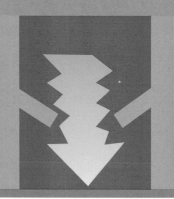

Decreased blood flow

Low blood flow through a stenotic valve can cause a murmur. The valves can't open or close properly because they're thickened, fibrotic, or calcified. Common examples include aortic and mitral stenosis.

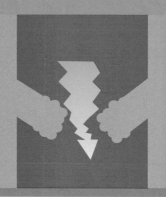

Backflow of blood

A backflow of blood through an insufficient or incompetent valve can cause a murmur. Because the valve can't close properly, blood can leak back or regurgitate into the heart chamber from which it came. Common examples include aortic and mitral insufficiency.

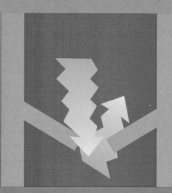

Corneal light reflex

To assess the corneal light reflex, ask the patient to look straight ahead; then shine a penlight on the bridge of his nose from about 12″ to 15″ (30.5 cm to 38 cm) away. The light should fall at the same spot on each cornea. If it doesn't, the eyes aren't being held in the same plane by the extraocular muscles. This lack of muscle coordination is known as *strabismus.*

Cardinal positions of gaze

Cardinal positions of gaze evaluate the oculomotor, trigeminal, and abducent nerves as well as the extraocular muscles. To perform this test, ask the patient to remain still while you hold a pencil or other small object directly in front of his nose at a distance of about 18″ (45 cm).

Eyeballs on the move

Ask him to follow the object with his eyes, without moving his head. Then move the object to each of the six cardinal positions (left superior, left lateral, left inferior, right superior, right lateral, and right inferior), returning to the midpoint after each movement. The patient's eyes should remain parallel as they move.

Examining intraocular structures

The ophthalmoscope allows you to directly observe the eye's internal structures. Use the green, positive numbers on the lens disc to focus on near objects such as the patient's lens. Use the red, minus numbers to focus on distant objects such as the retina.

Mood lighting

Before the examination, have the patient remove his contact lenses (if they're tinted) or eyeglasses, and darken the room to dilate his pupils and make your examination easier. Ask the patient to focus on a point behind you. Tell him that you'll be moving into his visual field and blocking his view. Also, explain that you'll be shining a bright light into his eye, which may be uncomfortable but not harmful. (See *Seeing eye to eye.*)

Closing in on the cornea

Set the lens disc at zero, hold the ophthalmoscope about 4″ (10 cm) from the patient's eye, and direct the light through the pupil to elicit the red reflex, a reflection of light off the choroid. Check the red reflex for depth of color.

Seeing eye to eye

This illustration shows the correct position for the examiner and the patient when an ophthalmoscope is used to examine the eye's internal structures.

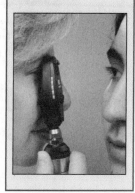

Now, move the ophthalmoscope closer to the eye. Adjust the lens disc so you can focus on the anterior chamber and lens. Look for clouding, foreign matter, or opacities. If the lens is opaque, indicating cataracts, you may not be able to complete the examination.

Rotating to the retinal structures

To examine the retina, start with the dial turned to zero. Rotate the lens-power disc to observe the vitreous body for clarity. Rotating the dial into the negative numbers will bring the blood vessels into focus. The arteries will look thinner and brighter than the veins.

Follow one of the vessels along its path toward the nose until you reach the optic disk, where all vessels in the eye originate. Examine arteriovenous crossings for arteriovenous nicking (localized constrictions in the retinal vessels), which might be a sign of hypertension.

Diggin' the disc and depression

The optic disk is a creamy pink to yellow-orange structure with clear borders and a round-to-oval shape. Identify the physiologic cup, a small depression that occupies about one-third of the disk's diameter. The disk may fill or exceed your field of vision. If you don't see it, follow a blood vessel toward the center until you do. The nasal border of the disk may be somewhat blurred.

Riveting on the retina

Completely scan the retina by following the four blood vessels that extend from the optic disk to different peripheral areas. The retina should have a uniform color and be free from scars and pigmentation. As you scan, note any lesions or hemorrhages.

Movin' in on the macula

Finally, move the light laterally from the optic disk to locate the macula, the part of the eye most sensitive to light. It appears as a darker structure, free from blood vessels. Most patients can't tolerate having a beam of light fall on the macula. If you locate it, ask the patient to shift his gaze into the light.

Assessing the ears, nose, and throat

To investigate a complaint about the ears, nose, or throat, ask about the onset, location, duration, and characteristics of the symptom as well as what aggravates and relieves it.

Initial ear, nose, and throat questions

When you ask the patient about his ear complaint, include the following questions:
• Do you have any associated symptoms such as ear discharge?
• Have you ever had a head injury?
• Do you have any feelings of abnormal movement or vertigo (spinning)? (If so, determine when and how frequently the episodes occur and whether they're associated with nausea, vomiting, or tinnitus.)
• Have you ever had an ear problem or injury?
• Does anyone in your family have ear or hearing problems?
• Have you been ill recently, or do you have a chronic disorder, such as diabetes or hypertension?
• Are you currently being treated for a health condition or taking any medications?
• Do you have allergies?
• Do you have nasal stuffiness, nasal discharge, or epistaxis (nosebleed)?
• Do you get colds frequently?
• Do you suffer from hay fever, headaches, or sinus trouble? Do certain conditions or places seem to cause or aggravate the problem?
• Have you ever suffered trauma to the nose or head? (If so, inquire about the color and consistency of the discharge.)
• Have you ever had bleeding or sore gums, mouth or tongue ulcers, a bad taste in your mouth, bad breath, toothaches, loose teeth, frequent sore throats, hoarseness, or facial swelling?
• Do you smoke or use other types of tobacco?
• Do you have neck pain or tenderness, neck swelling, or trouble moving your neck?

Hear ye, hear ye! His majesty doth decree that ye shall ask about onset, location, duration, and characteristics when assessing ear complaints.

Examining the ears

Use the techniques of inspection, palpation, and auscultation to examine the patient's ears. An ear assessment also requires the use of an otoscope.

External observations

Begin by observing the ears for position and symmetry. Inspect the auricle for lesions, drainage, nodules, or redness. Pull the helix back and note whether it's tender. If pulling the ear back hurts the patient, he may have otitis externa. Then inspect and palpate the mastoid area behind each auricle, noting tenderness, redness, or warmth. Finally, inspect the opening of the ear canal, noting discharge, redness, odor, or the presence of nodules or cysts.

Otoscopic examination

The next part of an ear assessment involves using an otoscope to examine the patient's auditory canal and inner ear structures. Before beginning, palpate the tragus — the cartilaginous projection anterior to the external opening of the ear — and pull the auricle up. If this area is tender, don't insert the speculum. The patient could have otitis externa, and inserting the speculum could be painful. The external canal should be free from inflammation and scaling. Next, check the canal for foreign bodies. If a foreign body is present, don't insert the speculum because you might push the foreign body deeper into the ear canal. (See *Using an otoscope.*)

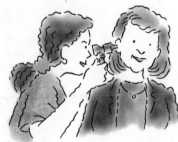

Use an otoscope to examine your patient's inner ear.

Go gently into that good ear canal

Now you're ready to perform the otoscopic examination. To insert the speculum of the otoscope, tilt the patient's head away from you. Then grasp the superior posterior auricle with your thumb and index finger and pull it up and back to straighten the canal. Insert the speculum to about one-third its length. Insert it gently, because the inner two-thirds of the canal are sensitive to pressure. Vary the angle of the speculum until you can see the tympanic membrane. (If the patient is younger than age 3, pull the auricle down to get a good view of the membrane.) Lean your hand holding the otoscope against the patient's head to keep the otoscope steady.

As the speculum turns

As you inspect the inner canal, note the cerumen's color. The elderly patient may have harder, drier cerumen because of rigid cilia in the ear canal. You may need to carefully rotate the speculum for a complete view of the tympanic membrane. The membrane should be pearl gray, glistening, and transparent. The annulus should be white and denser than the rest of the membrane. Inspect the membrane carefully for bulging, retraction, bleeding, lesions, and perforations, especially at the periphery. The elderly patient's eardrum may appear cloudy.

"Timing" the light reflex?

Now, examine the membrane for the light reflex. In the right ear, this reflex should be between 4 and 6 o'clock; in the left ear, between 6 and 8 o'clock. If the reflex is displaced or absent, the patient's tympanic membrane may be bulging, inflamed, or retracted.

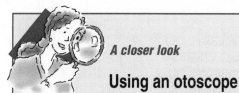

A closer look

Using an otoscope

Here's how to use an otoscope to examine the ears.

Inserting the speculum
Before insertion, straighten the ear canal by grasping the auricle and pulling it up and back.

Positioning the scope
To examine the ear's external canal, hold the otoscope with the handle parallel to the patient's head, as shown below. Brace your hand firmly against his head to avoid hitting the canal with the speculum.

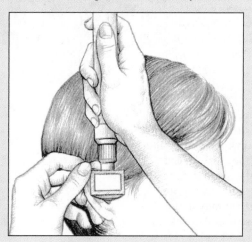

Viewing the structures
When the otoscope is positioned properly, you should see the tympanic membrane structures shown here.

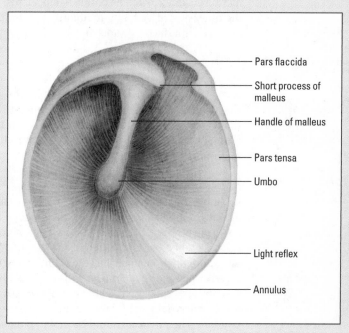

- Pars flaccida
- Short process of malleus
- Handle of malleus
- Pars tensa
- Umbo
- Light reflex
- Annulus

Finally, look for the bony landmarks. The malleus will appear as a dense, white streak at the 12 o'clock position. At the top of the light reflex, you'll find the umbo, the inferior point of the malleus.

Examining the nose and sinuses

A complete examination of the nose also includes checking the sinuses using the techniques of inspection and palpation.

Inspecting and palpating the nose

Begin by observing the patient's nose for position, symmetry, and color. Note variations, such as discoloration, swelling, or deformity. Observe for nasal discharge or flaring. If discharge is present, note the color, quantity, and consistency. If you notice flaring, observe for other signs of respiratory distress.

Name that smell...

To test nasal patency and olfactory nerve (cranial nerve I) function, ask the patient to block one nostril and inhale a familiar aromatic substance, such as coffee, soap, citrus, or nutmeg, through the other nostril. Ask him to identify the aroma. Then repeat the process with the other nostril, using a different aroma.

Test your patient's sense of smell by asking him to identify a familiar aroma.

Turn up the patient's nose

Inspect the nasal cavity. Ask the patient to tilt his head back slightly, and then push up the tip of the patient's nose. Use the light from the otoscope to illuminate his nasal cavities. Check for severe deviation or perforation of the nasal septum. Examine the vestibule and turbinates for redness, softness, swelling, and discharge.

Light at the end of the speculum

Examine the nostrils by direct inspection, using a nasal speculum, a penlight or small flashlight, or an otoscope with a short, wide-tip attachment. Have the patient sit in front of you with his head tilted back. Put on gloves, and then insert the tip of the closed nasal speculum into one nostril to the point where the blade widens. Slowly open the speculum as wide as possible without causing discomfort. Shine the flashlight in the nostril to illuminate the area. Observe the color and patency of the nostril, and check for exudate. The mucosa should be moist, pink to light red, and free from lesions and polyps. After inspecting one nostril, close the speculum, remove it, and inspect the other nostril.

Thumb his nose

Finally, palpate the patient's nose with your thumb and forefinger, assessing for pain, tenderness, swelling, and deformity.

Examining the sinuses

Next, examine the sinuses. Remember, only the frontal and maxillary sinuses are accessible; you won't be able to palpate the ethmoidal or sphenoidal sinuses. However, if the frontal and maxillary sinuses are infected, you can assume that the other sinuses are as well.

Tell me if it hurts

To begin, check for swelling around the eyes, especially over the sinus area. Then palpate the sinuses, checking for tenderness. To palpate the frontal sinuses, place your thumbs above the patient's eyes, just under the bony ridges of the upper orbits, and place your fingertips on his forehead. Apply gentle pressure. Next, palpate the maxillary sinuses. If the patient complains of tenderness during palpation of the sinuses, use transillumination to see whether they're filled with fluid or pus.

Examining the mouth and throat

Assessing the mouth and throat requires the techniques of inspection and palpation.

Assessing the mouth

Inspect the patient's lips, which should be pink, moist, symmetrical, and without lesions. Put on gloves, and then palpate the lips for lumps or surface abnormalities.

Use a tongue blade and a bright light to inspect the oral mucosa. Have the patient open his mouth; then place the tongue blade on top of his tongue. The oral mucosa should be pink, smooth, moist, and free from lesions and unusual odors. Increased pigmentation is seen in dark-skinned patients.

Sum up the gums

Next, observe the gingivae, or gums. They should be pink, moist, and have clearly defined margins at each tooth. They shouldn't be retracted. Inspect the teeth, noting their number, condition, and whether any are missing or crowded. If the patient is wearing dentures, ask him to remove them so you can inspect the gums underneath.

Give the tongue the once-over

Finally, inspect the tongue. It should be midline, moist, pink, and free from lesions. The posterior surface should be smooth, and the anterior surface should be slightly rough with small fissures. Ask the patient to raise the tip of his tongue and touch his palate directly behind his front teeth. Inspect the ventral surface of the tongue and the floor of the mouth. Next, wrap a piece of gauze around the tip of the tongue and move the tongue first to one side then the other to inspect the lateral borders. They should be smooth and even-textured.

Assessing the throat

To inspect the patient's oropharynx, ask him to open his mouth while you shine the penlight on the uvula and palate. You may need to insert a tongue blade into the mouth and depress the tongue. Place the tongue blade slightly off center to avoid eliciting the gag reflex. The uvula and oropharynx should be pink and moist, without inflammation or exudates. The tonsils should be pink and shouldn't be hypertrophied. Ask the patient to say, "Ahhh." Observe for movement of the soft palate and uvula.

Gag order

Palpate the lips, tongue, and oropharynx. Assess the patient's gag reflex by gently touching the back of the pharynx with a cotton-tipped applicator or the tongue blade. Doing so should produce a bilateral response.

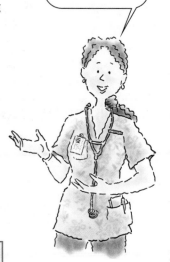

The tongue doesn't mind being depressed. It helps inspection of the oropharynx.

A closer look

Locating the thyroid gland

This illustration shows the structure and location of the thyroid gland.

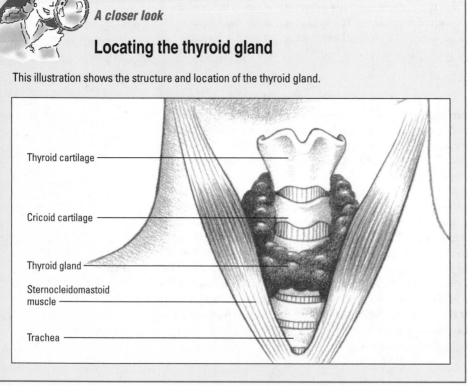

Thyroid cartilage

Cricoid cartilage

Thyroid gland

Sternocleidomastoid muscle

Trachea

By the throat

Palpate the trachea, which is normally located midline in the neck. Place your thumbs along each side of the trachea near the lower part of the neck. Assess whether the distance between the trachea's outer edge and the sternocleidomastoid muscle is equal on both sides.

Hard to swallow

To palpate the thyroid, stand behind the patient and put your hands around his neck, with the fingers of both hands over the lower trachea. Ask him to swallow as you feel the thyroid isthmus. The isthmus should rise with swallowing because it lies across the trachea, just below the cricoid cartilage.

Displace the thyroid to the right and then to the left, palpating both lobes for enlargement, nodules, tenderness, or a gritty sensation. (See *Locating the thyroid gland.*) If you detect an enlarged thyroid gland, also auscultate the thyroid area with the bell. Check for a bruit or a soft rushing sound, which indicates a hypermetabolic state.

Assessing the respiratory system

When you obtain the health history of a patient with a respiratory disorder, first ask questions pertinent to the respiratory system. Remember to look at the patient's medical and family history, being particularly watchful for a smoking habit, allergies, previous operations, and respiratory diseases, such as pneumonia and tuberculosis. Ask about environmental exposure to irritants such as asbestos.

Initial respiratory questions

Ask the patient to rate his usual level of dyspnea on a scale of 0 to 10, in which 0 means no dyspnea and 10 means the worst he has experienced. Then ask him to rate the level that day. Ask what he does to relieve the dyspnea and how well it works. (See *Grading dyspnea.*) Then ask these questions:
• How many pillows do you use? (The answer describes the severity of orthopnea, or shortness of breath when lying down.)
• Do you have a cough? Is your cough productive? If it's a chronic problem, has it changed recently? If so, how? What makes the cough better? What makes it worse?
• If you produce sputum (phlegm), about how many teaspoons (or some other common measurement) of sputum are produced?

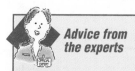

Advice from the experts

Grading dyspnea

To assess dyspnea as objectively as possible, ask your patient to briefly describe how various activities affect his breathing. Then document his response using this grading system:
• *Grade 0:* not troubled by breathlessness except with strenuous exercise
• *Grade 1:* troubled by shortness of breath when hurrying on a level path or walking up a slight hill
• *Grade 2:* walks more slowly on a level path than people of the same age because of breathlessness or has to stop to breathe when walking on a level path at his own pace
• *Grade 3:* stops to breathe after walking about 100 yards (91 m) on a level path
• *Grade 4:* too breathless to leave the house or breathless when dressing or undressing.

What's the color and consistency of the sputum? If sputum is a chronic problem, has it changed recently? If so, how?
• At what time of day do you cough most often? Do you cough up blood (hemoptysis)? If so, how much and how often?
• If you wheeze, when does wheezing occur? What makes you wheeze? Do you wheeze loudly enough for others to hear it? What helps stop your wheezing?
• If you have chest pain, where's the pain? What does it feel like? Is it sharp, stabbing, burning, or aching? Does it move to another area? How long does it last? What causes it to occur? What makes it better?

Inspecting the chest

A physical examination of the respiratory system follows four steps: inspection, palpation, percussion, and auscultation.

Back, then front

Examine the back of the chest. Always compare one side with the other. Then examine the front of the chest. Note masses or scars that indicate trauma or surgery. Look for chest wall symmetry. As the patient inhales, both sides of the chest should be equal at rest and should expand equally. The diameter of the chest, from front to back, should be about half the width of the chest.

A new angle

Also, look at the costal angle between the ribs and the sternum at the point immediately above the xiphoid process. In an adult, this angle should be less than 90 degrees. The angle will be larger if the chest wall is chronically expanded because of an enlargement of the intercostal muscles, as can happen with COPD.

Every breath you take

To find the patient's respiratory rate, count for a full minute — longer if you note abnormalities. Adults normally breathe at a rate of 12 to 20 breaths/minute. An infant's respiratory rate ranges between 30 and 80 breaths/minute, depending on the age of the infant; for a child, a rate of 15 to 30 breaths/minute is considered normal. The respiratory pattern should be even, coordinated, and regular.

Raising a red flag

Watch for paradoxical, or uneven, movement of the chest wall. Paradoxical movement may appear as an abnormal collapse of part of the chest wall when the patient inhales or an abnormal ex-

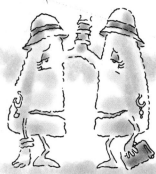

I love accessories, but using accessory muscles while breathing usually indicates a respiratory problem.

pansion when the patient exhales. Frequent use of accessory muscles may be normal in some athletes, but in most patients it indicates a respiratory problem.

Inspecting related structures

Inspection of the skin, tongue, mouth, fingers, and nail beds also may provide information about respiratory status.

Color clues

Patients with a bluish tint to their skin and mucous membranes are considered cyanotic. Cyanosis is a late sign of hypoxemia. The most reliable place to check for cyanosis is the tongue and mucous membranes of the mouth.

Clubbing clues

Check the fingers for clubbing, a possible sign of long-term hypoxia. When clubbing occurs, the angle at which the fingernail enters the skin is greater than or equal to 180 degrees.

Palpating the chest

The chest wall should feel smooth, warm, and dry. Crepitus indicates subcutaneous air in the chest, an abnormal condition. (See *Palpating the chest*, page 32.) If a patient has a chest tube, you may find a small amount of subcutaneous air around the insertion site.

Tender touch

Gentle palpation shouldn't cause the patient pain. Painful costochondral joints are typically located at the midclavicular line or next to the sternum. Rib or vertebral fractures will be quite painful over the fracture, though pain may radiate around the chest as well. Pain may also be caused by sore muscles as a result of protracted coughing. A collapsed lung may also cause pain.

Vibratin' fremitus

Also palpate for tactile fremitus, palpable vibrations caused by the transmission of air through the bronchopulmonary system. (See *Checking for tactile fremitus*, page 33.)

Equal measure

To evaluate the patient's chest wall symmetry and expansion, place your hands on the front of the chest wall with your thumbs touching each other at the second intercostal space. As the patient inhales deeply, watch your thumbs. They should separate simultaneously and equally to a distance several centimeters away from

Palpating the chest

To palpate the chest, place the palm of your hand (or hands) lightly over the thorax, as shown. Palpate for tenderness, alignment, bulging, and retractions of the chest and intercostal spaces. Assess the patient for crepitus, especially around drainage sites. Repeat this procedure on the patient's back.

Next, use the pads of your fingers, as shown, to palpate the front and back of the thorax. Pass your fingers over the ribs and any scars, lumps, lesions, or ulcerations. Note the skin temperature, turgor, and moisture. Also note tenderness and bony or subcutaneous crepitus. The muscles should feel firm and smooth.

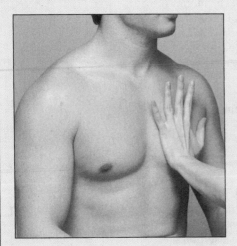
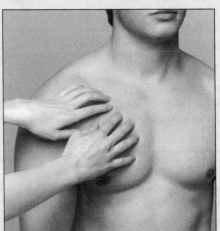

the sternum. Repeat the measurement at the fifth intercostal space. The same measurement may be made on the back of the chest near the tenth rib.

Warning signs

The patient's chest may expand asymmetrically if he has pleural effusion, atelectasis, pneumonia, or pneumothorax. Chest expansion may be decreased at the level of the diaphragm if the patient has emphysema, respiratory depression, diaphragm paralysis, atelectasis, obesity, or ascites.

Percussing the chest

You'll percuss the chest to find the boundaries of the lungs, to determine whether the lungs are filled with air or fluid or solid material, and to evaluate the distance the diaphragm travels between the patient's inhalation and exhalation. Percussion allows you to

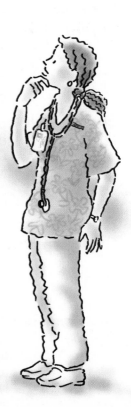

Checking for tactile fremitus

When you check the back of the thorax for tactile fremitus, ask the patient to fold his arms across his chest. This movement shifts the scapulae out of the way.

What to do
Check for tactile fremitus by lightly placing your open palms on both sides of the patient's back, as shown, without touching his back with your fingers. Ask the patient to repeat the phrase "ninety-nine" loud enough to produce palpable vibrations. Then palpate the front of the chest using the same hand positions.

What the results mean
Vibrations that feel more intense on one side than the other indicate tissue consolidation on that side. Less intense vibrations may indicate emphysema, pneumothorax, or pleural effu-

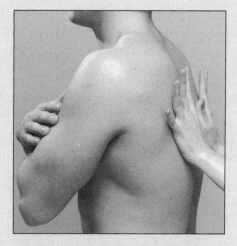

sion. Faint or no vibrations in the upper posterior thorax may indicate bronchial obstruction or a fluid-filled pleural space.

assess structures as deep as 3″ (7.6 cm). You'll hear different percussion sounds in different areas of the chest. (See *Identifying percussion sounds*, page 34.)

Auscultating the chest

To auscultate for breath sounds, you'll press the stethoscope firmly against the skin. Listen to a full inspiration and a full expiration at each site, using the diaphragm of the stethoscope. Ask the patient to breathe through his mouth because nose breathing alters the pitch of breath sounds.

Normal breath sounds

You'll hear four types of breath sounds over normal lungs. The type of sound you hear depends on where you listen. Classify each sound according to its intensity, location, pitch, duration, and characteristic. Note whether the sound occurs when the patient inhales, exhales, or both.

The normal breath sounds are chracterized as follows:

> Normal breath sounds vary significantly, depending on the auscultation site.

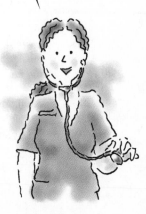

Identifying percussion sounds

Use this chart to help you become more comfortable with percussion and interpret percussion sounds quickly. Learn the different percussion sounds by practicing on yourself, your patients, and any other person willing to help.

Sound	Description	Clinical significance
Flat	Short, soft, high-pitched, extremely dull; found over the thigh	Consolidation, as in atelectasis and extensive pleural effusion
Dull	Medium in intensity and pitch, moderate length, thud-like; found over the liver	Solid area, as in lobar pneumonia
Resonant	Long, loud, low-pitched, hollow	Normal lung tissue; bronchitis
Hyperresonant	Very loud, lower-pitched; found over the stomach	Hyperinflated lung, as in emphysema or pneumothorax
Tympanic	Loud, high-pitched, moderate length, musical, drum-like; found over a puffed-out cheek	Air collection, as in a gastric air bubble, air in the intestines, or a large pneumothorax

Tracheal breath sounds, heard above the supraclavicular notch, are harsh, high-pitched, and discontinuous. They occur when a patient inhales or exhales.

Bronchial breath sounds, usually heard just above the clavicles on each side of the sternum, between the scapulae, and over the manubrium, are loud, high-pitched, and discontinuous. They're loudest when the patient exhales.

Bronchovesicular sounds, heard when the patient inhales or exhales, are medium-pitched and continuous. They're best heard over the upper third of the sternum and between the scapulae.

Vesicular sounds, heard over the rest of the lungs, are soft and low-pitched. They're prolonged during inhalation and shortened during exhalation.

Adventitious isn't advantageous

If you hear diminished but normal breath sounds in both lungs, the patient may have emphysema, atelectasis, severe bronchospasm, or shallow breathing. If you hear breath sounds in one lung only,

the patient may have pleural effusion, pneumothorax, a tumor, or mucus plugs in the airways. Adventitious sounds are abnormal no matter where you hear them in the lungs. Those sounds include:
• *crackles* — intermittent, nonmusical, crackling sounds heard during inspiration; classified as fine or coarse
• *wheezes* — high-pitched sounds caused by blocked airflow, heard mostly on expiration
• *rhonchi* — low-pitched snoring or rattling sound; heard primarily on exhalation
• *stridor* — loud high-pitched sound heard during inspiration
• *pleural friction rub* — low-pitched, grating sound heard during inspiration and expiration; typically accompanied by pain.

Assessing the cardiovascular system

Cardiovascular disease affects people of all ages and can take many forms. A consistent, methodical approach to your assessment will help you identify abnormalities. As always, the key to accurate assessment is regular practice, which helps to improve technique and efficiency.

Initial cardiovascular questions

As you conduct your cardiovascular assessment, make sure to ask the patient about:
• his family history and past medical history, including diabetes, chronic diseases of the lungs or kidneys, or liver disease (see *At risk for cardiovascular disease*)
• his level of stress and how he manages it
• his current health habits, such as smoking, alcohol and caffeine intake, exercise, and dietary intake of fat and sodium
• the medications he takes, including over-the-counter drugs and herbal preparations
• past surgeries
• environmental or occupational considerations
• ADLs.

The heart of the matter

In addition, ask the patient these questions:
• Do you have chest pain? How would you rate the pain on a scale of 0 to 10, in which 0 means no pain and 10 means the worst pain imaginable? (Reassess the patient's pain rating frequently during treatment to determine the effectiveness of interventions.)
• Do you experience irregular heartbeat or palpitations?

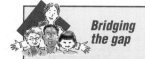

Bridging the gap

At risk for cardiovascular disease

As you analyze a patient's problems, remember that age, gender, and race are essential considerations in identifying patients at risk for cardiovascular disorders. For example, coronary artery disease most commonly affects white men between ages 40 and 60. Hypertension occurs most often in blacks.

Women are also vulnerable to heart disease, especially postmenopausal women and those with diabetes mellitus.

• Do you experience shortness of breath? If so, what activities cause it? Do you experience shortness of breath on exertion, lying down, or at night?
• Do you have a cough?
• Do you experience weakness, dizziness, or fatigue?
• Have you experienced unexplained weight loss or gain?
• Do you experience swelling of your extremities? How about pain in the extremities, such as leg pain or cramps?
• Do you experience dizziness or headaches?
• Do you experience high or low blood pressure?
• Have you noticed changes in your skin, decreased hair distribution, skin color changes, or a thin, shiny appearance to the skin?
• Do your rings or shoes feel tight?
• Do your ankles swell?
• Have you noticed changes in color or sensation in your legs? If so, what are those changes?
• If you have sores or ulcers, how quickly do they heal?
• Do you stand or sit in one place for long periods at work?

Inspecting the precordium

Before you begin your physical assessment, you'll need to obtain a stethoscope with a bell and a diaphragm, an appropriate-sized blood pressure cuff, a ruler, and a penlight or other flexible light source.

First, take a moment to assess the patient's general appearance. Note his skin color, temperature, turgor, and texture. Are his fingers clubbed? If the patient is dark-skinned, inspect his mucous membranes for pallor.

> Before beginning your assessment, be sure to gather the proper equipment.

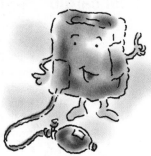

Checking out the chest

Next, inspect the chest. Note landmarks you can use to describe your findings as well as structures underlying the chest wall. (See *Identifying cardiovascular landmarks.*) Look for pulsations, symmetry of movement, retractions, or heaves. A heave is a strong outward thrust of the chest wall and occurs during systole.

Maximal impulse

Position a light source, such as a flashlight or gooseneck lamp, so that it casts a shadow on the patient's chest. Note the location of the apical impulse. This location is also usually the point of maximal impulse and should be located in the fifth intercostal space at or just medial to the left midclavicular line.

Identifying cardiovascular landmarks

These views show where to find critical landmarks used in cardiovascular assessment.

Anterior thorax

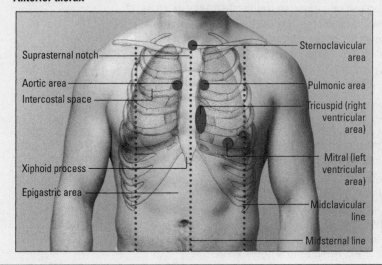

Suprasternal notch

Aortic area

Intercostal space

Xiphoid process

Epigastric area

Sternoclavicular area

Pulmonic area

Tricuspid (right ventricular area)

Mitral (left ventricular area)

Midclavicular line

Midsternal line

Lateral thorax

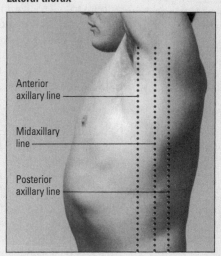

Anterior axillary line

Midaxillary line

Posterior axillary line

Auscultating for heart sounds

Begin by identifying the sites where you'll auscultate: over the four cardiac valves and at Erb's point, the third intercostal space at the left sternal border. Use the bell of your stethoscope to hear low-pitched sounds and the diaphragm to hear high-pitched sounds. Always identify first and second heart sounds (S_1 and S_2), and then listen for adventitious sounds, such as third and fourth heart sounds (S_3 and S_4), murmurs, and rubs.

Auscultate for heart sounds with the patient in three positions:

☝ lying on his back with the head of the bed raised 30 to 45 degrees

✌ sitting up

🖐 lying on his left side.

Listen for the "dub"

Start auscultating at the aortic area, where S_2 is loudest. S_2 is best heard at the base of the heart at the end of ventricular systole. This sound corresponds to closure of the pulmonic and aortic valves and is generally described as sounding like "dub." It's a shorter, higher-pitched, louder sound than S_1. When the pulmonic valve closes later than the aortic valve during inspiration, you'll hear a split S_2.

Listen for the "lub"

From the base of the heart, move to the pulmonic area and then down to the tricuspid area. Then move to the mitral area, where S_1 is the loudest. S_1 is best heard at the apex of the heart. This sound corresponds to closure of the mitral and tricuspid valves and is generally described as sounding like "lub." It's low-pitched and dull. S_1 occurs at the beginning of ventricular systole. It may be split if the mitral valve closes just before the tricuspid.

S_3: Classic sign of heart failure

A third heart sound, S_3, is a normal finding in children and young adults. In addition, S_3 is commonly heard in patients with high cardiac output. Called *ventricular gallop* when it occurs in adults, S_3 may be a cardinal sign of heart failure.

S_3 is best heard at the apex when the patient is lying on his left side. Often compared to the *y* sound in "Ken-tuck-y," S_3 is low-pitched and occurs when the ventricles fill rapidly. It follows S_2 in early ventricular diastole and probably results from vibrations caused by abrupt ventricular distention and resistance to filling. In addition to heart failure, S_3 may also be associated with such conditions as pulmonary edema, atrial septal defect, acute myocardial infarction (MI), and the last trimester of pregnancy.

S_4: An MI aftereffect

S_4 is an adventitious sound called an *atrial gallop* that's heard over the tricuspid or mitral areas with the patient on his left side. You may hear S_4 in patients who are elderly or in those with hypertension, aortic stenosis, or a history of MI. S_4, commonly described as sounding like "Ten-nes-see," occurs just before S_1, after atrial contraction.

The S_4 sound indicates increased resistance to ventricular filling. It results from vibrations caused by forceful atrial ejection of blood into ventricles that are enlarged or hypertrophied and don't move or expand as much as they should.

> The "lub" of the S_1 is loudest at the mitral area.

> The "dub" of the S_2 is loudest at the aortic area.

Auscultating for murmurs

Murmurs occur when structural defects in the heart's chambers or valves cause turbulent blood flow. Turbulence may also be caused by changes in the viscosity of blood or the speed of blood flow. Listen for murmurs over the same precordial areas used in auscultation for heart sounds.

Murmur variations

Murmurs can occur during systole or diastole and are described by several criteria. Their pitch can be high, medium, or low. They can vary in intensity, growing louder or softer. (See *Grading murmurs*.) They can vary by location, sound pattern (blowing, harsh, or musical), radiation (to the neck or axillae), and period during which they occur in the cardiac cycle (pansystolic or midsystolic).

Sit up, please

The best way to hear murmurs is to have the patient sit up and lean forward. Alternatively, you can ask the patient to lie on his left side.

Auscultating for pericardial friction rub

To listen for a pericardial friction rub, have the patient sit upright, lean forward, and exhale. Listen with the diaphragm of the stethoscope over the third intercostal space on the left side of the chest. A pericardial friction rub has a scratchy, rubbing quality. If you suspect a rub but have trouble hearing one, ask the patient to hold his breath.

Palpating arterial pulses

The first step in palpation is to assess skin temperature, texture, and turgor. Then check capillary refill by assessing the nail beds on the fingers and toes. Refill time should be no more than 3 seconds, or long enough to say "capillary refill."

Palpate the patient's arms and legs for temperature and edema. Edema is graded on a four-point scale. If your finger leaves a slight imprint, the edema is recorded as +1. If your finger leaves a deep imprint that only slowly returns to normal, the edema is recorded as +4.

Artery check!

Palpate for arterial pulses by gently pressing with the pads of your index and middle fingers. Start at the top of the patient's body at the temporal artery and work your way down. Check the carotid, brachial, radial, femoral, popliteal, posterior tibial, and dorsalis pedis pulses.

Palpate for the pulse on each side, comparing pulse volume and symmetry. Don't palpate both carotid arteries at the same time or press too firmly. If you do, the patient may faint or become bradycardic. All pulses should be regular in rhythm and equal in strength. Pulses are also graded on a four-point scale: 4+ is bounding, 3+ is increased, 2+ is normal, 1+ is weak, and 0 is absent.

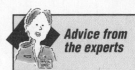

Advice from the experts

Grading murmurs

Use the system outlined here to describe the intensity of a murmur. When recording your findings, use roman numerals as part of a fraction, always with *VI* as the denominator. For example, a grade III murmur would be recorded as *grade III/VI*.
• *Grade I* is a barely audible murmur.
• *Grade II* is audible but quiet and soft.
• *Grade III* is moderately loud, without a thrust or thrill.
• *Grade IV* is loud, with a thrill.
• *Grade V* is very loud, with a thrust or a thrill.
• *Grade VI* is loud enough to be heard before the stethoscope comes into contact with the chest.

Assessing the neurologic system

The most common complaints about the neurologic system include headache, dizziness, faintness, confusion, impaired mental status, disturbances in balance or gait, and changes in level of consciousness (LOC).

Initial neurologic questions

Because many chronic diseases can affect the neurologic system, it's important that you ask the patient about his past health. Inquire about major illnesses, recurrent minor illnesses, accidents or injuries, surgical procedures, and allergies as well as what medications he's currently taking.

All in the family

Also, ask the patient about his family's medical history. Some genetic diseases are degenerative, and others cause muscle weakness. In addition, more than half of patients with migraine headaches have a family history of the disorder.

In the neuro know

Here are some specific questions to ask about the neurologic system:
• Do you have headaches? If so, how often? What seems to bring them on? When you have a headache, does light bother your eyes? Do other symptoms occur?
• Do you have dizziness, numbness, tingling, seizures, tremors, weakness, or paralysis?
• Do you have problems with any of your senses or walking, keeping your balance, swallowing, or urinating?
• How do you rate your memory and ability to concentrate?
• Do you ever have trouble speaking or understanding people?
• Do you have trouble reading or writing? If so, how much does it interfere with your daily activities?

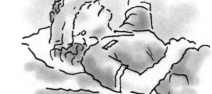

Not all inheritances are good fortune. Migraines are commonly passed from generation to generation.

Checking level of consciousness

A change in the patient's LOC is the earliest and most sensitive indicator that his neurologic status has changed. During your assessment, observe the patient's LOC. Is he alert, or is he falling asleep? Can he focus and maintain his attention, or is he easily distracted?

To avoid confusion, clearly describe the patient's response to various stimuli using these guidelines:
• *alert*—follows commands and responds completely and appropriately to stimuli
• *lethargic*—is drowsy; has delayed responses to verbal stimuli; may drift off to sleep during examination
• *stuporous*—requires vigorous stimulation for a response
• *comatose*—doesn't respond appropriately to verbal or painful stimuli; can't follow commands or communicate verbally.

More than a voice

If you need to use a stronger stimulus than your voice, record what it is and how strong it needs to be to get a response from the patient. The Glasgow Coma Scale offers a more objective way to assess the patient's LOC. (See *Glasgow Coma Scale*, page 42.)

Assessing cranial nerve function

There are 12 pairs of cranial nerves. These nerves transmit motor or sensory messages, or both, primarily between the brain and brain stem and the head and neck.

Something smells

To assess the olfactory nerve (cranial nerve I), have the patient block one nostril and inhale a familiar aromatic substance, such as coffee, citrus, or cinnamon, through the other nostril. Ask him to identify the aroma. Then repeat the process with the other nostril, using a different aroma. Avoid astringent odors, such as ammonia or peppermint, which stimulate the trigeminal nerve.

Seeing eye to eye

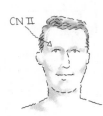

CN II

Next, assess the optic nerve (cranial nerve II). To test visual acuity, have the patient read a newspaper, starting with large headlines and moving to small print.

Test visual fields with a technique called *confrontation*. To do this, stand 2′ (0.6 m) in front of the patient, and have him cover one eye. Then close your eye on the side directly facing the patient's closed eye and bring your moving fingers into the patient's visual field from the periphery. Ask him to tell you when he sees the object. Test each quadrant of the patient's visual field, and compare his results with your own. Chart any defects you find. Finally, examine the fundus of the optic nerve. Blurring of the optic disc may indicate increased intracranial pressure (ICP).

Glasgow Coma Scale

The Glasgow Coma Scale provides an easy way to describe the patient's baseline mental status and to help detect and interpret changes from baseline findings. To use the Glasgow Coma Scale, test the patient's ability to respond to verbal, motor, and sensory stimulation, and grade your findings according to the scale. If a patient is alert, can follow simple commands, and is oriented to person, place, and time, his score will total 15 points. A decreased score in one or more categories may signal an impending neurologic crisis. A total score of 7 or less indicates severe neurologic damage.

Test	Score	Patient's response
Eye-opening response		
Spontaneously	4	Opens eyes spontaneously
To speech	3	Opens eyes when told to
To pain	2	Opens eyes only on painful stimulus
None	1	Doesn't open eyes in response to stimulus
Motor response		
Obeys	6	Shows two fingers when asked
Localizes	5	Reaches toward painful stimulus and tries to remove it
Withdraws	4	Moves away from painful stimulus
Abnormal flexion	3	Assumes a decorticate posture (below)
Abnormal extension	2	Assumes a decerebrate posture (below)
None	1	No response; just lies flaccid—an ominous sign
Verbal response		
Oriented	5	Tells current date
Confused	4	Tells incorrect year
Inappropriate words	3	Replies randomly with incorrect word
Incomprehensible	2	Moans or screams
None	1	No response
Total score		

Three real lookers

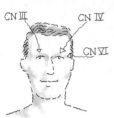

CN III CN IV

CN VI

The oculomotor nerve (cranial nerve III) controls most extraocular movement; it's also responsible for elevation of the eyelid and pupillary constriction. Abnormalities include ptosis (drooping of the upper lid) and pupil inequality. Make sure that the patient's pupils constrict when exposed to light and that his eyes accommodate for seeing objects at various distances.

The trochlear nerve (cranial nerve IV) is responsible for downward and inward eye movement, whereas the abducent nerve (cranial nerve VI) is responsible for lateral eye movement. To assess the oculomotor nerve, the trochlear nerve, and the abducent nerve, ask the patient to follow your finger through the six cardinal positions of gaze. Pause slightly before you move from one position to the next; this pause helps to assess the patient for involuntary eye movement (nystagmus) and the ability to hold the gaze in that particular position.

"Tri" chewing without this nerve

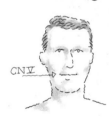

CN V

The trigeminal nerve (cranial nerve V) is a sensory and a motor nerve. It supplies sensation to the corneas, nasal and oral mucosa, and facial skin and also supplies motor function for the jaw and all chewing muscles.

To assess the sensory component, check the patient's ability to feel light touch on his face. Ask him to close his eyes; then touch him with a wisp of cotton on his forehead, cheek, and jaw on each side. Next, test pain perception by touching the tip of a safety pin to the same three areas. Ask the patient to describe and compare both sensations.

Alternate the touches between sharp and dull to test the patient's reliability in comparing sensations. Proper assessment of the nerve requires that the patient identify sharp stimuli. To test the motor component of cranial nerve V, ask the patient to clench his teeth while you palpate the temporal and masseter muscles.

Taking a taste test

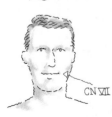

CN VII

The facial nerve (cranial nerve VII) also has a sensory and motor component. The sensory component controls taste perception on the anterior part of the tongue. Assess taste by placing items with various tastes on the anterior portion of the patient's tongue—for example, sugar (sweet), salt, lemon juice (sour), and quinine (bitter). Have the patient wash away each taste with a sip of water before moving on to the next.

The motor component is responsible for the facial muscles. Assess it by observing the patient's face for symmetry at rest and while he smiles, frowns, and raises his eyebrows. If a weakness caused by a stroke or other condition damages the cortex, the patient will be able to raise his eyebrows and wrinkle his forehead. If the weakness is due to an interruption of the facial nerve or other peripheral nerve involvement, one side of the face will be immobile.

Let's hear it for the acoustic nerve!

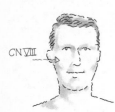

The acoustic nerve (cranial nerve VIII) is responsible for hearing and equilibrium. The cochlear division controls hearing, and the vestibular division controls balance.

To test hearing, ask the patient to cover one ear; then stand on his opposite side and whisper a few words. See whether he can repeat what you said. Test the other ear the same way.

To test the vestibular portion of this nerve, observe the patient for nystagmus and disturbed balance, and note reports of dizziness or a sensation of the room spinning.

Not so hard to swallow

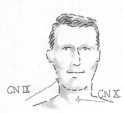

The glossopharyngeal nerve (cranial nerve IX) and the vagus nerve (cranial nerve X) are tested together because their innervation overlaps in the pharynx. The glossopharyngeal nerve is responsible for swallowing, salivation, and taste perception on the posterior one-third of the tongue. The vagus nerve controls swallowing and is also responsible for voice quality.

Start your assessment by listening to the patient's voice. Then check his gag reflex by touching the tip of a tongue blade against his posterior pharynx and asking him to open wide and say "Ahhh." Watch for the symmetrical upward movement of the soft palate and uvula and for the midline position of the uvula.

A very important accessory

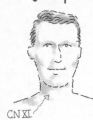

The spinal accessory nerve (cranial nerve XI) is a motor nerve that controls the sternocleidomastoid muscles and the upper portion of the trapezius muscle. To assess this nerve, test the strength of both muscles. First, place your palm against the patient's cheek; then ask him to turn his head against your resistance.

Test the trapezius muscle by placing your hands on the patient's shoulder and asking him to shrug his shoulders against your resistance. Repeat each test on the other side, comparing muscle strength.

Speaking about the tongue

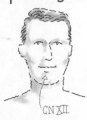

The hypoglossal nerve (cranial nerve XII) controls tongue movement involved in swallowing and speech. The tongue should be midline, without tremors or fasciculations. Test tongue strength by asking the patient to push his tongue against his cheek as you apply resistance. Observe his tongue for symmetry.

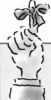

Memory jogger

Cranial nerves I, II, and VIII have sensory functions. Cranial nerves III, IV, VI, XI, and XII have motor functions. Cranial nerves V, VII, IX, and X have sensory and motor functions. How will you ever remember which does what?

Use the following mnemonic to help you remember which cranial nerves have sensory functions (S), motor functions (M), or both (B). The mnemonic begins with cranial nerve I and ends with cranial nerve XII.

I: Some
II: Say
III: Marry
IV: Money
V: But
VI: My
VII: Brother
VIII: Says
IX: Bad
X: Business
XI: Marries
XII: Money

Assessing sensory function

To test the patient for pain sensation, have him close his eyes; then touch all the major dermatomes, first with the sharp end of a safety pin and then with the dull end. Proceed in this order: fingers, shoulders, toes, thighs, and trunk. Ask him to identify when he feels the sharp stimulus.

If the patient has major deficits, start in the area with the least sensation and move toward the area with the most sensation to help you determine the level of deficit.

Getting in touch

To test for the sense of light touch, follow the same routine as above but use a wisp of cotton. Lightly touch the patient's skin—don't swab or sweep the cotton because you might miss an area of loss. A patient with a peripheral neuropathy may retain his sensation for light touch after he has lost pain sensation.

Good vibrations

To test vibratory sense, apply a tuning fork over certain bony prominences while the patient keeps his eyes closed. Start at the distal interphalangeal joint of the index finger and move proximally. Test only until the patient feels the vibration because everything above that level will be intact. If vibratory sense is intact, you won't have to check position sense because the same pathway carries both.

Fingers and toes on the move

To assess position sense, have the patient close his eyes. Then grasp the sides of his big toe, move the toe up and down, and ask him what position it's in. To be tested for position sense, the patient needs intact vestibular and cerebellar function. To perform the same test on the patient's upper extremities, grasp the sides of his index finger and move it back and forth.

Rate ability to discriminate

Discrimination testing assesses the ability of the cerebral cortex to interpret and integrate information. *Stereognosis* is the ability to discriminate the shape, size, weight, texture, and form of an object by touching and manipulating it. To test this, ask the patient to close his eyes and open his hand. Then place a common object, such as a key, in his hand and ask him to identify it.

If he can't identify the object, test graphesthesia by having the patient keep his eyes closed and hold out his hand while you draw a large number on his palm. Ask him to identify the number. Both of these tests assess the ability of the cortex to integrate sensory input.

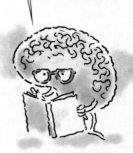

The pressure is on. Discrimination testing assesses the ability of the cerebral cortex to interpret and integrate information.

To test point localization, have the patient close his eyes; then touch one of his limbs, and ask him where you touched him. Test two-point discrimination by touching the patient simultaneously in two contralateral areas. He should be able to identify both touches. Failure to perceive touch on one side is called *extinction*.

Assessing motor function

Assessing the motor system includes inspecting the muscles and testing muscle tone and muscle strength.

Muscle tone

Muscle tone represents muscular resistance to passive stretching. To test arm muscle tone, move the patient's shoulder through passive range-of-motion (ROM) exercises. You should feel a slight resistance. Then let the arm drop to the patient's side. It should fall easily.

To test leg muscle tone, guide the hip through passive ROM exercises; then let the leg fall to the bed. The leg shouldn't fall into an externally rotated position; this finding is considered abnormal and may suggest myasthenia gravis or multiple sclerosis.

Muscle strength

To perform a general examination of muscle strength, observe the patient's gait and motor activities. To evaluate muscle strength, ask the patient to move major muscles and muscle groups against resistance. For instance, to test shoulder girdle strength, have him extend his arms with his palms up and maintain this position for 30 seconds.

If he can't maintain this position, test further by pushing down on his outstretched arms. If he does lift both arms equally, look for pronation of the hand and downward drift of the arm on the weaker side.

Assessing reflexes

Evaluating reflexes involves testing deep tendon and superficial reflexes and observing for primitive reflexes.

Deep tendon reflexes

The key to testing deep tendon reflexes is to make sure the patient is relaxed and the joint is flexed appropriately. First, distract the patient by asking him to focus on a point across the room. Always test deep tendon reflexes by moving from head to toe and comparing side to side. (See *Assessing deep tendon reflexes*.)

Assessing deep tendon reflexes

During a neurologic examination, you'll assess the patient's deep tendon reflexes. Test the biceps, triceps, brachioradialis, patellar or quadriceps, and Achilles reflexes.

Biceps reflex

Position the patient's arm so his elbow is flexed at a 45-degree angle and his arm is relaxed. Place your thumb or index finger over the biceps tendon and your remaining fingers loosely over the triceps muscle. Strike your finger with the pointed end of the reflex hammer, and watch and feel for the contraction of the biceps muscle and flexion of the forearm.

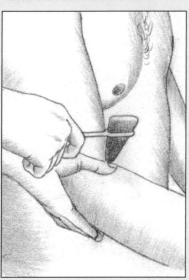

Triceps reflex

Have the patient adduct his arm and place his forearm across his chest. Strike the triceps tendon about 2" (5 cm) above the olecranon process on the extensor surface of the upper arm. Watch for contraction of the triceps muscle and extension of the forearm.

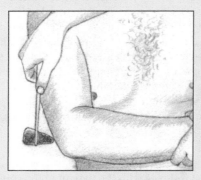

Brachioradialis reflex

Ask the patient to rest the ulnar surface of his hand on his abdomen or lap with the elbow partially flexed. Strike the radius, and watch for supination of the hand and flexion of the forearm at the elbow.

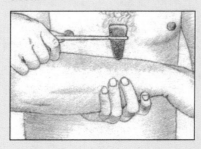

Patellar reflex

Have the patient sit with his legs dangling freely. If he can't sit up, flex his knee at a 45-degree angle and place your nondominant hand behind it for support. Strike the patellar tendon just below the patella, and look for contraction of the quadriceps muscle in the thigh with extension of the leg.

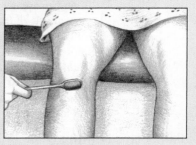

Achilles reflex

Have the patient flex his foot. Then support the plantar surface. Strike the Achilles tendon, and watch for plantar flexion of the foot at the ankle.

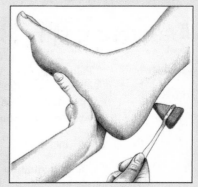

Grade deep tendon reflexes using the following scale:
- 0—absent impulses
- +1—diminished impulses
- +2—normal impulses
- +3—increased impulses (may be normal)
- +4—hyperactive impulses.

Superficial reflexes

Stimulating the skin or mucous membranes is a method of testing superficial reflexes. Because these reflexes are cutaneous, the more you try to elicit them in succession, the less response you'll get. So observe carefully the first time you stimulate.

Tickling the feet

Using an applicator stick, tongue blade, or key, slowly stroke the lateral side of the patient's sole from the heel to the great toe. The normal response in an adult is plantar flexion of the toes. Upward movement of the great toe and fanning of the little toes—called *Babinski's reflex*—is abnormal. Babinski's reflex indicates corticospinal damage, which may be present with amyotrophic lateral sclerosis, brain tumor, head trauma, multiple sclerosis, meningitis, rabies, or stroke.

Tickling the tummy

Test the abdominal reflexes with the patient in the supine position with his arms at his sides and his knees slightly flexed. Briskly stroke both sides of the abdomen above and below the umbilicus, moving from the periphery toward the midline. Movement of the umbilicus toward the stimulus is normal.

Assessing the GI system

Palpating or percussing the abdomen before you auscultate can change the character of the patient's bowel sounds and lead to an inaccurate assessment. Therefore, to perform an abdominal assessment, use this sequence:

 inspection

 auscultation

 percussion

 palpation.

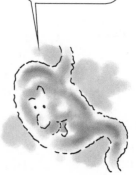

When performing a GI assessment, be sure to auscultate before you percuss.

Initial GI questions

If the patient has a GI problem, he'll usually complain about pain, heartburn, nausea, vomiting, or altered bowel habits. To investigate these and other signs and symptoms, ask him about the location, quality, onset, duration, frequency, and severity of each.

Also ask the patient about his occupation, home life, stress level, and recent life changes as well as alcohol, caffeine, and tobacco use; food consumption; exercise habits; sleep patterns; and oral hygiene. Here are some other questions to ask about his GI symptoms:

• Have you had a GI illness in the past, such as an ulcer; liver, pancreas, or gallbladder disease; inflammatory bowel disease; rectal or GI bleeding; hiatal hernia; irritable bowel syndrome; diverticulitis; gastroesophageal reflux disease; or cancer? (Ask this question to determine whether the patient's problem is new or recurring.)

• Does anyone in your family have a GI disorder? (Some GI conditions are hereditary.)

• Have you had abdominal surgery or trauma?

• Are you taking any medications, including laxatives? (Habitual laxative use may cause constipation.)

• Are you allergic to medications or foods?

• Have you noticed changes in appetite, difficulty chewing or swallowing, or changes in bowel habits?

• Do you have excessive belching or passing of gas?

• Have you noticed a change in the color, amount, and appearance of your stool? Have you ever seen blood in your stool?

• Have you recently traveled abroad? (Ask this question if the patient is seeking care for diarrhea because diarrhea, hepatitis, and parasitic infections can result from ingesting contaminated food or water.)

Inspecting the abdomen

Begin your inspection of the abdomen by mentally dividing the abdomen into four quadrants and then imagining the organs in each quadrant. (See *Abdominal quadrants*, page 50.)

Checking for a bulge

Observe the abdomen for symmetry, checking for bumps, bulges, or masses. Assess the umbilicus, which should be inverted and located midline in the abdomen. Conditions such as pregnancy, ascites, or an underlying mass can cause the umbilicus to protrude. Have the patient raise his head and shoulders. If his umbilicus protrudes, he may have an umbilical hernia.

Abdominal quadrants

To perform a systematic GI assessment, try to visualize the abdominal structures by dividing the abdomen into four quadrants, as shown here.

Right upper quadrant
• Right lobe of liver
• Gallbladder
• Pylorus
• Duodenum
• Head of the pancreas
• Hepatic flexure of the colon
• Portions of the ascending and transverse colon

Left upper quadrant
• Left lobe of the liver
• Stomach
• Body of the pancreas
• Splenic flexure of the colon
• Portions of the transverse and descending colon

Right lower quadrant
• Cecum and appendix
• Portion of the ascending colon

Left lower quadrant
• Sigmoid colon
• Portion of the descending colon

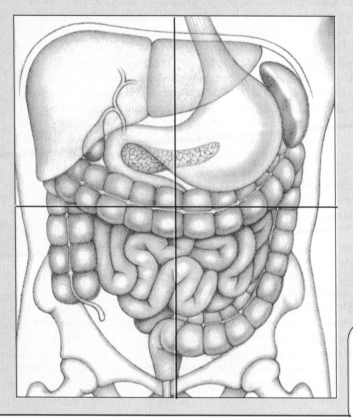

Watch out! Visibility of the wavelike movements of peristalsis may signal a bowel obstruction.

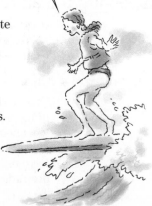

Scouring the skin

The abdominal skin should be smooth and uniform in color. Note dilated veins. Record the length of any surgical scars on the abdomen.

Riding the peristaltic wave

Note abdominal movements and pulsations. Usually, peristalsis can't be seen; if it's visible, it looks like slight, wavelike motions. Visible rippling waves may indicate bowel obstruction and should be reported immediately. Marked pulsations may occur with hypertension, aortic insufficiency, aortic aneurysm, and other conditions causing widening pulse pressure.

Auscultating the abdomen

Lightly place the stethoscope diaphragm in the right lower quadrant, slightly below and to the right of the umbilicus. Auscultate in a clockwise fashion in each of the four quadrants. Note the character and quality of bowel sounds in each quadrant. In some cases, you may need to auscultate for 5 minutes before you hear sounds.

Before auscultating the abdomen of a patient with a nasogastric tube or another abdominal tube connected to suction, briefly clamp the tube or turn off the suction. Suction noises can obscure or mimic actual bowel sounds.

Pardon my borborygmus

Normal bowel sounds are high-pitched, gurgling noises caused by air mixing with fluid during peristalsis. The rumbling noises, called *borborygmus*, vary in frequency, pitch, and intensity and occur irregularly from 5 to 34 times per minute. Bowel sounds are classified as normal, hypoactive, or hyperactive.

Voice of the vessels

Auscultate for vascular sounds with the bell of the stethoscope. Using firm pressure, listen over the aorta and renal, iliac, and femoral arteries for bruits, venous hums, and friction rubs.

Percussing the abdomen

Direct or indirect percussion is used to detect the size and location of abdominal organs and to detect air or fluid in the abdomen, stomach, or bowel.

In direct percussion, strike your hand or finger directly against the patient's abdomen. With indirect percussion, use the middle finger of your dominant hand or a percussion hammer to strike a finger resting on the patient's abdomen. Begin percussion in the right lower quadrant and proceed clockwise, covering all four quadrants.

Don't percuss the abdomen of a patient with an abdominal aortic aneurysm or a transplanted abdominal organ. Doing so can precipitate a rupture or organ rejection.

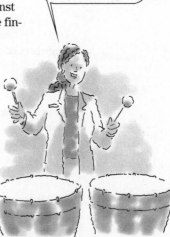

Percussion over hollow organs should reveal tympany, a drumlike sound.

Hollow or dull?

You normally hear two sounds during percussion of the abdomen: *tympany* and *dullness*. When you percuss over hollow organs, such as an empty stomach or bowel, you hear a clear, hollow sound like a drum beating. This sound, called *tympany*, predominates because air is normally present in the stomach and bowel. The degree of tympany depends on the amount of air and gastric dilation. When you percuss over solid organs, such as the liver, kidney, or feces-filled intestines, the sound changes to *dullness*. Note where percussed sounds change from tympany to dullness.

How large is the liver?

Percussion of the liver can help you estimate its size. Hepatomegaly (enlarged liver) is commonly associated with hepatitis and other liver diseases. Liver borders may be obscured and difficult to assess.

Splenic dullard

The spleen is located at about the level of the 10th rib, in the left midaxillary line. Percussion may produce a small area of dullness, generally 7″ (17.8 cm) or less in adults. However, the spleen usually can't be percussed because tympany from the colon masks the dullness of the spleen. To assess a patient for splenic enlargement, ask him to breathe deeply. Then percuss along the 9th to 11th intercostal spaces on the left, listening for a change from tympany to dullness. Measure the area of dullness. This change from tympany to dullness is called a *positive splenic percussion sign*.

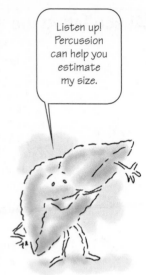

Listen up! Percussion can help you estimate my size.

Palpating the abdomen

Abdominal palpation includes light and deep touch to help determine the size, shape, position, and tenderness of major abdominal organs and detect masses and fluid accumulation. Palpate all four quadrants, leaving painful and tender areas for last.

Light touch

Light palpation helps identify muscle resistance and tenderness as well as the location of some superficial organs. To palpate, put the fingers of one hand close together, depress the skin about ½″ with your fingertips, and make gentle, rotating movements. Avoid short, quick jabs.

The abdomen should be soft and nontender. As you palpate the four quadrants, note organs, masses, and areas of tenderness or increased resistance. Determine whether resistance is caused by the patient being cold, tense, or ticklish, or whether it's due to involuntary guarding or rigidity from muscle spasms or peritoneal inflammation.

Pressing the issue

To perform deep palpation, push the abdomen down 2″ to 3″ (5 to 7.5 cm). In an obese patient, put one hand on top of the other and

Palpating the liver

These illustrations show the correct hand positions for two ways of palpating the liver: regular palpation and hooking.

Palpation

• Place the patient in the supine position. Stand at his right side, and place your left hand under his back at the approximate location of the liver, as shown below.
• Place your right hand slightly below the lower border of liver dullness. Point the fingers of your right hand toward the patient's head just under the right costal margin.
• As the patient inhales deeply, gently press in and up on the abdomen until the liver brushes under your right hand. The edge should be smooth, firm, and somewhat round. Note any tenderness.

Hooking

• Hooking is an alternative method for palpating the liver. To hook the liver, stand next to the patient's right shoulder, facing his feet. Place your hands side by side, and hook your fingertips over the right costal margin, below the lower border of liver dullness, as shown below.
• Ask the patient to take a deep breath as you push your fingertips in and up. If the liver is palpable, you may feel its edge as it slides down in the abdomen as he breathes in.

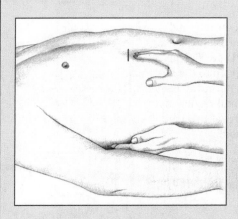
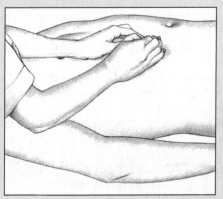

push. Palpate the entire abdomen in a clockwise direction, checking for tenderness, pulsations, organ enlargement, and masses.

If the patient's abdomen is rigid, don't palpate it. He could have peritoneal inflammation, and palpation could cause pain or could rupture an inflamed organ.

Palpating the liver and spleen

Palpate the patient's liver to check for enlargement and tenderness. (See *Palpating the liver*.) Unless the spleen is enlarged, it isn't

Palpating the spleen

Although a normal spleen isn't palpable, an enlarged spleen is. To palpate the spleen, stand on the patient's right side. Use your left hand to support his posterior left lower rib cage. Ask him to take a deep breath. Then, with your right hand on his abdomen, press up and in toward the spleen.

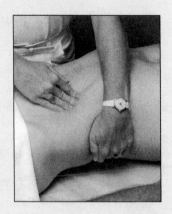

palpable. If you do feel the spleen, stop palpating immediately because compression can cause rupture. (See *Palpating the spleen*.)

On the rebound

When you suspect peritoneal inflammation, check for rebound tenderness at the end of your examination. To do so, choose a site away from the painful area and position your hand at a 90-degree angle to the abdomen. Push down slowly and deeply into the abdomen; then withdraw your hand quickly. Rapid withdrawal causes the underlying structures to rebound suddenly and results in a sharp, stabbing pain on the inflamed side. Don't repeat this maneuver because you may rupture an inflamed appendix.

Fluid overload

Ascites, a large accumulation of fluid in the peritoneal cavity, can be caused by advanced liver disease, heart failure, pancreatitis, or cancer. If ascities is present, use a tape measure to measure the fullest part of the abdomen. Mark this point on the patient's abdomen with indelible ink so you'll be sure to measure consistently. This measurement is important, especially if fluid removal or paracentesis is performed, because it can help you evaluate the effectiveness of the treatment.

Ascites is an accumulation of fluid in the peritoneal cavity.

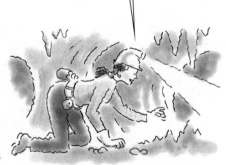

Assessing the urinary system

The most common complaints of the urinary system include output changes, such as polyuria, oliguria, and anuria; voiding pattern changes, such as hesitancy, frequency, urgency, nocturia, and incontinence; urine color changes; and pain. To perform a physical assessment of the urinary system, you'll use inspection, percussion, and palpation.

Initial urinary questions

During the assessment, be sure to ask the patient about:
• his medical history, especially the presence of diabetes or hypertension
• his family's health to get information on his risk of developing renal failure or kidney disease
• the medications he's currently taking, including over-the-counter drugs and herbal preparations as well as prescribed medications, because some drugs can affect the appearance of urine and nephrotoxic drugs can alter urinary function.

In addition, ask these questions:
• Do you have diabetes, cardiovascular disease, or hypertension?
• Have you ever had a kidney or bladder infection or an infection of the reproductive system? How about kidney or bladder trauma or kidney stones?
• Have you ever been catheterized?
• Have you noticed a change in the color or odor of your urine?
• Do you have pain or burning during urination?
• Do you have allergies? (Allergic reactions can cause tubular damage. A severe anaphylactic reaction can cause temporary renal failure and permanent tubular necrosis.)
• Do you have problems with incontinence or frequency? (See *Assessing urine appearance*, page 56.)

Inspecting the urethral meatus

In the male patient, check the penile shaft and glans for lesions, nodules, inflammations, and swelling. Then gently compress the tip of the glans to open the urethral meatus. It should be located in the center of the glans and be pink and smooth. Inspect it for swelling, discharge, lesions, inflammation and, especially, genital warts. If you note discharge, obtain a culture specimen. (See *Examining the urethral meatus*, page 56.)

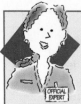

Advice from the experts

Assessing urine appearance

The appearance of your patient's urine can provide clues about his general health and the source of his genitourinary problem. During the health history, ask whether he has noticed any change in color. If he has, use this list to help interpret the changes:
• Pale and diluted—diabetes insipidus, diuretic therapy, excessive fluid intake
• Dark yellow or amber and concentrated—acute febrile disease, inadequate fluid intake, severe diarrhea or vomiting
• Blue-green—methylene blue ingestion
• Green-brown—bile duct obstruction
• Dark brown or black—acute glomerulonephritis, intake of such drugs as chlorpromazine
• Orange-red or orange-brown—obstructive jaundice, urobilinuria, intake of such drugs as rifampin or phenazopyridine
• Red or red-brown—hemorrhage, porphyria, intake of such drugs as phenazopyridine.

Examining the urethral meatus

To inspect the urethral meatus, compress the tip of the glans, as shown.

Urethral meatus

Glans penis

Scrotum

In the female patient, first put on a pair of gloves. Then spread the labia and locate the urethral meatus. It should be a pink, irregular, slitlike opening at the midline, just above the vagina. Note the presence of discharge (a sign of urethral infection) or ulcerations (a sign of a sexually transmitted disease [STD]).

Percussing the urinary organs

Kidney percussion checks for costovertebral angle tenderness that occurs with inflammation. To percuss over the kidneys, have the patient sit up. Place the ball of your nondominant hand on the patient's back at the costovertebral angle of the 12th rib. Strike the ball of that hand with the ulnar surface of your other hand. Use just enough force to cause a painless but perceptible thud.

To percuss the bladder, first ask the patient to empty it. Then have her lie in the supine position. Start at the symphysis pubis and percuss upward toward the bladder and over it. You should hear tympany. A dull sound signals retained urine.

Palpating the urinary organs

Because the kidneys lie behind other organs and are protected by muscle, they normally aren't palpable unless they're enlarged. However, in very thin patients, you may be able to feel the lower end of the right kidney as a smooth round mass that drops on inspiration.

Because I lie behind other organs and I'm protected by muscle, you may not be able to palpate me. That's fine because I'm ticklish anyway.

Assessing the male reproductive system

The male reproductive system includes the penis, scrotum, testicles, epididymis, vas deferens, seminal vesicles, and prostate gland.

Initial male reproductive questions

During your assessment, be sure to inquire about the patient's sexual preference and practices to assess risk-taking behaviors. Also ask these questions:
• Have you noticed sores, lumps, or ulcers on your penis?
• Do you have scrotal swelling? (This sign can indicate an inguinal hernia, a hematocele, epididymitis, or a testicular tumor.)
• Do you have penile discharge or bleeding?
• How many sexual partners do you currently have? How many have you had in the past?
• Have you ever had an STD? If so, did you receive treatment?
• What precautions do you take to prevent contracting STDs? Have you been tested for HIV? If so, what was your HIV status?
• What measures do you take for birth control? Have you had a vasectomy?
• Have you ever had trauma to your penis or scrotum?
• Have you ever been diagnosed with an undescended testicle?
• Have you ever been diagnosed with a low sperm count?

Inspecting and palpating the male genitalia

Make the patient as comfortable as possible, and explain what you're doing every step of the way. Put on gloves.

Inspection

Start by examining the penis. The penile skin should be slightly wrinkled and pink to light brown in white patients and light brown to dark brown in black patients. Check the penile shaft and glans for lesions, nodules, inflammations, and swelling. Inspect the glans of an uncircumcised penis by retracting the prepuce. Also check the glans for smegma, a cheesy secretion commonly found beneath the prepuce.

Pressing the point

Next, gently compress the tip of the glans to open the urethral meatus. It should be located in the center of the glans and be pink and smooth. Inspect it for swelling, discharge, lesions, inflammation and, especially, genital warts. If you note discharge, obtain a culture specimen.

Then inspect the scrotum and testicles. Have the patient hold his penis away from his scrotum so you can observe the scrotum's general size and appearance. Spread the surface of the scrotum, and examine the skin for swelling, nodules, redness, ulceration, and distended veins.

Finally, inspect the inguinal and femoral areas. Have the patient stand. Then ask him to hold his breath and bear down while you inspect the inguinal and femoral areas for bulges or hernias.

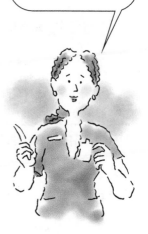

Assessment of the reproductive system can be uncomfortable for the patient. Explain what you're doing as you go along to reduce his anxiety.

Palpation

Palpate the penis, testicles, epididymides, spermatic cords, inguinal and femoral areas, and prostate gland.

Penis

Use your thumb and forefinger to palpate the entire penile shaft. It should be somewhat firm, and the skin should be smooth and movable. Note swelling, nodules, or indurations.

Testicles

Gently palpate both testicles between your thumb and first two fingers. Assess their size, shape, and response to pressure. A normal response is a deep visceral pain. The testicles should be equal in size, move freely in the scrotal sac, and feel firm, smooth, and rubbery. (See *Testicular self-examination*.)

Shed some light on the subject

If you note hard, irregular areas or lumps, transilluminate them by darkening the room and pressing the head of a flashlight against the scrotum, behind the lump. The testicle and any lumps, masses, warts, or blood-filled areas will appear as opaque shadows. Transilluminate the other testicle to compare your findings.

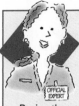

Advice from the experts

Testicular self-examination

During the patient history, ask your patient whether he performs monthly testicular self-examinations. If he doesn't, explain that testicular cancer, the most common cancer in men ages 20 to 35, can be treated successfully when it's detected early.

Teaching the technique

To perform this examination, the patient should hold his penis out of the way with one hand, then roll each testicle between the thumb and first two fingers of his other hand. A normal testicle should have no lumps, move freely in the scrotal sac, and feel firm, smooth, and rubbery. Both testicles should be the same size, although the left one is usually lower than the right because the left spermatic cord is longer.

If the patient finds any abnormalities, he should notify his doctor immediately.

Epididymides

Next, palpate the epididymides, which are usually located in the posterolateral area of the testicles. They should be smooth, discrete, nontender, and free from swelling and induration.

Spermatic cords

Palpate both spermatic cords, which are located above each testicle. Palpate from the base of the epididymis to the inguinal canal. The vas deferens is a smooth, movable cord inside the spermatic cord. If you feel swelling, irregularity, or nodules, transilluminate the problem area, as previously described. If serous fluid is present, you won't see a glow.

Inguinal area

To assess the patient for a direct inguinal hernia, place two fingers over each external inguinal ring and ask the patient to bear down. If he has a hernia, you'll feel a bulge.

To assess the patient for an indirect inguinal hernia, examine him while he's standing and then while he's in a supine position with his knee flexed on the side you're examining.

Prostate gland

Tell the patient that you need to examine his prostate gland, and warn him that he'll feel some pressure or urgency during the examination. Have him stand and lean over the examination table. If he can't do this, have him lie on his left side, with his right knee and hip flexed or with both knees drawn toward his chest. Inspect the skin of the perineal, anal, and posterior scrotal areas. It should be smooth and unbroken, with no protruding masses.

Then lubricate the gloved index finger of your dominant hand and insert it into the rectum. If the patient is having difficulty relaxing the anal sphincter, ask him to bear down as if having a bowel movement while you gently insert your finger. With your finger pad, palpate the prostate gland on the anterior rectal wall just past the anorectal ring. The gland should feel smooth, rubbery, and about the size of a walnut. (See *Palpating the prostate gland.*)

If the prostate gland protrudes into the rectal lumen, it's probably enlarged. An enlarged prostate gland is classified from grade 1 (protruding less than $3/8''$ [1 cm] into the rectal lumen) to grade 4 (protruding more than 1" [3.2 cm] into the rectal lumen). Also, note tenderness or nodules.

Palpating the prostate gland

To palpate the prostate gland, insert your lubricated, gloved index finger into the rectum. Palpate the prostate on the anterior rectal wall, just past the anorectal ring.

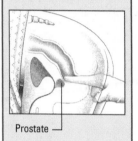

Prostate

Assessing the female reproductive system

The most common reproductive system complaints are pain, vaginal discharge, abnormal uterine bleeding, pruritus, and infertility.

Initial female reproductive questions

Throughout the assessment, ask the female patient to describe her symptoms in her own words, encouraging her to speak freely. If she's sexually active, talk to her about the importance of safer sex and the prevention of STDs and HIV. Also ask these questions:
• How old were you when you began to menstruate?
• How long does your period usually last? How often does it occur? Do you have cramps, spotting, or an unusually heavy or light flow?
• Have you ever been pregnant? If so, how many times and how many times did you give birth? Did you have vaginal or cesarean deliveries?
• Have you had any miscarriages or therapeutic abortions?
• How many sexual partners do you currently have?
• What kind of birth control, if any, do you use?
• Do you experience pain with intercourse?
• Have you ever had an STD?
• Have you ever been tested for HIV?
• When was your last Pap test, and what was the result?
  If the patient is postmenopausal, also ask:

• What is the date of your last menses? Are you having hot flashes, night sweats, mood swings, flushing, or vaginal dryness or itching?
• Have you ever had breast lumps, biopsy, or surgery, including enlargement or reduction?
• Have you ever had breast cancer, fibroadenoma, or fibrocystic disease? (If so, ask for more information — for example, if she had cancer, ask when, which breast, and what treatment she received; if a fibroadenoma, ask which breast was affected, when it was found, and whether surgical excision was necessary; if fibrocystic breast disease, ask whether she underwent any treatment.)

Inspecting the female genitalia

Before the examination, ask the patient to void. Have her disrobe and put on an examination gown. Help her into the dorsal lithotomy position, and drape all areas not being examined. Make sure you explain the procedure to her before the examination.

Inspecting the external genitalia

First, put on a pair of gloves. Spread the labia and locate the urethral meatus. It should be a pink, irregular, slitlike opening at the midline, just above the vagina. Note the presence of discharge or ulcerations. You may detect a normal discharge that varies from clear and stretchy before ovulation to white and opaque after ovulation. The discharge should be odorless and nonirritating to the mucosa.

Vestibule

Then examine the vestibule, especially the area around the Bartholin's and Skene's glands. Check for swelling, redness, lesions, discharge, and unusual odor. Finally, inspect the vaginal opening, noting whether the hymen is intact or perforated.

Labia

Spread the labia with one hand and palpate with the other. The labia should feel soft, and the patient shouldn't feel any pain. Note swelling, hardness, or tenderness. If you detect a mass or lesion, palpate it to determine its size, shape, and consistency.

Inspecting and palpating the internal genitalia

Nurses don't routinely inspect internal genitalia unless they're in advanced practice. However, you may be asked to assist with this examination.

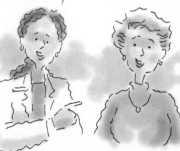

The reproductive system is the source of most health complaints in women.

If you are involved with the examination, hold the speculum under warm, running water to lubricate and warm the blades. Don't use other lubricants because many of them are bacteriostatic and can alter Pap test results.

Tell her about it

Sit or stand at the foot of the examination table. Tell the patient she'll feel internal pressure and possibly some slight, transient discomfort as the speculum is inserted and opened. The person performing the inspection will look for lesions or abnormal discharge.

After the speculum is removed, the internal genitalia are palpated. To palpate the internal genitalia, lubricate the index and middle fingers of your gloved dominant hand. Use the thumb and index finger of your other hand to spread the labia majora. Insert your two lubricated fingers into the vagina, exerting pressure posteriorly to avoid irritating the anterior wall and urethra.

Note a little tenderness

When your fingers are fully inserted, note tenderness or nodularity in the vaginal wall. Ask the patient to bear down so you can assess the support of the vaginal outlet. Bulging of the vaginal wall may indicate a cystocele or a rectocele.

Next stop, cervix

To palpate the cervix, sweep your fingers from side to side across the cervix and around the os. The cervix should be smooth and firm and should protrude ¼″ to 1¼″ (0.5 to 3 cm) into the vagina. If you palpate nodules or irregularities, the patient may have cysts, tumors, or other lesions.

Next, place your fingers into the recessed area around the cervix. The cervix should move in all directions. If the patient reports pain during this part of the examination, she may have inflammation of the uterus or adnexa (ovaries, fallopian tubes, and ligaments of the uterus).

Get ready for the rectum

Rectovaginal palpation examines the posterior part of the uterus and the pelvic cavity. Put on a new pair of gloves, and apply water-soluble lubricant to the index and middle fingers of your dominant hand. Instruct the patient to bear down with her vaginal and rectal muscles; then insert your index finger a short way into her vagina and your middle finger into her rectum. Use your middle finger to assess rectal muscle and sphincter tone. Insert your finger deeper into the rectum, and palpate the rectal wall with your middle finger. Sweep the rectum with your fingers, assessing for masses or nodules.

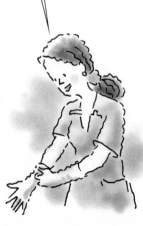

Before performing a rectovaginal exam, put on a clean pair of gloves.

Palpate the posterior wall of the uterus through the anterior wall of the rectum, evaluating the uterus for size, shape, tenderness, and masses. The rectovaginal septum, the wall between the rectum and the vagina, should feel smooth and springy.

Place your nondominant hand on the patient's abdomen at the symphysis pubis. With your index finger in the vagina, palpate deeply to feel the posterior edge of the cervix and the lower posterior wall of the uterus.

Wrapping up

When you're finished, discard the gloves and wash your hands. Help the patient to a sitting position, and provide privacy for dressing and personal hygiene.

Inspecting and palpating the breasts and axillae

Have the patient disrobe from the waist up and sit with her arms at her sides. Keep both breasts uncovered so you can observe them simultaneously to detect differences.

Breast skin should be smooth, undimpled, and the same color as the rest of the skin. Check for edema, which can accompany lymphatic obstruction and may signal cancer. Note breast size and symmetry. Asymmetry may occur normally in some adult women, with the left breast usually larger than the right. Inspect the nipples, noting their size and shape. If a nipple is inverted (dimpled or creased), ask the patient when she first noticed the inversion.

Changing positions

Next, inspect the patient's breasts while she holds her arms over her head, and then again while she has her hands on her hips. Having the patient assume these positions will help you detect skin or nipple dimpling that might not have been obvious before.

If the patient has large or pendulous breasts, have her stand with her hands on the back of a chair and lean forward. This position helps reveal subtle breast or nipple asymmetry.

Before palpating the breasts, ask the patient to lie in a supine position, and place a small pillow under her shoulder on the side you're examining. This causes the breast on that side to protrude. (See *Palpating the breast*, page 64.)

Have the patient put her hand behind her head on the side you're examining. To perform palpation, place your fingers flat on the breast and compress the tissues gently against the chest wall, palpating in concentric circles outward from the nipple. Palpate the entire breast, including the periphery, tail of Spence, and areola. For a patient with pendulous breasts, palpate down or across the breast with the patient sitting upright.

Palpating the breast

Use your three middle fingers to palpate the breast systematically. Rotating your fingers gently against the chest wall, move in concentric circles. Make sure you include the tail of Spence in your examination.

Examining the areola and nipple
After palpating the breast, palpate the areola and nipple. Gently squeeze the nipple between your thumb and index finger to check for discharge.

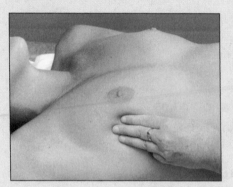

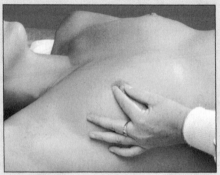

Watch for inconsistencies

As you palpate, note the consistency of the breast tissue. Normal consistency varies widely, depending in part on the proportions of fat and glandular tissue. Check for nodules and unusual tenderness. Tenderness may be related to cysts and cancer. However, nodularity, fullness, and mild tenderness are also premenstrual symptoms. Be sure to ask the patient where she is in her menstrual cycle.

A lump or mass that feels different from the rest of the breast tissue may indicate a pathologic change and warrants further investigation by a doctor. If you find what you think is an abnormality, check the other breast, too.

Get a smear

Finally, palpate the nipple, noting its elasticity. It should be rough, elastic, and round. The nipple also typically protrudes from the breast. Compress the nipple and areola to detect discharge. If discharge is present and the patient isn't pregnant or lactating, assess the color, consistency, and quantity of the discharge. If possible, obtain a cytologic smear.

On to the axillae

To examine the axillae, use the techniques of inspection and palpation. Before palpating, ask the patient to relax her arm on the

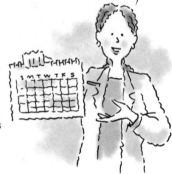

Find out where the woman is in her menstrual cycle to help you differentiate abnormalities from premenstrual symptoms.

side you're examining. Support her elbow with one of your hands. Cup the fingers of your other hand, and reach high into the apex of the axilla. Place your fingers directly behind the pectoral muscles, pointing toward the midclavicle.

Assessing the musculoskeletal system

During a musculoskeletal assessment, you'll use sight, hearing, and touch to determine the health of the patient's muscles, bones, joints, tendons, and ligaments. Because many musculoskeletal injuries are emergencies, you might not have time for a thorough assessment.

Initial musculoskeletal questions

Ask the patient about his past and current health, occupation, and hobbies as well as whether his ADLs have been affected by his condition. Also ask the following:
• Have you experienced a recent blunt or penetrating trauma? If so, how did it happen? (This information can help guide your assessment and predict hidden trauma.)
• Do you carry a heavy knapsack or purse? (Habitually carrying heavy bags can cause injury or increase muscle size.)
• Have you noticed grating sounds when you move certain parts of your body? Do you use ice, heat, or other remedies to treat the problem?
• Have you been diagnosed with gout, arthritis, tuberculosis, cancer (which may cause bony metastases), or osteoporosis? (See *Biocultural variations in bone density*.)
• Do you use a cane, walker, brace, or other assistive device? (If so, watch him use the device to assess how he moves.)
• What medications do you take regularly, including over-the-counter and herbal treatments?

Assessing the bones and joints

Perform a complete examination if the patient has generalized symptoms such as aching in several joints. Perform an abbreviated examination if he has pain in only one body area. The only special equipment you'll need is a tape measure.

Head and neck

Inspect and palpate the patient's neck, noting muscle asymmetry or masses. Palpate the spinous processes of the cervical vertebrae

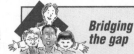
Bridging the gap

Biocultural variations in bone density

Studies of bone density have shown that Black males have the densest bones. They also have a relatively low incidence of osteoporosis, a bone disorder characterized by a decrease in bone mass that leaves bones porous, brittle, and prone to being fractured. Although the bone density of Whites falls below that of Blacks, Whites tend to have higher bone densities than Chinese, Japanese, and Inuit patients. Use this information to help you identify patients at risk for osteoporosis.

and the areas above each clavicle for tenderness, swelling, or nodules.

Check ROM in the neck by asking the patient to try touching his right ear to his right shoulder and his left ear to his left shoulder. The usual ROM is 40 degrees on each side. Next, ask him to touch his chin to his chest and then to point his chin toward the ceiling. The neck should flex forward 45 degrees and extend backward 55 degrees. Assess rotation by having the patient turn his head to each side without moving his trunk. His chin should be parallel to his shoulders. Finally, ask him to move his head in a circle; normal rotation is 70 degrees.

Spine

Have the patient stand in profile. In this position, the spine has a reverse "S" shape. Next, observe the spine posteriorly. It should be in midline position, without deviation to either side. Lateral deviation suggests scoliosis. Normally, the spine remains at midline. (See *Testing for scoliosis*.)

Spine-tingling procedure

Finally, palpate the spinal processes and the areas lateral to the spine. Have the patient bend at the waist and let his arms hang loosely at his sides. Palpate the spine with your fingertips. Then repeat the palpation using the side of your hand, lightly striking the areas lateral to the spine. Note tenderness, swelling, or spasms.

Shoulders and elbows

Inspect the patient's shoulders, noting asymmetry, muscle atrophy, or deformity. Palpate the shoulders to locate bony landmarks; note crepitus or tenderness. Palpate the shoulder muscles for firmness and symmetry. Also palpate the elbow and the ulna for subcutaneous nodules that occur with rheumatoid arthritis.

Lift and rotate

If the patient's shoulders don't appear to be dislocated, assess rotation. Start with the patient's arm straight at his side. Ask him to lift his arm straight up from his side to shoulder level and then to bend his elbow horizontally until his forearm is at a 90-degree angle to his upper arm. His arm should be parallel to the floor, and his fingers should be extended with palms down.

To assess external rotation, have him bring up his forearm until his fingers point toward the ceiling. To assess internal rotation, have him lower his forearm until his fingers point toward the floor. Normal ROM is 90 degrees in each direction.

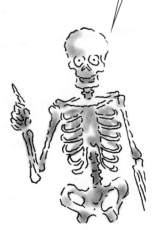

If the patient's condition isn't an emergency, perform a complete musculoskeletal examination.

Flex and extend

To assess flexion and extension, start with the patient's arm in the neutral position (at his side). To assess flexion, ask him to move his arm anteriorly over his head, as if reaching for the sky. Full flexion is 180 degrees. To assess extension, have him move his arm from the neutral position posteriorly as far as possible. Normal extension ranges from 30 to 50 degrees.

Swing into position

To assess abduction, ask the patient to move his arm from the neutral position laterally as far as possible. Normal ROM is 180 degrees. To assess adduction, have the patient move his arm from the neutral position across the front of his body as far as possible. Normal ROM is 50 degrees.

Up to his elbows

Next, assess the elbows for flexion and extension. Have the patient rest his arm at his side. Ask him to flex his elbow from this position and then extend it. Normal ROM is 90 degrees for both flexion and extension. To assess supination and pronation of the elbow, have the patient place the side of his hand on a flat surface with the thumb on top. Ask him to rotate his palm down toward the table for pronation and upward for supination. The normal angle of elbow rotation is 90 degrees in each direction.

Wrists

Inspect the wrists for contour, and compare them for symmetry. Use your thumb and index finger to palpate both wrists. Note any tenderness, nodules, or bogginess.

Assess ROM in the wrists. Ask the patient to rotate each wrist by moving his entire hand—first laterally, then medially—as if he's waxing a car. Normal ROM is 55 degrees laterally and 20 degrees medially.

Hips and knees

Inspect the hip area for contour and symmetry. Inspect the position of the knees, noting whether the patient is bowlegged, with knees that point out, or knock-kneed, with knees that turn in. Palpate each hip over the iliac crest and trochanteric area for tenderness or instability. Palpate both knees. They should feel smooth, and the tissues should feel solid.

Hip, hip, hooray!

Assess ROM in the hip with the patient in a supine position. To assess hip flexion, place your hand under the patient's lower back

---

Testing for scoliosis

When testing for scoliosis, have the patient remove her shirt and stand as straight as possible with her back to you. Look for:
• uneven shoulder height and shoulder blade prominence
• unequal distance between the arms and the body
• asymmetrical waistline
• uneven hip height
• sideways lean.

Bent over
Next, have the patient bend forward, keeping her head down and palms together. Look for:
• asymmetrical thoracic spine or prominent rib cage (rib hump) on either side
• asymmetrical waistline.

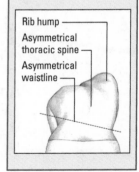

Rib hump
Asymmetrical thoracic spine
Asymmetrical waistline

and have the patient bend one knee and pull it toward his abdomen and chest as far as possible. You'll feel the patient's back touch your hand as the normal lumbar lordosis of the spine flattens. As the patient flexes his knee, the opposite hip and thigh should remain flat on the bed. Repeat on the opposite side.

To assess hip abduction, stand alongside the patient while he remains in the supine position. Press down on the superior iliac spine of the opposite hip with one hand to stabilize the pelvis. With your other hand, hold the patient's leg by the ankle and gently abduct the hip until you feel the iliac spine move. That movement indicates the limit of hip abduction. Then, while continuing to stabilize the pelvis, move the ankle medially across the patient's body to assess hip adduction. Repeat on the other side. Normal ROM is about 45 degrees for abduction and 30 degrees for adduction.

To assess hip extension, have the patient lie prone (facedown), and gently extend the thigh upward. Repeat on the other thigh.

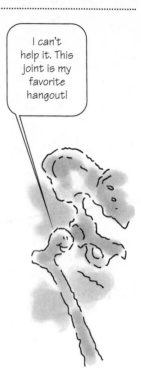

I can't help it. This joint is my favorite hangout!

As the hip turns

To assess internal and external rotation of the hip, ask the patient to lift one leg up and, keeping his knee straight, turn his leg and foot medially and laterally. Normal ROM for internal rotation is 40 degrees; for external rotation, 45 degrees.

On bended knee

Assess ROM in the knee. If the patient is standing, ask him to bend his knee as if trying to touch his heel to his buttocks. Normal ROM for flexion is 120 to 130 degrees. If the patient is lying down, have him draw his knee up to his chest. His calf should touch his thigh.

Knee extension returns the knee to a neutral position of 0 degrees; however, some knees may normally be hyperextended up to 15 degrees. If the patient can't extend his leg fully or his knee pops audibly and painfully, consider the response abnormal. Other abnormalities include pronounced crepitus, which may signal a degenerative disease of the knee, and sudden buckling, which may indicate a ligament injury.

Ankles and feet

Inspect the ankles and feet for swelling, redness, nodules, and other deformities. Check the arch of the foot and look for toe deformities. Also note edema, calluses, bunions, corns, ingrown toenails, plantar warts, trophic ulcers, hair loss, or unusual pigmentation.

Use your fingertips to palpate the bony and muscular structures of the ankles and feet.

The ankle angle

To examine the ankle, have the patient sit in a chair or on the side of a bed. To test plantar flexion, ask him to point his toes toward the floor. Test dorsiflexion by asking him to point his toes toward the ceiling. Normal ROM for plantar flexion is about 45 degrees; for dorsiflexion, 20 degrees.

Next, assess ROM in the ankle. Ask the patient to demonstrate inversion by turning his feet inward, and eversion by turning his feet outward. Normal ROM for inversion is 45 degrees; for eversion, 30 degrees.

To assess the metatarsophalangeal joints, ask the patient to flex his toes and then straighten them.

Assessing the muscles

Inspect all major muscle groups for tone, strength, and symmetry. If a muscle appears atrophied or hypertrophied, measure it by wrapping a tape measure around the largest circumference of the muscle on each side of the body and comparing the two numbers.

Other abnormalities of muscle appearance include contracture and abnormal movements, such as spasms, tics, tremors, and fasciculation.

Tuning in to muscle tone

To test the patient's arm muscle tone, move his shoulder through passive ROM exercises. You should feel a slight resistance. Then let his arm drop. It should fall easily to his side. Test leg muscle tone by putting the patient's hip through passive ROM exercises and then letting the leg fall to the examination table or bed. Like the arm, the leg should fall easily.

Abnormal findings include muscle rigidity and flaccidity. Rigidity indicates increased muscle tone, possibly caused by an upper motor neuron lesion such as from a stroke. Flaccidity may result from a lower motor neuron lesion.

Wrestling with muscle strength

Observe the patient's gait and movements to form an idea of his general muscle strength. Grade muscle strength on a scale of 0 to 5, with 0 representing no strength and 5 representing maximum strength. Document the results as a fraction, with the score as the numerator and maximum strength as the denominator. (See *Grading muscle strength*, page 70.)

To test specific muscle groups, ask the patient to move the muscles while you apply resistance; then compare the contralateral (opposing) muscle groups.

Grading muscle strength

The chart below outlines how to grade muscle strength on a scale of zero to five.

Grade	Evaluation	Requirement
5/5	Normal	Patient moves joint through full range of motion (ROM) and against gravity with full resistance.
4/5	Good	Patient completes ROM against gravity with moderate resistance.
3/5	Fair	Patient completes ROM against gravity only.
2/5	Poor	Patient completes full ROM with gravity eliminated (passive motion).
1/5	Trace	Patient's attempt at muscle contraction is palpable but without joint movement.
0/5	Zero	Patient shows no evidence of muscle contraction.

Nutritional assessment

A patient's nutritional health can influence his body's response to illness and treatment, and nutritional problems may be associated with various disorders or risk factors. (See *Detecting nutritional problems*.) A better understanding of the patient's nutritional status can help you plan his care more effectively.

Initial nutrition questions

To start the nutritional assessment, obtain the patient's nutritional health history. Ask him about past medical problems and surgeries, and whether he has a family history of obesity, diabetes, stomach or GI disturbances, or metabolic disorders such as hypercholesterolemia. Also ask the following questions:
• What do you normally eat in a typical day?
• Do you have any dietary restrictions?
• Have you recently lost or gained weight?
• What medications do you take, including over-the-counter medications, vitamins, and herbal preparations?
• Do you have any allergies, including food allergies?
• Do you smoke? If so, how much?
• Do you drink alcohol or use drugs? If so, how much and how often?

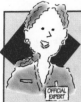

Advice from the experts

Detecting nutritional problems

Nutritional problems may stem from physical conditions, drugs, diet, or lifestyle factors. The list below will help you find out whether your patient is particularly susceptible to nutritional problems.

Physical condition
• Chronic illnesses, such as diabetes and neurologic, cardiac, or thyroid problems
• Family history of diabetes or heart disease
• Draining wounds or fistulas
• Obesity or a weight gain of 20% above normal body weight
• Unplanned weight loss of 20% below normal body weight
• Cystic fibrosis
• History of GI disturbances
• Anorexia or bulimia
• Depression or anxiety
• Severe trauma

• Recent chemotherapy, radiation therapy, or bone marrow transplantation
• Physical limitations, such as paresis or paralysis
• Recent major surgery
• Pregnancy, especially teen or multiple-birth pregnancy
• Burns

Drugs and diet
• Fad diets
• Steroid, diuretic, or antacid use
• Mouth, tooth, or denture problems
• Excessive alcohol intake
• Strict vegetarian diet
• Liquid diet or nothing by mouth for more than 3 days

Lifestyle factors
• Lack of support from family or friends
• Financial problems

Anthropometric measurements

If the patient can stand without assistance, measure his height using the height bar on a scale and weigh him using a calibrated balance beam scale. If he's weak or bedridden, measure his height with a measuring stick or tape and weigh him using a bed scale.

To obtain weight as a percentage of ideal body weight, divide the patient's true weight by an ideal body weight, found on an ideal body weight chart, and multiply that number by 100. A body weight of 120% or more of the ideal body weight indicates obesity. Below 90% indicates less-than-adequate weight.

Ask your patient to describe what he eats in a typical day.

Weighty terms

Here are some weight-related definitions:
• *seriously underweight*—20% or more below ideal weight
• *underweight*—10% to 20% below ideal weight
• *normal weight*—10% above or below ideal weight
• *overweight*—10% to 20% above ideal weight
• *obese*—20% or more above ideal weight.

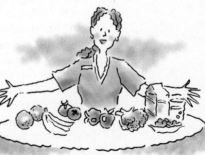

A "mass"ing weight data

Another way to evaluate a patient's weight is to use body mass index (BMI). BMI is a measure of body fat based on height and weight. To determine a patient's BMI, consult a BMI chart or use this formula:

$$\text{BMI} = \left(\frac{\text{Weight in pounds}}{\text{Height in inches} \times \text{Height in inches}} \right) \times 703$$

Here are some weight definitions based on BMI:
- *underweight* — BMI less than 18.5
- *normal weight* — BMI between 18.5 and 24.9
- *overweight* — BMI between 25 and 29.9
- *obese* — BMI of 30 or greater.

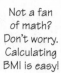

Not a fan of math? Don't worry. Calculating BMI is easy!

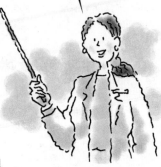

Anthropometric alternatives

Other anthropometric measurements include midarm circumference, midarm muscle circumference, and skin-fold thickness. These measurements are used to evaluate muscle mass and subcutaneous fat, both of which relate to nutritional status. (See *Taking anthropometric arm measurements*.)

Laboratory studies

Here are some common biochemical tests that may be performed as part of a nutritional assessment, along with possible outcomes and interpretations:
- *Serum albumin level* assesses protein levels in the body, helps maintain plasma osmotic pressure, and functions as a carrier protein for various substances such as iron. The serum albumin level is decreased with serious protein deficiency and loss of blood protein resulting from burns, malnutrition, liver or renal disease, heart failure, major surgery, infections, or cancer.
- *Hemoglobin level* is a measure of the main component of red blood cells (RBCs). It helps assess the blood's oxygen-carrying capacity and is useful in diagnosing anemia, protein deficiency, and hydration status. A decreased hemoglobin level suggests iron deficiency anemia, protein deficiency, excessive blood loss, or overhydration; increased hemoglobin level suggests dehydration or polycythemia.
- *Hematocrit* reflects the proportion of RBCs in a whole blood sample. Decreased values suggest iron deficiency anemia, excessive fluid intake, or excessive blood loss. Increased values suggest severe dehydration or polycythemia.
- *Transferrin level* is a measure of the carrier protein that transports iron and reflects the patient's protein status more accurately than the serum albumin level. Decreased values may indicate in-

Taking anthropometric arm measurements

Follow these steps to determine the triceps skin-fold thickness, midarm circumference, and midarm muscle circumference.

Triceps skin-fold thickness

1. Find the arm's midpoint circumference by placing the tape measure halfway between the axilla and the elbow. Then grasp the patient's skin with your thumb and forefinger, about ⅜" (1 cm) above the midpoint, as shown below.

2. Place the calipers at the midpoint and squeeze for 3 seconds.

3. Record the measurement to the nearest millimeter.

4. Take two more readings and use the average.

Midarm circumference and midarm muscle circumference

1. At the midpoint, measure the midarm circumference, as shown below. Record the measurement in centimeters.

2. Calculate the midarm muscle circumference by multiplying the triceps skin-fold thickness—measured in millimeters—by 3.14.

3. Subtract this number from the midarm circumference.

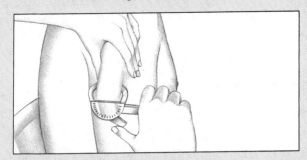 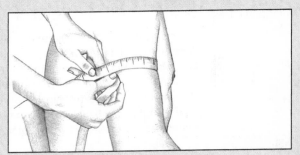

Recording the measurements

Record all three measurements as a percentage of the standard measurements (see chart below), using this formula:

$$\frac{\text{Actual measurement}}{\text{Standard measurement}} \times 100 = \%$$

After you've taken all the measurements, apply these rules:

• A measurement less than 90% of the standard indicates caloric deprivation.

• A measurement 90% or more indicates adequate or more than adequate energy reserves.

Measurement	Standard	90%
Triceps skin-fold thickness	Men: 12.5 mm Women: 16.5 mm	Men: 11.3 mm Women: 14.9 mm
Midarm circumference	Men: 29.3 cm Women: 28.5 cm	Men: 26.4 cm Women: 25.7 cm
Midarm muscle circumference	Men: 25.3 cm Women: 23.3 cm	Men: 22.8 cm Women: 20.9 cm

adequate protein production resulting from liver damage, protein loss from renal disease, acute or chronic infection, or cancer. Elevated levels may indicate severe iron deficiency.

• *Nitrogen balance test* involves collecting all urine during a 24-hour period to determine the adequacy of a patient's protein intake. Proteins contain nitrogen. Nitrogen intake and excretion should be equal.
• *Triglyceride levels* are a measure of the main storage form of lipids. These levels can help identify hyperlipidemia early. Decreased triglyceride levels commonly occur in those who are malnourished.
• *Total cholesterol test* measures circulating levels of free cholesterol and cholesterol esters. Increased levels indicate an increased risk of coronary artery disease. Decreased levels are commonly associated with malnutrition.

Mental health assessment

Effective patient care requires consideration of the psychological as well as the physiologic aspects of health. For this assessment to be effective, you need to establish a therapeutic relationship with the patient that's built on trust. You must communicate to him that his thoughts and behaviors are important. (See *Therapeutic communication techniques.*)

Don't skip the introductions

If you're meeting the patient for the first time, introduce yourself and explain the interview's purpose. If you're interviewing a patient who has cognitive or memory losses, you may need to reorient him before beginning the interview.

Remember, the patient may not be a reliable source of information, particularly if he has a mental illness or other mental impairment. If possible, verify his responses with family members, friends, or health care personnel. Also, check hospital records for previous admissions, if possible, and compare the patient's past and present behavior, symptoms, and circumstances.

Initial mental health questions

To establish a baseline and confirm that the patient's record is correct, ask the patient for demographic data, including his age, ethnic origin, primary language, birthplace, religion, occupation, and marital status. Gathering socioeconomic data (educational level, family, housing conditions, income, and employment status) also may provide clues to his current problem.

Sorry I have to put you on the couch, but a mental health assessment is an important part of patient care.

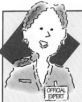

Advice from the experts

Therapeutic communication techniques

Therapeutic communication is the foundation of a good nurse-patient relationship. The techniques below can help you develop that relationship.

Listening
Listening intently enables you to hear and analyze everything the patient is saying, alerting you to his communication patterns.

Rephrasing
Succinct rephrasing of the patient's key statements helps ensure that you understand and emphasize the important points in his message. For example, you might say, "You're feeling angry and you say it's because of the way your friend treated you yesterday."

Broad openings and general statements
Using broad openings and general statements to initiate conversation encourages the patient to talk about any subject that comes to mind, allows him to focus the conversation, and demonstrates your willingness to interact. For example, you might say, "Is there something you would like to talk about?"

Clarification
Asking the patient to clarify a confusing or vague statement shows the patient that you want to understand what he's saying. It can also elicit precise information crucial to his recovery. For example, to ask for clarification, you might say, "I'm not sure I understood what you said."

Focusing
In employing a focusing technique, you help the patient redirect attention toward something specific. It fosters his self-control and helps avoid vague generalizations, so he can accept responsibility for his problems. One example of focusing might be, "Let's go back to what we were just talking about."

Silence
Silence gives the patient time to talk, think, and gain insight into problems. It also allows you to gather more information. Use this technique judiciously, however; you don't want to give the impression that you're disinterested or judgmental.

Suggesting collaboration
Suggesting collaboration gives the patient the opportunity to explore the pros and cons of a suggested approach. It must be used carefully to avoid directing the patient. For example, you might say, "Perhaps we can meet with your parents to discuss the matter."

Sharing impressions
When sharing impressions, you attempt to describe the patient's feelings, then seek his corrective feedback. Doing so allows him to clarify any misperceptions and gives you a better understanding of his true feelings. For example, you might say, "Does what I said sound like what you're feeling?"

Disorder distortion

In addition, find out if the patient has a history of medical disorders that may cause distorted thought processes, disorientation, depression, or other symptoms of mental illness. These medical disorders include renal or hepatic failure, infection, thyroid disease, increased intracranial pressure, or a metabolic disorder.

Finally, keep in mind that a patient's cultural and religious beliefs can affect how he responds to illness and adapts to care. Certain questions and behaviors considered acceptable in one culture may be inappropriate in another.

Chief complaint

Begin by asking about the patient's chief complaint. Note that the patient may not directly voice this complaint. Instead, you or others may note that he is having difficulty coping or is exhibiting unusual behavior. If you note a problem, determine whether the patient is aware of it. When documenting the patient's response, write it word for word and enclose it in quotation marks.

Symptom specifics

If the patient is aware of his symptoms, ask these questions:
• Why are you here today?
• When did your current symptoms begin?
• How severe or persistent are they?
• Did they occur suddenly or develop over time?

History of psychiatric illnesses

Next, determine whether the patient has a history of psychiatric illness by asking:
• Is there a history of psychiatric illness or substance abuse in your family?
• Have you experienced any emotional disturbances in the past, including episodes of delusions, violence, attempted suicides, drug or alcohol abuse, or depression? If so, did you receive psychiatric treatment?

Medication history

Then ask these questions about medications the patient is taking or has taken:
• Are you taking medications, including over-the-counter preparations? If so, how much do you take and how often do you take them? Do you use home remedies, herbal preparations, or dietary supplements?
• Are you currently taking a psychiatric drug? If so, are you taking it as prescribed and have you had any adverse reactions? Have your symptoms improved?

Initial observations

As you make your assessment, keep in mind that you can determine much about a patient's mental state simply by observing his appearance and how he handles himself in your presence. Record your observations of the patient's appearance, behavior, mood, thought processes and cognitive function, coping mechanisms, and potential for self-destructive behavior.

Appearance

Appearance is an important indicator of emotional and mental status. Is he clean, and is his appearance appropriate for his age, sex, and situation? Is his posture erect or slouched? Is his head lowered? Does he walk normally? Does he look alert, or does he stare blankly? Does he appear sad or angry? Does he maintain eye contact? Does he stare at you for long periods?

You seem distracted. Would you like to talk about it?

Behavior

Note the patient's demeanor and overall attitude as well as any extraordinary behavior such as speaking to a person who isn't present. Also, record his mannerisms. Does he bite his nails, fidget, or pace? Does he display any tics or tremors? How does he respond to you? Is he cooperative, friendly, hostile, or indifferent?

Mood

Does the patient appear anxious or depressed? Is he crying, sweating, breathing heavily, or trembling? Ask him to describe his current feelings in concrete terms and to suggest possible reasons for these feelings. Note inconsistencies between body language and mood (such as smiling when discussing an anger-provoking situation).

Thought processes and cognitive function

Evaluate the patient's orientation to time, place, and person, noting any confusion or disorientation. Listen for any indication that he might be having delusions, hallucinations, obsessions, compulsions, fantasies, or daydreams.

Attention, please

Assess the patient's attention span and ability to recall events in both the distant and recent past. For example, to assess immediate recall, ask him to repeat a series of five or six objects.

Hypothetically speaking

Test his intellectual functioning by asking him to add a series of numbers, and test his sensory perception and coordination by having him copy a simple drawing. Keep in mind that the patient's cultural background will influence his answers.

Spee-eech

Note any speech characteristics that may indicate altered thought processes, including monosyllabic responses, irrelevant or illogical replies to questions, convoluted or excessively detailed speech, slurred speech, repetitious speech patterns, a flight of ideas, and sudden silence without obvious reason.

Assess the patient's insight by asking whether he understands the significance of his illness, the plan of treatment, and the effect the illness will have on his life.

Coping mechanisms

The patient who's faced with a stressful situation may adopt coping, or defense, mechanisms — behaviors that operate on an unconscious level to protect the ego. Examples include denial, displacement, fantasy, identification, projection, and repression. Listen for an excessive reliance on these coping mechanisms. (See *Exploring coping mechanisms*.)

Potential for self-destructive behavior

Assess the patient for suicidal tendencies, particularly if he reports symptoms of depression. Not all such patients want to die; however, the incidence of suicide is higher in depressed patients than in patients with other diagnoses. If the patient is actively planning suicide, be prepared to take immediate action to prevent the act from occurring.

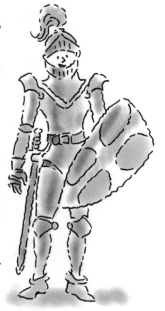

Patients faced with stressful situations may adopt defensive behaviors.

Psychological and mental status testing

You can do most of a mental status assessment during an interview. However, you'll also need to evaluate other aspects of the

---

Exploring coping mechanisms

The use of coping, or defense, mechanisms helps to relieve anxiety. Common coping strategies include:
• *denial*—refusal to admit truth or reality
• *displacement*—transferring an emotion from its original object to a substitute
• *fantasy*—creation of unrealistic or improbable images to escape from daily pressures and responsibilities
• *identification*—unconscious adoption of another person's personality characteristics, attitudes, values, and behaviors
• *projection*—displacement of negative feelings onto another person
• *rationalization*—substitution of acceptable reasons for the real or actual reasons motivating behavior
• *reaction formation*—behaving in a manner opposite from the way the person feels
• *regression*—return to behavior of an earlier, more comfortable time
• *repression*—exclusion of unacceptable thoughts and feelings from the conscious mind, leaving them to operate in the subconscious.

patient's mental status with psychological and mental status tests. Commonly used tests include:

• *Mini-Mental Status Examination*, which measures orientation, registration, recall, calculation, language, and graphomotor function
• *Cognitive Capacity Screening Examination*, which measures orientation, memory, calculation, and language
• *Cognitive Assessment Scale*, which measures orientation, general knowledge, mental ability, and psychomotor function
• *Beck Depression Inventory*, which helps diagnose depression, determine its severity, and monitor the patient's response during treatment
• *Global Deterioration Scale*, which assesses and stages primary degenerative dementia based on orientation, memory, and neurologic function
• *Minnesota Multiphasic Personality Inventory*, which helps assess personality traits and ego function in adolescents and adults and the results of which include information on coping strategies, defenses, strengths, gender identification, and self-esteem. (The test pattern may strongly suggest a diagnostic category, point to a suicide risk, or indicate potential violence.)

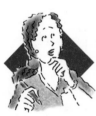

Quick quiz

1. When assessing the abdomen, the proper sequence of techniques is:
    A.   inspection, palpation, percussion, auscultation.
    B.   inspection, auscultation, percussion, palpation.
    C.   palpation, percussion, inspection, auscultation.
    D.   percussion, palpation, auscultation, inspection.

Answer: B. Because palpation and percussion can alter bowel sounds, perform inspection and auscultation first.

2. If a patient doesn't blink during a corneal sensitivity test, this may indicate damage to the sensory fibers of cranial nerve:
    A.   II.
    B.   III.
    C.   V.
    D.   VI.

Answer: C. Testing corneal sensitivity reflects the sensory fibers of cranial nerve V and the motor fibers of cranial nerve VI.

3. The breath sounds that are medium in loudness and pitch are called:

    A.   tracheal.
    B.   bronchial.
    C.   bronchovesicular.
    D.   vesicular.

Answer: C. Bronchovesicular sounds, heard when the patient inhales or exhales, are medium-pitched and continuous.

4. When auscultating heart sounds, S_1, the first heart sound, is loudest at which area of the heart?

    A.   Pulmonic
    B.   Tricuspid
    C.   Aortic
    D.   Mitral

Answer: D. S_1, which corresponds to the closure of the mitral and tricuspid valves, is loudest at the mitral area.

5. Examples of fluid-filled skin lesions would be:

    A.   macules.
    B.   bullae.
    C.   nodules.
    D.   wheals.

Answer: B. Bullae, along with vesicles, pustules, and cysts, are fluid-filled lesions and will transilluminate with a red glow when you shine a flashlight at right angles to them.

Scoring

☆☆☆ If you answered all five questions correctly, look up to the sky! You're the galaxy's brightest nursing star.

  ☆☆ If you answered four questions correctly, congratulations! You're more dazzling than a meteor shower.

    ☆ If you answered fewer than four questions correctly, don't worry! You're exploring a whole new universe of assessment skills.

ECG interpretation

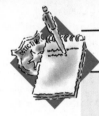

Just the facts

In this chapter, you'll learn:

♦ the normal components of a rhythm strip

♦ ways to identify a normal sinus rhythm

♦ rhythm strip interpretation

♦ ways to identify arrhythmias.

Observing the cardiac rhythm

Before you begin ECG interpretation, you must make sure that the leads are in their proper positions. Electrode placement is different for each lead, and different leads provide different views of the heart. A lead may be chosen to highlight a particular part of the ECG complex or the electrical events of a specific cardiac cycle. (See *Electrode placements*, page 82.)

After the electrodes are in their proper positions, the monitor is on, and the necessary cables are attached, observe the

Memory jogger

To help you remember where to place electrodes in a five-electrode configuration, think of the phrase, "White to the upper right." Then think of snow over trees (white electrode above green electrode) and smoke over fire (black electrode above red electrode). And, of course, chocolate (brown electrode) lies close to the heart.

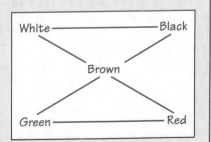

Electrode placements

This chart shows the correct electrode positions for some of the leads you'll use most often—the five-leadwire and telemetry systems. The chart uses the abbreviations RA for the right arm, LA for the left arm, RL for the right leg, LL for the left leg, C for chest, and G for the ground.

Electrode positions

In the five-leadwire system, electrode position for one lead may be identical to those for another lead. When two electrode positions are identical, change the lead selector switch to the setting that corresponds to the lead you want. In some cases, you'll need to reposition the electrodes.

Telemetry

In a telemetry monitoring system, you can create the same leads as the other systems with just two electrodes (+ and −) and a ground wire.

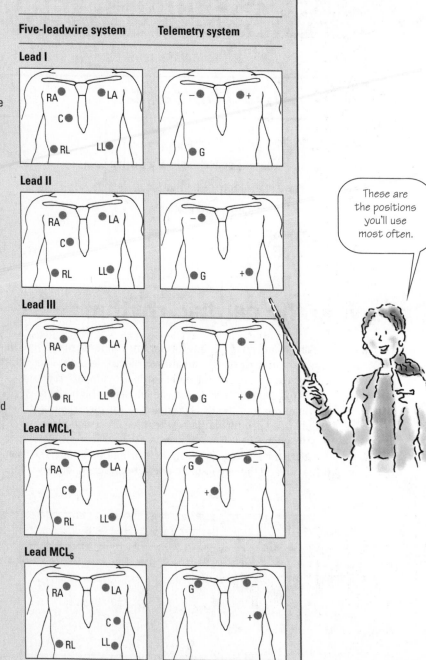

These are the positions you'll use most often.

screen. You should see the patient's ECG waveform. To get a print-out of the patient's cardiac rhythm, press the record control on the monitor. The ECG strip will be printed at the central console.

It's all on paper

Waveforms produced by the heart's electric current are recorded on ECG paper. ECG paper consists of horizontal and vertical lines forming a grid. A piece of ECG paper is call an *ECG strip* or *tracing*. (See *ECG grid*.)

Timepiece

The horizontal axis of the ECG strip represents time. Each small block equals 0.04 second, and five small blocks form a large block, which equals 0.20 second. To determine this time increment, mul-tiply 0.04 second (for one small block) by 5, the number of small blocks that compose a large block. Five large blocks equal 1 sec-ond. When measuring or calculating a patient's heart rate, a 6-second strip consisting of 30 large blocks is used.

Ample voltage

The ECG strip's vertical axis measures amplitude in millimeters (mm) or electrical voltage in millivolts (mV). Each small block represents 1 mm or 0.1 mV; each large block, 5 mm or 0.5 mV. To determine the amplitude of a wave, segment, or interval, count the number of small blocks from the baseline to the highest or lowest point of the wave, segment, or interval.

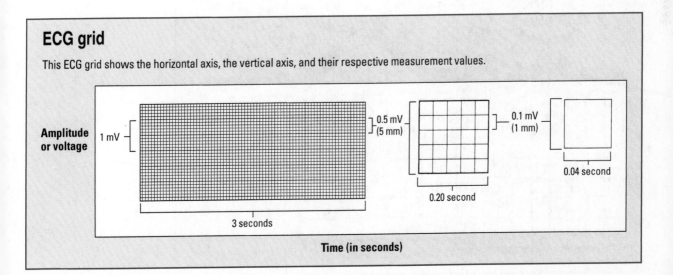

ECG grid

This ECG grid shows the horizontal axis, the vertical axis, and their respective measurement values.

A look at ECG components

An ECG complex represents the electrical events occurring in one cardiac cycle. A complex consists of five waveforms labeled with the letters *P, Q, R, S,* and *T.* The middle three letters—*Q, R,* and *S*— are referred to as a unit, the *QRS complex.* ECG tracings represent the conduction of electrical impulses from the atria to the ventricles. (See *Normal ECG.*)

Normal ECG

This strip shows the components of a normal ECG waveform.

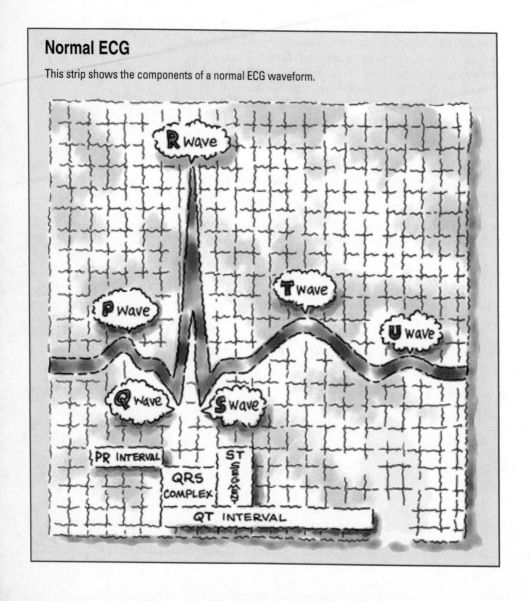

The P wave

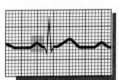

The P wave is the first component of a normal ECG waveform. It represents atrial depolarization—conduction of an electrical impulse through the atria. When you evaluate a P wave, look closely at its characteristics, especially its location, configuration, and deflection. A normal P wave has the following characteristics:
- *location*—precedes the QRS complex
- *amplitude*—2 to 3 mm high
- *duration*—0.06 to 0.12 second
- *configuration*—usually rounded and upright
- *deflection*—positive or upright in leads I, II, aV_F, and V_2 to V_6; usually positive but variable in leads III and aV_L; negative or inverted in lead aV_R; and biphasic or variable in lead V_1.

Pretty Ps

If the deflection and configuration of a P wave are normal—for example, if the P wave is upright in lead II and is rounded and smooth—and if the P wave precedes each QRS complex, you can assume that this electrical impulse originated in the sinoatrial (SA) node. The atria start to contract partway through the P wave, but you won't see this on the ECG. Remember, the ECG records electrical activity only, not mechanical activity or contraction.

Problem Ps

Varying P waves indicate that the impulse may be coming from different sites, as with a wandering pacemaker rhythm, irritable atrial tissue, or damage near the SA node. Absent P waves may signify conduction by a route other than the SA node, as with a junctional or atrial fibrillation rhythm.

I deduce that if atrial depolarization is absent, so is the P wave.

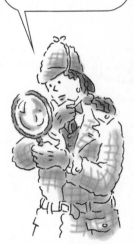

The PR interval

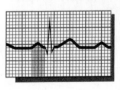

The PR interval tracks the atrial impulse from the atria through the atrioventricular (AV) node, bundle of His, and right and left bundle branches. When evaluating a PR interval, look especially at its duration. Changes in the PR interval indicate an altered impulse formation or a conduction delay, as seen in AV block. A normal PR interval has the following characteristics (amplitude, configuration, and deflection aren't measured):
- *location*—from the beginning of the P wave to the beginning of the QRS complex
- *duration*—0.12 to 0.20 second.

The short and long of it

Short PR intervals (less than 0.12 second) indicate that the impulse originated somewhere other than the SA node. This variation is associated with junctional arrhythmias and preexcitation syndromes. Prolonged PR intervals (greater than 0.20 second) may represent a conduction delay through the atria or AV junction stemming from digoxin toxicity or heart block — slowing related to ischemia or conduction tissue disease.

The QRS complex

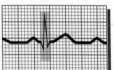

The QRS complex follows the P wave and represents depolarization of the ventricles. Immediately after the ventricles depolarize, as represented by the QRS complex, they contract. That contraction ejects blood from the ventricles and pumps it through the arteries, creating a pulse.

Not necessarily mechanical

Whenever you monitor cardiac rhythm, remember that the waveform you see represents the heart's electrical activity only. It doesn't guarantee a mechanical contraction of the heart and a subsequent pulse. The contraction could be weak, as happens with premature ventricular contractions, or absent, as happens with pulseless electrical activity. So before you treat the strip, check the patient.

It's all normal

Pay special attention to the duration and configuration when evaluating a QRS complex. A normal complex has the following characteristics:
- *amplitude* — 5 to 30 mm high but differs for each lead used
- *duration* — 0.06 to 0.10 second, or one-half of the PR interval. Duration is measured from the beginning of the Q wave to the end of the S wave or from the beginning of the R wave if the Q wave is absent.
- *configuration* — consists of the Q wave (the first negative deflection after the P wave), the R wave (the first positive deflection after the P wave or the Q wave), and the S wave (the first negative deflection after the R wave). You may not always see all three waves. The ventricles depolarize quickly, so the QRS complex typically appears thinner than other ECG components. It may also look different in each lead.
- *deflection* — positive in leads I, II, III, aV_L, aV_F, and V_4 to V_6 and negative in leads aV_R and V_1 to V_3.

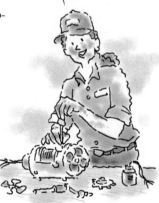

Remember that the mechanical activity of the heart may not match up with the electrical activity represented on the ECG waveform.

Crucial I.D.

Remember that the QRS complex represents intraventricular conduction time. That's why identifying and correctly interpreting it is so crucial. If no P wave appears with the QRS complex, then the impulse may have originated in the ventricles, indicating a ventricular arrhythmia. (See *Older adult ECGs.*)

Complex complexes

Deep, wide Q waves may represent myocardial infarction (MI). A notched R wave may signify a bundle-branch block. A widened QRS complex (greater than 0.12 second) may signify a ventricular conduction delay. A missing QRS complex may indicate AV block or ventricular standstill.

Ages and stages

Older adult ECGs

Always keep the patient's age in mind when interpreting the ECG. Differences in the ECG of an older adult include increased PR, QRS, and QT intervals, decreased amplitude of the QRS complex, and a shift of the QRS axis to the left.

The ST segment

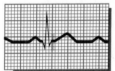

The ST segment represents the end of ventricular conduction or depolarization and the beginning of ventricular recovery or repolarization. The point that marks the end of the QRS complex and the beginning of the ST segment is known as the *J point*.

Pay special attention to the deflection of an ST segment. A normal ST segment has the following characteristics (amplitude, duration, and configuration aren't observed):
- *location* — extends from the S wave to the beginning of the T wave
- *deflection* — usually isoelectric (neither positive nor negative); may vary from − 0.5 to + 1 mm in some precordial leads.

Not-so-normal ST

A change in the ST segment may indicate myocardial damage. An ST segment may become either elevated or depressed. (See *Changes in the ST segment*, page 88.)

The T wave

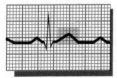

The T wave represents ventricular recovery or repolarization. When evaluating a T wave, look at the amplitude, configuration, and deflection. Normal T waves have the following characteristics (duration isn't measured):
- *location* — follows the S wave
- *amplitude* — 0.5 mm in leads I, II, and III and up to 10 mm in the precordial leads
- *configuration* — typically round and smooth
- *deflection* — usually upright in leads I, II, and V_3 to V_6; inverted in lead aV_R; and variable in all other leads.

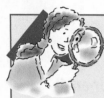

A closer look

Changes in the ST segment

Closely monitoring the ST segment on a patient's ECG can help you detect ischemia or injury before infarction develops.

ST-segment depression
An ST segment is considered depressed when it's 0.5 mm or more below the baseline. A depressed ST segment may indicate myocardial ischemia or digoxin toxicity.

ST-segment elevation
An ST segment is considered elevated when it's 1 mm or more above the baseline. An elevated ST segment may indicate myocardial injury.

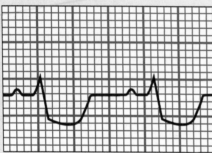
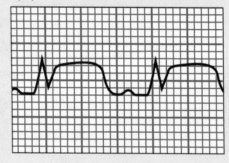

Why is that T so bumpy?

A T wave's peak represents the relative refractory period of ventricular repolarization, a period during which cells are especially vulnerable to extra stimuli. Bumps in a T wave may indicate that a P wave is hidden in it. If a P wave is hidden, atrial depolarization has occurred, the impulse having originated at a site above the ventricles.

Tall, inverted, or pointy T's

Tall, peaked, or tented T waves indicate myocardial injury or hyperkalemia. Inverted T waves in leads I, II, or V_3 through V_6 may represent myocardial ischemia. Heavily notched or pointed T waves in an adult may mean pericarditis.

The QT interval

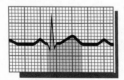

The QT interval measures ventricular depolarization and repolarization. The length of the QT interval varies as a result of the patient's changing heart rate. The faster the heart rate, the shorter the QT interval. When checking the QT interval, look closely at the duration.

A normal QT interval has the following characteristics (amplitude, configuration, and deflection aren't observed):
- *location* — extends from the beginning of the QRS complex to the end of the T wave
- *duration* — varies according to age, sex, and heart rate; usually lasts from 0.36 to 0.44 second; shouldn't be greater than one-half the distance between consecutive R waves when the rhythm is regular.

The importance of QT

An abnormality in QT interval duration may indicate myocardial problems. Prolonged QT intervals indicate that the relative refractory period is longer. A prolonged QT interval increases the risk of a life-threatening arrhythmia known as *torsades de pointes*. Prolonged QT syndrome is a congenital conduction-system defect present in certain families. Short QT intervals may result from digoxin toxicity or hypercalcemia.

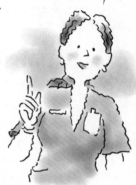

Keep in mind that the U wave isn't present on every ECG.

The U wave

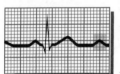

The U wave represents the recovery period of the Purkinje or ventricular conduction fibers. It isn't present on every rhythm strip. The configuration is the most important characteristic of the U wave.

When present, a normal U wave has the following characteristics (amplitude and duration aren't measured):
- *location* — follows the T wave
- *deflection* — upright.

A prominent U wave may be due to hypercalcemia, hypokalemia, or digoxin toxicity.

8-step strip analysis

Rhythm strip analysis requires a sequential and systematic approach such as the eight steps outlined here.

Step 1: Determine the rhythm.

To determine the heart's atrial and ventricular rhythms, use either the paper-and-pencil method or the caliper method. (See *Methods of measuring rhythm*, page 90.)

For atrial rhythm, measure the P-P interval (the interval between two consecutive P waves). These intervals should occur regularly with only small variations associated with respirations. Then compare the P-P intervals in several cycles. Consistently

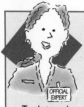

Advice from the experts

Methods of measuring rhythm

To determine the atrial and ventricular rhythms, you can either use the paper-and-pencil method or the caliper method.

Paper-and-pencil method

Place the ECG strip on a flat surface. Then position the straight edge of a piece of paper along the strip's baseline. Move the paper up slightly so the straight edge is near the peak of the R wave. With a pencil, mark the paper at the R waves of two consecutive QRS complexes, as shown at right. This is the R-R interval.

Next, move the paper across the strip, aligning the two marks with succeeding R-R intervals. If the distance for each R-R interval is the same, the ventricular rhythm is regular. If the distance varies, the rhythm is irregular.

Use the same method to measure the distance between the P waves (the P-P interval) and determine whether the atrial rhythm is regular or irregular.

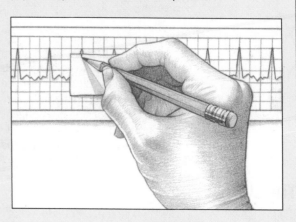

Caliper method

With the ECG on a flat surface, place one point of the caliper on the peak of the first R wave of two consecutive QRS complexes. Then adjust the caliper legs so the other point is on the peak of the next R wave, as shown at right. This distance is the R-R interval.

Now pivot the first point of the caliper toward the third R wave and note whether it falls on the peak of that wave. Check succeeding R-R intervals in the same way. If they're all the same, the ventricular rhythm is regular. If they vary, the rhythm is irregular.

Use the same method to measure the P-P intervals to determine whether the atrial rhythm is regular or irregular.

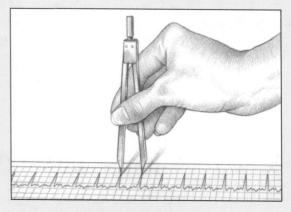

similar P-P intervals indicate regular atrial rhythm; dissimilar P-P intervals indicate irregular atrial rhythm.

To determine the ventricular rhythm, measure the intervals between two consecutive R waves in the QRS complexes. If an R wave isn't present, use the Q wave of consecutive QRS complexes. The R-R intervals should occur regularly. Then compare R-R intervals in several cycles. As with atrial rhythms, consistently similar intervals mean a regular rhythm; dissimilar intervals point to an irregular rhythm.

Ask yourself these questions when evaluating the rhythm: Is the rhythm irregular? If so, is it slightly irregular or markedly so? Does the irregularity occur in a pattern (a regularly irregular pattern)?

Step 2: Determine the rate.

You can use one of three methods to determine atrial and ventricular heart rate. Remember, don't rely on those methods alone. Always check a pulse to correlate it with the heart rate on the ECG.

10-times method

The easiest way to calculate rate is the 10-times method, especially if the rhythm is irregular. You'll notice that ECG paper is marked in increments of 3 seconds, or 15 large boxes. To figure the atrial rate, obtain a 6-second strip, count the number of P waves, and multiply by 10. Ten 6-second strips represent 1 minute. Calculate ventricular rate the same way, using the R waves.

1,500 method

If the heart rhythm is regular, use the 1,500 method, so named because 1,500 small squares represent 1 minute. Count the small squares between identical points on two consecutive P waves and then divide 1,500 by that number to calculate the atrial rate. To obtain the ventricular rate, use the same method with two consecutive R waves.

Sequence method

The third method of estimating heart rate is the sequence method, which requires that you memorize a sequence of numbers. To get the atrial rate, find a P wave that peaks on a heavy black line and assign the following numbers to the next six heavy black lines: 300, 150, 100, 75, 60, and 50. Then find the next P wave peak and estimate the atrial rate, based on the number assigned to the nearest heavy black line. Estimate the ventricular rate the same way, using the R wave.

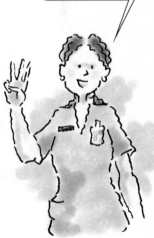

Although you can use three different methods to determine heart rate from an ECG, you should always check the patient's pulse to verify the rate.

Step 3: Evaluate the P wave.

When you examine a rhythm strip for P waves, ask yourself: Are P waves present? Do they all have normal configurations? Do they all have a similar size and shape? Does every P wave have a QRS complex?

Step 4: Determine the duration of the PR interval.

To measure the PR interval, count the small squares between the start of the P wave and the start of the QRS complex; then multiply the number of squares by 0.04 second. Now ask yourself: Is the duration a normal 0.12 to 0.20 second? Is the PR interval constant?

Step 5: Determine the duration of the QRS complex.

When determining QRS duration, be sure to measure straight across from the end of the PR interval to the end of the S wave, not just to the peak. Remember, the QRS has no horizontal components. To calculate duration, count the number of small squares between the beginning and end of the QRS complex and multiply this number by 0.04 second. Then ask yourself: Is the duration a normal 0.06 to 0.10 second? Are all QRS complexes the same size and shape? (If not, measure each one and describe it individually.) Does a QRS complex appear after every P wave?

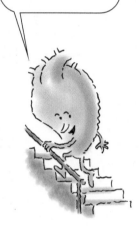

Talk about steps in the right direction. A sequential and systematic approach can simplify strip interpretation.

Step 6: Evaluate the T waves.

Examine the strip for T waves. Then ask yourself: Are T waves present? Do they all have a normal shape? Do they all have normal amplitude? Do they all have the same amplitude as the QRS complexes?

Step 7: Determine the duration of the QT interval.

Count the number of small squares between the beginning of the QRS complex and the end of the T wave, where the T wave returns to the baseline. Multiply this number by 0.04 second. Ask yourself: Is the duration a normal 0.36 to 0.44 second?

Step 8: Evaluate any other components.

Check for ectopic beats and other abnormalities. Also check the ST segment for abnormalities, and look for the presence of a U wave. Note your findings, and then interpret them by naming the rhythm strip according to one or all of these findings:

- origin of the rhythm (for example, sinus node, atria, AV node, or ventricles)
- rate characteristics (for example, bradycardia or tachycardia)
- rhythm abnormalities (for example, flutter, fibrillation, heart block, escape rhythm, or other arrhythmias).

Recognizing normal sinus rhythm

Normal sinus rhythm records an impulse that starts in the sinus node and progresses to the ventricles through a normal conduction pathway—from the sinus node to the atria and AV node, through the bundle of His, to the bundle branches, and on to the Purkinje fibers. Normal sinus rhythm is the standard against which all other rhythms are compared. (See *Normal sinus rhythm.*)

What makes for normal?

These are the characteristics of normal sinus rhythm:
- Atrial and ventricular rhythms are regular.
- Atrial and ventricular rates fall between 60 and 100 beats/minute, the SA node's normal firing rate, and all impulses are conducted to the ventricles.

Normal sinus rhythm

Normal sinus rhythm, shown in the rhythm strip below, represents normal impulse conduction through the heart. Notice its distinguishing characteristics.

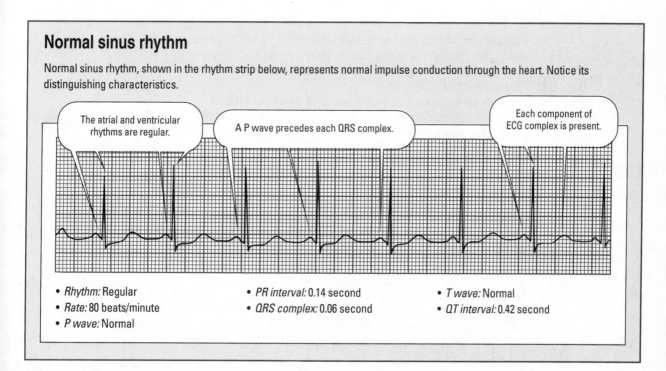

The atrial and ventricular rhythms are regular.

A P wave precedes each QRS complex.

Each component of ECG complex is present.

- *Rhythm:* Regular
- *Rate:* 80 beats/minute
- *P wave:* Normal

- *PR interval:* 0.14 second
- *QRS complex:* 0.06 second

- *T wave:* Normal
- *QT interval:* 0.42 second

- P waves are rounded, smooth, and upright in lead II, signaling that a sinus impulse has reached the atria.
- The PR interval is normal (0.12 to 0.20 second), indicating that the impulse is following normal conduction pathways.
- The QRS complex is of normal duration (less than 0.12 second), representing normal ventricular impulse conduction and recovery.
- The T wave is upright in lead II, confirming that normal repolarization has taken place.
- The QT interval is within normal limits (0.36 to 0.44 second).
- No ectopic or aberrant beats occur.

Sinus node arrhythmias

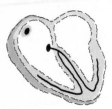

When a heart is functioning normally, the SA node, also called the *sinus node*, acts as the primary pacemaker. The sinus node assumes this role because its automatic firing rate exceeds that of the heart's other pacemakers. In an adult at rest, the sinus node has an inherent firing rate of 60 to 100 times per minute. Types of sinus node arrhythmias include sinus arrhythmia, sinus bradycardia, sinus tachycardia, sinus arrest, and sick sinus syndrome.

Sinus arrhythmia

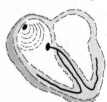

In sinus arrhythmia, the pacemaker cells of the SA node fire irregularly. The cardiac rate stays within normal limits, but the rhythm is irregular and corresponds to the respiratory cycle. (See *Recognizing sinus arrhythmia*.)

Sinus arrhythmias commonly occur in athletes, children, and elderly people but rarely in infants. Conditions unrelated to respiration may also produce sinus arrhythmia, including inferior-wall MI, advanced age, use of digoxin or morphine, and increased intracranial pressure.

How you intervene

Unless the patient is symptomatic, treatment usually isn't necessary. If sinus arrhythmia is unrelated to respiration, the underlying cause may require treatment.

Pharmaco cause

If sinus arrhythmia is caused by drugs, such as morphine or other sedatives, the doctor may decide to discontinue those medications. If a patient taking digoxin suddenly develops sinus arrhythmia, the patient may be experiencing digoxin toxicity.

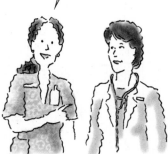

Notify the doctor if sinus arrhythmia suddenly develops in a patient taking digoxin.

Recognizing sinus arrhythmia

To identify sinus arrhythmia, observe the patient's heart rhythm during respiration. The atrial and ventricular rates should be within normal limits (60 to 100 beats/minute), but increase during inspiration and slow with expiration. ECG complexes fall closer together during inspiration, shortening the P-P interval, which is the time elapsed between two consecutive P waves. During expiration, the P-P interval lengthens. The difference between the shortest and longest P-P interval exceeds 0.12 second. This rhythm strip illustrates sinus arrhythmia. Notice its distinguishing characteristics.

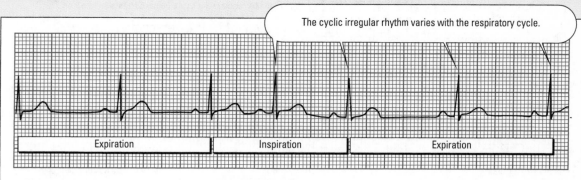

The cyclic irregular rhythm varies with the respiratory cycle.

Expiration — Inspiration — Expiration

- *Rhythm:* Irregular
- *Rate:* 60 beats/minute
- *P wave:* Normal

- *PR interval:* 0.16 second
- *QRS complex:* 0.06 second
- *T wave:* Normal

- *QT interval:* 0.36 second
- *Other:* Phasic slowing and quickening

Sinus bradycardia

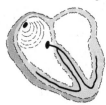

In sinus bradycardia, the sinus rate falls below 60 beats/minute while the rhythm remains regular. (See *Recognizing sinus bradycardia,* page 96.) It may occur normally during sleep. It may also be normal in an athletic person because a well-conditioned heart can pump more blood with each contraction, maintaining a normal cardiac output with fewer beats. Sinus bradycardia usually occurs as a normal response to a reduced demand for blood flow.

Causes for concern?

Sinus bradycardia commonly occurs after an inferior-wall MI involving the right coronary artery, which supplies blood to the SA node. Numerous other conditions and the use of certain drugs may also cause sinus bradycardia.

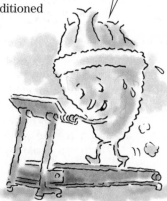

Sinus bradycardia may be normal in a well-conditioned heart because it can pump more blood with each contraction.

Recognizing sinus bradycardia

In sinus bradycardia, the heartbeat is regular with a rate less than 60 beats/minute. All other ECG findings are normal: a P wave precedes each QRS complex, and the PR interval, QRS complex, T wave, and QT interval are all normal. The clinical significance of sinus bradycardia depends on whether the patient is symptomatic. This rhythm strip illustrates sinus bradycardia. Notice its distinguishing characteristics.

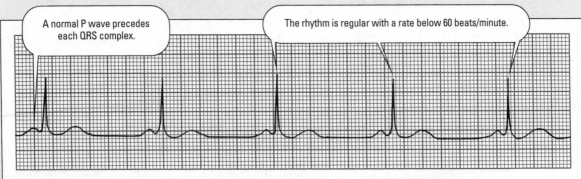

> A normal P wave precedes each QRS complex.

> The rhythm is regular with a rate below 60 beats/minute.

- *Rhythm:* Regular
- *Rate:* 48 beats/minute
- *P wave:* Normal

- *PR interval:* 0.16 second
- *QRS complex:* 0.08 second
- *T wave:* Normal

- *QT interval:* 0.50 second
- *Other:* None

How you intervene

If the patient is asymptomatic and his vital signs are stable, treatment isn't necessary. Continue to observe his heart rhythm, monitoring the progression and duration of bradycardia. Check with the doctor about stopping medications that may be depressing the SA node, such as digoxin, beta-adrenergic blockers, and calcium channel blockers.

Identify and correct

If the patient is symptomatic, treatment aims to identify and correct the underlying cause. Meanwhile, such drugs as atropine, epinephrine, and dopamine or a temporary pacemaker can help maintain an adequate heart rate. Patients with chronic, symptom-producing sinus bradycardia may require insertion of a permanent pacemaker. (See *Treating symptom-producing bradycardia.*)

> Drugs may be used to maintain an adequate heart rate until the underlying cause is identified.

Check the ABCs

If the patient abruptly develops significant sinus bradycardia, assess his airway, breathing, and circulation (ABCs). If these are adequate, determine whether the patient has an effective cardiac output.

Treating symptom-producing bradycardia

This algorithm shows the steps for treating bradycardia in a patient who isn't in cardiac arrest.

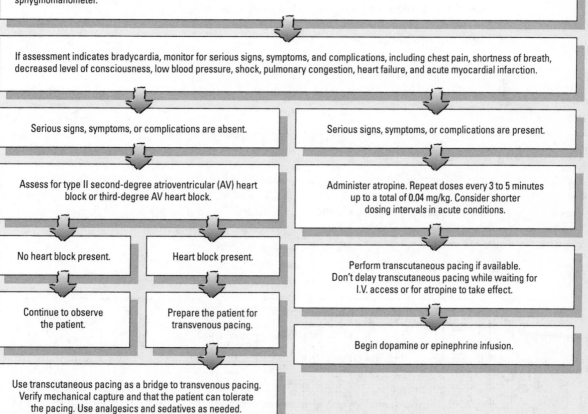

Perform initial assessment and early interventions:

- Assess airway, breathing, and circulation.
- Secure the patient's airway noninvasively.
- Make sure a monitor defibrillator is available.
- Assess whether invasive airway management is needed.
- Administer oxygen.
- Start an I.V. line, attach a monitor, and give I.V. fluids.
- Assess vital signs, and apply a pulse oximeter and an automatic sphygmomanometer.

- Obtain and review a 12-lead electrocardiogram.
- Obtain and review a portable chest X-ray.
- Review the patient's health history.
- Perform a physical examination.
- Develop a differential diagnosis.

If assessment indicates bradycardia, monitor for serious signs, symptoms, and complications, including chest pain, shortness of breath, decreased level of consciousness, low blood pressure, shock, pulmonary congestion, heart failure, and acute myocardial infarction.

Serious signs, symptoms, or complications are absent.

Serious signs, symptoms, or complications are present.

Assess for type II second-degree atrioventricular (AV) heart block or third-degree AV heart block.

Administer atropine. Repeat doses every 3 to 5 minutes up to a total of 0.04 mg/kg. Consider shorter dosing intervals in acute conditions.

No heart block present.

Heart block present.

Perform transcutaneous pacing if available. Don't delay transcutaneous pacing while waiting for I.V. access or for atropine to take effect.

Continue to observe the patient.

Prepare the patient for transvenous pacing.

Begin dopamine or epinephrine infusion.

Use transcutaneous pacing as a bridge to transvenous pacing. Verify mechanical capture and that the patient can tolerate the pacing. Use analgesics and sedatives as needed.

Sinus tachycardia

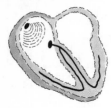

Sinus tachycardia in an adult is characterized by a sinus rate greater than 100 beats/minute. The rate rarely exceeds 180 beats/minute except during strenuous exercise. (See *Recognizing sinus tachycardia.*)

The clinical significance of sinus tachycardia depends on the underlying cause. Sinus tachycardia may be a normal response to exercise, pain, stress, fever, or strong emotion. It can also occur with certain cardiac conditions, as a compensatory mechanism, or when taking certain drugs. Sinus tachycardia in a patient who has had an acute MI suggests massive heart damage and is a sign of a poor prognosis. Persistent tachycardia may also signal impending heart failure or cardiogenic shock.

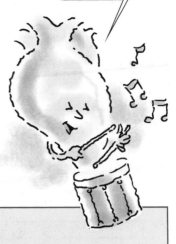

I know I'm supposed to be a regular guy, but sometimes I just get a crazy beat.

Recognizing sinus tachycardia

In sinus tachycardia, atrial and ventricular rhythms are regular. Both rates are equal, generally 100 to 160 beats/minute. The P wave is of normal size and shape and precedes each QRS complex, but it may increase in amplitude. As the heart rate increases, the P wave may be superimposed on the preceding T wave and difficult to identify. The PR interval, QRS complex, and T wave are normal. The QT interval normally shortens with tachycardia. This rhythm strip illustrates sinus tachycardia. Notice its distinguishing characteristics.

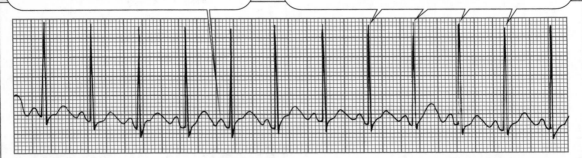

A normal P wave precedes each QRS complex.

The rhythm is regular with a rate above 100 beats/minute.

- *Rhythm:* Regular
- *Rate:* 120 beats/minute
- *P wave:* Normal

- *PR interval:* 0.14 second
- *QRS complex:* 0.06 second
- *T wave:* Normal

- *QT interval:* 0.34 second
- *Other:* None

How you intervene

No treatment of sinus tachycardia is necessary if the patient is otherwise healthy and asymptomatic or if the rhythm is the result of physical exertion. In other cases, the underlying cause may be treated, which usually resolves the arrhythmia. (For example, if tachycardia is caused by hemorrhage, treatment measures include stopping the bleeding and replacing blood and fluid.) The goal of treatment for a patient with sinus tachycardia is to maintain adequate cardiac output and tissue perfusion and to identify and correct the underlying cause.

If tachycardia leads to cardiac ischemia, treatment may include medications to slow the heart rate. The most commonly used drugs include beta-adrenergic blockers, such as metoprolol and atenolol, and calcium channel blockers such as verapamil.

Solving the mystery with the history

Check the patient's medication history. Over-the-counter sympathomimetic drugs, which mimic the effects of the sympathetic nervous system, may contribute to sinus tachycardia. These agents may be contained in nose drops and cold formulas.

You should also ask about the patient's use of caffeine, nicotine, alcohol, and such illicit drugs as cocaine and amphetamines — any of which can trigger tachycardia. Advise him to avoid these substances. Be aware that a sudden onset of sinus tachycardia after an MI may signal extension of the infarction.

Sinus arrest

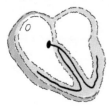

A disorder of impulse formation, sinus arrest results from a lack of electrical activity in the atrium (atrial standstill). During atrial standstill, the atria aren't stimulated and an entire PQRST complex is missing from the ECG strip. Except for this missing complex, or pause, the ECG usually remains normal. (See *Recognizing sinus arrest*, page 100.)

Atrial standstill is called *sinus pause* when one or two beats aren't formed and *sinus arrest* when three or more beats aren't formed. Sinus arrest closely resembles third-degree SA block, also called *exit block*, on the ECG strip. (See *Understanding sinoatrial blocks*, pages 101 and 102.)

Lack of impulsiveness

Sinus arrest occurs when the SA node fails to generate an impulse. Such failure may result from several conditions, including acute infection, heart disease, and vagal stimulation. Pauses of

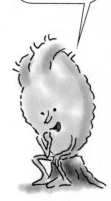

I can't help it if I need to pause and reflect. I'm a thinker!

Recognizing sinus arrest

In sinus arrest, you'll find on the ECG that atrial and ventricular rhythms are regular except for a missing complex at the onset of atrial standstill. Atrial and ventricular rates are equal and are usually within normal limits. However, the rate may vary as a result of the pauses.

A P wave of normal size and shape precedes each QRS complex, but the P wave is absent during a pause. The PR interval is normal and constant when the P wave is present. The QRS complex, the T wave, and the QT interval are normal when present, and they're absent during a pause.

Junctional escape beats, including premature atrial, junctional, or ventricular contractions, may also be present. With sinus arrest, the length of the pause isn't a multiple of the previous R-R intervals. This rhythm strip illustrates sinus arrest. Notice its distinguishing characteristics.

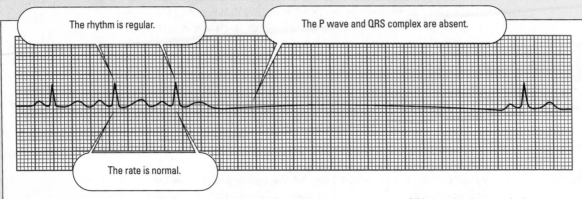

The rhythm is regular.

The P wave and QRS complex are absent.

The rate is normal.

- *Rhythm:* Regular, except for the missing PQRST complexes
- *Rate:* 40 beats/minute
- *P wave:* Normal, absent during pause
- *PR interval:* 0.20 second
- *QRS complex:* 0.08 second, absent during pause
- *T wave:* Normal, absent during pause
- *QT interval:* 0.40 second, absent during pause
- *Other:* None

2 to 3 seconds normally occur in healthy adults during sleep and occasionally in patients with increased vagal tone or hypersensitive carotid sinus disease. Sinus arrest may be associated with sick sinus syndrome.

How you intervene

The goal for treating the patient with sinus arrest is to maintain adequate cardiac output and perfusion. An asymptomatic patient needs no treatment. For a patient displaying mild symptoms, identify and treat the cause of the sinus arrest.

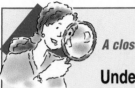

A closer look

Understanding sinoatrial blocks

In sinoatrial (SA) block, the SA node discharges impulses at regular intervals. However, some of those impulses are delayed on the way to the atria. Based on the length of the delay, SA blocks are divided into three categories: first-, second-, and third-degree. Second-degree block is further divided into type I and type II.

First-degree SA block consists of a delay between the firing of the sinus node and the depolarization of the atria. Because the ECG doesn't show sinus node activity, you can't detect first-degree SA block. However, you can detect the other types of SA block.

Second-degree block type I

In type I block, conduction time between the sinus node and the surrounding atrial tissue becomes progressively longer until an entire cycle is dropped. The pause is less than twice the length of the shortest P-P interval.

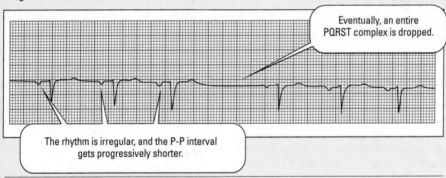

Eventually, an entire PQRST complex is dropped.

The rhythm is irregular, and the P-P interval gets progressively shorter.

Second-degree block type II

In type II block, conduction time between the sinus node and atrial tissue is normal until an impulse is blocked. The duration of the pause is a multiple of the P-P interval.

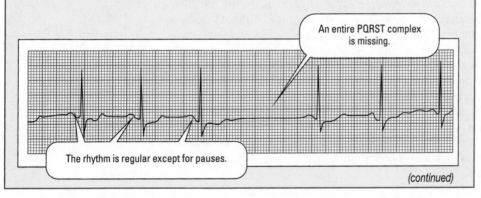

An entire PQRST complex is missing.

The rhythm is regular except for pauses.

(continued)

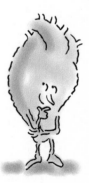

Understanding sinoatrial blocks (continued)

Third-degree block

In third-degree block, some impulses are obstructed, causing long sinus pauses. The pause isn't a multiple of the sinus rhythm. On an ECG, third-degree SA block looks similar to sinus arrest but results from a different cause.

Third-degree SA block is caused by a failure to conduct impulses; sinus arrest results from failure to form impulses. Failure in each case causes atrial activity to stop.

In sinus arrest, the pause commonly ends with a junctional escape beat. In third-degree block, the pause lasts for an indefinite period and ends with a sinus beat.

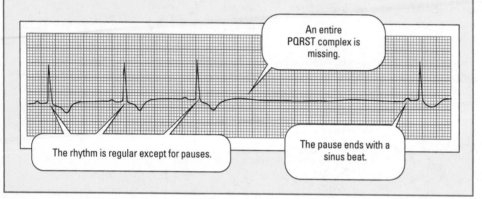

An entire PQRST complex is missing.

The rhythm is regular except for pauses.

The pause ends with a sinus beat.

Pause for concern

If sinus pauses are recurrent, assess the patient for evidence of decreased cardiac output, such as altered mental status, low blood pressure, and cool, clammy skin. Ask him whether he's dizzy or light-headed or has blurred vision. Does he feel as if he has passed out? If so, he may be experiencing syncope from a prolonged sinus arrest.

Assess for a progression of the arrhythmia. Notify the doctor immediately if the patient becomes unstable. Withhold medications that may contribute to sinus pauses or SA node suppression, such as digoxin, beta-adrenergic blockers, and calcium channel blockers, and check with the doctor about whether those drugs should be continued. A patient who develops signs of circulatory collapse needs immediate treatment.

Document the patient's vital signs and how he feels during pauses as well as what activities he was involved in when they occurred. Activities that increase vagal stimulation, such as Valsalva's maneuver or vomiting, increase the likelihood of sinus pauses.

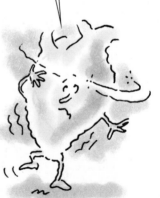

If the patient is dizzy or light-headed, he may be experiencing syncope.

Sick sinus syndrome

Also called *sinus nodal dysfunction*, sick sinus syndrome refers to a wide spectrum of SA node abnormalities. The syndrome is caused by disturbances in the way impulses are generated or the inability to conduct impulses to the atrium.

The brady-tachy bunch

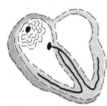

Sick sinus syndrome usually shows up as bradycardia, with episodes of sinus arrest and SA block interspersed with sudden, brief periods of rapid atrial fibrillation. Patients are also prone to paroxysms of other atrial tachyarrhythmias, such as atrial flutter and ectopic atrial tachycardia, a condition sometimes referred to as *bradycardia-tachycardia (or brady-tachy) syndrome.* (See *Recognizing sick sinus syndrome.*)

Recognizing sick sinus syndrome

To identify patients with sick sinus syndrome, look for an irregular rhythm with sinus pauses and abrupt rate changes. Atrial and ventricular rates may be fast, slow, or alternating periods of fast rates and slow rates interrupted by pauses.

The P wave varies with the rhythm and usually precedes each QRS complex. The PR interval is usually within normal limits but varies with changes in the rhythm. The QRS complex and T wave are usually normal, as is the QT interval, which may vary with rhythm changes.

The patient's pulse rate may be fast, slow, or normal, and the rhythm may be regular or irregular. This rhythm strip illustrates sick sinus syndrome. Notice its distinguishing characteristics.

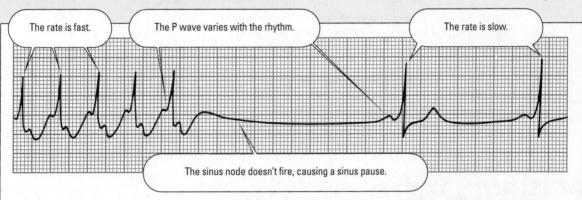

The rate is fast.

The P wave varies with the rhythm.

The rate is slow.

The sinus node doesn't fire, causing a sinus pause.

- *Rhythm:* Irregular
- *Rate:* Atrial—60 beats/minute; ventricular—70 beats/minute
- *P wave:* Configuration varies
- *PR interval:* Varies with rhythm
- *QRS complex:* 0.10 second
- *T wave:* Configuration varies
- *QT interval:* Varies with rhythm changes
- *Other:* None

Sinus headache

The onset is progressive, insidious, and chronic. Sick sinus syndrome results either from a dysfunction of the sinus node's automaticity or from abnormal conduction or blockages of impulses coming out of the nodal region. These conditions, in turn, stem from a degeneration of the area's autonomic nervous system and partial destruction of the sinus node, as may occur with an interrupted blood supply after an inferior-wall MI.

How you intervene

As with other sinus node arrhythmias, no treatment is necessary if the patient is asymptomatic. If the patient is symptomatic, however, treatment aims to alleviate signs and symptoms and correct the underlying cause of the arrhythmia.

Atropine or epinephrine may be given initially for an acute attack. A pacemaker may be used until the underlying disorder resolves. Tachyarrhythmias may be treated with antiarrhythmic medications, such as metoprolol and digoxin.

When the solution is part of the problem

Unfortunately, medications used to suppress tachyarrhythmias may worsen an underlying SA node disease and bradyarrhythmias. The patient may need anticoagulants if he develops sudden bursts, or paroxysms, of atrial fibrillation. The anticoagulants help prevent thromboembolism and stroke, a complication of the condition. Because the syndrome is progressive and chronic, a symptomatic patient needs lifelong treatment.

Keep a running total

When caring for a patient with sick sinus syndrome, monitor and document all arrhythmias he experiences and signs or symptoms he develops. Assess how his rhythm responds to activity and pain and look for changes in the rhythm.

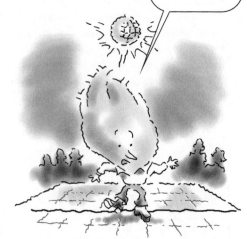

Atrial arrhythmias are the most common reason I lose my rhythm.

Atrial arrhythmias

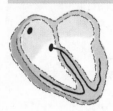

Atrial arrhythmias are caused by impulses that originate in areas outside the SA node. These arrhythmias can affect ventricular filling time and diminish the strength of atrial kick, a contraction that normally provides the ventricles with about 30% of their blood. Atrial arrhythmias are thought to result from three mechanisms:

altered automaticity, circus reentry, and afterdepolarization. Types of atrial arrhythmias include premature atrial contractions, atrial flutter, atrial fibrillation, and atrial tachycardia.

Premature atrial contractions

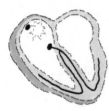

Premature atrial contractions (PACs) originate outside the SA node and usually result from an irritable spot, or focus, in the atria that takes over as pacemaker for one or more beats. The SA node fires an impulse, but then an irritable focus jumps in, firing its own impulse before the SA node can fire again.

PACs may not be conducted through the AV node and the rest of the heart, depending on their prematurity and the status of the AV and intraventricular conduction system. Nonconducted or blocked PACs don't trigger a QRS complex. (See *Recognizing PACs*.)

Recognizing PACs

When examining a premature atrial contraction (PAC) on an ECG, look for irregular atrial and ventricular rates. The underlying rhythm may be regular. The P wave is premature and abnormally shaped and may be lost in the previous T wave, distorting that wave's configuration. (The T wave might be bigger or have an extra bump.) Varying configurations of the P wave indicate more than one ectopic site.

The PR interval is usually normal but may be shortened or slightly prolonged, depending on the origin of the ectopic focus. If no QRS complex follows the premature P wave, a nonconducted PAC has occurred.

PACs may occur in bigeminy (every other beat is a PAC), trigeminy (every third beat is a PAC), or couplets (two PACs at a time). This rhythm strip illustrates PACs. Notice their distinguishing characteristics.

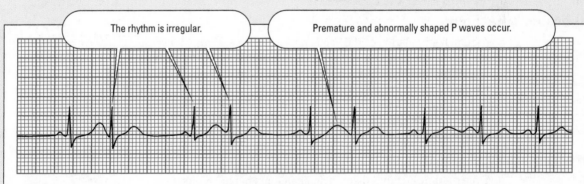

The rhythm is irregular.

Premature and abnormally shaped P waves occur.

- *Rhythm:* Irregular
- *Rate:* 90 beats/minute
- *P wave:* Abnormal with PAC; some lost in previous T wave
- *PR interval:* 0.20 second
- *QRS complex:* 0.08 second
- *T wave:* Abnormal with some embedded P waves
- *QT interval:* 0.32 second
- *Other:* Noncompensatory pause

How you intervene

Most patients with PACs are asymptomatic and don't need treatment. However, if the patient is symptomatic, treatment focuses on eliminating the cause, such as caffeine and alcohol intake. People who have frequent PACs may be treated with drugs that prolong the refractory period of the atria. Those drugs include digoxin, procainamide, and quinidine. If the patient has ischemic or valvular heart disease, monitor for signs and symptoms of heart failure, electrolyte imbalances, and the development of more severe atrial arrhythmias.

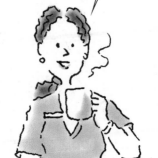

PACs may be caused by excessive intake of caffeine or alcohol.

Atrial flutter

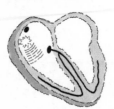

Atrial flutter, a supraventricular tachycardia, is characterized by an atrial rate of 250 to 400 beats/minute. It's generally around 300 beats/minute. Originating in a single atrial focus, this rhythm results from circus reentry and, possibly, increased automaticity.

On an ECG, the P waves lose their distinction due to the rapid atrial rate. The waves blend together in a saw-toothed appearance and are called *flutter waves*. These waves are the hallmark of atrial flutter. (See *Recognizing atrial flutter*.)

How you intervene

Atrial flutter with a rapid ventricular response and reduced cardiac output requires immediate intervention. Therapy aims to control the ventricular rate and convert the atrial ectopic rhythm to a normal sinus rhythm.

A shocking treatment

Although stimulation of the vagus nerve may temporarily increase the block ratio and slow the ventricular rate, the effects won't last. Therefore, cardioversion remains the treatment of choice. Synchronized cardioversion involves the delivery of an electrical stimulus during depolarization. The stimulus makes part of the myocardium refractory to ectopic impulses and terminates circus reentry movements.

Fluttering away

Drug therapy includes digoxin and calcium channel blockers, which decrease AV conduction time. Quinidine may be given to convert flutter to fibrillation, an easier arrhythmia to treat. If digoxin and quinidine therapy is used, the patient must first be given a loading dose of digoxin. Ibutilide may be used to convert recent-onset atrial flutter to sinus rhythm. If possible, the underlying cause of the atrial flutter should be treated.

Recognizing atrial flutter

Atrial flutter is characterized by abnormal P waves that produce a saw-toothed appearance. Varying degrees of AV block produce ventricular rates one-half to one-fourth of the atrial rate. The QRS complex is usually normal but may be widened if flutter waves are buried in the complex. You won't be able to identify a T wave, nor will you be able to measure the QT interval.

The clinical significance of atrial flutter is determined by the number of impulses conducted through the node—expressed as a conduction ratio, for example, 2:1 or 4:1—and the resulting ventricular rate. If the ventricular rate is too slow (less than 40 beats/minute) or too fast (more than 150 beats/minute), cardiac output can be seriously compromised.

This rhythm strip illustrates atrial flutter. Notice its distinguishing characteristics.

Classic, saw-toothed flutter waves occur.

The atrial rate is greater than the ventricular rate.

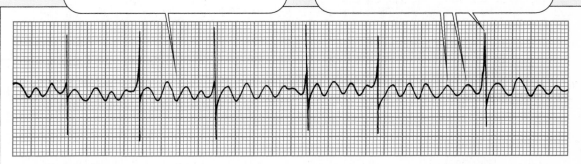

- *Rhythm:* Atrial—regular; ventricular—irregular
- *Rate:* Atrial—280 beats/minute; ventricular—60 beats/minute
- *P wave:* Classic, saw-toothed appearance
- *PR interval:* Unmeasurable
- *QRS complex:* 0.08 second
- *T wave:* Unidentifiable
- *QT interval:* Unidentifiable
- *Other:* None

Atrial fibrillation

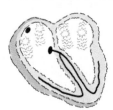

Atrial fibrillation, sometimes called *A-fib*, is defined as chaotic, asynchronous, electrical activity in atrial tissue. The ectopic impulses may fire at a rate of 400 to 600 times/minute, causing the atria to quiver instead of contract. The ventricles respond only to those impulses that make it through the AV node.

On an ECG, atrial activity is no longer represented by P waves but by erratic baseline waves called *fibrillatory waves.* This rhythm may either be sustained or paroxysmal (occurring in bursts). It can be preceded by, or result from, PACs. (See *Recognizing atrial fibrillation,* page 108.)

Recognizing atrial fibrillation

In atrial fibrillation, the atrial rate is almost indiscernible but is usually greater than 400 beats/minute. The ventricular rate usually varies from 100 to 150 beats/minute but can be lower. Atrial fibrillation is called *coarse* if the fibrillatory waves are pronounced and *fine* if they aren't. Atrial fibrillation and flutter may also occur simultaneously. Look for a configuration that varies between fibrillatory waves and flutter waves.

If the ventricular response is greater than 100 beats/minute — a condition called *uncontrolled atrial fibrillation* — the patient may develop heart failure, angina, or syncope. This rhythm strip illustrates atrial fibrillation. Notice its distinguishing characteristics.

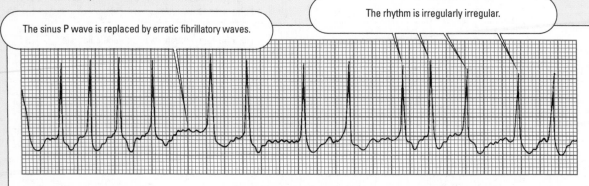

The sinus P wave is replaced by erratic fibrillatory waves.

The rhythm is irregularly irregular.

- *Rhythm:* Irregularly irregular
- *Rate:* Atrial—indiscernible; ventricular—130 beats/minute
- *P wave:* Absent; replaced by fine fibrillatory waves
- *PR interval:* Indiscernible
- *QRS complex:* 0.08 second
- *T wave:* Indiscernible
- *QT interval:* Unmeasurable
- *Other:* None

How you intervene

Assess the peripheral and apical pulses. You may find that the radial pulse rate is slower than the apical rate because the weaker contractions of the heart don't produce a palpable peripheral pulse.

Keep your eyes on the prize

The major therapeutic goal in treating atrial fibrillation is to reduce the ventricular response rate to less than 100 beats/minute. When the onset of atrial fibrillation is acute and the patient can cooperate, vagal maneuvers or carotid sinus massage may slow the ventricular response but won't convert the arrhythmia.

Bring in the drugs

The ventricular rate may be controlled with such drugs as diltiazem, verapamil, digoxin, and beta-adrenergic blockers. Ibutilide may be used to convert new-onset atrial fibrillation to sinus rhythm. Quinidine and procainamide can also convert atrial fibrillation to normal sinus rhythm, usually after anticoagulation.

Symptoms need synchrony

If the patient is symptomatic, immediate synchronized cardioversion is necessary. Cardioversion is most successful if used within the first 3 days of onset and less successful if the rhythm has existed for a long time. If possible, anticoagulants should be administered first because conversion to normal sinus rhythm causes forceful atrial contractions to resume abruptly. If a thrombus has formed in the atria, the resumption of contractions can result in systemic emboli.

Such drugs as digoxin, procainamide, propranolol, quinidine, amiodarone, and verapamil can be given after successful cardioversion to maintain normal sinus rhythm and control the ventricular rate in chronic atrial fibrillation. If drug therapy is used, monitor serum drug levels and observe the patient for evidence of toxicity.

Radio days

Symptom-producing atrial fibrillation that doesn't respond to routine treatment may be treated with *radiofrequency ablation therapy*. A transvenous catheter is used to locate the area within the heart that participates in initiating or perpetuating certain tachyarrhythmias. Radiofrequency energy is then delivered to the myocardium through this catheter to produce a small area of necrosis. The damaged tissue can no longer cause or participate in the tachyarrhythmia. However, if the energy is delivered close to the AV node, bundle of His, or bundle branches, a block can occur.

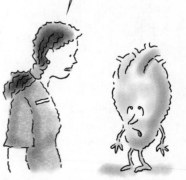

I hate to say it, but sometimes a little necrosis can be a good thing. Radiofrequency ablation is used to damage tissue that is causing a tachyarrhythmia.

Atrial tachycardia

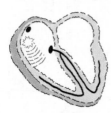

Atrial tachycardia is characterized by an atrial rate of 150 to 250 beats/minute. The rapid rate shortens diastole, resulting in a loss of atrial kick, reduced cardiac output, reduced coronary perfusion, and ischemic myocardial changes. (See *Recognizing atrial tachycardia*, page 110, and *Identifying types of atrial tachycardia*, page 111.)

How you intervene

Treatment depends on the type of tachycardia and the severity of the patient's symptoms. Because one of the most common causes of atrial tachycardia is digoxin toxicity, be sure to monitor levels of this drug.

Made to maneuver

Valsalva's maneuver and carotid sinus massage may be used to treat paroxysmal atrial tachycardia. Both of these types of vagal maneuvers are particularly effective when the tachycardia is caused by circus reentry, which is signaled by frequent PACs.

Recognizing atrial tachycardia

When assessing a rhythm strip for atrial tachycardia, you'll see that atrial rhythm is always regular. Ventricular rhythm is regular when the block is constant and irregular when it isn't. The rate consists of three or more successive ectopic atrial beats at a rate of 140 to 250 beats/minute. The ventricular rate varies according to the AV conduction ratio.

The P wave has a 1:1 ratio with the QRS complex unless a block is present. The P wave may not be discernible because of the rapid rate and may be hidden in the previous ST segment or T wave. You may not be able to measure the PR interval if the P wave can't be distinguished from the preceding T wave.

The QRS complex is usually normal, unless the impulses are being conducted abnormally through the ventricles. The T wave may be normal or inverted if ischemia is present. The QT interval is usually within normal limits but may be shorter because of the rapid rate. Changes in the ST-segment and T-wave may appear if ischemia occurs with a prolonged arrhythmia. This rhythm strip illustrates atrial tachycardia. Notice its distinguishing characteristics.

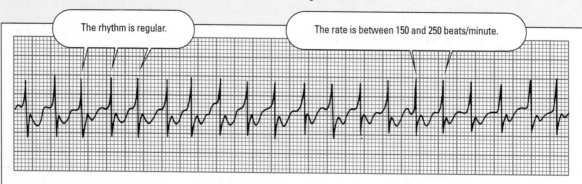

> The rhythm is regular.

> The rate is between 150 and 250 beats/minute.

- *Rhythm:* Regular
- *Rate:* 210 beats/minute
- *P wave:* Almost hidden in T wave
- *PR interval:* 0.12 second
- *QRS complex:* 0.10 second
- *T wave:* Distorted by P wave
- *QT interval:* 0.20 second
- *Other:* None

Drugs do decrease

Other treatment options include drugs that increase the degree of AV block, which in turn decreases the ventricular response and slows the rate. Such drugs include digoxin, beta-adrenergic blockers, and calcium channel blockers.

In addition, adenosine can be used to stop atrial tachycardia, and procainamide can be used to establish normal sinus rhythm. When other treatments fail, synchronized cardioversion may be used.

Identifying types of atrial tachycardia

Atrial tachycardia comes in three varieties.

Atrial tachycardia with block

Atrial tachycardia with block is caused by increased automaticity of the atrial tissue. As the atrial rate speeds up and atrioventricular conduction becomes impaired, a 2:1 block typically occurs. Occasionally, a type 1 (Wenckebach) second-degree heart block may be seen.

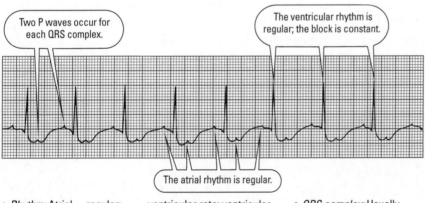

Two P waves occur for each QRS complex.

The ventricular rhythm is regular; the block is constant.

The atrial rhythm is regular.

• *Rhythm:* Atrial—regular; ventricular—regular if block is constant; irregular if block is variable
• *Rate:* Atrial—140 to 250 beats/minute, multiple of ventricular rate; ventricular —varies with block
• *P wave:* Slightly abnormal
• *PR interval:* Usually normal; may be hidden

• *QRS complex:* Usually normal
• *Other:* More than one P wave for each QRS complex

(continued)

Identifying types of atrial tachycardia *(continued)*

Multifocal atrial tachycardia

In multifocal atrial tachycardia (MAT), atrial tachycardia occurs with numerous atrial foci firing intermittently. MAT produces varying P waves on the strip and occurs most commonly in patients with chronic pulmonary disease. The irregular baseline in this strip is caused by movement of the chest wall.

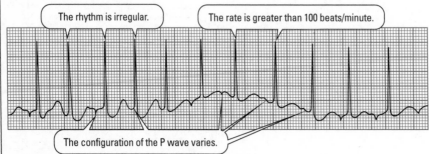

The rhythm is irregular.

The rate is greater than 100 beats/minute.

The configuration of the P wave varies.

- *Rhythm:* Both irregular
- *Rate:* Atrial—100 to 250 beats/minute; usually under 160; ventricular—100 to 250 beats/minute

- *P wave:* Configuration varies; must see at least three different P wave shapes

- *PR interval:* Varies
- *Other:* None

Paroxysmal atrial tachycardia

A type of paroxysmal supraventricular tachycardia, paroxysmal atrial tachycardia (PAT) features brief periods of tachycardia that alternate with periods of normal sinus rhythm. PAT starts and stops suddenly as a result of rapid firing of an ectopic focus. It commonly follows frequent premature atrial contractions (PACs), one of which initiates the tachycardia.

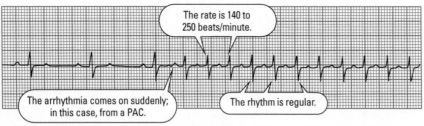

The rate is 140 to 250 beats/minute.

The arrhythmia comes on suddenly; in this case, from a PAC.

The rhythm is regular.

- *Rhythm:* Regular
- *Rate:* 140 to 250 beats/minute

- *P wave:* Abnormal, possibly hidden in the previous T wave
- *PR interval:* Identical for each cycle

- *QRS complex:* Possibly aberrantly conducted
- *Other:* A single P wave for each QRS complex

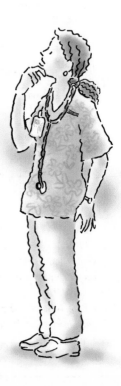

Shifting into overdrive

Atrial overdrive pacing (also called *burst pacing* or *rapid atrial pacing*) can also be used to stop the arrhythmia. In this procedure, the patient's atrial rate is electronically paced slightly higher than the intrinsic arterial rate. The pacing interferes with the conduction circuit and renders part of it unresponsive to the reentrant impulse. Atrial tachycardia stops, and the SA node resumes its normal role as pacemaker.

Junctional arrhythmias

Junctional arrhythmias originate in the AV junction—the area around the AV node and the bundle of His. These arrhythmias occur when the SA node is suppressed and fails to conduct impulses or when a block occurs in conduction. Electrical impulses may then be initiated by pacemaker cells in the AV junction.

Which way did the impulse go?

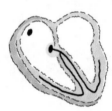

Because the AV junction is located in the middle of the heart, impulses generated in this area cause the heart to be depolarized in an abnormal way. The impulse moves upward and causes backward, or retrograde, depolarization of the atria. This depolarization results in inverted P waves in leads II, III, and aV$_F$, in which you would usually see upright P waves. The impulse also moves down toward the ventricles, causing forward, or antegrade, depolarization of the ventricles and an upright QRS complex.

Types of junctional arrhythmias include premature junctional contraction (PJC) junctional escape rhythm, accelerated junctional rhythm, and junctional tachycardia.

Premature junctional contraction

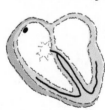

A PJC is a beat that occurs before a normal beat and causes an irregular rhythm. This ectopic beat occurs when an irritable location within the AV junction acts as a pacemaker and fires either prematurely or out of sequence.

With PJC, as with all junctional arrhythmias, the atria depolarize in retrograde fashion, causing an inverted P wave on the ECG. The ventricles depolarize normally. (See *Recognizing a PJC*, page 114.)

How you intervene

Although PJCs themselves aren't usually dangerous, you'll need to monitor the patient carefully and assess him for other signs of in-

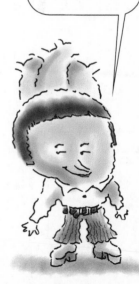

In junctional arrhythmias, the atria depolarize in a retrograde fashion.

114

Recognizing a PJC

A premature junctional contraction (PJC) appears on a rhythm strip as an early beat that causes an irregularity. The rest of the strip may show regular atrial and ventricular rhythms, depending on the patient's underlying rhythm.

Look for an inverted P wave in leads II, III, and aV$_F$. Depending on when the impulse occurs, the P wave may fall before, during, or after the QRS complex. If it falls during the QRS complex, it's hidden. If it comes before the QRS complex, the PR interval is less than 0.12 second.

Because the ventricles usually depolarize normally, the QRS complex has a normal configuration and a normal duration of less than 0.12 second. The T wave and the QT interval are usually normal. This rhythm strip shows a premature junctional contraction. Notice its distinguishing characteristics.

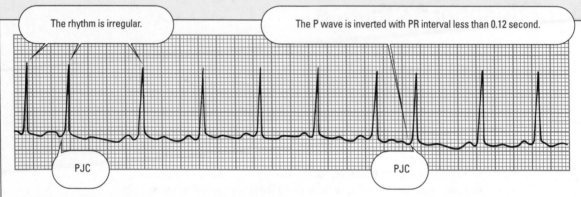

The rhythm is irregular.

The P wave is inverted with PR interval less than 0.12 second.

PJC

PJC

- *Rhythm:* Irregular atrial and ventricular rhythms
- *Rate:* 100 beats/minute
- *P wave:* Inverted and precedes the QRS complex
- *PR interval:* 0.14 second for the underlying rhythm and 0.06 second for the PJC
- *QRS complex:* 0.06 second
- *T wave:* Normal configuration
- *QT interval:* 0.36 second
- *Other:* Pause after PJC

trinsic pacemaker failure. If digoxin toxicity is the culprit, check with the patient's doctor about discontinuing the medication and monitoring serum drug levels. You should also monitor the patient for hemodynamic instability. If ectopic beats are frequent, the patient should decrease or eliminate his caffeine intake.

Junctional escape rhythm

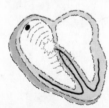

A junctional escape rhythm shows a regular rhythm of 40 to 60 beats/minute. The atria depolarize by retrograde conduction. P waves are inverted, and impulse conduction through the ventricles is normal. (See *Recognizing junctional escape rhythm.*)

Recognizing junctional escape rhythm

A junctional escape rhythm shows a regular rhythm of 40 to 60 beats/minute on the ECG strip. Look for inverted P waves in leads II, III, and aV$_F$.

The P waves will occur before, after, or hidden within the QRS complex. The PR interval is less than 0.12 second and is measurable only if the P wave comes before the QRS complex.

The rest of the ECG waveform—including the QRS complex, T wave, and QT interval—should appear normal because impulses through the ventricles are usually conducted normally.

This rhythm strip shows a junctional escape rhythm. Note the inverted P wave.

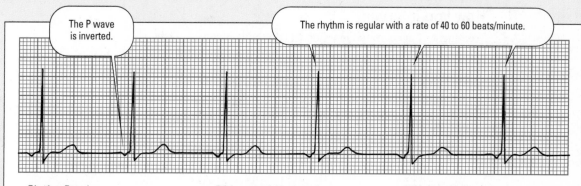

The P wave is inverted.

The rhythm is regular with a rate of 40 to 60 beats/minute.

- *Rhythm:* Regular
- *Rate:* 60 beats/minute
- *P wave:* Inverted and preceding each QRS complex

- *PR interval:* 0.10 second
- *QRS complex:* 0.10 second
- *T wave:* Normal

- *QT interval:* 0.44 second
- *Other:* None

The great escape

Remember that the AV junction can take over as the heart's pacemaker if higher pacemaker sites slow down or fail to fire or conduct. The junctional escape beat is an example of this compensatory mechanism. Because junctional escape beats prevent ventricular standstill, they should never be suppressed.

How you intervene

Treatment of a junctional escape rhythm involves correcting the underlying cause. Atropine may be given to increase the heart rate, or a temporary or permanent pacemaker may be inserted if the patient is symptomatic.

Monitor the patient's serum digoxin and electrolyte levels and watch for signs of decreased cardiac output, such as hypotension, syncope, and blurred vision. If the patient is hypotensive, lower the head of his bed as far as he can tolerate and keep atropine at the bedside.

Accelerated junctional rhythm

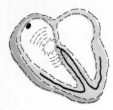

An accelerated junctional rhythm results when an irritable focus in the AV junction speeds up and takes over as the heart's pacemaker. The atria depolarize by retrograde conduction, whereas the ventricles depolarize normally. The accelerated rate is usually between 60 and 100 beats/minute. (See *Recognizing accelerated junctional rhythm.*)

How you intervene

Treatment of accelerated junctional arrhythmia involves correcting the underlying cause. Nursing interventions include observing the patient for signs of decreased cardiac output and monitoring his vital signs for hemodynamic instability. You should also assess the levels of potassium and other electrolytes and administer supplements as ordered. Finally, monitor the patient's digoxin level and withhold digoxin as ordered.

(Text continues on page 117.)

Recognizing accelerated junctional rhythm

To identify an accelerated junctional rhythm, look for a regular rhythm and a rate of 60 to 100 beats/minute. If a P wave is present, it's inverted in leads II, III, and aV$_F$ and occurs before or after the QRS complex or may be hidden in it. If the P wave comes before the QRS complex, the PR interval is less than 0.12 second. The QRS complex, T wave, and QT interval appear normal.

This rhythm strip illustrates accelerated junctional rhythm. Notice its distinguishing characteristics.

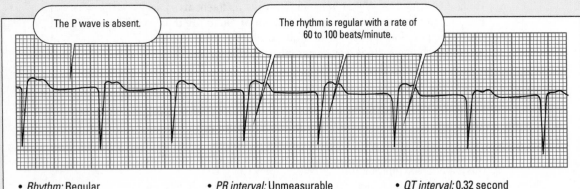

The P wave is absent.

The rhythm is regular with a rate of 60 to 100 beats/minute.

- *Rhythm:* Regular
- *Rate:* 80 beats/minute
- *P wave:* Absent

- *PR interval:* Unmeasurable
- *QRS complex:* 0.10 second
- *T wave:* Normal

- *QT interval:* 0.32 second
- *Other:* None

How electrolyte imbalances affect ECGs

Electrical impulses move through the heart's conduction system to create rhythmic contractions. Normal electrical activity in the heart depends on normal serum electrolyte concentrations.

The electrolytes sodium, potassium, and calcium, with the help of magnesium, shift back and forth across myocardial cell membranes. This shifting of electrolytes causes alternating periods of activity (depolarization) and rest (repolarization), which allow for normal myocardial function. Electrolyte imbalances cause trademark changes in electrocardiogram (ECG) readings and myocardial function. This special section details changes in two critical electrolytes: magnesium and potassium.

Hypermagnesemia

Magnesium

Hypermagnesemia (serum magnesium > 2.5 mEq/L) can be caused by excessive magnesium administration or renal failure. The condition can cause a prolonged PR interval and the ECG changes shown below. If left untreated, hypermagnesemia can lead to sinoatrial or atrioventricular (AV) heart block and, eventually, cardiac arrest.

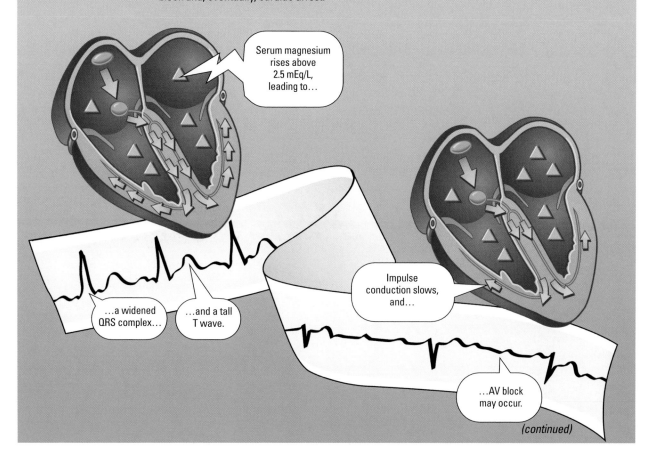

(continued)

Hyperkalemia

Potassium

Hyperkalemia (serum potassium > 5.5 mEq/L) may be caused by renal failure or excessive potassium administration. Excess potassium alters the heart's electrical activity and leads to depressed conduction. Among the earliest signs of hyperkalemia is a tall, tented T wave, as shown below. AV or ventricular block may develop. Other possible ECG abnormalities include a flattened P wave, a prolonged PR interval, a widened QRS complex as ventricular conduction slows, and a depressed ST segment.

If left untreated, severe hyperkalemia (serum potassium > 9 mEq/L) occurs, causing the the P wave to disappear, the QRS complex to widen, and sine waves to form. Hyperkalemia may end in lethal arrhythmias.

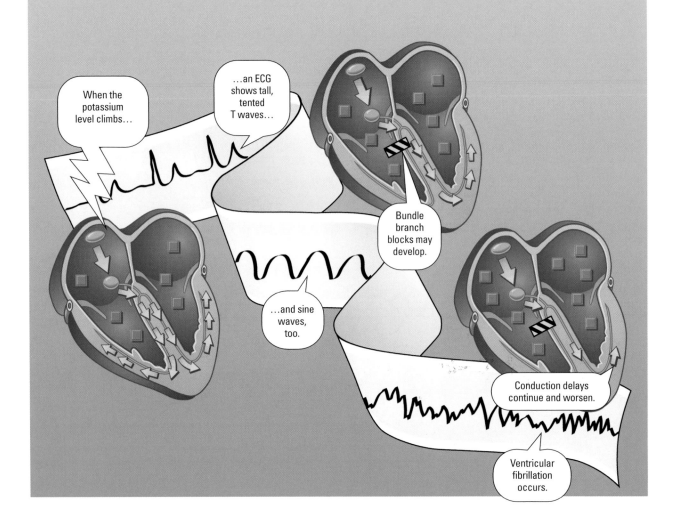

Hypokalemia

Potassium

Hypokalemia (serum potassium < 3.5 mEq/L) can be caused by diuresis or loss of other body fluids. An abnormally low potassium level affects the heart's electrical activity. Ventricular repolarization is prolonged. ECG changes include a prominent U wave — a hallmark of hypokalemia.

As the potassium level decreases, ectopic impulses form and conduction disturbances increase. Atrial and ventricular arrhythmias may develop. As ectopy becomes more frequent, the patient is at risk for potentially fatal arrhythmias. Examples of hypokalemic ECG changes are shown here.

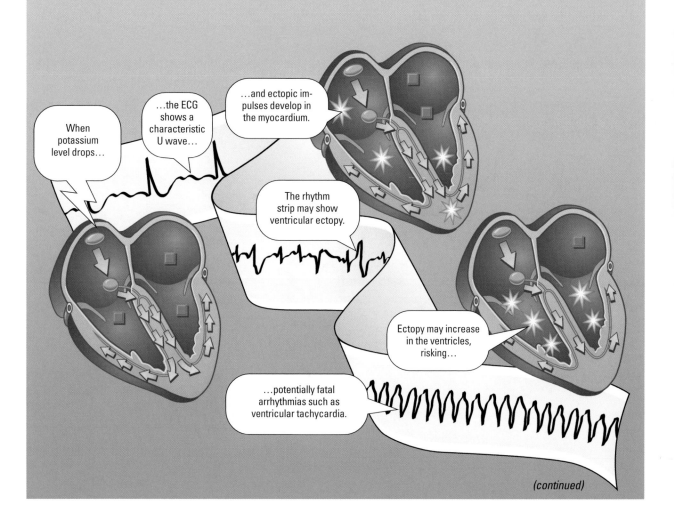

(continued)

Hypomagnesemia

Magnesium

Hypomagnesemia (serum magnesium < 1.5 mEq/L) may be caused by malnutrition or excessive loss of body fluids. Its effects on the electrical activity of the heart include ECG changes (shown below), such as a slightly widened QRS complex, a prolonged QT interval (which increases myocardial vulnerability to a stimulus), and a depressed ST segment.

Dangerously low magnesium levels make myocardial cells more excitable, which can trigger such life-threatening arrhythmias as ventricular tachycardia, torsades de pointes, and ventricular fibrillation.

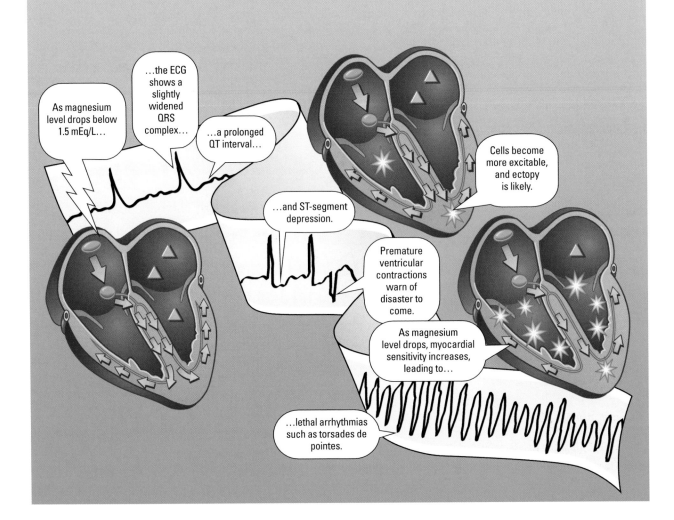

Junctional tachycardia

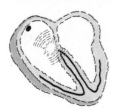

In junctional tachycardia, three or more premature junctional contractions occur in a row. The rate is usually 100 to 200 beats/minute. (See *Recognizing junctional tachycardia.*)

How you intervene

The underlying cause of junctional tachycardia should be treated. If the cause is digoxin toxicity, digoxin should be discontinued. Vagal maneuvers and medications such as verapamil may slow the heart rate for the symptomatic patient.

Keeping pace

If the patient recently had an MI or heart surgery, he may need a temporary pacemaker to reset the heart's rhythm. Children with permanent arrhythmias may be resistant to drug therapy and require surgery. Patients with recurrent junctional tachycardia may

---

Recognizing junctional tachycardia

When assessing a rhythm strip for junctional tachycardia, look for a rate of 100 to 200 beats/minute. The P wave is inverted in leads II, III, and aV$_F$ and can occur before, during (hidden P wave), or after the QRS complex. If it comes before the QRS complex, the only time the PR interval can be measured, it's always less than 0.12 second. The QRS complexes look normal, as does the T wave, unless a P wave occurs in it or the rate is so fast that the T wave can't be detected.

This rhythm strip illustrates junctional tachycardia. Notice its distinguishing characteristics.

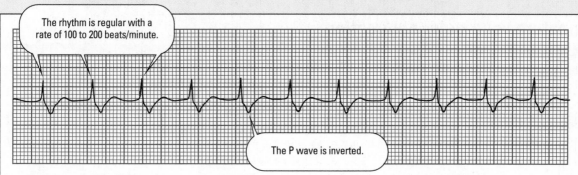

The rhythm is regular with a rate of 100 to 200 beats/minute.

The P wave is inverted.

- *Rhythm:* Regular atrial and ventricular rhythms
- *Rate:* Atrial and ventricular rates of 115 beats/minute
- *P wave:* Inverted, follows QRS complex
- *PR interval:* Unmeasurable
- *QRS complex:* 0.08 second
- *T wave:* Normal
- *QT interval:* 0.36 second
- *Other:* None

be treated with ablation therapy, followed by permanent pacemaker insertion.

Monitor patients with junctional tachycardia for signs of decreased cardiac output. Also check digoxin and potassium levels and administer potassium supplements, as ordered. If symptoms are severe and digoxin is the culprit, the doctor may order digoxin immune Fab, a digoxin-binding drug.

Ventricular arrhythmias

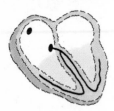

Ventricular arrhythmias originate in the ventricles below the bundle of His. They occur when electrical impulses depolarize the myocardium using a different pathway than the one used by normal impulses.

On an ECG, the QRS complex is wider than normal because of the prolonged conduction time through the ventricles. The T wave and the QRS complex deflect in opposite directions because of the difference in the action potential during ventricular depolarization and repolarization. Also, the P wave is absent because atrial depolarization doesn't occur.

Potential to kill

Although ventricular arrhythmias may be benign, they're potentially deadly because the ventricles are ultimately responsible for cardiac output. Types of ventricular arrhythmia include premature ventricular contraction (PVC), ventricular tachycardia, ventricular fibrillation, idioventricular rhythms, and asystole.

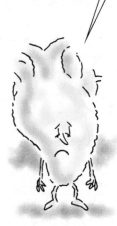

My atria have no spark left, so my ventricles are generating my electrical impulses now.

Premature ventricular contraction

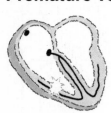

PVC is an ectopic beat originating low in the ventricles and occurring earlier than normal. PVCs may occur in healthy people without causing problems. They may also occur singly, in clusters of two or more, or in repeating patterns, such as bigeminy or trigeminy. When PVCs occur in patients with underlying heart disease, they may indicate impending lethal ventricular arrhythmias. (See *Recognizing PVCs.*)

How you intervene

If the patient is asymptomatic and doesn't have heart disease, the arrhythmia probably won't require treatment. If he has symptoms or a dangerous form of PVCs, the type of treatment depends on the cause of the problem.

Recognizing PVCs

On the ECG strip, premature ventricular contractions (PVCs) look wide and bizarre and appear as early beats that cause atrial and ventricular irregularity. The rate follows the underlying rhythm, which is usually regular. The P wave is usually absent. A PVC may trigger retrograde P waves, which can distort the ST segment. The PR interval and QT interval aren't measurable on a premature beat, only on the normal beats.

Early QRS

The QRS complex occurs early. Configuration of the QRS complex is usually normal in the underlying rhythm. The duration of the QRS complex in the premature beat exceeds 0.12 second. The T wave in the premature beat has a deflection opposite that of the QRS complex. When a PVC strikes on the downslope of the preceding normal T wave—the R-on-T phenomenon—it can trigger more serious rhythm disturbances.

Compensatory pause

A horizontal baseline called a *compensatory pause* may follow the T wave of the PVC. When a compensatory pause appears, the interval between two normal sinus beats containing a PVC equals two normal sinus intervals. This pause occurs because the ventricle is refractory and can't respond to the next regularly timed P wave from the sinus node. When a compensatory pause doesn't occur, the PVC is referred to as *interpolated*.

PVC look-alikes

PVCs that look alike are called *unifocal* and originate from the same ectopic focus. PVCs that don't look alike are called *multifocal* and originate from different foci.

This rhythm strip shows unifocal PVCs on beats 1, 6, and 11. Note the wide and bizarre appearance of the QRS complex.

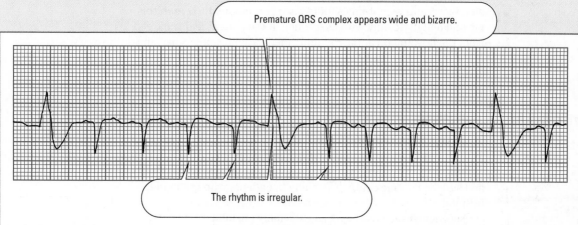

Premature QRS complex appears wide and bizarre.

The rhythm is irregular.

- *Rhythm:* Irregular
- *Rate:* 120 beats/minute
- *P wave:* None with PVC, but P wave present with other QRS complexes
- *PR interval:* 0.12 second in underlying rhythm

- *QRS complex:* Early, with bizarre configuration and duration of 0.14 second in PVC; QRS complexes are 0.08 second in underlying rhythm

- *T wave:* Normal; opposite direction from QRS complex
- *QT interval:* 0.28 second with underlying rhythm
- *Other:* None

From the heart

If the PVCs have a cardiac origin, the doctor may order such drugs as procainamide or lidocaine to suppress ventricular irritability. Procainamide may be given by infusion at a maintenance dose of 1 to 4 mg/minute. After an I.V. bolus of 1 to 1.5 mg/kg of lidocaine, you may give an infusion of 1 to 4 mg/minute.

The outsiders

When PVCs have a noncardiac origin, treatment aims to correct the cause. For example, you might adjust drug therapy or correct acidosis, electrolyte imbalances, hypothermia, or hypoxia.

Stat patient stats

Patients who have recently developed PVCs need prompt assessment, especially if they have underlying heart disease or complex medical problems. Those with chronic PVCs should be observed closely for the development of more frequent PVCs or more dangerous PVC patterns.

Until effective treatment begins, patients with PVCs accompanied by serious symptoms should have continuous ECG monitoring and ambulate only with assistance. If the patient is discharged from the hospital on antiarrhythmic medications, make sure family members know how to obtain emergency medical assistance and how to perform cardiopulmonary resuscitation (CPR).

Ventricular tachycardia

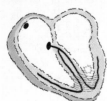

In ventricular tachycardia, commonly called *V-tach*, three or more PVCs occur in a row and the ventricular rate exceeds 100 beats/minute. This arrhythmia usually precedes ventricular fibrillation and sudden cardiac death, especially in patients who aren't in the hospital.

Ventricular tachycardia is an extremely unstable rhythm. It can occur in short, paroxysmal bursts that last less than 30 seconds and cause few or no symptoms. Alternatively, it can be sustained, requiring immediate treatment to prevent death, even in patients initially able to maintain adequate cardiac output. (See *Recognizing ventricular tachycardia* and *Understanding torsades de pointes*, page 122.)

How you intervene

Treatment depends on whether the patient's pulse is detectable or undetectable. Patients with pulseless ventricular tachycardia require immediate resuscitation using the same methods as those used for ventricular fibrillation. Treatment of patients with a de-

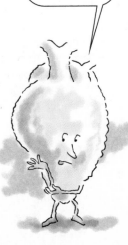

V-tach is extremely dangerous because it usually precedes V-fib.

Recognizing ventricular tachycardia

In ventricular tachycardia, the atrial rhythm and rate can't be determined on the ECG strip. The ventricular rhythm is usually regular but may be slightly irregular. The ventricular rate is usually rapid (100 to 200 beats/minute).

Absent P

The P wave is usually absent but may be obscured by the QRS complex. Retrograde P waves may be present. Because the P wave can seldom be seen, you can't measure the PR interval.

Bizarre QRS

The QRS complex has a bizarre configuration, usually with increased amplitude and duration of longer than 0.14 second.

QRS complexes in monomorphic ventricular tachycardia have a uniform shape. In polymorphic ventricular tachycardia, the shape of the QRS complex constantly changes. If the T wave is visible, it occurs opposite the QRS complex. The QT interval isn't measurable.

This rhythm strip illustrates ventricular tachycardia. Notice its distinguishing characteristics.

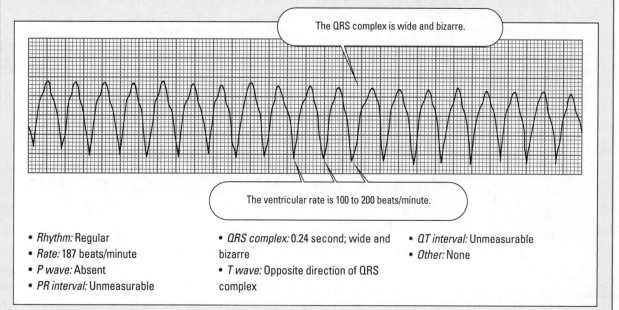

The QRS complex is wide and bizarre.

The ventricular rate is 100 to 200 beats/minute.

- *Rhythm:* Regular
- *Rate:* 187 beats/minute
- *P wave:* Absent
- *PR interval:* Unmeasurable

- *QRS complex:* 0.24 second; wide and bizarre
- *T wave:* Opposite direction of QRS complex

- *QT interval:* Unmeasurable
- *Other:* None

tectable pulse depends on whether their condition is stable or unstable. Unstable patients generally have heart rates greater than 150 beats/minute. They may also have hypotension, shortness of breath, an altered level of consciousness, heart failure, angina, or MI. These patients are treated immediately with direct-current synchronized cardioversion.

Complex treatments

A stable patient with a wide QRS complex tachycardia and no signs of cardiac decompensation is treated differently. First, if the patient has monomorphic ventricular tachycardia, procainamide

Understanding torsades de pointes

Torsades de pointes, which means "twisting about the points," is a special form of polymorphic ventricular tachycardia. The hallmark characteristics of this rhythm (shown below) are QRS complexes that rotate about the baseline, deflecting downward and upward for several beats. The rate is 150 to 250 beats/minute, usually with an irregular rhythm, and the QRS complexes are wide. The P wave is usually absent.

Paroxysmal rhythm

This arrhythmia may be paroxysmal, starting and stopping suddenly, and may deteriorate into ventricular fibrillation. It should be considered when ventricular tachycardia doesn't respond to antiarrhythmic therapy or other treatments.

Reversible causes

Causes of this form of ventricular tachycardia are usually reversible. The most common causes are drugs that lengthen the QT interval, such as the antiarrhythmics quinidine, procainamide, and sotalol. Other causes include myocardial ischemia and electrolyte abnormalities, such as hypokalemia, hypomagnesemia, and hypocalcemia.

Going into overdrive

Torsades de pointes is treated by correcting the underlying cause, especially if the cause is related to specific drug therapy. The doctor may order mechanical overdrive pacing, which overrides the ventricular rate and breaks the triggered mechanism for the arrhythmia. Magnesium may also be effective. Electrical cardioversion may be used when torsades de pointes doesn't respond to other treatment.

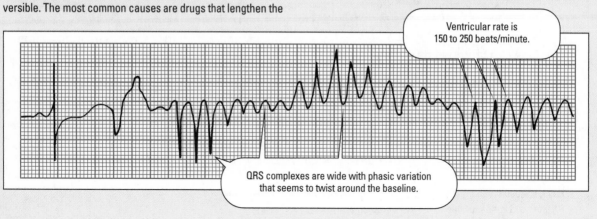

Ventricular rate is 150 to 250 beats/minute.

QRS complexes are wide with phasic variation that seems to twist around the baseline.

is given to try to correct the rhythm disturbance; then other drugs, such as amiodarone, are used. If the patient becomes unstable, immediate synchronized cardioversion is performed. If the patient has polymorphic ventricular tachycardia, a beta-adrenergic blocker, amiodarone, or procainamide may be given.

Patients with chronic, recurrent episodes of ventricular tachycardia who are unresponsive to drug therapy may have a cardioverter-defibrillator implanted. This device is a more permanent solution to recurrent episodes of ventricular tachycardia.

Assume the worst

Any wide QRS complex tachycardia should be treated as ventricular tachycardia until definitive evidence is found to establish another diagnosis, such as supraventricular tachycardia with abnormal ventricular conduction. Always assume that the patient has ventricular tachycardia and treat him accordingly. Rapid intervention will prevent cardiac decompensation or the onset of more lethal arrhythmias.

Ventricular fibrillation

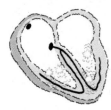

Ventricular fibrillation, commonly called *V-fib*, is a chaotic pattern of electrical activity in the ventricles in which electrical impulses arise from many different foci. It produces no effective muscular contraction and no cardiac output. Untreated ventricular fibrillation causes most cases of sudden cardiac death in people outside of a hospital. (See *Recognizing ventricular fibrillation*, page 124.)

CPR must be performed on a patient in V-fib until a defibrillator arrives.

How you intervene

Defibrillation is the most effective treatment for ventricular fibrillation. CPR must be performed until the defibrillator arrives to preserve oxygen supply to the brain and other vital organs. Such drugs as epinephrine or vasopressin may help the heart respond better to defibrillation. Amiodarone and magnesium may be given to decrease heart irritability and prevent a recurrence of ventricular fibrillation.

Jump start

During defibrillation, electrode paddles direct an electric current through the patient's heart. The current causes the myocardium to depolarize which, in turn, encourages the SA node to resume normal control of the heart's electrical activity. During cardiac surgery, internal paddles are placed directly on the myocardium.

Automated external defibrillators are used increasingly to provide early defibrillation. In this method, electrode pads are placed on the patient's chest and a microcomputer in the unit interprets the cardiac rhythm, providing the caregiver with step-by-step instructions on how to proceed. These defibrillators can be used by people without medical experience.

Need for speed

For patients with ventricular fibrillation, successful resuscitation requires rapid recognition of the problem and prompt defibrilla-

Recognizing ventricular fibrillation

In ventricular fibrillation, ventricular activity appears on the ECG strip as fibrillatory waves with no recognizable pattern. Atrial rate and rhythm can't be determined, nor can ventricular rhythm because no pattern or regularity occurs. As a result, the ventricular rate, P wave, PR interval, QRS complex, T wave, and QT interval can't be determined.

This first rhythm strip shows coarse ventricular fibrillation; the second shows fine ventricular fibrillation. Fine ventricular fibrillation sometimes resembles asystole.

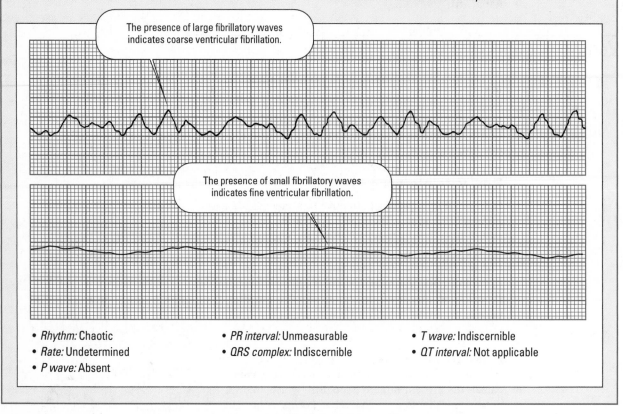

- *Rhythm:* Chaotic
- *Rate:* Undetermined
- *P wave:* Absent
- *PR interval:* Unmeasurable
- *QRS complex:* Indiscernible
- *T wave:* Indiscernible
- *QT interval:* Not applicable

tion. Many health care facilities and emergency medical systems have established protocols to help health care workers initiate prompt treatment. Make sure you know where your facility keeps its emergency equipment and how to recognize and deal with potentially lethal arrhythmias.

Idioventricular rhythms

Called the *rhythms of last resort*, idioventricular rhythms act as safety mechanisms to prevent ventricular standstill when no impulses are conducted to the ventricles from above the bundle of

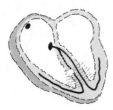

His. The cells of the His-Purkinje system take over and act as the heart's pacemaker to generate electrical impulses.

Idioventricular rhythms can occur as ventricular escape beats (only one idioventricular beat is generated late in the conduction cycle), idioventricular rhythm, or accelerated idioventricular rhythm. (See *Recognizing idioventricular rhythm.*)

> Bizarre QRS complexes characterize idioventricular rhythms.

How you intervene

Treatment should be initiated immediately to increase the patient's heart rate, improve cardiac output, and establish a normal rhythm. Atropine may be prescribed to increase the heart rate. If atropine isn't effective or if the patient develops hypotension or other signs

Recognizing idioventricular rhythm

Consecutive ventricular beats on the ECG strip make up idioventricular rhythm. When this arrhythmia occurs, atrial rhythm and rate can't be determined. The ventricular rhythm is usually regular at 20 to 40 beats/minute, the inherent rate of the ventricles. If the rate is faster, it's called an *accelerated idioventricular rhythm.*

Distinguishing characteristics of idioventricular rhythm include an absent P wave or one that has no relationship to the QRS complex. This makes the PR interval unmeasurable.

Because of abnormal ventricular depolarization, the QRS complex has a duration of longer than 0.12 second, with a wide and bizarre configuration. The T-wave deflection may be opposite the QRS complex. The QT interval is usually prolonged, indicating delayed depolarization and repolarization.

This rhythm strip illustrates idioventricular rhythm. Notice its distinguishing characteristics.

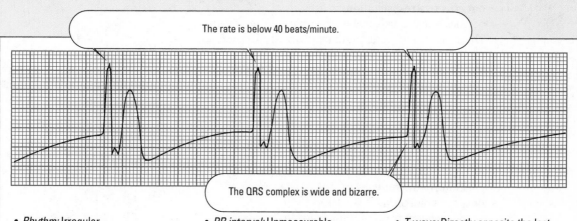

The rate is below 40 beats/minute.

The QRS complex is wide and bizarre.

- *Rhythm:* Irregular
- *Rate:* Atrial—can't be determined; ventricular—30 beats/minute
- *P wave:* Absent
- *PR interval:* Unmeasurable
- *QRS complex:* 0.20 second and bizarre
- *T wave:* Directly opposite the last part of QRS complex
- *QT interval:* 0.46 second
- *Other:* None

of instability, a pacemaker may be needed to reestablish a heart rate that provides enough cardiac output to perfuse organs properly. A transcutaneous pacemaker may be used in an emergency until a temporary or permanent transvenous pacemaker can be inserted.

Don't fight it

Remember that the goal of treatment doesn't include suppressing the idioventricular rhythm because that rhythm acts as a safety mechanism to protect the heart from standstill. Idioventricular rhythm should never be treated with lidocaine or other antiarrhythmics that would suppress that safety mechanism.

Electronic surveillance

Patients with idioventricular rhythms need continuous ECG monitoring and constant assessment until treatment restores hemodynamic stability. Keep atropine and pacemaker equipment at the bedside. Enforce bed rest until a permanent system is in place for maintaining an effective heart rate.

Asystole

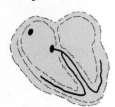

Asystole is ventricular standstill. The patient is completely unresponsive, with no electrical activity in the heart and no cardiac output. This arrhythmia results most commonly from a prolonged period of cardiac emergency, such as ventricular fibrillation, without effective resuscitation.

Asystole has been called the *arrhythmia of death*. The patient is in cardiopulmonary arrest. Without rapid initiation of CPR and appropriate treatment, the situation quickly becomes irreversible. (See *Recognizing asystole.*)

How you intervene

The immediate treatment for asystole is CPR. Start CPR as soon as you determine that the patient has no pulse. Then verify the presence of asystole by checking two different ECG leads. Give repeated doses of epinephrine as ordered.

Subsequent treatment for asystole focuses on identifying and either treating or removing the underlying cause. Transcutaneous pacing may also be considered.

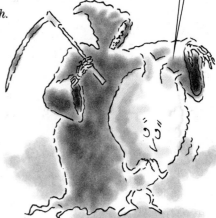

Asystole is also known as the arrhythmia of death. I sure hope death takes a holiday!

Recognizing asystole

This rhythm strip shows asystole, the absence of electrical activity in the ventricles. Except for a few P waves or pacer spikes, nothing appears on the waveform and the line is almost flat.

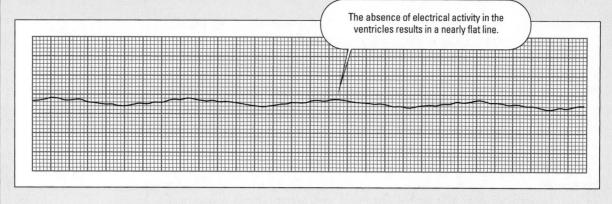

The absence of electrical activity in the ventricles results in a nearly flat line.

Start me up

Your job is to recognize this life-threatening arrhythmia and start resuscitation right away. Unfortunately, most patients with asystole can't be resuscitated, especially after a prolonged period of cardiac arrest.

You should also be aware that pulseless electrical activity can lead to asystole. Know how to recognize this problem and treat it. (See *Pulseless electrical activity*, page 128.)

Atrioventricular blocks

AV heart block results from an interruption in the conduction of impulses between the atria and ventricles. AV block can be total or partial or it may delay conduction. The block can occur at the AV node, the bundle of His, or the bundle branches.

The clinical effect of the block depends on how many impulses are completely blocked, how slow the ventricular rate is as a result, and how the block ultimately affects the heart. A slow ventricular rate can decrease cardiac output, possibly causing light-headedness, hypotension, and confusion.

The cause before the block

Various factors may lead to AV block, including underlying heart conditions, use of certain drugs, congenital anomalies, and conditions that disrupt the cardiac conduction system.

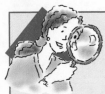

A closer look

Pulseless electrical activity

In pulseless electrical activity, the heart muscle loses its ability to contract even though electrical activity is preserved. As a result, the patient goes into cardiac arrest.

On an ECG, you'll see evidence of organized electrical activity, but you won't be able to palpate a pulse or measure the blood pressure. This condition requires rapid identification and treatment.

Causes
Causes include hypovolemia, hypoxia, acidosis, tension pneumothorax, cardiac tamponade, massive pulmonary embolism, hypothermia, hyperkalemia, massive acute myocardial infarction, and an overdose of drugs such as tricyclic antidepressants.

Treatment
Cardiopulmonary resuscitation is the immediate treatment, along with epinephrine. Atropine may be given to patients with bradycardia. Subsequent treatment focuses on identifying and correcting the underlying cause.

Under the knife

AV block can also be caused by inadvertent damage to the heart's conduction system during cardiac surgery. Similar disruption of the conduction system can occur from radiofrequency ablation therapy.

Class consciousness

AV block is classified according to its severity, not its location. That severity is measured according to how well the node conducts impulses, and a block is classified by degrees: first, second, and third.

First-degree AV block

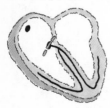

First-degree AV block occurs when impulses from the atria are consistently delayed during conduction through the AV node. Conduction eventually occurs; it just takes longer than normal. It's as if people are walking in a line through a doorway, but each person hesitates before crossing the threshold. (See *Recognizing first-degree AV block.*)

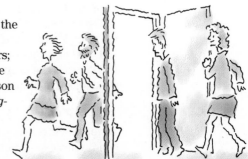

Recognizing first-degree AV block

In general, a rhythm strip with first-degree atrioventricular (AV) block looks like a normal sinus rhythm except that the PR interval is longer than normal. The rhythm is regular, with one normal P wave for every QRS complex. The PR interval is greater than 0.20 second and is consistent for each beat. The QRS complex is usually normal, although sometimes a bundle-branch block may occur along with first-degree AV block and cause a widening of the QRS complex. This rhythm strip illustrates first-degree AV block. Notice its distinguishing characteristics.

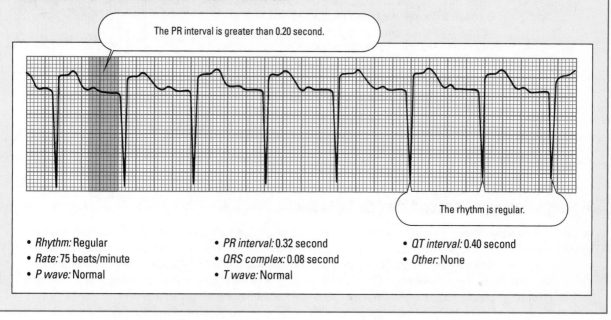

The PR interval is greater than 0.20 second.

The rhythm is regular.

- *Rhythm:* Regular
- *Rate:* 75 beats/minute
- *P wave:* Normal
- *PR interval:* 0.32 second
- *QRS complex:* 0.08 second
- *T wave:* Normal
- *QT interval:* 0.40 second
- *Other:* None

How you intervene

In most cases, only the underlying cause is treated, not the conduction disturbance itself. For example, if a medication is causing the block, the dosage may be reduced or the medication discontinued. Close monitoring helps to detect progression of first-degree AV block to a more serious form of block.

When caring for a patient with first-degree AV block, evaluate him for underlying causes that can be corrected, such as medications he may be taking or ischemia. Observe the ECG for progression of the block to a more severe form of block. Administer digoxin, calcium channel blockers, or beta-adrenergic blockers cautiously.

Type I second-degree AV block

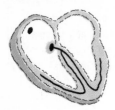

Also called *Wenckebach* or *Mobitz type I block*, type I second-degree AV block occurs when each successive impulse from the SA node is delayed slightly longer than the previous impulse. That pattern continues until an impulse fails to be conducted to the ventricles, and the cycle then repeats. It's like a line of people trying to get through a doorway, each taking longer and longer until finally one person can't get through. (See *Recognizing type I second-degree AV block.*)

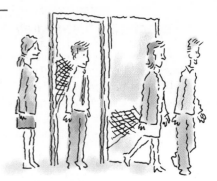

How you intervene

No treatment is needed for type I AV block if the patient is asymptomatic. For a symptomatic patient, atropine may improve AV node conduction. A temporary pacemaker may be required for long-term relief of symptoms until the rhythm resolves.

Recognizing type I second-degree AV block

In type I second-degree atrioventricular (AV) block, the atrial rhythm is normal. The PR interval gets gradually longer with each successive beat until a P wave finally fails to conduct to the ventricles. This failure makes the ventricular rhythm irregular, with a repeating pattern of groups of QRS complexes followed by a dropped beat in which the P wave isn't followed by a QRS complex. The QRS complexes are usually normal because the delays occur in the AV node.

This rhythm strip illustrates type I second-degree AV block. Notice its distinguishing characteristics.

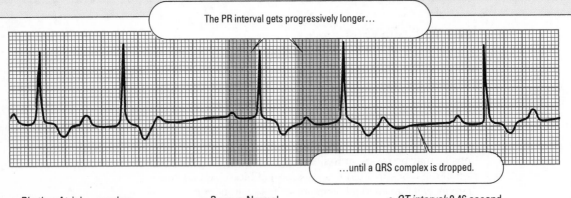

The PR interval gets progressively longer...

...until a QRS complex is dropped.

- *Rhythm:* Atrial—regular; ventricular—irregular
- *Rate:* Atrial—80 beats/minute; ventricular—50 beats/minute
- *P wave:* Normal
- *PR interval:* Progressively prolonged
- *QRS complex:* 0.08 second
- *T wave:* Normal
- *QT interval:* 0.46 second
- *Other:* Wenckebach pattern of grouped beats

When caring for a patient with this block, assess his tolerance for the rhythm and the need for treatment to improve cardiac output. Evaluate the patient for possible causes of the block, including the use of certain medications or the presence of ischemia.

Keep an eye on the ECG

Check the ECG frequently to see if a more severe type of AV block develops. Make sure the patient has a patent I.V. line. Teach him about his temporary pacemaker if indicated.

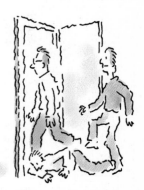

> **Memory jogger**
>
> When you're trying to identify type I second-degree AV block, think of the phrase "longer, longer, drop," which describes the progressively prolonged PR intervals and the missing QRS complex.

Type II second-degree AV block

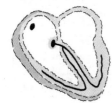

Type II second-degree AV block, also known as *Mobitz type II block*, is less common than type I but more serious. It occurs when occasional impulses from the SA node fail to conduct to the ventricles.

On an ECG, you won't see the PR interval lengthen before the impulse fails to conduct, as you do with type I second-degree AV block. Instead, you'll see consistent AV node conduction and an occasional dropped beat. This block is like a line of people passing through a doorway at the same speed, except that, periodically, one of them just can't get through. (See *Recognizing type II second-degree AV block*, page 132.)

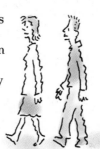

How you intervene

If the dropped beats are infrequent and the patient shows no symptoms of decreased cardiac output, the doctor may choose only to observe the rhythm, particularly if the cause is thought to be reversible. If the patient is hypotensive, treatment aims to improve cardiac output by increasing the heart rate. Because the conduction block occurs in the His-Purkinje system, transcutaneous pacing should be initiated quickly.

Pacemaker place

Type II second-degree AV block commonly requires placement of a pacemaker. A temporary pacemaker may be used until a permanent pacemaker can be placed.

When caring for a patient with type II second-degree block, assess his tolerance for the rhythm and the need for treatment to improve cardiac output. Evaluate for possible correctable causes such as ischemia. Observe the patient for progression to a more severe form of AV block. If the patient receives a pacemaker, teach him and his family about its use.

Recognizing type II second-degree AV block

With type II second-degree atrioventricular (AV) block, look for an atrial rhythm that's regular and a ventricular rhythm that may be regular or irregular, depending on the block. If the block is intermittent, the rhythm is irregular. If the block is constant, such as 2:1 or 3:1, the rhythm is regular.

Overall, the strip will look as if someone erased some QRS complexes. The PR interval will be constant for all conducted beats but may be prolonged in some cases. The QRS complex is usually wide, but normal complexes may occur.

This rhythm strip illustrates type II second-degree AV block. Notice its distinguishing characteristics.

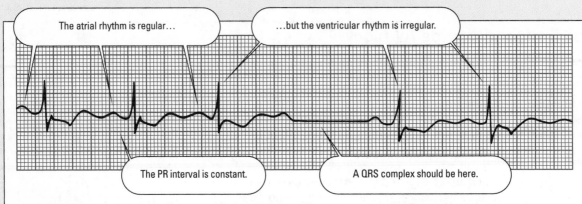

> The atrial rhythm is regular…

> …but the ventricular rhythm is irregular.

> The PR interval is constant.

> A QRS complex should be here.

- *Rhythm:* Atrial — regular; ventricular — irregular
- *Rate:* Atrial — 60 beats/minute; ventricular — 50 beats/minute
- *P wave:* Normal
- *PR interval:* 0.28 second
- *QRS complex:* 0.10 second
- *T wave:* Normal
- *QT interval:* 0.60 second
- *Other:* None

Third-degree AV block

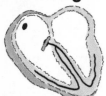

Also called *complete heart block*, third-degree AV block occurs when impulses from the atria are completely blocked at the AV node and can't be conducted to the ventricles. Maintaining our doorway analogy, this form of block is like a line of people waiting to go through a doorway, but no one can go through.

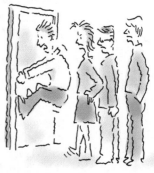

Beats of different drummers

Acting independently, the atria, generally under the control of the SA node, tend to maintain a regular rate of 60 to 100 beats/minute. The ventricular rhythm can originate from the AV node and maintain a rate of 40 to 60 beats/minute or from the Purkinje system in the ventricles and maintain a rate of 20 to 40 beats/minute. (See *Recognizing third-degree AV block.*) Third-degree block is a similar rhythm to complete AV dissociation;

Recognizing third-degree AV block

When analyzing an ECG for third-degree atrioventricular (AV) block, you'll note regular atrial and ventricular rhythms. However, because the atria and ventricles beat independently of each other, PR intervals vary with no pattern or regularity.

Some P waves may be buried in QRS complexes or T waves. In fact, the rhythm strip of a patient with third-degree AV block looks like a strip of P waves laid independently over a strip of QRS complexes.

The site of the escape rhythm determines the appearance of the QRS complex. If it originates in the AV node, the QRS complex is normal and the ventricular rate is 40 to 60 beats/minute. If the escape rhythm originates in the Purkinje system, the QRS complex is wide, with a ventricular rate below 40 beats/minute. This rhythm strip illustrates third-degree AV block. Notice its distinguishing characteristics.

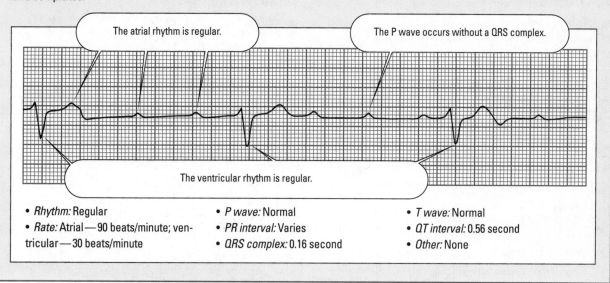

The atrial rhythm is regular.

The P wave occurs without a QRS complex.

The ventricular rhythm is regular.

- *Rhythm:* Regular
- *Rate:* Atrial—90 beats/minute; ventricular—30 beats/minute
- *P wave:* Normal
- *PR interval:* Varies
- *QRS complex:* 0.16 second
- *T wave:* Normal
- *QT interval:* 0.56 second
- *Other:* None

however, there are some key differences. (See *Recognizing complete AV dissociation*, page 134.)

How you intervene

When caring for a patient with third-degree heart block, immediately assess the patient's tolerance of the rhythm and the need for treatment to support cardiac output and relieve symptoms. Make sure the patient has a patent I.V. line. Administer oxygen therapy as ordered. Evaluate for possible correctable causes of the arrhythmia, such as medications or ischemia. Minimize the patient's activity and maintain his bed rest.

If cardiac output isn't adequate or the patient's condition seems to be deteriorating, therapy aims to improve the ventricular rate. Atropine may be given, or a temporary pacemaker may be used to restore adequate cardiac output. Temporary pacing may

Recognizing complete AV dissociation

With third-degree atrioventricular (AV) block and complete AV dissociation, the atria and ventricles beat independently, each controlled by its own pacemaker.

However, there's a key difference between these two arrhythmias: In third-degree AV block, the atrial rate is faster than the ventricular rate. With complete AV dissociation, the two rates are usually about the same, with the ventricular rate slightly faster.

Rhythm disturbances

Never the primary problem, complete AV dissociation results from one of three underlying rhythm disturbances:

 slowed or impaired sinus impulse formation or sinoatrial conduction, as in sinus bradycardia or sinus arrest

accelerated impulse formation in the AV junction or the ventricular pacemaker, as in junctional or ventricular tachycardia

AV conduction disturbance, as in complete AV block.

When to treat

The clinical significance of complete AV dissociation—as well as treatment for the arrhythmia—depends on the underlying cause and its effects on the patient. If the underlying rhythm decreases cardiac output, the patient needs treatment to correct the arrhythmia.

Depending on the underlying cause, the patient may be treated with an antiarrhythmic, such as atropine, to restore synchrony. Alternatively, the patient may be given a pacemaker to support a slow ventricular rate. If drug toxicity caused the original disturbance, the drug should be discontinued.

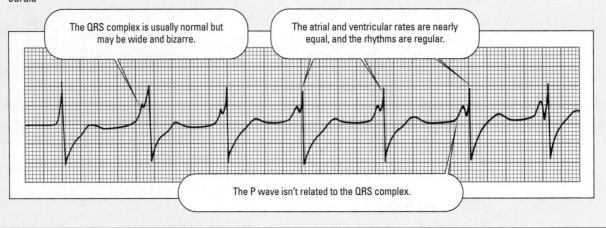

The QRS complex is usually normal but may be wide and bizarre.

The atrial and ventricular rates are nearly equal, and the rhythms are regular.

The P wave isn't related to the QRS complex.

continue until the cause of the block resolves or until a permanent pacemaker can be inserted. A permanent block requires placement of a permanent pacemaker.

Bundles of troubles

The patient with an anterior-wall MI is more likely to have permanent third-degree AV block if the MI involved the bundle of His or the bundle branches than if it involved other areas of the myocardium. Those patients commonly require prompt placement of a permanent pacemaker.

An AV block in a patient with an inferior-wall MI is more likely to be temporary, as a result of injury to the AV node. Placement of a permanent pacemaker is commonly delayed in such cases to evaluate recovery of the conduction system.

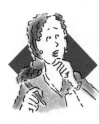

Quick quiz

1. To determine whether an arrhythmia is atrial or junctional in nature, observe the:
    A.   P wave.
    B.   PR interval.
    C.   QRS complex.
    D.   T wave.

Answer: B. Looking at the PR interval helps you determine whether an arrhythmia is atrial or junctional. An arrhythmia with an inverted P wave before the QRS complex and a normal PR interval originated in the atria. An arrhythmia with a PR interval less than 0.12 second originated in the AV junction.

2. On an ECG, the QRS complex represents:
    A.   ventricular depolarization.
    B.   ventricular repolarization.
    C.   atrial depolarization.
    D.   atrial repolarization.

Answer: A. The ECG represents the electrical events occurring in one cardiac cycle. The QRS complex represents the depolarization of the ventricles.

3. The normal duration of the PR interval is:
    A.   0.6 to 0.10 second.
    B.   0.10 to 0.12 second.
    C.   0.12 to 0.20 second.
    D.   0.20 to 0.24 second.

Answer: C. The PR interval tracks the atrial impulses from the atria through the AV node, bundle of His, and right and left bundle branches. Normal duration is 0.12 to 0.20 second. Changes in the PR interval indicate an altered impulse formation or a conduction delay.

4. A serious potential complication of sick sinus syndrome is:
A. tachycardia.
B. bradycardia.
C. heart failure.
D. thromboembolism.

Answer: D. If the patient with sick sinus syndrome develops sudden bursts of atrial fibrillation, he may develop thromboembolism and possible stroke. Anticoagulants may be administered to help prevent this complication.

5. The AV block with the increasingly longer PR interval is:
A. first-degree.
B. type I second-degree.
C. type II second-degree.
D. third-degree.

Answer: B. When you're trying to identify type I second-degree AV block, think of the phrase "longer, longer, drop," which describes the progressively prolonged PR intervals and the missing QRS complex.

Scoring

☆☆☆ If you answered all five questions correctly, sensational! Don't get a complex, but we think you have ECG interpretation down pat.

☆☆ If you answered four questions correctly, good job! It may seem impulsive, but we think that at this junction, you're ready to move on.

☆ If you answered fewer than four questions correctly, don't worry. It can take a while to get into the rhythm of understanding arrhythmias. Take a break, review the chapter, and then try the quick quiz again.

Laboratory tests

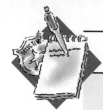

Just the facts

In this chapter, you'll learn:

♦ the normal results of select laboratory tests

♦ possible implications of abnormal test results

♦ techniques for obtaining laboratory tests

♦ associated symptoms of abnormal test results.

A look at laboratory tests

Laboratory tests are used for screening, confirming or ruling out a diagnosis, and managing disease, all of which are important elements in providing quality patient care.

Explain and reassure

The first step in preparing a patient for a laboratory test is to explain it. Your patient should always know what's happening to him and why. Use simple, direct language and avoid jargon. If the patient is a child, is elderly, or is otherwise unable to understand your instructions, you may also need to explain the test to a parent or caregiver.

Get to the point

If a blood sample is required, keep in mind that some patients may be uneasy about needles. Before taking a blood sample, explain that brief discomfort may accompany the needle puncture or the application of a tourniquet. Try to use a large-gauge needle when you draw a blood sample, and handle the sample carefully to prevent the breakdown of red blood cells (RBCs), the main component of blood. This breakdown (hemolysis) may interfere with test results. (See *Special people, special techniques*, page 138.)

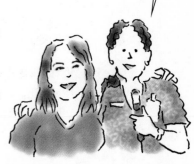

Testing, testing, 1, 2. The first step in preparing a patient for a laboratory test is to explain the test.

Ages and stages

Special people, special techniques

Special blood-drawing techniques may be employed for pediatric and elderly patients as well as those with specific needs. For example, pediatric sample tubes may be used for pediatric and elderly patients as well as those patients who have low hemoglobin levels. The amount of blood required to fill the tube is much less than required by larger adult tubes. Therefore, patients experience less blood loss from the venipuncture.

You can also alter your blood-drawing technique to make it less traumatic. Simply avoid using the tourniquet. This technique prevents vessel damage from excess pressure caused by tourniquet application.

Handle with care

Always follow standard precautions. Also, after obtaining a blood sample, check the venipuncture site for bleeding. If a hematoma develops at the venipuncture site, apply warm soaks.

Common laboratory tests

Many laboratory tests are commonly used. This chapter covers the most common tests, along with possible results, interfering factors, and nursing interventions for each.

Alanine aminotransferase

Alanine aminotransferase (ALT) is one of two enzymes that catalyze a reversible amino group transfer reaction in the Krebs cycle (tricarboxylic acid or citric acid cycle). This enzyme is necessary for tissue energy production. ALT is found primarily in the liver with lesser amounts in the kidneys, heart, pancreas, and skeletal muscles. It's a relatively specific indicator of acute hepatocellular damage.

What results mean

Normally, serum ALT levels range from 8 to 50 IU/L (SI, 0.14 to 0.85 μkat/L).

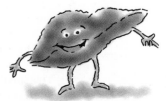

ALT primarily lives in the liver. I wonder if I should collect rent.

Highs and lows

Very high ALT levels (up to 50 times the normal level) suggest viral or severe drug-induced hepatitis or another hepatic disease with extensive necrosis. In these cases, aspartate aminotransferase (AST) levels are also elevated but usually to a lesser degree. Moderate to high levels may indicate infectious mononucleosis, chronic hepatitis, intrahepatic cholestasis (arrest of bile secretion) or cholecystitis, early or improving acute viral hepatitis, or severe hepatic congestion associated with heart failure.

Slight to moderate ALT elevations, usually with higher increases in AST levels, may appear in any condition that produces acute hepatocellular injury, such as active cirrhosis and drug-induced or alcoholic hepatitis. Marginal elevations occasionally occur in association with acute myocardial infarction (MI), reflecting secondary hepatic congestion or the release of small amounts of ALT from myocardial tissue. (See *ALT test interference*.)

What needs to be done

• Tell the patient that he should avoid hepatotoxic or cholestatic drugs, such as methotrexate, chlorpromazine, salicylates, and opioids, before the test. If they must be continued, note this on the laboratory request.
• Perform a venipuncture and collect the sample in a 7-ml tube without additives.
• Be aware that ALT activity is stable in serum for up to 3 days at room temperature.
• Resume medications that were withheld before the test, as ordered.

Ammonia, plasma

The plasma ammonia test measures plasma levels of ammonia, a nonprotein nitrogen compound that helps maintain acid-base balance. Most ammonia is absorbed from the intestinal tract, where it's produced by bacterial action on protein; a smaller amount of ammonia is produced in the kidneys from hydrolysis of glutamine. Normally, the body uses the nitrogen fraction of ammonia to rebuild amino acids and then converts the ammonia to urea in the liver for excretion by the kidneys. In such diseases as cirrhosis of the liver, ammonia can bypass the liver and accumulate in the blood. Therefore, plasma ammonia levels may help indicate the severity of hepatocellular damage.

ALT test interference

Falsely elevated ALT levels can result from:
• barbiturates
• chlorpromazine
• exposure to carbon tetrachloride
• griseofulvin
• ingestion of lead
• isoniazid
• methotrexate
• methyldopa
• nitrofurantoin
• opioid analgesics
• phenothiazines
• phenytoin
• salicylates
• tetracycline.

Ammonia is a nitrogen compound that helps to maintain acid-base balance.

BASES   ACIDS

What results mean

Normally, plasma ammonia levels are 15 to 45 µg/dl (SI, 11 to 32 µmol/L). Elevated plasma ammonia levels are common in patients with severe hepatic disease, such as cirrhosis and acute hepatic necrosis, and may lead to hepatic coma. Elevated levels are also possible in patients with Reye's syndrome, severe heart failure, GI hemorrhage, and erythroblastosis fetalis (a type of hemolytic anemia in neonates). (See *Plasma ammonia test interference.*)

What needs to be done

• Tell the patient that he must fast the night before the test because plasma ammonia levels may vary with protein intake.
• Notify the laboratory before performing the venipuncture so that preliminary preparations can begin.
• Perform a venipuncture and collect the sample in a 10-ml heparinized tube.
• Make sure bleeding has stopped before removing pressure from the venipuncture site.
• Handle the sample gently, pack it in ice, and send it to the laboratory immediately. Don't use a chilled container.
• Watch for signs of impending or established hepatic coma, if plasma ammonia levels are high.

> ### Plasma ammonia test interference
>
> Such drugs as acetazolamide, thiazides, ammonium salts, neomycin, and furosemide can raise ammonia levels. Total parenteral nutrition and a portacaval shunt can also raise levels.
>
> Lactulose, neomycin, and kanamycin depress ammonia levels.

Amylase, serum

Amylase is an enzyme that helps the body digest starch and glycogen in the mouth, stomach, and intestine. In cases of suspected acute pancreatic disease, measurement of serum amylase is the most important laboratory test.

What results mean

Serum amylase levels for adults age 18 and older normally range from 25 to 85 units/L (SI, 0.39 to 1.45 µkat/L). After the onset of acute pancreatitis, serum amylase levels begin to rise in 2 hours, peak at 12 to 48 hours, and return to normal in 3 to 4 days.

Elevations and depressions

Moderate serum elevations may accompany pancreatic injury from perforated peptic ulcer, pancreatic cancer, acute salivary gland disease, impaired renal function, or obstruction of the common bile duct, the pancreatic duct, or the ampulla of Vater. Levels may be slightly elevated in a patient who's asymptomatic or who has an unusual response to therapy.

> Serum amylase is the most important test for acute pancreatic disease.

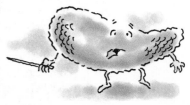

Serum amylase test interference

Elevated serum levels of amylase may occur with the use of:
- aminosalicylic acid
- azathioprine
- bethanechol
- chloride salts
- cholinergics
- corticosteroids
- ethacrynic acid
- ethyl alcohol
- fluoride salts
- furosemide
- hormonal contraceptives
- indomethacin
- mercaptopurine
- opioids
- rifampin,
- sulfasalazine
- thiazide diuretics.

Decreased serum levels of amylase may occur with:
- recent pancreatic surgery
- perforated ulcer or intestine
- abscess
- spasm of the sphincter of Oddi.

Depressed amylase levels can occur in patients with chronic pancreatitis, pancreatic cancer, cirrhosis, hepatitis, advanced cystic fibrosis, and toxemia of pregnancy. (See *Serum amylase test interference.*)

What needs to be done
- Tell the patient that he must abstain from alcohol for 24 hours before the test.
- If the patient has severe abdominal pain, draw a sample before diagnostic or therapeutic intervention. For accurate results, it's important to obtain an early sample.
- Perform a venipuncture and collect the sample in a 7-ml clot-activator tube.
- Handle the sample gently to prevent hemolysis.
- Resume administration of drugs discontinued before the test, as ordered.

Anion gap

The anion gap reflects anion-cation balance in the serum and helps distinguish types of metabolic acidosis without expensive, time-consuming measurement of all serum electrolytes. The anion gap test uses serum levels of routinely measured electrolytes (sodium, chloride, and bicarbonate) for a quick calculation based on a simple physical principle: Total concentrations of cations and anions are normally equal, thereby maintaining electrical neutrality in serum.

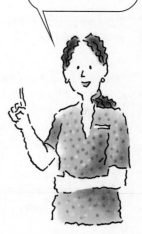

The anion gap can be used to distinguish between different types of metabolic acidosis.

Sodium accounts for more than 90% of circulating cations, whereas chloride and bicarbonate together account for 85% of the counterbalancing anions. So the gap between measured cation and anion levels represents those anions not routinely measured, including sulfates, phosphates, proteins, and organic acids, such as ketone bodies and lactic acid.

What results mean

Normally, the anion gap ranges from 8 to 14 mEq/L (SI, 8 to 14 mmol/L). A normal anion gap doesn't rule out metabolic acidosis.

Bye-bye bicarbonate; hello chloride

When acidosis results from loss of bicarbonate in the urine or other body fluids, renal reabsorption of sodium promotes retention of chloride, and the anion gap remains unchanged. Thus, metabolic acidosis associated with excessive chloride levels is known as *normal anion gap acidosis.*

Many metabolic acids

When acidosis results from accumulation of metabolic acids, as with lactic acidosis, the anion gap increases above 14 mEq/L (SI, 14 mmol/L) with the increase being in unmeasured anions. Metabolic acidosis caused by such accumulation is known as *high anion gap acidosis.* (See *Understanding anion gap and metabolic acidosis.*)

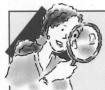

A closer look

Understanding anion gap and metabolic acidosis

Metabolic acidosis may occur with a normal or increased anion gap.

Normal

Metabolic acidosis with a normal anion gap (8 to 14 mEq/L [SI, 8 to 14 µmol/L]) occurs with bicarbonate loss, such as from:

• hypokalemic acidosis associated with renal tubular acidosis, diarrhea, or ureteral diversions
• hyperkalemic acidosis caused by acidifying agents (for example, ammonium chloride or hydrochloric acid), hydronephrosis, or sickle cell nephropathy.

Increased

Metabolic acidosis with an increased anion gap (greater than 14 mEq/L [SI, greater than 14 mmol/L]) occurs with accumulation of organic acids, sulfates, or phosphates from such causes as:

• renal failure
• ketoacidosis associated with starvation, diabetes mellitus, or alcohol abuse
• lactic acidosis
• ingestion of toxins, such as salicylates, methanol, ethylene glycol (antifreeze), and paraldehyde.

Because the anion gap determines only total anion-cation balance, it doesn't necessarily reflect abnormal values for individual electrolytes. Further investigation and diagnostic tests are usually necessary to determine the specific cause of metabolic acidosis.

A decreased anion gap (less than 8 mEq/L [SI, 8 mmol/L]) is rare but may occur in hypermagnesemia and in paraproteinemic states, such as multiple myeloma and Waldenström's macroglobulinemia. (See *Anion gap test interference*.)

What needs to be done

• Perform a venipuncture and collect the sample in a 7-ml clot-activator tube.
• Instruct the patient to resume use of any drugs discontinued for the test, as ordered.

Arterial blood gas analysis

Arterial blood gas (ABG) analysis evaluates gas exchange in the lungs by measuring the partial pressures of arterial oxygen (PaO_2) and arterial carbon dioxide ($PaCO_2$) as well as the pH of an arterial sample:
• PaO_2 measures the pressure exerted by the oxygen dissolved in the blood and evaluates the lungs' ability to oxygenate the blood.
• $PaCO_2$ measures the pressure exerted by carbon dioxide dissolved in the blood and reflects the adequacy of ventilation by the lungs.
• pH measures the blood's hydrogen ion concentration. It's the best way to tell whether blood is too acidic or too alkaline.
• Bicarbonate (HCO_3^-) is a measure of the bicarbonate ion concentration in the blood, which is regulated by the kidneys.
• Oxygen saturation (SaO_2) is the oxygen content of the blood expressed as a percentage of the oxygen capacity (the amount of oxygen the blood is capable of carrying if all of the hemoglobin [Hb] is fully saturated).
• Oxygen content (O_2CT) measures the actual amount of oxygen in the blood and isn't commonly used in blood gas evaluation.

What results mean

Normal ABG values fall within the following ranges:
• *pH:* 7.35 to 7.45 (SI, 7.35 to 7.45)
• *$PaCO_2$:* 35 to 45 mm Hg (SI, 4.7 to 5.3 kPa)
• *PaO_2:* 80 to 100 mm Hg (SI, 10.6 to 13.3 kPa)
• *HCO_3^-:* 22 to 26 mEq/L (SI, 22 to 26 mmol/L)
• *SaO_2:* 94% to 100% (SI, 0.94 to 1)
• *O_2CT:* 15% to 23% (SI, 0.15 to 0.23).

Anion gap test interference

The use of certain drugs can increase the anion gap. These drugs include:
• ammonium chloride
• antihypertensives
• bicarbonates
• corticosteroids
• ethacrynic acid
• furosemide
• prolonged infusion of dextrose 5% in water
• salicylates
• thiazide diuretics.
  Other drugs and substances can decrease the anion gap, including:
• chlorothiazide diuretics
• chlorpropamide
• cortisone
• diuretics
• excessive ingestion of alkalis or licorice
• lithium
• vasopressin.

Anything but normal

Low PaO_2, O_2CT, and SaO_2 levels in combination with a high $PaCO_2$ may occur with:

• respiratory muscle weakness or paralysis (as in Guillain-Barré syndrome or myasthenia gravis)
• respiratory center inhibition (from head injury, brain tumor, or drug abuse) or airway obstruction (possibly from a mucus plug or tumor)
• bronchiole obstruction associated with asthma or emphysema
• abnormal ventilation-perfusion ratio.

When inspired air contains insufficient oxygen, PaO_2, O_2CT, and SaO_2 also decrease, but $PaCO_2$ may be normal. Such findings are common with:

• pneumothorax
• impaired diffusion between alveoli and blood (such as that caused by interstitial fibrosis)
• an arteriovenous shunt that permits blood to bypass the lungs.

Low O_2CT with normal PaO_2, SaO_2, and possibly $PaCO_2$ may result from severe anemia, decreased blood volume, and reduced oxygen-carrying capacity of Hb. In addition to clarifying blood oxygen disorders, ABG values can provide considerable information about acid-base disorders. (See *ABG interference.*)

What needs to be done

• Wait at least 20 minutes before drawing an ABG sample after:
  – initiating, changing, or discontinuing oxygen therapy
  – initiating or changing settings of mechanical ventilation
  – extubation.
• Tell the patient which site—radial, brachial, or femoral artery—has been selected for the puncture.
• Instruct the patient to breathe normally during the test, and warn him that he may feel brief cramping or throbbing pain at the puncture site. (See *Obtaining an ABG sample.*)
• Include the following information on the laboratory form:
  – room air or amount of oxygen and method of delivery (for example, 40% aerosol face mask)
  – ventilator settings if on mechanical ventilation (fraction of inspired oxygen, tidal volume, mode, respiratory rate, and positive-end respiratory pressure)
  – patient's temperature.
• Monitor vital signs and observe for signs of circulatory impairment, such as swelling, discoloration, pain, numbness, and tingling in the arm or leg in which the puncture was performed.

ABG interference

Bicarbonate, ethacrynic acid, hydrocortisone, metolazone, prednisone, and thiazides may elevate $PaCO_2$.

Acetazolamide, methicillin, nitrofurantoin, and tetracycline may decrease $PaCO_2$.

False highs and lows
Fever may cause false-high PaO_2 and $PaCO_2$ levels.

Hypothermia may cause false-low PaO_2 and $PaCO_2$ levels.

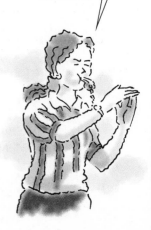

Timeout! Certain situations require you to wait 20 minutes before drawing an ABG sample.

Aspartate aminotransferase

AST is one of two enzymes that catalyze the conversion of the nitrogenous portion of an amino acid to an amino acid residue. This enzyme is essential to energy production in the Krebs cycle. AST is found in the cytoplasm and mitochondria of many cells, primarily in the liver, heart, skeletal muscles, kidneys, and pancreas and, to a lesser extent, in RBCs. It's released into serum in proportion to cellular damage. The change in AST values over time is a reliable monitoring mechanism.

What results mean

AST levels range from 8 to 46 U/L (SI, 0.14 to 0.78 µkat/L) in males and from 7 to 34 U/L (SI, 0.12 to 0.58 µkat/L) in females. Values for children are typically higher.

AST levels fluctuate in response to the extent of cellular necrosis and therefore may be temporarily and slightly elevated early in the disease process and extremely elevated during the most acute phase. Also, depending on when during the course of the disease the initial sample was drawn, AST levels can rise, indicating increasing disease severity and tissue damage, or fall, indicating disease resolution and tissue repair. Thus, the relative change in AST values serves as a reliable monitoring mechanism.

From top to bottom

Very high AST levels (more than 20 times normal) may indicate acute viral hepatitis, severe skeletal muscle trauma, extensive surgery, drug-induced hepatic injury, or severe passive liver congestion.

High levels (ranging from 10 to 20 times normal) may indicate severe MI, severe infectious mononucleosis, or alcoholic cirrhosis. High levels also occur during the initial or resolving stages of conditions listed above that cause very high elevations.

Moderate to high levels (ranging from 5 to 10 times normal) may indicate Duchenne's muscular dystrophy, dermatomyositis, or chronic hepatitis. They also occur during initial and resolving stages of diseases that cause high elevations.

Low to moderate levels (ranging from 2 to 5 times normal) may indicate hemolytic anemia, metastatic hepatic tumors, acute pancreatitis, pulmonary emboli, alcohol withdrawal syndrome, or fatty liver. AST levels also rise slightly after the first few days of biliary duct obstruction. (See *AST test interference*, page 146.)

What needs to be done

• Tell the patient that the test usually requires three venipunctures — one at admission and one each day for the next 2 days.

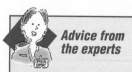

Advice from the experts

Obtaining an ABG sample

Follow the steps below to obtain a sample for an arterial blood gas (ABG) analysis:

• After Allen's test, perform a cutaneous arterial puncture (or, if an arterial line is in place, draw blood from the arterial line).

• Use a heparinized blood gas syringe to draw the sample.

• Eliminate all air from the sample, place it on ice immediately, and transport it for analysis.

• Apply pressure to the puncture site for 3 to 5 minutes. If the patient is receiving anticoagulants or has a coagulopathy, hold the puncture site longer than 5 minutes, if necessary.

• Tape a gauze pad firmly over the puncture site. If the puncture site is on the arm, don't tape the entire circumference because this may restrict circulation.

- Tell the patient that he must refrain from taking morphine, codeine, meperidine, chlorpropamide, methyldopa, phenazopyridine, and antituberculosis drugs (such as isoniazid and pyrazinamide) as ordered. If any of these medications must be continued, note this on the laboratory request.
- To avoid missing peak AST levels, draw serum samples at the same time each day.
- Perform a venipuncture and collect the sample in a 7-ml clot-activator tube.
- Resume medications discontinued before the test, as ordered.

AST test interference

Elevated levels of AST may result from use of:
- antituberculosis agents
- chlorpropamide
- erythromycin
- large doses of acetaminophen, salicylates, or vitamin A
- methyldopa
- opiates
- pyridoxine
- sulfonamides.

Decreased levels of AST may result from:
- muscle trauma associated with I.M. injections
- strenuous exercise.

Bilirubin

The serum bilirubin test measures serum levels of bilirubin. The main pigment in bile, bilirubin is the major product of Hb catabolism. Serum bilirubin values are especially significant in neonates because excessive unconjugated bilirubin can accumulate in the brain, causing irreversible damage.

What results mean

In adults, indirect serum bilirubin measures 1.1 mg/dl (SI, 19 µmol/L) or less; direct serum bilirubin measures less than 0.5 mg/dl (SI, less than 6.8 µmol/L). In neonates, total serum bilirubin measures 2 to 12 mg/dl (SI, 34 to 205 µmol/L).

Indirectly speaking

Elevated indirect serum bilirubin levels commonly indicate hepatic damage in which the cells can no longer conjugate bilirubin. Consequently, indirect bilirubin reenters the bloodstream. High levels of indirect bilirubin are also common in patients with severe hemolytic anemia, when excessive indirect bilirubin overwhelms the liver's conjugating mechanism. If hemolysis continues, both direct and indirect bilirubin may rise. Other causes of elevated indirect bilirubin levels include congenital enzyme deficiency, such as Gilbert's disease and Crigler-Najjar syndrome.

But what I really want to do is direct

Elevated direct serum bilirubin levels usually indicate biliary obstruction, in which direct bilirubin, blocked from its normal pathway from the liver into the biliary tree, overflows into the bloodstream. If the obstruction continues, direct and indirect bilirubin eventually may be elevated because of hepatic damage. In severe chronic hepatic damage, direct bilirubin concentrations may return to normal or near-normal levels, but elevated indirect bilirubin levels persist.

Exchange rate

In neonates, total bilirubin levels that reach or exceed 15 mg/dl (SI, 257 µmol/L) indicate the need for an exchange transfusion. Notify the doctor immediately of the results so prompt action can be taken. (See *Bilirubin test interference*.)

What needs to be done

• Instruct the adult patient to fast for at least 4 hours before the test, although he may drink fluids. (Fasting isn't necessary for neonates.)
• If the patient is an adult, perform a venipuncture and collect the sample in a 7-ml clot-activator tube.
• If the patient is a neonate, perform a heelstick and fill the microcapillary tube to the designated level with blood.
• Protect the sample from strong sunlight and ultraviolet light because bilirubin breaks down when exposed to light.
• Send the sample to the laboratory immediately.

> ### Bilirubin test interference
> Exposure of the sample to direct sunlight or ultraviolet light may cause a decrease in bilirubin levels. Rough handling of the sample may cause hemolysis.

Blood urea nitrogen

The blood urea nitrogen (BUN) test measures the nitrogen fraction of urea. Urea is the chief end product of protein metabolism. Formed in the liver from ammonia and excreted by the kidneys, urea constitutes 40% to 50% of the blood's nonprotein nitrogen. Because the level of reabsorption of urea in the renal tubules is directly related to the rate of urine flow through the kidneys, the BUN level is a less reliable indicator of uremia than the serum creatine level.

What results mean

BUN values normally range from 8 to 20 mg/dl (SI, 2.9 to 7.5 mmol/L), with slightly higher values in elderly patients. Elevated BUN levels occur in renal disease, reduced renal blood flow (such as with dehydration), urinary tract obstruction, and increased protein catabolism (such as occurs in burns).

Depressed BUN levels occur in severe hepatic damage, malnutrition, and overhydration. (See *BUN test interference*.)

What needs to be done

• Tell the patient to avoid a diet high in meat.
• Perform a venipuncture and collect the sample in a 7-ml clot-activator tube.

> ### BUN test interference
> Chloramphenicol can depress BUN levels.
> Nephrotoxic drugs, such as aminoglycosides, amphotericin B, corticosteroids, methicillin, and nafcillin can elevate BUN levels.

B-type natriuretic peptide assay

B-type natriuretic peptide is a neurohormone produced predominantly by the heart ventricle. It's released from the heart in response to ventricle distention caused by blood volume expansion or pressure overload.

What results mean

The normal value of B-type natriuretic peptide is less than 100 pg/ml (SI, 100 ng/L). Plasma B-type natriuretic peptide increases with the severity of heart failure. Studies have demonstrated that the heart is the major source of circulating B-type natriuretic peptide. Measurement of this peptide is an excellent hormonal marker of ventricular systolic and diastolic dysfunction. Blood concentrations greater than 100 pg/ml are an accurate predictor of heart failure. (See *B-type natriuretic peptide assay interference.*)

What needs to be done

• Perform a venipuncture and collect the sample in a 3.5-ml EDTA tube.

> **B-type natriuretic peptide assay interference**
>
> Hemolysis can occur as a result of rough handling of the sample.

Calcium

Total calcium measurement is the most commonly performed test for evaluation of serum calcium levels. Approximately 1% of the total calcium in the body circulates in the blood. Of this, about 50% is bound to plasma proteins and 40% is ionized, or free.

Calcium gets around

Evaluation of serum calcium levels measures the total amount of calcium circulating in the blood. Evaluation of ionized calcium levels measures the fraction of serum calcium that's in the ionized form, which is the most physiologically active form of serum calcium. The other 99% of the calcium in the body is stored in the bones and teeth.

Many laboratories don't have the equipment to measure ionized calcium levels. Because of this lack, serum albumin should be measured at the same time serum calcium is measured because the serum calcium level decreases 0.8 mg/dl for every 1-g decrease in the serum albumin level. The measured serum calcium is then adjusted upward by the amount of decrease in serum albumin. Ionized calcium is estimated to be approximately half of the adjusted calcium value.

What results mean

Normal calcium values are:
- *total calcium*—8.2 to 10.2 mg/dl (SI, 2.05 to 2.54 mmol/L) in adults; 8.6 to 11.2 mg/dl (SI, 2.15 to 2.79 mmol/L) in children
- *ionized calcium*—4.65 to 5.28 mg/dl (SI, 1.1 to 1.32 mmol/L).

> Total calcium levels range from 8.2 to 10.2 mg/dl in adults.

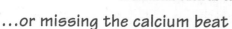

Going overboard with calcium...

Hypercalcemia may occur in patients with hyperparathyroidism and parathyroid tumors (because of oversecretion of parathyroid hormone), Paget's disease of the bone, multiple myeloma, metastatic carcinoma, multiple fractures, or prolonged immobilization. Elevated serum calcium levels may also result from inadequate excretion of calcium, such as in adrenal insufficiency and renal disease; from excessive calcium ingestion; or from overuse of antacids such as calcium carbonate.

...or missing the calcium beat

Hypocalcemia may result from hypoparathyroidism, total parathyroidectomy, or malabsorption. Decreased serum levels of calcium may follow calcium loss in patients with Cushing's syndrome, renal failure, acute pancreatitis, or peritonitis. (See *Calcium test interference*.)

What needs to be done

- Perform a venipuncture (without using a tourniquet, if possible), and collect the sample in a 7-ml clot-activator tube.

Calcium test interference

Excessive ingestion of vitamin D or its derivatives (dihydrotachysterol, calcitriol) may increase calcium levels. Use of certain drugs, such as androgens, calciferol-activated calcium salts, progestins-estrogens, and thiazide diuretics, can also elevate levels.

Chronic laxative use and the administration of acetazolamide, corticosteroids, or mithramycin can alter test results. Excessive transfusions of citrated blood can lower serum calcium levels.

Prolonged application of a tourniquet causes venous stasis and may falsely increase calcium levels.

Cerebrospinal fluid analysis

For qualitative analysis, cerebrospinal fluid (CSF) is most commonly obtained by lumbar puncture (usually between the third and fourth lumbar vertebrae) or, rarely, by cisternal or ventricular puncture. A CSF specimen may also be obtained during other neurologic tests such as myelography.

What results mean

For a summary of normal and abnormal findings in CSF analysis, see *Findings in CSF analysis.*)

Normally, the CSF pressure is recorded and the appearance of the specimen is checked. Three tubes are collected routinely and are sent to the laboratory for analysis of protein, sugar, and cells as well as for serologic testing, such as the Venereal Disease Research Laboratory testing for neurosyphilis. A specimen is also sent to the laboratory for culture and sensitivity testing. Electrolyte analysis and Gram stain may be ordered as supplementary tests. CSF electrolyte levels are of special interest in patients with abnormal serum electrolyte levels or CSF infection and in those receiving hyperosmolar agents. (See *CSF analysis interference.*)

What needs to be done

• Position the patient on his side at the edge of the bed with his knees drawn up to his abdomen and his chin on his chest. Alternately, the patient may assume a sitting position, bending his chest and head toward his knees. Help the patient maintain the position throughout the procedure.
• Use sterile technique for the procedure.

Puncture, pain, pulse, pallor...

• An anesthetic is injected and the spinal needle is inserted in the midline, between the spinous processes of the vertebrae, usually between the third and fourth lumbar vertebrae. At this point, initial CSF pressure is measured and a specimen is obtained.
• During the procedure, observe closely for adverse reactions, such as elevated pulse rate, pallor, or clammy skin. Report significant changes immediately.

...and postpunctural procedures

• After the specimen is collected, label the containers in the order in which they were filled.
• Take a final pressure reading just before the needle is removed. After needle removal, clean the puncture site and apply an adhesive bandage.

CSF analysis interference

Several factors can alter CSF test results:
• Patient position and activity may increase or decrease CSF pressure.
• Crying, coughing, or straining may increase CSF pressure.
• Delay between collection time and laboratory testing may result in possible invalidation of test results, especially cell counts.

Findings in CSF analysis

The table below outlines the normal and abnormal results of cerebrospinal fluid (CSF) analysis, along with their implications.

Test	Normal	Abnormal	Implications
Pressure	50 to 180 mm H_2O	Increase	Increased intracranial pressure
		Decrease	Spinal subarachnoid obstruction above puncture site
Appearance	Clear, colorless	Cloudy	Infection
		Xanthochromic or bloody	Subarachnoid, intracerebral, or intraventricular hemorrhage; spinal cord obstruction; traumatic tap (usually noted only in initial specimen)
		Brown, orange, or yellow	Elevated protein levels, red blood cell (RBC) breakdown (blood present for at least 3 days)
Protein	15 to 50 mg/dl (SI, 0.15 to 0.5 q/L)	Marked increase	Tumors, trauma, hemorrhage, diabetes mellitus, polyneuritis, blood in CSF
		Marked decrease	Rapid CSF production
Gamma globulin	3% to 12% of total protein	Increase	Demyelinating disease, neurosyphilis, Guillain-Barré syndrome
Glucose	50 to 80 mg/dl (SI, 2.8 to 4.4 mmol/L)	Increase	Systemic hyperglycemia
		Decrease	Systemic hypoglycemia, bacterial or fungal infection, meningitis, mumps, postsubarachnoid hemorrhage
Cell count	0 to 5 white blood cells	Increase	Active disease: meningitis, acute infection, onset of chronic illness, tumor, abscess, infarction, demyelinating disease
	No RBCs	RBCs	Hemorrhage or traumatic lumbar puncture
Venereal Disease Research Laboratory test for syphilis, and other serologic tests	Nonreactive	Positive	Neurosyphilis
Chloride	118 to 130 mEq/L (SI, 118 to 130 mmol/L)	Decrease	Infected meninges
Gram stain	No organisms	Gram-positive or gram-negative organisms	Bacterial meningitis

Resting reminders

• Generally, the patient lies flat or has his head slightly elevated for 8 hours after the lumbar puncture. He may turn side to side but may not raise his head during this time.

Red alert

• Infection at the puncture site contraindicates removal of CSF; in a patient with increased intracranial pressure, CSF should be removed with extreme caution because the rapid reduction in pressure that follows withdrawal of fluid can cause cerebellar tonsillar herniation and medullary compression.
• Watch for complications of lumbar puncture, such as reaction to the anesthetic, meningitis, bleeding into the spinal canal, cerebellar tonsillar herniation, and medullary compression. Signs of meningitis include fever, neck rigidity, and irritability. Signs of herniation include decreased level of consciousness, changes in pupil size, reaction to light, and equality, altered vital signs (including widened pulse pressure, decreased pulse rate, and irregular respirations), or respiratory failure.

Chloride

The serum chloride test, a quantitative analysis, measures serum levels of chloride, the major extracellular fluid anion. Interacting with sodium, chloride helps maintain the osmotic pressure of blood and, therefore, helps regulate blood volume and arterial pressure. Chloride levels also affect acid-base balance. Serum concentrations of this electrolyte are regulated by aldosterone secondarily to regulation of sodium. Chloride is absorbed from the intestines and is excreted primarily by the kidneys.

What results mean

Normal serum chloride levels range from 100 to 108 mEq/L (SI, 100 to 108 mmol/L).

Chloride levels relate inversely to those of bicarbonate and thus reflect acid-base balance. Excessive loss of gastric juices or of other secretions containing chloride may cause hypochloremic metabolic alkalosis. Excessive chloride retention or ingestion may lead to hyperchloremic metabolic acidosis.

Level with me

Elevated serum chloride levels (hyperchloremia) may result from bicarbonate loss caused by diarrhea, severe dehydration, complete renal shutdown, head injury (producing neurogenic hyperventilation), or primary aldosteronism.

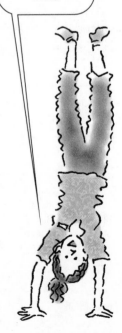

Chloride levels are inversely related to bicarbonate levels.

Low chloride levels (hypochloremia) are usually associated with low sodium and potassium levels. Possible underlying causes include prolonged vomiting, gastric suctioning, intestinal fistula, chronic renal failure, diabetic ketoacidosis, burns, Cushing's syndrome, and Addison's disease. Heart failure or edema resulting in excess extracellular fluid can cause dilutional hypochloremia. (See *Chloride test interference.*)

What needs to be done

Perform a venipuncture and collect the sample in a 7-ml clot-activator tube.

Cholesterol, total

The total serum cholesterol test measures the circulating levels of free cholesterol and cholesterol esters; it reflects the level of the two forms in which this biochemical compound appears in the body.

What results mean

Total cholesterol levels vary with age and sex.

Adults
- *Normal*—less than 200 mg/dl (SI, less than 5 mmol/L) for women and less than 190 mg/dl (SI, less than 4.9 mmol/L) for men
- *Borderline-high*—200 to 240 mg/dl (SI, 5 to 6.2 mmol/L)
- *High*—greater than 240 mg/dl (SI, greater than 6.2 mmol/L)

Children ages 12 to 18
- *Normal*—less than 170 mg/dl (SI, less than 4.4 mmol/L)
- *High*—greater than 200 mg/dl (SI, greater than 5.15 mmol/L)

Keeping the context

The cholesterol level must be evaluated in the context of the entire risk factor analysis for each patient. If the level is abnormal, a second cholesterol test should be completed 1 week later to verify the results. Marked fluctuations can occur from day to day. A decision to begin treatment will be based on the number of risk factors and a patient's prior cardiovascular history.

Danger signs

An elevated serum cholesterol level (hypercholesterolemia) may indicate an increased risk of coronary artery disease (CAD) as well as impend-

> **Chloride test interference**
>
> Ammonium chloride, cholestyramine, or excessive I.V. infusion of sodium chloride may elevate serum chloride levels.
>
> Thiazide diuretics, ethacrynic acid, furosemide, bicarbonates, or prolonged I.V. infusion of dextrose 5% in water may decrease serum chloride levels.

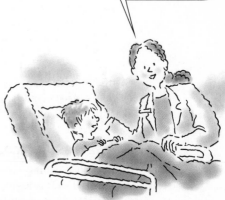

Normal total cholesterol levels for children, which should be less than 170 mg/dl, are lower than those for adults.

ing hepatitis, lipid disorders, bile duct blockage, nephrotic syndrome, obstructive jaundice, pancreatitis, and hypothyroidism. Hypercholesterolemia associated with increased intake of fats and cholesterol-rich foods requires dietary changes and, possibly, medication to slow absorption of cholesterol.

A low serum cholesterol level (hypocholesterolemia) is commonly associated with malnutrition, cellular necrosis of the liver, and hyperthyroidism.

Getting to the heart of the matter

Abnormal cholesterol levels commonly require further testing to pinpoint the causative disorder, depending on the type of abnormality and the presence of overt signs. Abnormal levels associated with cardiovascular disease, for example, may require lipoprotein phenotyping. (See *Total cholesterol test interference.*)

What needs to be done

• Fasting isn't needed for isolated cholesterol checks or screening but is required if the test is part of a lipid profile. If fasting is required, instruct the patient to abstain from food and drink for 12 hours before the test.
• Perform a venipuncture and collect the sample in a 7-ml tube containing EDTA. The patient should be in a sitting position for 5 minutes before the blood is drawn. Fingersticks can also be used for initial screening when using an automated analyzer. Document any drugs the patient is taking.
• Send the sample to the laboratory immediately.

C-reactive protein

C-reactive protein (CRP) is a specific abnormal protein that appears in the blood during an inflammatory process. It's absent from the serum of healthy people. This nonspecific protein is mainly synthesized in the liver and is found in many body fluids (pleural, peritoneal, pericardial, and synovial). It appears in the blood 18 to 24 hours after the onset of tissue damage, with levels that increase up to 1,000-fold and then decline rapidly when the inflammatory process regresses. CRP has been found to increase before rises in antibody titers and erythrocyte sedimentation rate (ESR) levels occur, and also decreases sooner than ESR levels.

What results mean

Reference values usually aren't present. In adults, results may be reported as less than 0.8 mg/dl (SI, less than 8 mg/L). An elevated level may be present in rheumatoid arthritis, rheumatic fever, MI,

---

Total cholesterol test interference

Various factors can influence total cholesterol test results:
• Cholestyramine, clofibrate, colestipol, dextrothyroxine, haloperidol, neomycin, niacin, and chlortetracycline lower cholesterol levels.
• Epinephrine, chlorpromazine, trifluoperazine, hormonal contraceptives, and trimethadione raise cholesterol levels.
• Androgens may have a variable effect on cholesterol level.
• Certain vitamins (such as vitamin E) may cause false elevations.
• Pregnancy may increase levels.
• Myocardial infarction may produce false-low readings.

cancer (active, widespread), acute bacterial and viral infections, inflammatory bowel disease, Hodgkin's disease, systemic lupus erythematosus, and postoperatively (declines after the fourth day). (See *C-reactive protein test interference.*)

What needs to be done

• Perform a venipuncture and collect the sample in a 5-ml clot-activator tube.
• Inform the patient that he must restrict all fluids except for water for 8 to 12 hours before the test.
• Steroids, salicylates, and hormonal contraceptives may need to be restricted before the test.

Creatine kinase

Creatine kinase (CK) is an enzyme that catalyzes the creatine-creatinine metabolic pathway in muscle cells and brain tissue. Because of its important role in energy production, CK levels reflect normal tissue catabolism. Above-normal serum levels indicate trauma to cells with high CK content.

A triad of isoenzymes

CK may be separated into three isoenzymes with distinct molecular structures:
• CK-BB (CK_1), found primarily in brain tissue
• CK-MB (CK_2), found primarily in cardiac muscle (a small amount also appears in skeletal muscle)
• CK-MM (CK_3), found mainly in skeletal muscle.

Getting specific

Total serum CK levels were once widely used to detect acute MI, but elevated levels caused by skeletal muscle damage reduce the test's specificity for this disorder. Fractionation and measurement of CK isoenzymes has replaced total CK assay to accurately localize the site of increased tissue destruction. In addition, subunits of CK-MM and CK-MB, called *isoforms*, can be assayed to increase the sensitivity of the test.

What results mean

Total CK values normally range from 55 to 170 U/L (SI, 0.94 to 2.89 µkat/L) for men and from 30 to 135 U/L (SI, 0.51 to 2.3 µkat/L) for women. CK levels may be significantly higher in very muscular people. Infants up to age 1 year have levels two to four times higher than adults, possibly reflecting birth trauma and striated muscle development.

C-reactive protein test interference

Several factors can alter C-reactive protein test results:
• Steroids and salicylates may cause a false-normal level.
• Hormonal contraceptives may cause a false increase.
• Pregnancy (third trimester) and intrauterine contraceptive devices increase levels.

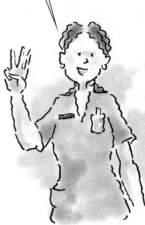

The three isoenzymes of CK — BB, MB, and MM — have distinct molecular structures.

The normal ranges for isoenzyme levels are:
- CK-BB, undetectable
- CK-MB, less than 6% (SI, less than 0.06)
- CK-MM, 90% to 100% (SI, 0.9 to 1).

Detectable CK-BB

CK-MM constitutes over 99% (SI, over 0.99) of total CK normally present in serum. Detectable CK-BB levels may indicate brain tissue injury, certain widespread malignant tumors, severe shock, or renal failure. However, such elevations don't confirm a specific diagnosis.

High CK-MB

CK-MB levels greater than 5% of total CK indicate MI, especially if the lactate dehydrogenase 1 and 2 (LD_1-LD_2) isoenzyme ratio is greater than 1 (flipped LD). In acute MI and after cardiac surgery, CK-MB levels begin to rise in 2 to 4 hours, peak in 12 to 24 hours, and usually return to normal in 24 to 48 hours; persistent elevations or increasing levels indicate ongoing myocardial damage. (See *Serum protein and isoenzyme levels after MI.*) Total CK follows roughly the same pattern but rises slightly later.

Serious skeletal muscle injury that occurs in certain muscular dystrophies, polymyositis, and severe myoglobinuria may produce mildly elevated CK-MB levels because a small amount of this isoenzyme is present in some skeletal muscles.

Rising CK-MM

Rising CK-MM values follow skeletal muscle damage from trauma, such as surgery and I.M. injections, or diseases, such as dermatomyositis and muscular dystrophy (values may be 50 to 100 times normal). A moderate rise in CK-MM levels develops in patients with hypothyroidism; sharp elevations occur with muscular activity caused by agitation such as an acute psychotic episode.

Total CK

Total CK levels may be elevated in patients with severe hypokalemia, carbon monoxide poisoning, malignant hyperthermia, or alcoholic cardiomyopathy; in patients who have recently had a seizure; and, occasionally, in patients who have suffered pulmonary or cerebral infarctions. (See *Creatine kinase test interference.*)

What needs to be done
- If the patient is being evaluated for skeletal muscle disorders, advise him to avoid exercising for 24 hours before the test.
- Advise the patient that, before the test, he must refrain from ingesting alcohol, aminocaproic acid, lithium, clofibrate, codeine,

Creatine kinase test interference

The following factors may raise total CK values:
- alcohol
- aminocaproic acid (large doses)
- cardioversion
- halothane
- I.M. injections
- invasive diagnostic procedures
- lithium
- muscle massage
- recent vigorous exercise
- severe coughing and trauma
- succinylcholine
- surgery through skeletal muscle.

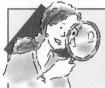

A closer look

Serum protein and isoenzyme levels after MI

Because they're released by damaged tissue, serum proteins and isoenzymes (catalytic proteins that vary in concentration in specific organs) can help identify the compromised organ and assess the extent of damage after myocardial infarction (MI). The serum protein and isoenzyme determinations listed here are most significant after MI.

Isoenzymes

• Creatine kinase-MB (CK-MB): in the heart muscle and a small amount in skeletal muscle
• Lactate dehydrogenase 1 and 2 (LD_1, LD_2): in the heart, brain, kidneys, liver, skeletal muscles, and red blood cells

Proteins

• Troponin-I and troponin-T (the cardiac contractile proteins) have greater sensitivity than CK-MB in detecting myocardial injury.

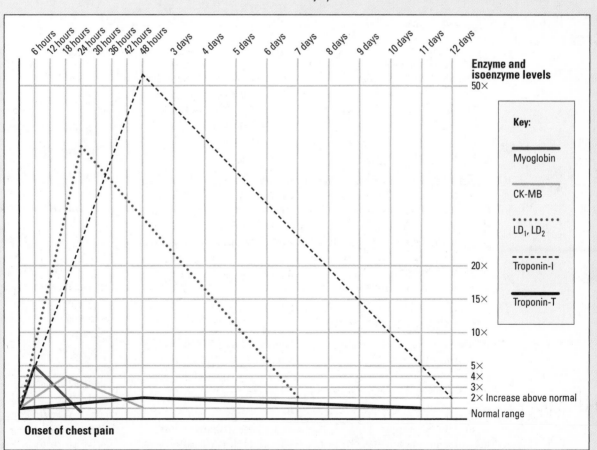

dexamethasone, digoxin, lithium, morphine, succinylcholine, furosemide, glutethimide, halothane, heroin, imipramine, meperidine, and phenobarbital. If these substances must be continued, note this on the laboratory request.
• Obtain the sample as scheduled. Because timing is important to the diagnosis, be sure to record the date and time the sample was drawn and the number of hours that elapsed since the onset of chest pain.
• Draw the sample before giving an I.M. injection, or wait at least 1 hour after the injection, because muscle trauma raises total CK levels.
• Perform a venipuncture and collect the sample in a 7-ml tube without additives.
• Send the sample to the laboratory immediately because CK activity diminishes significantly after 2 hours at room temperature.
• Resume medications discontinued before the test, as ordered.

Creatinine

A quantitative analysis of serum creatinine levels, the serum creatinine test provides a more sensitive measure of renal damage than BUN levels because renal impairment is virtually the only cause of creatinine elevation. Because creatinine levels normally remain constant, elevated levels usually indicate diminished renal function.

What results mean

Serum creatinine levels in males normally range from 0.8 to 1.2 mg/dl (SI, 62 to 115 µmol/L); in females, they range from 0.6 to 0.9 mg/dl (SI, 53 to 97 µmol/L). Elevated serum creatinine levels generally indicate renal disease that has seriously damaged 50% or more of the nephrons. They may also be associated with gigantism and acromegaly (a metabolic condition characterized by enlargement and elongation of facial bones and extremities). (See *Creatinine test interference*.)

What needs to be done

Perform a venipuncture and collect the sample in a 7-ml clot-activator tube.

D-dimer

A D-dimer is an asymmetrical carbon compound fragment formed after thrombin converts fibrinogen to fibrin, factor XIIIa stabilizes it into a clot, and plasma acts on the cross-linked, or *clotted*, fib-

---

Creatinine test interference

Several factors can alter creatinine test results:
• Ascorbic acid, barbiturates, and diuretics may raise serum creatinine levels.
• Sulfobromophthalein or phenolsulfonphthalein given within the previous 24 hours can elevate creatinine levels.
• Exceptionally large muscle mass (for example, in athletes) may cause above-average creatinine levels, even with normal renal function.

rin. The test is specific for fibrinolysis because it confirms the presence of fibrin split products.

What results mean

Normal D-dimer test results are negative or less than 250 ug/L (SI, less than 250 ug/L). Increased D-dimer values may indicate disseminated intravascular disease, pulmonary embolism, arterial or venous thrombosis, neoplastic disease, pregnancy (late and postpartum), surgery occurring up to 2 days before testing, subarachnoid hemorrhage (spinal fluid only), or secondary fibrinolysis. (See *D-dimer test interference.*)

What needs to be done

• Perform a venipuncture and collect the sample in a 4.5-ml tube with sodium citrate added.
• For spinal fluid analysis, the sample is collected during a lumbar puncture and placed in a plastic vial. See "Cerebrospinal fluid analysis," page 150, for details about lumbar puncture.

Erythrocyte sedimentation rate

ESR measures the degree of erythrocyte, or RBC, settling during a specified time period. As the RBCs descend in the tube, they displace an equal volume of plasma upward, which slows the downward progress of other settling blood elements.

Early indicator

ESR is a sensitive but nonspecific test that's commonly the earliest indicator of disease when other chemical or physical signs are normal. ESR typically rises significantly in widespread inflammatory disorders caused by infection or autoimmune mechanisms; such elevations may be prolonged in localized inflammation and malignancy.

What results mean

Normal ESR ranges from 0 to 10 mm/hour (SI, 0 to 10 mm/hour) in males and from 0 to 20 mm/hour (SI, 0 to 20 mm/hour) in females; rates gradually increase with age.

On the rise

The ESR rises in pregnancy, acute or chronic inflammation, tuberculosis, blood cell dyscrasias, rheumatic fever, rheumatoid arthritis, and some cancers. Anemia also tends to raise ESR because

---

D-dimer test interference

Failure to fill the collection tube completely or to send the sample to the laboratory immediately may alter D-dimer test results.

These factors can also influence test results:
• High rheumatoid factor titers or increased CA-125 levels result in a possible false-positive result.
• Spinal fluid analysis in infants younger than age 6 months may produce a false-negative result.
• Rough handling of the sample may cause hemolysis.

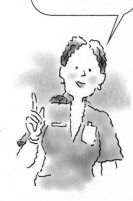

ESR is commonly the earliest indicator of disease when other chemical or physical signs are normal.

less upward displacement of plasma occurs to retard the relatively few sedimenting RBCs.

How depresssing

Polycythemia, sickle cell anemia, hyperviscosity (excessively thick blood), or low plasma fibrinogen or globulin levels tend to depress ESR. (See *ESR test interference.*)

What needs to be done

• Perform a venipuncture and collect the sample in a 7-ml tube containing EDTA or a 4.5-ml tube with sodium citrate added. (Check with the laboratory to determine preference.)
• Completely fill the collection tube, and invert it gently several times to adequately mix the sample and anticoagulant.
• Send the sample to the laboratory immediately after examining it for clots or clumps. The sample must be tested within 2 hours.

Glucose, fasting plasma

Commonly used to screen for diabetes mellitus, the fasting plasma glucose test (also known as the *fasting blood sugar test*) measures plasma glucose levels following a 12- to 14-hour fast.

What results mean

The normal range for fasting plasma glucose varies according to the laboratory procedure. Generally, normal values after at least an 8-hour fast are 70 to 110 mg (SI, 3.9 to 6.1 mmol/L) of true glucose per deciliter of blood.

Diabetes detector

A fasting plasma glucose level of 126 mg/dl (SI, 7 mmol/L) or higher obtained on two or more occasions confirms provisional diabetes mellitus. An impaired blood glucose level is 125 mg/dl (SI, 6.9 mmol/L). A borderline or transiently elevated level requires the 2-hour postprandial plasma glucose test or the oral glucose tolerance test to confirm the diagnosis.

Boosting levels

Increased fasting plasma glucose levels can also result from pancreatitis, recent acute illness (such as MI), Cushing's syndrome, acromegaly, and pheochromocytoma (a tumor of the adrenal medulla). Hyperglycemia may also stem from hyperlipoproteinemia (especially type III, IV, or V), chronic hepatic disease, nephrotic syndrome, brain tumor, sepsis, or gastrectomy with dumping

---

ESR test interference

Several factors can alter ESR:
• Failure to use the proper anticoagulant and inadequate mixing of the sample and anticoagulant may produce inaccurate results.
• Failure to send the sample to the laboratory immediately may alter test results.
• Hemolysis caused by rough handling or excessive mixing of the sample may alter test results.
• Prolonged tourniquet constriction may cause hemoconcentration.
• Testing delayed more than 2 hours after sample collection may decrease values.

syndrome and is typical in eclampsia, anoxia, and seizure disorders.

Depressed levels

Depressed plasma glucose levels can result from hyperinsulinism, insulinoma, von Gierke's disease (glycogen storage disease), functional or reactive hypoglycemia, myxedema, adrenal insufficiency, congenital adrenal hyperplasia, hypopituitarism, malabsorption syndrome, or some cases of hepatic insufficiency.

Diabetes downer

When using fasting plasma glucose tests to monitor drug or diet therapy in patients with diabetes mellitus, results can be obtained that require immediate action. Most patients develop symptoms when blood glucose is between 50 to 60 mg/dl (SI, 2.8 to 3 mmol/L). Symptoms include fatigue, malaise, nervousness, mood changes, irritability, trembling, tension, headache, hunger, cold sweats, rapid heart rate, and palpitations. Without immediate reversal of the hypoglycemia with parenteral or I.V. glucose, the blood glucose level will continue to fall. Evidence of progressive central nervous system (CNS) disturbance includes blurry or double vision, inability to concentrate, confusion, motor weakness, hemiplegia, seizures, loss of consciousness, irreversible brain damage, and death.

Rapid response required

Plasma glucose levels higher than 300 mg/dl (SI, 15 mmol/L) can also be an urgent situation. Treatment with appropriate insulin dosages can correct the hyperglycemia. (See *Fasting plasma glucose test interference*, page 162.)

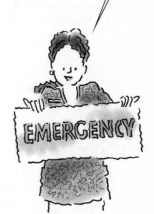

Plasma glucose levels above 300 mg/dl indicate severe hyperglycemia. Urgent treatment may be indicated.

What needs to be done

- Tell the patient he must fast for 12 to 14 hours before the test.
- Advise the patient to avoid drugs that affect test results, as ordered. Advise the patient with diabetes that he'll receive his medication after the test.
- Instruct the patient to report the symptoms of hypoglycemia (weakness, restlessness, nervousness, hunger, and sweating).
- Perform a venipuncture and collect the sample in a 5-ml clot-activator tube.
- Specify on the laboratory request the time the patient last ate, the sample collection time, and the time he received the last pretest dose of insulin or oral antidiabetic drug (if applicable).
- Send the sample to the laboratory immediately because blood glucose levels decrease when the sample is left at room temperature. If transport is delayed, refrigerate the sample.

Fasting plasma glucose test interference

Factors that may increase plasma glucose levels include:
- acetaminophen (may cause false-positive findings)
- arginine
- benzodiazepines
- chlorthalidone
- corticosteroids
- dextrothyroxine
- diazoxide
- epinephrine
- ethacrynic acid (may also cause hyperglycemia or, in large doses, hypoglycemia in patients with uremia)
- furosemide
- hormonal contraceptives (estrogen-progestogen combination)
- hydrochlorothiazide
- lithium
- nicotinic acid (large doses)
- phenolphthalein
- phenothiazines
- phenytoin
- thiazide diuretics
- triamterene
- recent illness, infection, or pregnancy
- recent I.V. glucose infusions.
    Factors that may decrease plasma glucose levels include:
- beta-adrenergic blockers
- clofibrate
- ethanol
- insulin
- monoamine oxidase inhibitors
- oral antidiabetic agents
- strenuous exercise.

- Provide a balanced meal or a snack. As ordered, resume administration of medications withheld before the test.

Hematocrit

Hematocrit (HCT) levels reflect the proportion of blood occupied by RBCs. The HCT test is a common, reliable test that measures the percentage by volume of packed RBCs in a whole-blood sample. For example, an HCT of 40% (SI, 0.40) means that a 100-ml sample contains 40 ml of packed RBCs. The packing of RBCs is achieved by centrifugation of anticoagulated whole blood in a capillary tube, which tightly packs RBCs without causing hemolysis.

What results mean

HCT values vary depending on the patient's sex and age, the type of sample, and the laboratory performing the test. (See *HCT reference values* and *HCT test interference*.)

Ages and stages

HCT reference values

The following ranges represent normal hematocrit (HCT) values for different age-groups:
- *neonates:* 55% to 68% (SI, 0.55 to 0.68)
- *1 week:* 47% to 65% (SI, 0.47 to 0.65)
- *1 month:* 37% to 49% (SI, 0.37 to 0.49)
- *3 months:* 30% to 36% (SI, 0.3 to 0.36)
- *1 year:* 29% to 41% (SI, 0.29 to 0.41)
- *10 years:* 36% to 40% (SI, 0.36 to 0.4)
- *adult males:* 42% to 52% (SI, 0.42 to 0.52)
- *adult females:* 36% to 48% (SI, 0.36 to 0.48).

Low HCT suggests anemia, hemodilution, or massive blood loss; high HCT indicates polycythemia or hemoconcentration resulting from blood loss and dehydration.

What needs to be done

• For adults, perform a venipuncture and collect the sample in a 7-ml tube containing EDTA. For younger children and infants, collect the sample by fingerstick or heelstick in a microcollection device containing EDTA.
• Completely fill the collection tube, and invert it gently several times to adequately mix the sample and anticoagulant.
• Send the sample to the laboratory immediately.

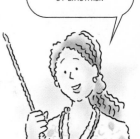

> **HCT test interference**
>
> Hemoconcentration caused by tourniquet constriction for longer than 1 minute typically raises HCT by 2.5% to 5% and may alter HCT test results.

Hemoglobin

Hb, which transports oxygen, is the main component of an RBC. Each RBC contains about 250 million molecules of Hb. Therefore, Hb concentration correlates closely with the RBC count. Hb level is a good indicator of anemia.

> Hemoglobin concentration correlates closely with RBC count and, therefore, is a reliable indicator of anemia.

What results mean

Hb concentration varies depending on the patient's age and sex and on the type of blood sample drawn. (See *Hb reference values.*)

Ages and stages

Hb reference values

The following values reflect normal hemoglobin (Hb) concentrations (in number of grams per deciliter) for different age-groups:
• *neonates:* 17 to 22 g/dl (SI, 170 to 220 g/L)
• *1 week:* 15 to 20 g/dl (SI, 150 to 200 g/L)
• *1 month:* 11 to 15 g/dl (SI, 110 to 150 g/L)
• *children:* 11 to 13 g/dl (SI, 110 to 130 g/L)
• *adult males:* 14 to 17.4 g/dl (SI, 140 to 174 g/L)
• *males after middle age:* 12.4 to 14.9 g/dl (SI, 124 to 149 g/L)
• *females:* 12 to 16 g/dl (SI, 120 to 160 g/L)
• *females after middle age:* 11.7 to 13.8 g/dl (SI, 117 to 138 g/L).

A low point

Low Hb concentration may indicate anemia, recent hemorrhage, or fluid retention, which can cause hemodilution. Elevated Hb levels suggest hemoconcentration from polycythemia or dehydration. (See *Hb test interference.*)

What needs to be done

• For adults and older children, perform a venipuncture and collect the sample in a 7-ml tube containing EDTA. For younger children and infants, collect the sample by fingerstick or heelstick in a microcollection device containing EDTA.
• Completely fill the collection tube, and invert it gently several times to adequately mix the sample and anticoagulant.

Hemoglobin, glycosylated

The glycosylated Hb test, also known as the *total fasting Hb* or *glycohemoglobin test*, helps monitor the effectiveness of diabetes therapy. Glycosylated Hb levels reflect the average blood glucose level during the preceding 2 to 3 months. This test requires only one venipuncture every 6 to 8 weeks and can, therefore, be used for evaluating long-term effectiveness of diabetes therapy.

What results mean

Glycosylated Hb values are reported as a percentage of the total Hb within an RBC. Because Hb A_{1c} is present in a larger quantity than the other minor Hbs, it's commonly measured and reported separately. Hb A_{1a} and Hb A_{1b} account for about 1.6% and 0.8% of total Hb, respectively; Hb A_{1c} accounts for approximately 5%; and total glycosylated Hb accounts for 4% to 7%.

Under control or out of control

Good diabetic control is indicated when the glycosylated Hb value is less than 8%. A value greater than 10% indicates poor control. Glycosylated Hb levels approach normal range as therapy begins to control diabetes. (See *Glycosylated Hb test interference.*)

What needs to be done

• Perform a venipuncture and collect the sample in a 5-ml tube containing EDTA.
• Fill the collection tube completely, and invert it gently several times to adequately mix the sample and anticoagulant.
• Schedule the patient for an appointment in 6 to 8 weeks for appropriate follow-up testing.

Hb test interference

Very high white blood cell counts or RBCs that resist lysis may falsely elevate Hb values.

Glycosylated Hb test interference

Hemolytic anemia, chronic blood loss, or abnormal hemoglobins (S, C, or D) may lower results.

Hyperglycemia, thalassemia, chronic renal failure, dialysis, a recent splenectomy, or elevated triglyceride or Hb F levels may elevate results.

Human chorionic gonadotropin, serum

Human chorionic gonadotropin (hCG) is a hormone produced by the trophoblastic cells of the placenta. When conception occurs, the hCG assay may detect this hormone in the blood as early as 9 days after ovulation. This interval coincides with implantation of the fertilized ovum into the uterine wall.

hCG comes early

Although the precise function of this hormone is still unclear, hCG, along with progesterone, appears to maintain the corpus luteum during early pregnancy. Production of hCG increases steadily during the first trimester, peaking around the 10th week of gestation. (See *Production of hCG during pregnancy*.) This serum immunoassay is more sensitive (and costly) than the routine pregnancy test using a urine specimen.

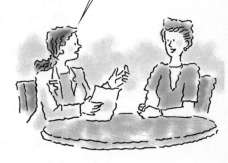

I've got good news. Increased hCG level is a good indicator of pregnancy during the first trimester.

Production of hCG during pregnancy

Production of human chorionic gonadotropin (hCG) increases steadily during the first trimester, peaking around the 10th week of gestation, as shown below. Levels then fall to less than 10% of the first-trimester levels during the remainder of pregnancy.

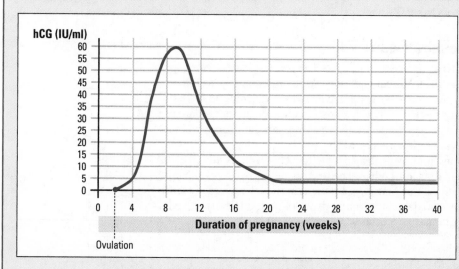

What results mean

Normal values for hCG are less than 4 mIU/L (SI, 4 IU/L). During pregnancy, hCG levels are quite variable and depend partially on the number of days since the last normal menses.

High and Lois

Elevated hCG levels indicate pregnancy; significantly higher concentrations are present in a multiple pregnancy. Increased levels may also suggest hydatidiform mole, trophoblastic neoplasm of the placenta, or nontrophoblastic carcinomas that secrete hCG (including gastric, pancreatic, and ovarian adenocarcinomas). Because levels are high in both conditions, hCG levels can't differentiate between pregnancy and tumor recurrence.

Low hCG levels can occur in ectopic pregnancy or pregnancy of fewer than 9 days. (See *hCG test interference.*)

What needs to be done

- Perform a venipuncture and collect the sample in a 7-ml clot-activator tube.
- Send the sample to the laboratory immediately.

Human immunodeficiency virus testing

The human immunodeficiency virus (HIV) antibodies test detects antibodies to HIV in serum. HIV is the virus that causes acquired immunodeficiency syndrome (AIDS). Initial identification of HIV is usually achieved through enzyme immunoassay. Positive findings are confirmed by Western blot test and immunofluorescence. (See *Testing for HIV.*)

What results mean

Test results are normally negative. The test detects previous exposure to the virus. However, it doesn't identify patients who have been exposed to the virus but haven't yet made antibodies. A positive test for the HIV antibody doesn't indicate whether a patient harbors an actively replicating virus or when the patient will manifest signs and symptoms of AIDS.

Many apparently healthy people have been exposed to HIV and have circulating antibodies. The test results for such people aren't false-positives. Furthermore, a patient in the later stages of AIDS may exhibit no detectable antibody in his serum because he can no longer mount an antibody response.

hCG test interference

Heparin anticoagulants and EDTA depress plasma hCG levels.

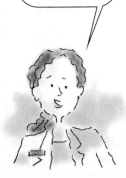

HIV testing detects HIV antibodies, which indicate previous exposure to the virus.

Testing for HIV

Newer tests are available to help identify human immunodeficiency virus (HIV) antibodies more quickly, including those listed below. There are no known factors that interfere with HIV testing.

Oraquick Rapid HIV1 Antibody test
Oraquick Rapid HIV1 Antibody test allows results to be obtained in less than 20 minutes using one drop of blood. A color indicator similar to the indicator in a home pregnancy test is used. If results are positive, a confirmatory test must be done to validate the results.

Nucleic acid test
The nucleic acid test is a test used to screen donated plasma for HIV and hepatitis C. This test has dramatically reduced the waiting time involved until blood and blood products may be used.

Gene-based tests
Spikes of HIV virus in the bloodstream commonly mean that the individual being treated for HIV is growing resistant to the drug treatment being used. A gene-based test can help determine whether an HIV infected person's virus is mutating, causing therapy to fail. Test results can guide the doctor in selecting a better treatment plan.

What needs to be done

- Make sure that informed consent has been signed, according to facility policy.
- Perform a venipuncture and collect the sample in a 10-ml barrier tube. Barrier tubes help prevent contamination when pouring the serum in the laboratory.
- Keep test results confidential.

Human leukocyte antigen typing

The human leukocyte antigen (HLA) test identifies a group of antigens that are present on the surface of all nucleated cells but are most easily detected on lymphocytes. These antigens are essential to immunity and determine the degree of histocompatibility between transplant recipients and donors. HLA typing has also been used for paternity testing.

Antiserum breakup

Three types of HLA (HLA-A, HLA-B, and HLA-C) are measured with a lymphocytotoxicity assay. A lymphocyte sample is mixed with known antisera to these antigens and complement. Lymphocytes react with a specific antiserum, which causes them to break up and allow a dye to enter; they may then be detected by a microscope.

Mixed reaction

A fourth type of HLA (HLA-D) is measured by a mixed lymphocyte reaction. Leukocytes from the recipient and the donor are combined in culture to determine HLA-D compatibility.

What results mean

In HLA-A, HLA-B, and HLA-C testing, lymphocytes that react with the test antiserum break up and are detected by phase microscopy. In HLA-D testing, leukocyte incompatibility is marked by blast formation, deoxyribonucleic acid synthesis, and reproduction.

Incompatible HLA-A, HLA-B, HLA-C, and HLA-D groups may cause unsuccessful tissue transplantation.

Strong association

Many diseases have a strong association with certain types of HLAs. For example, HLA-DR5 (a specific HLA type) is associated with Hashimoto's thyroiditis. B8 and Dw3 are associated with Graves' disease, whereas B8 alone is associated with chronic autoimmune hepatitis, celiac disease, and myasthenia gravis. Dw3 alone is associated with Addison's disease, Sjögren's syndrome, dermatitis herpetiformis, and systemic lupus erythematosus. (See *HLA typing interference.*)

What needs to be done

• Perform a venipuncture and collect the sample in a tube containing acid citrate dextrose solution.
• Check the patient's history for recent blood transfusions. HLA testing may need to be postponed if he has recently undergone a transfusion.

> ### HLA typing interference
>
> HLA from blood transfusion within 72 hours before sample collection can affect the accuracy of test results. In addition, rough handling of the sample can cause hemolysis.

International Normalized Ratio

The International Normalized Ratio (INR) system is the best means of standardizing measurement of prothrombin time to monitor oral anticoagulant therapy.

What results mean

Normal INR for those receiving warfarin therapy is 2.0 to 3.0 (SI, 2.0 to 3.0). For those with mechanical prosthetic heart valves, an INR of 2.5 to 3.5 (SI, 2.5 to 3.5) is suggested.

Increased INR values may indicate disseminated intravascular coagulation, cirrhosis, hepatitis, vitamin K deficiency, salicylate intoxication, uncontrolled oral anticoagulation, or massive blood transfusion. (See *INR interference.*)

What needs to be done

• Perform a venipuncture and collect the sample in a 7-ml tube with sodium citrate added.
• Completely fill the collection tube; otherwise, excess citrate will appear in the sample.
• Gently invert the tube several times to thoroughly mix the sample and anticoagulant.
• Put the sample on ice, and send it to the laboratory promptly.

Lactate dehydrogenase

Lactate dehydrogenase (LD) speeds up the chemical reaction of (catalyzes) the reversible conversion of muscle lactic acid into pyruvic acid, which ultimately produces cellular energy.

Gimme five

Because LD is present in almost all body tissues, cellular damage causes an elevation of total serum LD, thus limiting its diagnostic usefulness. However, five tissue-specific isoenzymes can be identified and measured. Two of these isoenzymes, LD_1 and LD_2, appear primarily in the heart, RBCs, and kidneys; LD_3, primarily in the lungs; and LD_4 and LD_5, in the liver and the skeletal muscles. Also, the midzone fractions (LD_2, LD_3, and LD_4) can be elevated in granulocytic leukemia, lymphomas, and platelet disorders.

I spy MI

The specificity of LD isoenzymes and their distribution pattern are useful in diagnosing hepatic, pulmonary, and erythrocytic damage. However, their widest use is in aiding diagnosis of acute MI. (See *LD isoenzyme variations in disease,* page 170.) An LD isoenzyme assay is helpful when CK hasn't been measured within 24 hours of an acute MI. The myocardial LD level rises later than CK (12 to 48 hours after infarction begins), peaks in 2 to 5 days, and drops to normal in 7 to 10 days if tissue necrosis doesn't persist.

What results mean

Total LD levels normally range from 71 to 207 units/L (SI, 1.2 to 3.52 µkat/L), depending on the method used. Normal isoenzyme distribution is:
• *LD_1:* 14% to 26% (SI, 0.14 to 0.26) of total
• *LD_2:* 29% to 39% (SI, 0.29 to 0.39) of total
• *LD_3:* 20% to 26% (SI, 0.2 to 0.26) of total

> **INR interference**
>
> Failure to fill the collection tube completely, adequately mix the sample and the anticoagulant, or send the sample to the laboratory immediately may result in inaccurate test results.
>
> Hemolysis may occur as a result of excessive probing at the venipuncture site or rough handling of the sample.

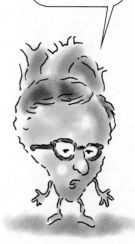

My, oh my! LD isoenzymes are most commonly used to diagnose acute MI.

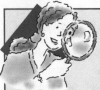

A closer look

LD isoenzyme variations in disease

In some instances, total lactate dehydrogenase (LD) levels may be normal but there may be abnormal proportions of individual enzymes, indicating damage to a specific organ. The chart below shows the variations in each enzyme level that may occur with some common diseases. The black areas denote normal enzyme levels; the colored shading represents levels that are diagnostic for the specific disorder, and the white areas show that levels aren't diagnostic for the disorder.

Disease	LD_1	LD_2	LD_3	LD_4	LD_5
Cardiovascular					
Myocardial infarction (MI)	Normal	Normal	Not diagnostic	Not diagnostic	Not diagnostic
MI with hepatic congestion	Normal	Normal	Not diagnostic	Not diagnostic	Diagnostic
Rheumatic carditis	Normal	Normal	Not diagnostic	Not diagnostic	Not diagnostic
Myocarditis	Normal	Normal	Not diagnostic	Not diagnostic	Not diagnostic
Heart failure (decompensated)	Not diagnostic	Not diagnostic	Not diagnostic	Not diagnostic	Diagnostic
Shock	Normal	Diagnostic	Diagnostic	Diagnostic	Diagnostic
Angina pectoris	Normal	Not diagnostic	Not diagnostic	Not diagnostic	Not diagnostic
Pulmonary					
Pulmonary embolism	Normal	Not diagnostic	Not diagnostic	Not diagnostic	Not diagnostic
Pulmonary infarction	Not diagnostic	Not diagnostic	Diagnostic	Not diagnostic	Not diagnostic
Hematologic					
Pernicious anemia	Diagnostic	Diagnostic	Not diagnostic	Not diagnostic	Not diagnostic
Hemolytic anemia	Diagnostic	Diagnostic	Not diagnostic	Not diagnostic	Not diagnostic
Sickle cell anemia	Diagnostic	Diagnostic	Not diagnostic	Not diagnostic	Not diagnostic
Hepatobiliary					
Hepatitis	Not diagnostic	Not diagnostic	Not diagnostic	Not diagnostic	Diagnostic
Active cirrhosis	Not diagnostic	Not diagnostic	Not diagnostic	Not diagnostic	Diagnostic
Hepatic congestion	Not diagnostic	Not diagnostic	Not diagnostic	Not diagnostic	Diagnostic

Key: ● Normal   ● Diagnostic   ○ Not diagnostic

- LD_4: 8% to 16% (SI, 0.08 to 0.16) of total
- LD_5: 6% to 16% (SI, 0.06 to 0.16) of total.

Because many common diseases cause elevations in total LD levels, isoenzyme electrophoresis is usually necessary for diagnosis. In some disorders, total LD may be within normal limits, but abnormal proportions of each isoenzyme indicate specific organ tissue damage. For instance, in acute MI, the concentration of LD_1 is greater than LD_2 within 12 to 48 hours after onset of symptoms (that is, the LD_1-LD_2 ratio is greater than 1). This reversal of normal isoenzyme patterns is typical of myocardial damage and is referred to as "flipped LD." (See *LD test interference*.)

What needs to be done

- Tell the patient that, if an MI is suspected, the test will likely be be repeated for the next few mornings to monitor progressive changes.
- Draw the samples on schedule to avoid missing peak levels, and mark the collection time on the laboratory request.
- Perform a venipuncture and collect the sample in a 7-ml clot-activator tube.
- Send the sample to the laboratory immediately or, if transport is delayed, keep the sample at room temperature. Changes in temperature reportedly inactivate LD_5, thus altering isoenzyme patterns.

> **LD test interference**
>
> Recent surgery or pregnancy can cause elevated LD levels. Prosthetic heart valves can also increase LD levels because of chronic hemolysis.

Lipoprotein-cholesterol fractionation

Lipoprotein fractionation tests are used to isolate and measure the types of cholesterol in serum, low-density lipoproteins (LDLs), and high-density lipoproteins (HDLs). The HDL level is inversely related to the risk of CAD; the higher the HDL level, the lower the incidence of CAD. Conversely, the higher the LDL level, the higher the incidence of CAD. (See *Apolipoproteins and CAD*, page 172.)

What results mean

LDL cholesterol level in an individual who doesn't have CAD is considered *normal* if it's less than 130 mg/dl (SI, less than 3.36 mmol/L), *borderline-high* if it's in the range of 130 to 159 mg/dl (SI, 3.36 to 4.1 mmol/L), and *high* if it's more than 160 mg/dl (SI, more than 4.1 mmol/L). For an individual who has CAD, an optimal level is less than 100 mg/dl (SI, less than 2.6 mmol/L), and a higher-than-optimal level is more than 100 mg/dl (SI, more than 2.6 mmol/L).

> How am I doing? The lipoprotein-cholesterol fractionation test assesses the risk of CAD and the efficacy of lipid-lowering drugs.

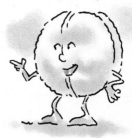

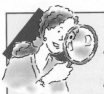

A closer look

Apolipoproteins and CAD

Mounting evidence suggests that apolipoproteins—the protein fractions of lipoprotein molecules—may have important clinical applications. Because apolipoprotein levels can be measured directly in serum, they may indicate an individual's risk of coronary artery disease (CAD) more accurately than levels of high-density lipoproteins (HDLs) or low-density lipoproteins (LDLs), which must be measured indirectly.

Eight apolipoproteins have been identified. Of these, apolipoprotein A (ApoA)—the major protein component of HDL—and apolipoprotein B (ApoB)—the major component of LDL—are most clinically significant. Decreased ApoA levels occur with ischemic heart disease; increased ApoB levels, with hyperlipidemia, angina pectoris, and myocardial infarction.

Optimal HDL cholesterol values range from 37 to 70 mg/dl (SI, 0.96 to 1.8 mmol/L) in males and from 40 to 85 mg/dl (SI, 1.03 to 2.2 mmol/L) in females.

Low and behold

Decreased LDL levels can occur during acute stress (illness, burns, MI), inflammatory joint disease, chronic pulmonary disease, and myeloma. Decreased HDL levels are commonly seen in patients with hypertriglyceridemia. The HDL level may increase if the elevated triglyceride level is treated.

High and healthy?

High LDL levels increase the risk of CAD. Elevated HDL levels generally reflect a healthy state, but they can also indicate chronic hepatitis, early-stage primary biliary cirrhosis, or alcohol consumption. Rarely, a sharp rise (to as high as 100 mg/dl [SI, 2.58 mmol/L]) indicates a second type of HDL (alpha-HDL) that may signal CAD.

Normal levels but increased risk

Studies show that 3% of males in the United States have low HDL levels for unknown reasons even though their total cholesterol and triglyceride levels are normal. These males are at increased risk for CAD. Risk levels of CAD associated with HDL values are:
• *dangerously high*—less than 25 mg/dl (SI, less than 0.64 mmol/L)
• *high*—26 to 35 mg/dl (SI, 0.67 to 0.9 mmol/L)
• *moderate*—36 to 44 mg/dl (SI, 0.93 to 1.1 mmol/L)

Lipoprotein-cholesterol fractionation test interference

Several factors can alter lipoprotein-cholesterol fractionation test results:
• Antilipemic medications, such as clofibrate, cholestyramine, colestipol, niacin, and gemfibrozil, lower values.
• Hormonal contraceptives, disulfiram, alcohol, miconazole, and high doses of phenothiazines increase values.
• Estrogens, bilirubin, Hb, salicylates, iodine, vitamins A and D, and concurrent illness also may alter test results, making them inaccurate.

- *average* — 45 to 59 mg/dl (SI, 1.16 to 1.5 mmol/L)
- *below average* — 60 to 74 mg/dl (SI, 1.55 to 1.91 mmol/L)
- *probable protection* — greater than 75 mg/dl (SI, greater than 1.93 mmol/L). (See *Lipoprotein-cholesterol fractionation test interference.*)

What needs to be done

- Tell the patient to maintain a normal diet for 2 weeks before the test.
- Tell him to abstain from alcohol for 24 hours before the test and to fast and avoid exercise for 12 to 14 hours before the test.
- As ordered, tell the patient to discontinue use of thyroid hormone, hormonal contraceptives, and antilipemic agents until after the test because they alter test results.
- Perform a venipuncture and collect the sample in a 7-ml tube containing EDTA.
- Send the sample to the laboratory immediately to avoid spontaneous redistribution among the lipoproteins. If the sample can't be transported immediately, refrigerate it but don't allow it to freeze.

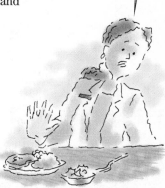

The patient should fast for 12 to 14 hours before the lipoprotein-cholesterol fractionation test.

Lyme disease serology

Serologic tests for Lyme disease — indirect immunofluorescent and enzyme-linked immunosorbent assays — measure antibody response to this spirochete and indicate current infection or past exposure. Serologic tests can identify 50% of patients with early-stage Lyme disease and all patients tested later when such complications as carditis, neuritis, and arthritis occur.

What results mean

Normal serum values are nonreactive.

I cannot tell a Lyme

A positive Lyme serology can help confirm diagnosis but isn't definitive. Other treponemal diseases and high rheumatoid factor titers can cause false-positive results. More than 15% of patients with Lyme disease fail to develop antibodies. (See *Lyme disease serology interference.*)

What needs to be done

- Instruct the patient to fast for 12 hours before the sample is drawn, but to drink fluids as usual.

Lyme disease serology interference

Several factors can alter Lyme disease serology test results:

- High serum lipid levels may cause inaccurate results that require repetition of the test after a period of restricted fat intake.
- Samples contaminated with other bacteria may cause a false-positive result.
- Rough handling of the sample may cause hemolysis.

• Perform a venipuncture and collect the sample in a 7-ml clot-activator tube.

Magnesium

Magnesium is a commonly overlooked electrolyte vital to neuromuscular function. Magnesium activates many essential enzymes and affects the metabolism of nucleic acids and proteins. It also helps transport sodium and potassium across cell membranes and, through its effect on the secretion of parathyroid hormone, influences intracellular calcium levels.

Magnesium is measured to evaluate electrolyte status and assess neuromuscular or renal function. The serum magnesium test, a quantitative analysis, measures serum levels of magnesium, which is (after potassium) the most abundant intracellular cation.

Magnesium is necessary for protein production.

An absorbing topic

Most magnesium is found in bone and intracellular fluid; a small amount is found in extracellular fluid. Magnesium is absorbed by the small intestine and is excreted in the urine and feces.

What results mean

Normally, serum magnesium levels range from 1.3 to 2.1 mg/dl (SI, 0.65 to 1.05 mmol/L).

Rise from kidney compromise

Elevated serum magnesium levels (hypermagnesemia) that aren't caused by magnesium administration or ingestion most commonly occur in renal failure, when the kidneys excrete inadequate amounts of magnesium. Adrenal insufficiency (Addison's disease) can also elevate serum magnesium levels.

Need magnesium?

Decreased serum magnesium levels (hypomagnesemia) most commonly result from chronic alcoholism. Other causes include malabsorption syndrome, diabetic ketoacidosis, diarrhea, faulty absorption after bowel resection, prolonged bowel or gastric aspiration, acute pancreatitis, preeclampsia, primary aldosteronism, severe burns, hypercalcemic conditions (including hyperparathyroidism), and use of certain diuretics. (See *Magnesium test interference*.)

What needs to be done

• Tell the patient he shouldn't use magnesium salts, such as milk of magnesia and Epsom salts, for at least 3 days before the test.

Magnesium test interference

Several factors can alter magnesium levels:
• Excessive use of antacids or cathartics or excessive infusion of magnesium sulfate raises magnesium levels.
• Prolonged I.V. infusions without magnesium suppress levels. (Excessive use of diuretics decreases magnesium levels.)
• I.V. administration of calcium gluconate may falsely decrease serum magnesium levels.

• Perform a venipuncture (without a tourniquet, if possible) and collect the sample in a 7-ml clot-activator tube.
• Educate patients at risk for hypermagnesemia about antacids, laxatives, and mineral supplements that contain magnesium.

Myoglobin

Myoglobin, which is normally found in skeletal and cardiac muscle, functions as an oxygen-binding muscle protein. It's released into the bloodstream in ischemia, trauma, and inflammation of the muscle.

What results mean

Normal myoglobin values are 0 to 0.09 µg/ml (SI, 5 to 70 µ/L). In addition to occurring in MI, increased myoglobin levels may occur in acute alcohol intoxication, dermatomyositis, hypothermia (with prolonged shivering), muscular dystrophy, polymyositis, severe burn injuries, trauma, severe renal failure, and systemic lupus erythematosus. (See *Myoglobin test interference*.)

What needs to be done

• Expect to collect blood samples 4 to 8 hours after the onset of an acute MI.
• Tell the patient that the results of this test must be correlated with other tests for a definitive diagnosis.
• Perform a venipuncture and collect the sample in a 5-ml tube with no additives.
• Send the sample to the laboratory immediately.

Partial thromboplastin time

The partial thromboplastin time (PTT) test evaluates all of the clotting factors of the intrinsic pathway, except platelets, by measuring the time it takes a clot to form after adding calcium and phospholipid emulsion to a plasma sample. The PTT test also helps monitor a patient's response to heparin therapy.

What results mean

Normally, a fibrin clot forms 21 to 35 seconds (SI, 21 to 35 s) after the addition of reagents. For a patient on anticoagulant therapy, check with the attending doctor to find out the desirable values for the therapy being delivered.

Myoglobin test interference

Several factors can alter myoglobin test results:
• Radioactive scans performed within 1 week of the test may interfere with test results.
• Recent angina, cardioversion, or improper timing of the test may increase levels.
• An I.M. injection may cause a false-positive result.

May signal deficiency

Prolonged PTT may indicate a deficiency of certain plasma clotting factors, the presence of heparin, or the presence of fibrin split products, fibrinolysins, or circulating anticoagulants that are antibodies to specific clotting factors. (See *PTT test interference*.)

What needs to be done

• Tell the patient receiving heparin therapy that this test may be repeated at regular intervals to assess his response to treatment.
• Perform a venipuncture and collect the sample in a 7-ml tube with sodium citrate added.
• Completely fill the collection tube, invert it gently several times, and send it to the laboratory on ice.
• For a patient on anticoagulant therapy, additional pressure may be needed at the venipuncture site to control bleeding.

Phosphates

Phosphates are essential in the storage and utilization of energy, calcium regulation, RBC function, acid-base balance, bone formation, and metabolism of carbohydrates, protein, and fat. Tests for phosphates measure serum levels of phosphates, the dominant cellular anions.

Linked to calcium

The intestine absorbs a considerable amount of phosphates from dietary sources, but adequate levels of vitamin D are necessary for their absorption. The kidneys regulate phosphate excretion and retention. Because calcium and phosphates interact in a reciprocal relationship, urinary excretion of phosphates increases or decreases in inverse proportion to serum calcium levels.

Abnormal phosphate levels result more commonly from improper excretion than from abnormal ingestion or absorption from dietary sources.

What results mean

Normally, serum phosphate levels in adults range from 2.7 to 4.5 mg/dl (SI, 0.87 to 1.45 mmol/L). In children, the normal range is 4.5 to 6.7 mg/dl (SI, 1.45 to 1.78 mmol/L).

Leveling factor

Decreased phosphate levels (hypophosphatemia) may result from malnutrition, malabsorption syndromes, hyperparathyroidism, re-

---

PTT test interference

Several factors can alter PTT:
• Failure to use the proper anticoagulant, fill the collection tube completely, or mix the sample and the anticoagulant adequately may alter test results.
• Hemolysis may occur as a result of rough handling of the sample or excessive probing at the venipuncture site.
• Failure to send the sample to the laboratory immediately or place it on ice may alter test results.

nal tubular acidosis, or treatment of diabetic acidosis. In children, low phosphate levels can suppress normal growth.

Elevated phosphate levels (hyperphosphatemia) may result from skeletal disease, healing fractures, hypoparathyroidism, acromegaly, diabetic acidosis, high intestinal obstruction, and renal failure. Elevated phosphate levels are rarely clinically significant; however, if prolonged, they can alter bone metabolism by causing abnormal calcium phosphate deposits. (See *Phosphate test interference*.)

What needs to be done

• Perform a venipuncture (without a tourniquet, if possible) and collect the sample in a 7-ml clot-activator tube.

Platelet count

Platelets, or thrombocytes, are the smallest formed elements in the blood. Platelets promote coagulation by supplying phospholipids to the intrinsic clotting pathway, helping to form a hemostatic plug for vascular injuries.

The platelet count is one of the most important screening tests of platelet function. Accurate counts are vital for monitoring severe increases or decreases in the number of platelets in the blood. A platelet count that falls below 50,000/µl (SI, 50×10^9/L) can cause spontaneous bleeding; when the count drops below 5,000/µl (SI, 5×10^9/L), fatal CNS bleeding or massive GI hemorrhage is possible.

What results mean

A normal platelet count ranges from 140,000 to 400,000/µl (SI, 140 to 400×10^9/L) in adults and from 150,000 to 450,000/µl (SI, 150 to 450×10^9/L) in children.

Too many? Too few? What's a platelet to do?

An increased platelet count (thrombocytosis) can result from hemorrhage, infectious disorders, cancers, iron deficiency anemia, or inflammatory disease as well as from recent surgery, pregnancy, or splenectomy. In such cases, the platelet count returns to normal after the patient recovers from the primary disorder. However, the count remains high in primary thrombocytosis, myelofibrosis with myeloid metaplasia, polycythemia vera, and chronic myelogenous leukemia.

Phosphate test interference

Extended I.V. infusion of dextrose 5% in water, the use of phosphate-binding antacids, and the use of acetazolamide, insulin, and epinephrine may alter test results. In addition, excessive vitamin D intake and use of anabolic corticosteroids or androgens may elevate serum phosphate levels.

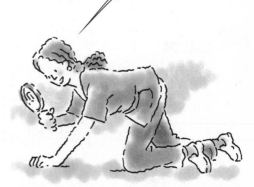

Platelets are the smallest formed elements in blood.

Platelet count test interference

Various conditions and activities can increase platelet count, including:
- excitement
- high altitudes
- persistent cold temperatures
- strenuous exercise.

Platelet count may decrease as a result of menstruation or use of drugs, including:
- acetazolamide
- acetohexamide
- antineoplastics
- brompheniramine maleate
- carbamazepine
- chloramphenicol
- ethacrynic acid
- furosemide
- gold salts
- indomethacin
- isoniazid
- mephenytoin
- oral diazoxide
- phenytoin
- salicylates
- thiazide and thiazide-like diuretics
- tricyclic antidepressants.

A decreased platelet count (thrombocytopenia) can result from aplastic (undeveloped) or hypoplastic (underdeveloped) bone marrow; infiltrative bone marrow disease, such as leukemia or disseminated infection; ineffective platelet development caused by folic acid or vitamin B_{12} deficiency; pooling of platelets in an enlarged spleen; increased platelet destruction caused by drugs or immune disorders; disseminated intravascular coagulation; or mechanical injury to platelets. (See *Platelet count test interference*.)

What needs to be done

- Perform a venipuncture and collect the sample in a 7-ml tube containing EDTA.
- Completely fill the collection tube, and invert it gently several times to adequately mix the sample and anticoagulant.

Potassium

Potassium is the major intracellular cation. The intracellular concentration of potassium is 150 to 160 mEq/L (SI, 150 to 160 mmol/L), and the extracellular concentration is 3.5 to 5 mEq/L (SI, 3.5 to 5 mmol/L). Evaluation of serum potassium measures the extracellular levels of this electrolyte.

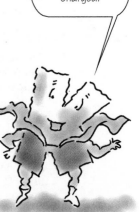

Potassium is the major intracellular cation. That means I'm positively charged!

Potassium is important in maintaining cellular electrical neutrality. The sodium-potassium active transport pump maintains the ratio of intracellular potassium to extracellular potassium, which determines the resting membrane potential necessary for nerve impulse transmission. Disturbances in this ratio alter cardiac rhythms, transmission and conduction of nerve impulses, and muscle contraction.

What results mean

Normally, serum potassium levels range from 3.5 to 5 mEq/L (SI, 3.5 to 5 mmol/L).

A mess of potassium...

Hyperkalemia (elevated potassium level) occurs with:
- acidosis
- burns
- crushing injuries
- decreased renal excretion
- diabetic ketoacidosis
- extensive surgery
- increased potassium intake
- infusion of stored whole blood
- insulin deficiency
- MI
- penicillin G
- renal failure
- replacement potassium
- shift in the concentration from intracellular to extracellular fluid.

...or less of potassium?

Hypokalemia (decreased potassium level) occurs with depletion of total body potassium caused by shifts from extracellular fluid to intracellular fluid. Depletion of total body potassium occurs with:
- diabetic ketoacidosis and insulin administration without potassium supplements
- diarrhea
- diuretics
- excessive aldosterone secretion
- excessive licorice ingestion
- gastric suctioning
- GI and renal disorders
- vomiting. (See *Potassium test interference.*)

Potassium test interference

The following factors may cause elevated potassium levels:
- repeated fist clenching before venipuncture
- excessive or rapid potassium infusion, spironolactone or penicillin G potassium therapy, or renal toxicity from administration of amphotericin B, methicillin, or tetracycline.

What needs to be done

• Perform a venipuncture and collect the sample in a 7-ml clot-activator tube.
• Draw the sample immediately after applying the tourniquet because a delay may elevate the potassium level by allowing intracellular potassium to leak into the serum.
• Educate patients at risk for hypokalemia about increasing dietary intake of potassium-rich foods.

Prostate-specific antigen

Until recently, digital rectal examination and measurement of prostatic acid phosphatase were the primary methods of monitoring the progression of prostate cancer. Now, measurement of prostate-specific antigen (PSA) helps track the course of this disease and evaluates response to treatment.

What results mean

Normal PSA values are:
• *ages 40 to 50:* 2 to 2.8 ng/ml (SI, 2 to 2.8 µg/L)
• *ages 51 to 60:* 2.9 to 3.8 ng/ml (SI, 2.9 to 3.8 µg/L)
• *ages 61 to 70:* 4 to 5.3 ng/ml (SI, 4 to 5.3 µg/L)
• *age 71 and older:* 5.6 to 7.2 ng/ml (SI, 5.6 to 7.2 µg/L).

About 80% of patients with prostate cancer have pretreatment PSA values greater than 4 ng/ml (SI, 4 µg/L). This percentage is higher in advanced stages and lower in early stages.

Not a solo act

PSA results alone shouldn't be considered diagnostic for prostate cancer because approximately 20% of patients with benign prostatic hyperplasia also have levels over 4 ng/ml. Further testing, including tissue biopsy and digital rectal examination, is needed to confirm a diagnosis of cancer. (See *PSA test interference.*)

What needs to be done

• Collect the sample before a digital rectal examination or at least 48 hours after one to avoid falsely elevated PSA levels.
• Perform a venipuncture and collect the sample in a 7-ml clot-activator tube.
• Send the sample, on ice, to the laboratory immediately.

PSA test interference

Excessive doses of chemotherapeutic drugs, such as cyclophosphamide, diethylstilbestrol, and methotrexate, may alter PSA test results.

Protein electrophoresis

Protein electrophoresis measures serum albumin and globulins, the major blood proteins, by separating the proteins into five distinct fractions: albumin and alpha$_1$, alpha$_2$, beta, and gamma globulins.

What results mean

Normal protein values are:
- *total serum protein:* 6.4 to 8.3 g/dl (SI, 64 to 83 g/L)
- *albumin:* 3.5 to 5 g/dl (SI, 35 to 50 g/L)
- *alpha$_1$-globulin:* 0.1 to 0.3 g/dl (SI, 1 to 3 g/L)
- *alpha$_2$-globulin:* 0.6 to 1 g/dl (SI, 6 to 10 g/L)
- *beta globulin:* 0.7 to 1.1 g/dl (SI, 7 to 11 g/L)
- *gamma globulin:* 0.8 to 1.6 g/dl (SI, 8 to 16 g/L). (See *Clinical implications of abnormal protein levels,* page 182, and *Protein electrophoresis test interference.*)

What needs to be done

- This test must be performed on a serum sample to avoid measuring the fibrinogen fraction. (The fibrinogen fraction, if present, would be indistinguishable from certain monoclonal gammopathies.)
- Perform a venipuncture and collect the sample in a 7-ml clot-activator tube.

Protein electrophoresis test interference

Pretest administration of a contrast agent falsely elevates protein test results.

Cytotoxic drug use and pregnancy can lower serum albumin levels.

Prothrombin time

Prothrombin, or factor II, is a plasma protein produced by the liver. The prothrombin time test (commonly known as *pro time,* or *PT*) measures the time required for a fibrin clot to form in a citrated plasma sample after the addition of calcium ions and tissue thromboplastin (factor III). It's an excellent screening procedure for overall evaluation of prothrombin, fibrinogen, and extrinsic coagulation factors V, VII, and X. PT and INR are the tests of choice for monitoring oral anticoagulant therapy.

What results mean

Normally, PT ranges from 10 to 14 seconds (SI, 10 to 14 s). In a patient receiving warfarin therapy, PT is usually maintained between 1½ and 2 times the normal control value. (See "International Normalized Ratio," page 168.)

Clinical implications of abnormal protein levels

Abnormal levels of albumin or globulins occur in many pathologic states, including those listed here.

Increased levels

Total proteins
- Dehydration
- Vomiting, diarrhea
- Diabetic acidosis
- Fulminating and chronic infections
- Multiple myeloma
- Monocytic leukemia
- Chronic inflammatory disease (such as rheumatoid arthritis or early-stage Laënnec's cirrhosis)

Albumin
- Multiple myeloma

Globulins
- Multiple myeloma
- Chronic syphilis
- Tuberculosis
- Subacute bacterial endocarditis
- Collagen diseases
- Systemic lupus erythematosus
- Rheumatoid arthritis
- Diabetes mellitus
- Hodgkin's disease

Decreased levels

Total proteins
- Malnutrition
- GI disease
- Blood dyscrasias
- Essential hypertension
- Hodgkin's disease
- Uncontrolled diabetes mellitus
- Malabsorption
- Hepatic dysfunction
- Toxemia of pregnancy
- Nephrosis
- Surgical and traumatic shock
- Severe burns
- Hemorrhage
- Hyperthyroidism
- Benzene and carbon tetrachloride poisoning
- Heart failure

Albumin
- Malnutrition
- Nephritis, nephrosis
- Diarrhea
- Plasma loss from burns
- Hepatic disease
- Hodgkin's disease
- Hypogammaglobulinemia
- Peptic ulcer
- Acute cholecystitis
- Sarcoidosis
- Collagen diseases
- Systemic lupus erythematosus
- Rheumatoid arthritis
- Essential hypertension
- Metastatic cancer
- Hyperthyroidism

Globulins
- Variable levels in neoplastic and renal diseases, hepatic dysfunction, and blood dyscrasias

PT test interference

The following drugs may shorten PT:
- antihistamines
- corticosteroids
- digoxin
- diuretics
- glutethimide
- progestin-estrogen combinations
- pyrazinamide
- vitamin K
- xanthines.

The following drugs may prolong PT:
- alcohol overuse
- administration of corticotropin
- anabolic steroids
- heparin I.V.
- indomethacin
- methimazole
- phenylbutazone
- phenytoin
- propylthiouracil
- quinidine
- thyroid hormones
- vitamin A.

I think it's gonna be a long, long time

Prolonged PT may indicate hepatic disease or deficiencies in fibrinogen, prothrombin, vitamin K, or factors V, VII, or X. (Specific assays can pinpoint such deficiencies.) Alternatively, it may result from ongoing oral anticoagulant therapy. Prolonged PT that exceeds 2½ times the control value is commonly associated with abnormal bleeding. (See *PT test interference*.)

What needs to be done

- Check the patient history for use of medications that may affect test results, such as vitamin K or antibiotics.
- Perform a venipuncture and collect the sample in a 7-ml siliconized tube.
- Completely fill the collection tube, and invert it gently several times to adequately mix the sample and anticoagulant. If the tube isn't filled to the correct volume, an excess of citrate appears in the sample.

We RBCs have quite a load to carry. RBC count helps assess the blood's oxygen-carrying capacity.

Red blood cell count

The RBC count helps assess the blood's oxygen-carrying capacity and can be useful in diagnosing anemia, protein deficiency, and dehydration. An RBC count, also known as an *erythrocyte count*, is used to find the number of RBCs in a microliter (cubic milliliter) of whole blood. RBCs are commonly counted with electronic devices, which provide fast, accurate results. The RBC count itself provides no information about the size, shape, or concentration of Hb within the cells, but it may be used to calculate two erythrocyte indices: mean corpuscular volume and mean corpuscular Hb.

What results mean

Normal RBC values vary depending on a number of factors. In adult males, the RBC count ranges from 4.5 to 5.5 million/µl (SI, 4.5 to 5.5×10^{12}/L) of venous blood; in adult females, the count ranges from 4 to 5 million/µl (SI, 4 to 5×10^{12}/L) of venous blood; and, in children, from 4.6 to 4.8 million/µl (SI, 4.6 to 4.8×10^{12}/L) of venous blood. In full-term neonates, values range from 4.4 to 5.8 million/µl (SI, 4.4 to 5.8×10^{12}/L) of capillary blood at birth, fall to 3 to 3.8 million/µl (SI, 3 to 3.8×10^{12}/L) at age 2 months, and increase slowly thereafter. Values are also generally higher in people living at high altitudes.

Ups and downs

An elevated RBC count may indicate absolute or relative polycythemia. A depressed count may indicate anemia, fluid overload, or hemorrhage lasting more than 24 hours. (See *RBC test interference*.)

What needs to be done

• For adults and older children, draw venous blood into a 7-ml tube containing EDTA. For younger children, collect capillary blood in a microcollection device.
• Completely fill the collection tube, and invert it gently several times to mix the sample and anticoagulant.

Red cell indices

There are three main red cell indices, which are ascertained through the use of other blood tests. Using the results of the RBC count, HCT, and total Hb test, the red cell indices (also known as *erythrocyte indices*) provide important information about Hb concentration and weight and the size of an average RBC. The red cell indices include:
• mean corpuscular volume (MCV)
• mean corpuscular Hb (MCH)
• mean corpuscular Hb concentration (MCHC).

RBC test interference

A high white blood cell count falsely elevates the RBC count in semi-automated and automated counters.

Diseases that cause RBCs to clump, such as sickle cell anemia, lead to a falsely decreased RBC count.

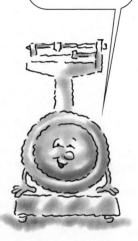

RBC indices can help you obtain important information about the size and weight of RBCs.

Eyes on the size

MCV, the ratio of HCT (packed cell volume) to the RBC count, expresses the average size of the erythrocytes and indicates whether they're undersized (microcytic), oversized (macrocytic), or normal (normocytic).

A weighty issue

MCH, the ratio of Hb weight to the RBC count, gives the weight of Hb in an average RBC.

Rating the ratio

MCHC, the ratio of Hb weight to HCT, defines the Hb concentration in 100 ml of packed RBCs. It helps distinguish normally colored (normochromic) RBCs from paler (hypochromic) RBCs.

What results mean

The range of normal red cell indices is as follows:
- *MCV:* 82 to 98 mm^3 (SI, 82 to 98 fl)
- *MCH:* 26 to 34 pg (SI, 26 to 34 pg)
- *MCHC:* 31 to 37 g/dl (SI, 310 to 370 g/L).

Anemia exposé

The red cell indices help classify anemias. Low MCV and MCHC indicate microcytic, hypochromic anemias caused by iron deficiency anemia, pyridoxine-responsive anemia, or thalassemia. A high MCV suggests macrocytic anemias caused by megaloblastic anemias that are, in turn, caused by folic acid or vitamin B_{12} deficiency, inherited disorders of deoxyribonucleic acid synthesis, or reticulocytosis.

Because MCV reflects the average volume of many cells, a value within the normal range can encompass RBCs of varying size, from microcytic to macrocytic. (See *Red cell indices test interference.*)

What needs to be done

- Perform a venipuncture and collect the sample in a 7-ml tube containing EDTA.
- Completely fill the collection tube, and invert it gently several times to adequately mix the sample and anticoagulant.

Red cell indices test interference

Several factors can alter red cell indices test results:
- Falsely elevated RBC count caused by a high white blood cell count in semiautomated and automated counters invalidates MCV and MCH results.
- Falsely elevated Hb values invalidate MCH and MCHC results.
- Diseases that cause RBCs to clump together falsely decrease RBC count.

Sodium

The serum sodium test measures serum levels of sodium, the major extracellular cation. Sodium affects body water distribution, maintains osmotic pressure of extracellular fluid, and helps promote neuromuscular function; it also helps maintain acid-base balance and influences chloride and potassium levels. Sodium is absorbed by the kidneys; a small amount is lost through the skin.

> Sodium imbalance can result from a change in water volume.

Relationship with water

Serum sodium levels are evaluated in relation to the amount of water in the body, which is affected by the cellular mechanics of sodium (decreased sodium levels promote water excretion, and increased levels promote retention). For example, a sodium deficit (hyponatremia) refers to a decreased level of sodium in relation to the body's water level.

What results mean

Normally, serum sodium levels range from 135 to 145 mEq/L (SI, 135 to 145 mmol/L). Sodium imbalance can result from a loss or gain of sodium or from a change in water volume. Remember, serum sodium results must be interpreted in light of the patient's state of hydration.

When it's high

Elevated serum sodium levels (hypernatremia) may be caused by inadequate water intake, water loss that exceeds sodium loss (as in diabetes insipidus, impaired renal function, prolonged hyperventilation and, occasionally, severe vomiting or diarrhea), and sodium retention (as in aldosteronism). Hypernatremia can also result from excessive sodium intake.

When it's low

Abnormally low serum sodium levels (hyponatremia) may result from inadequate sodium intake or excessive sodium loss caused by profuse sweating, GI suctioning, diuretic therapy, diarrhea, vomiting, adrenal insufficiency, burns, or chronic renal insufficiency with acidosis. Urine sodium determinations are commonly more sensitive to early changes in sodium balance and should always be evaluated simultaneously with serum sodium findings. (See *Sodium test interference.*)

What needs to be done

• Perform a venipuncture and collect the sample in a 7-ml clot-activator tube.

Sodium test interference

Sodium test results can be affected by certain drugs:
• Most diuretics, lithium, chlorpropamide, and vasopressin suppress serum sodium levels.
• Corticosteroids and antihypertensives (such as methyldopa, hydralazine, and reserpine) elevate serum sodium levels.

Thyroid-stimulating hormone

Thyroid-stimulating hormone (TSH) is a protein secreted by the anterior pituitary. It stimulates an increase in the size, number, and secretory activity of thyroid cells; heightens iodine "pump" activity, commonly raising the ratio of intracellular to extracellular iodine as much as 350:1; and stimulates the release of triiodothyronine (T_3) and thyroxine (T_4). These hormones affect total body metabolism and are essential for normal growth and development.

Gettin' hip to hypothyroidism

This test, also known as the *serum thyrotropin test*, measures serum TSH levels by immunoassay. It can detect primary hypothyroidism and can determine whether it results from thyroid gland failure or from pituitary or hypothalamic dysfunction. Normal serum TSH levels rule out primary hypothyroidism. This test may not distinguish between low-normal and subnormal levels, especially in secondary hypothyroidism.

The thyrotropin-releasing hormone (TRH) challenge test evaluates thyroid function and can be performed after a baseline TSH reading has been obtained.

What results mean

Normal values for adults and children range from undetectable to 15 µIU/ml (SI, 15 mU/L). TSH levels that exceed 20 µIU/ml (SI, 20 mU/L) suggest primary hypothyroidism or, possibly, an endemic goiter (associated with dietary iodine deficiency). TSH levels may be slightly elevated in patients with normal thyroid function who have thyroid cancer.

Low TSH

Low or undetectable TSH levels may be normal but may occasionally indicate secondary hypothyroidism. Low TSH levels may also result from hyperthyroidism (Graves' disease) or thyroiditis. Testing with thyrotropin-releasing hormone is necessary to confirm the diagnosis. (See *TRH challenge test*, page 188, and *TSH test interference*, page 188.)

What needs to be done

• Keep the patient relaxed and recumbent for 30 minutes before the test.
• As ordered, withhold steroids, thyroid hormones, aspirin, and other drugs that may influence test results. If these medications must be continued, note this on the laboratory request.

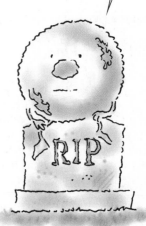

The TRH challenge test is a reliable indicator of Graves' disease.

TRH challenge test

The thyrotropin-releasing hormone (TRH) challenge test, which evaluates thyroid function and is the first direct test of pituitary reserve, is a reliable diagnostic tool for thyrotoxicosis (Graves' disease). The test requires an injection of TRH. Here's how the test is performed:

• Perform a venipuncture to obtain a baseline thyroid-stimulating hormone (TSH) reading.
• Administer synthetic TRH (protirelin) by I.V. bolus.
• Draw samples of 5 ml each at 5, 10, 15, 20, and 60 minutes after the TRH injection. (To facilitate blood collection, a saline lock catheter can be used.)

The results

A sudden spike above the baseline TSH reading indicates a normally functioning pituitary but suggests hypothalamic dysfunction. If the TSH level fails to rise or remains undetectable, pituitary failure is likely. With thyrotoxicosis and thyroiditis, TSH levels fail to rise when challenged by TRH.

TSH test interference

Failure to observe pretest restrictions may alter results.

• Between 6 a.m. and 8 a.m., perform a venipuncture, collect the sample in a 5-ml clot-activator tube, and send it to the laboratory immediately.

Thyroxine

T_4 is an amine secreted by the thyroid gland in response to TSH from the pituitary and, indirectly, to TRH from the hypothalamus. The rate of secretion is normally regulated by a complex system of negative and positive feedback involving three glands: the thyroid, anterior pituitary, and hypothalamus. The suspected precursor, or *prohormone*, of T_3 is T_4, which is converted to T_3 mainly in the liver and kidneys.

The T_4 that binds

Only a fraction of T_4 (about 0.3%) circulates freely in the blood; the rest binds strongly to plasma proteins, primarily to thyroxine-binding globulin (TBG). This minute fraction of free-circulating T_4 is responsible for the clinical effects of thyroid hormone. TBG binds so tenaciously that T_4 survives in the plasma for a relatively long time, with a half-life of about 6 days. This test measures the total circulating T_4 level when TBG is normal.

What results mean

Normal total T_4 levels range from 5 to 13.5 µg/dl (SI, 60 to 165 nmol/L). Normal T_4 levels don't guarantee normal thyroid functioning; for example, normal readings occur in T_3 thyrotoxicosis.

Abnormally elevated levels of T_4 are consistent with primary and secondary hyperthyroidism, including excessive T_4 (levothyroxine) replacement therapy. Subnormal levels of T_4 suggest primary or secondary hypothyroidism or T_4 suppression by normal, elevated, or replacement levels of T_3. Overt signs of hyperthyroidism require further testing and, in cases where hypothyroidism is unlikely, the TSH or TRH test may be indicated. (See *Thyroxine test interference.*)

What needs to be done

• As ordered, withhold any medications that may interfere with test results. If these medications must be continued, note this on the laboratory request. (If this test is being performed to monitor thyroid therapy, the patient continues to receive daily thyroid supplements.)
• Perform a venipuncture, collect the sample in a 7-ml clot-activator tube, and send the sample to the laboratory immediately.

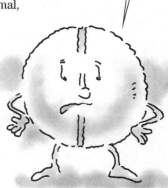

Always be sure to withhold any medications that may interfere with diagnostic test results.

Thyroxine, free, and free triiodothyronine

These tests measure serum levels of free thyroxine (FT_4) and free triiodothyronine (FT_3), the minute portions of T_4 and T_3 not bound to TBG, as well as other serum proteins.

Boundless hormones

As the active components of T_4 and T_3, these unbound hormones enter target cells and are responsible for the thyroid's effects on cellular metabolism. Measurement of free hormone levels is the best indicator of thyroid function because levels of circulating FT_4 and FT_3 are regulated by a feedback mechanism that compensates for changes in binding protein concentrations by adjusting total hormone levels. Of the two tests, FT_3 is the better indicator. This test may be useful for the 5% of patients in whom the standard T_3 or T_4 tests fail to produce diagnostic results.

Thyroxine test interference

Several factors can alter thyroxine test results:
• Estrogens, progestins, levothyroxine, and methadone increase T_4 levels.
• Free fatty acids, heparin, iodides, liothyronine sodium, lithium, phenytoin, propylthiouracil, salicylates (high doses), steroids, sulfonamides, and sulfonylureas decrease T_4.
• Clofibrate can increase or decrease T_4.

What results mean

Normal range for FT_4 is 0.9 to 2.3 ng/dl (SI, 10 to 30 nmol/L); for FT_3, 0.2 to 0.6 ng/dl (SI, 0.003 to 0.009 nmol/L). Values vary depending on the laboratory.

High TSH time

Elevated FT_4 and FT_3 levels typically indicate hyperthyroidism. A distinct form of hyperthyroidism called *T_3 toxicosis* yields high FT_3 levels with normal or low FT_4 values. Low FT_4 levels usually indicate hypothyroidism, except in patients receiving replacement therapy with T_3. Patients receiving thyroid hormone replacement therapy may have varying levels of FT_4 and FT_3, depending on the preparation used and the time of sample collection. (See *FT_3 and T_3 test interference*.)

What needs to be done

Perform a venipuncture, collect the sample in a 7-ml clot-activator tube, and send it to the laboratory immediately.

Triiodothyronine

This highly specific immunoassay measures total serum content of T_3 to investigate clinical indications of thyroid dysfunction. The more potent thyroid hormone, T_3 is derived primarily from T_4. At least 50% and as much as 90% of T_3 is thought to be derived from T_4. The remaining 10% or more is secreted directly by the thyroid gland. Like T_4 secretion, T_3 secretion occurs in response to TSH released by the pituitary and, secondarily, to TRH from the hypothalamus.

This test aids in the diagnosis of T_3 toxicosis, helps diagnose hypothyroidism or hyperthyroidism, and helps monitor the course of thyroid replacement therapy.

T_3 versus T_4

Although T_3 is present in the bloodstream in minute quantities and is metabolically active for only a short time, its impact on body metabolism dominates that of T_4. T_3 binds less firmly to TBG and, therefore, persists in the bloodstream for a short time — half of it disappears in about 1 day — whereas half of T_4 disappears in 6 days.

FT_3 and T_3 test interference

Depending on the dosage, thyroid medication may increase levels. However, these medications shouldn't be withheld.

What results mean

Normally, serum T_3 levels range from 80 to 200 ng/dl (SI, 1.2 to 3 nmol/L). Serum T_3 and T_4 levels usually rise and fall in tandem. However, in T_3 toxicosis, only T_3 levels rise, while total and free T_4 levels remain normal. T_3 toxicosis occurs in patients with Graves' disease, toxic adenoma, or toxic nodular goiter. T_3 levels also surpass T_4 levels in patients receiving thyroid replacement containing more T_3 than T_4. In iodine-deficient areas, the thyroid may produce larger amounts of the more cellularly active T_3 than T_4 in an effort to maintain the euthyroid state.

On the levels

Generally, T_3 levels appear to be a more accurate diagnostic indicator of hyperthyroidism than T_4 levels. Although hyperthyroidism increases T_3 and T_4 levels in about 90% of patients, it causes a disproportionate increase in T_3. In some patients with hypothyroidism, T_3 levels may fall within the normal range and may not be sufficient for diagnosis.

In pregnant patients, it's normal to see a rise in serum T_3 levels. Low T_3 levels may appear in euthyroid patients with systemic illness, during severe acute illness, or after trauma or major surgery; in such patients, however, TSH levels are within normal limits. Low serum T_3 levels are also sometimes found in euthyroid patients with malnutrition. (See *T_3 test interference*.)

> It's normal to see a rise in serum T_3 levels in pregnant patients.

What needs to be done

• As ordered, withhold medications that may influence thyroid function, such as steroids, propranolol, and cholestyramine. If such medications must be continued, record this information on the laboratory request.
• Perform a venipuncture, collect the sample in a 7-ml clot-activator tube, and send it to the laboratory immediately.
• If a patient must receive thyroid preparations, such as T_3 (liothyronine), note the time of drug administration on the laboratory request.

Triiodothyronine uptake

The T_3 uptake test measures FT_4 levels. It does so indirectly by demonstrating the availability of serum protein-binding sites for T_4. The results of T_3 uptake are commonly combined with a T_4 radioimmunoassay or T_4 (D) (competitive protein-binding) test to

T_3 test interference

Several factors can alter T_3 test results:
• Heparin, iodides, lithium, methimazole, phenylbutazone, phenytoin, propranolol, salicylates, steroids, and sulfonamides may alter results.
• Markedly increased or decreased TBG levels, regardless of cause, may interfere with accuracy of test results.
• Clofibrate, estrogen, liothyronine sodium, methadone, and progestins may alter results.

determine the FT_4 index, a mathematical calculation that's thought to reflect FT_4 by correcting for TBG abnormalities. The T_3 uptake test has become less popular recently because rapid tests for T_3, T_4, and TSH are readily available.

What results mean

Normal T_3 uptake values are 25% to 35%. In primary thyroid disease, T_3 uptake and T_4 uptake vary in the same direction: A high T_3 uptake percentage in the presence of elevated T_4 levels indicates hyperthyroidism. A low uptake percentage together with low T_4 levels indicates hypothyroidism.

Reading the variance

Abnormality of TBG is suggested when the variance in T_3 and T_4 uptake is conflicting. For example, a high T_3 uptake percentage with a low or normal FT_4 level suggests decreased TBG levels. Such decreased levels may result from protein loss (as in nephrotic syndrome), decreased production (because of androgen excess or genetic or idiopathic causes), or competition for T_4-binding sites by certain drugs (salicylates, phenylbutazone, and phenytoin).

Conversely, a low T_3 uptake percentage with a high or normal FT_4 level suggests increased TBG levels. Such increased levels may be caused by supplemental estrogen or estrogen produced by the body (pregnancy), or they may result from unknown causes. Thus, in primary disorders of TBG levels, measured T_4 and free sites change in the same direction. (See *T_3 uptake test interference.*)

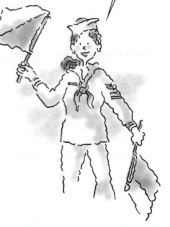

In primary disorders of TBG levels, measured T_4 and free sites change in the same direction.

What needs to be done

• Withhold medications, such as estrogens, androgens, phenytoin, salicylates, and thyroid preparations, that may interfere with test results. If they must be continued, note this on the laboratory request.
• Perform a venipuncture, collect the sample in a 7-ml clot-activator tube, and send it to the laboratory immediately.

Triglycerides, serum

Serum triglyceride testing provides quantitative analysis of triglycerides, the main storage form of lipids, which constitute about 95% of fatty tissue. Although not in itself diagnostic, serum triglyceride analysis permits early identification of hyperlipidemia (characteristic in nephrotic syndrome and other conditions) and determination of the risk of CAD.

T_3 uptake test interference

Markedly increased or decreased TBG levels, regardless of cause, can alter test results. Drugs such as steroids, clofibrate, and propranolol can also alter test results.

What results mean

Triglyceride values are age- and sex-related. Some controversy exists over the most appropriate normal ranges. Nonetheless, serum values of 40 to 180 mg/dl (SI, 0.11 to 2.01 mmol/L) for adult men and 10 to 190 mg/dl (SI, 0.11 to 2.21 mmol/L) for adult women are widely accepted.

Increased or decreased serum triglyceride levels merely suggest a clinical abnormality; additional tests are required for a definitive diagnosis. For example, measurement of cholesterol may also be necessary because cholesterol and triglyceride levels vary independently. High levels of triglyceride and cholesterol reflect an increased risk of CAD.

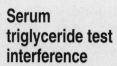

Remember that serum triglyceride levels vary by age and sex.

Increased levels: Mild, moderate, and severe

A mild to moderate increase in serum triglyceride levels may indicate biliary obstruction, diabetes, nephrotic syndrome, endocrine disorders, or overconsumption of alcohol. Diet changes and, possibly, drug therapy are recommended for patients whose fasting triglyceride level exceeds 500 mg/dl (SI, 5.46 mmol/L). The patient should start on a cardiac step 1 diet. Fish oils may also be used to lower triglyceride levels. Markedly increased levels without an identifiable cause reflect congenital hyperlipoproteinemia and necessitate lipoprotein phenotyping to confirm the diagnosis. Severe elevations (greater than 1,000 mg/dl [SI, greater than 11.29 mmol/L]) have a significant association with abdominal pain and pancreatitis.

In familial hypertriglyceridemia, patients may exhibit signs, such as eruptive xanthomas (slightly elevated, soft, rounded plaque, usually on the eyelid), corneal arcus (opaque, white ring about the periphery of the cornea), xanthelasma (yellowish tumor found on the eyelids), and lipemia retinalis (a condition in which retinal vessels appear reddish white or white).

Decreased levels

Decreased serum levels are rare, occurring mainly in malnutrition or abetalipoproteinemia (a rare inherited disease characterized by defective apoprotein B synthesis). In the latter, serum is virtually devoid of beta-lipoproteins and triglycerides because the body lacks the capacity to transport preformed triglycerides from the epithelial cells of the intestinal mucosa or from the liver. (See *Serum triglyceride test interference*.)

What needs to be done

• Be sure to inform the doctor if the patient has an acute illness, infection, fever, or other acute problem that might interfere with the laboratory result.

Serum triglyceride test interference

Long-term use of corticosteroids increases triglyceride levels, as do hormonal contraceptives, estrogen, ethyl alcohol, furosemide, and miconazole. Cholestyramine and colestipol hydrochloride may raise triglyceride levels. Alcohol ingestion within 24 hours of the test may also cause elevated triglyceride levels.

Clofibrate, dextrothyroxine, gemfibrozil, and niacin lower triglyceride levels.

- Because triglycerides are highly affected by a fat-containing meal, with levels rising and peaking 4 hours after ingesting a meal, tell the patient that he should abstain from food for 10 to 14 hours before the test and from alcohol for 24 hours but that he may drink water.
- Have the patient sit for 5 minutes before drawing blood.
- Perform a venipuncture, collect a sample in a 7-ml tube containing EDTA, and send the sample to the laboratory immediately.
- Avoid prolonged venous occlusion. Remove the tourniquet within 1 minute of application.

Troponin I and cardiac troponin T

Troponin I and cardiac troponin T are proteins in the striated cells, part of the calcium-binding complex of the thin myofilaments of myocardial tissue.

Troponins mark the spot

Troponins are extremely specific markers of cardiac damage. When injury occurs to the myocardial tissue, these proteins are released into the bloodstream, increasing from normally undetectable blood levels to levels of more than 50 µg/L (SI, 50 µg/L). Elevations in troponin levels can be seen within 1 hour of MI and will persist for 1 week or longer, making this a useful diagnostic tool.

What results mean

Laboratories may give varying results, with some calling a cardiac troponin test positive if it shows any detectable levels and others giving a range for abnormal results.

A gray zone

Normally, troponin I levels are less than 0.35 µg/L (SI, less than 0.35 µg/L). Cardiac troponin T levels are less than 0.1 µg/L (SI, less than 0.1 µg/L). Troponin I levels between 0 and 0.4 µg/L (SI, between 0 and 0.4 µg/L) don't suggest cardiac injury, and levels from 0.5 to 1.9 µg/L (SI, from 0.5 to 1.9 µg/L) are indeterminate for cardiac injury.

A hurtin' heart

Troponin I levels greater than 2 µg/L (SI, greater than 2 µg/L) suggest cardiac injury. Results of a qualitative cardiac troponin T rapid immunoassay that are greater than 0.2 µg/L (SI, greater than 0.2 µg/L) are considered positive for cardiac injury. When quantitative serum assays for cardiac troponin T are done, the upper limit for normal is 0.1 µg/L (SI, 0.1 µg/L). As long as tissue injury contin-

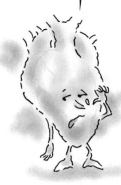

As long as tissue injury continues, troponin levels will remain high.

ues, the troponin levels will remain high. Troponin levels rise rapidly and are detectable within 1 hour of myocardial cell injury. Troponin I levels aren't detectable in people without cardiac injury. (See *Cardiac troponin test interference*.)

What needs to be done

• Tell the patient that this test helps assess myocardial injury and that multiple samples may be drawn to detect fluctuations in serum levels.
• Obtain each sample on schedule, and note the date and collection time on each.
• Perform a venipuncture and collect the sample in a 7-ml clot-activator tube.

Uric acid

Used primarily to detect gout, the uric acid test measures serum levels of uric acid, the major end metabolite of purine. Purine is a nitrogen-containing compound produced in the digestion of certain dietary proteins.

What results mean

Uric acid concentrations in men normally range from 3.4 to 7 mg/dl (SI, 202 to 416 µmol/L); in women, from 2.3 to 6 mg/dl (SI, 143 to 357 µmol/L).

The lowdown on levels

Increased serum uric acid levels may indicate gout or impaired renal function; however, levels don't correlate with the severity of disease. Levels may also rise in heart failure, glycogen storage disease (type I, von Gierke's disease), infections, hemolytic or sickle cell anemia, polycythemia, neoplasms, and psoriasis.

Depressed uric acid levels may indicate defective tubular absorption (as in Fanconi's syndrome and Wilson's disease) or acute hepatic atrophy. (See *Uric acid test interference*.)

What needs to be done

• Tell the patient that he must fast for 8 hours before the test.
• Perform a venipuncture and collect the sample in a 7-ml clot-activator tube.

Cardiac troponin test interference

Sustained vigorous exercise may increase troponin T levels in the absence of significant cardiac damage associated with noncardiac specific troponin T found in these skeletal muscles. Cardiotoxic drugs such as doxorubicin may also increase levels of troponin T.

Uric acid test interference

Several factors can alter uric acid test results:
• Starvation, a high-purine diet, stress, alcohol abuse, loop diuretics, ethambutol, vincristine, pyrazinamide, thiazides, and low aspirin doses may raise levels.
• Acetaminophen, ascorbic acid, and levodopa may cause false elevations.
• High aspirin doses may decrease levels.

Urinalysis

Routine urinalysis serves many functions. It can be used to screen patients for kidney and urinary tract disease and can help detect metabolic or systemic disease.

During the course of a routine urinalysis, you'll:
- evaluate the color, odor, and opacity of urine
- determine urine's specific gravity and pH

Normal findings in routine urinalysis

The table below lists the elements evaluated in urinalysis along with their normal findings.

Element	Findings
Macroscopic	
Color	Straw to dark yellow
Odor	Slightly aromatic
Appearance	Clear
Specific gravity	1.005 to 1.035
pH	4.5 to 8.0
Protein	None
Glucose	None
Ketones	None
Bilirubin	None
Urobilinogen	Normal
Hemoglobin	None
Red blood cells (RBCs)	None
Nitrite (bacteria)	None
White blood cells (WBCs)	None
Microscopic	
RBCs	0 to 2 per high-power field
WBCs	0 to 5 per high-power field
Epithelial cells	0 to 5 per high-power field
Casts	None, except 1 to 2 hyaline casts per low-power field
Crystals	Present
Bacteria	None
Yeast cells	None
Parasites	None

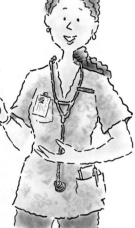

You're in for a treat. This chart lists normal findings in routine urinalysis.

- detect and measure protein, glucose, and ketone bodies
- examine urine sediment for blood cells, casts, and crystals.

What results mean

Results of urine tests are based on the elements that make up urine. Even with normal findings, these elements have certain characteristics. (See *Normal findings in routine urinalysis*.)

Pondering the pathologic

Abnormal findings show an alteration in the normal characteristics of urine. The following abnormal findings typically suggest a pathologic condition:

- *color change*—from diet, drugs, or disease
- *unusual odor*—due to ketone bodies, infection, or disease
- *turbidity* (cloudiness)—from kidney infection
- *low specific gravity* (less than 1.005)—from diabetes insipidus, acute tubular necrosis, or pyelonephritis
- *fixed specific gravity* (1.010 regardless of fluid intake)—from chronic glomerulonephritis with severe kidney damage
- *high specific gravity* (greater than 1.035)—from nephrotic syndrome, dehydration, acute glomerulonephritis, heart failure, liver failure, or shock
- *high pH* (alkaline urine)—from Fanconi's syndrome, urinary tract infection, or metabolic or respiratory alkalosis
- *low pH* (acidic urine)—from renal tuberculosis, pyrexia, phenylketonuria, alkaptonuria, or acidosis
- *proteinuria* (excess serum proteins in urine)—from renal failure or, possibly, multiple myeloma
- *sugars in urine*—usually from diabetes mellitus but possibly from pheochromocytoma (brain tumor), Cushing's syndrome, impaired tubular reabsorption, advanced kidney disease, increased intracranial pressure, or I.V. solutions containing glucose and total parenteral nutrition containing from 10% to 50% glucose
- *ketone bodies* (used as fuel by muscle and brain tissue)—from diabetes mellitus, starvation, pregnancy and lactation, or diarrhea or vomiting
- *bilirubin*—from liver disease or fibrosis of the biliary canaliculi (as in cirrhosis)
- *increased urobilinogen*—liver damage, hemolytic disease, or severe infection
- *decreased urobilinogen*—biliary obstruction, inflammatory disease, antimicrobial therapy, severe diarrhea, or renal insufficiency
- *blood cells*—infection, obstruction, inflammation, trauma, tumors, or other causes, such as low platelet count and surgery
- *excessive casts*—renal disease
- *calcium oxalate crystals*—hypercalcemia

- *cystine crystals* — inborn error of metabolism
- *bacteria, yeast cells, parasites* — genitourinary tract infection or contamination of external genitalia. (See *Urinalysis test interference.*)

What needs to be done

- Tell the patient to avoid stress and strenuous exercise before the test.
- Check for drugs that influence urinalysis.
- Collect a random urine specimen of at least 15 ml, preferably a first-voided morning specimen.
- If the patient is being evaluated for renal colic, strain the specimen to catch stones or stone fragments.
- Refrigerate the specimen if analysis will be delayed.

White blood cell count

The white blood cell (WBC), or *leukocyte,* count measures the number of WBCs in a microliter of whole blood. This measurement is done using electronic devices. A WBC count can be useful in diagnosing infection and inflammation as well as monitoring a patient's response to chemotherapy or radiation therapy. WBC counts can also help determine whether further tests are needed.

Counter culture

WBC counts can vary depending on a number of factors. On any given day, counts may vary by as much as 2,000 cells/μl (SI, 2 × 10^9/L) because of the effects of stress, strenuous exercise, or other factors. The count can also rise or fall significantly with certain diseases.

A WBC count is useful for diagnosing the severity of a disease process. However, the WBC differential gives more specific information about which type of WBC is being affected and is, therefore, more diagnostically useful.

What results mean

The WBC count normally ranges from 4,000 to 10,000/μl (SI, 4 to 10 × 10^9/L).

Serious numbers

An elevated WBC count (leukocytosis) commonly signals infection, such as an abscess, meningitis, appendicitis, or tonsillitis. A high count may also indicate leukemia or tissue necrosis caused by burns, MI, or gangrene.

Urinalysis test interference

Several factors can alter urinalysis results:
- Strenuous exercise before routine urinalysis may cause transient myoglobulinuria.
- Insufficient urinary volume (less than 2 ml) may limit the range of procedures.
- Failure to send the specimen to the laboratory immediately after the urine is collected may falsely lower urobilinogen.
- Foods, such as beets, berries, and rhubarb, may falsely change urine color.
- Highly dilute urine, as in diabetes insipidus, may alter results.
- Blood present from menstrual flow may falsely change color and reveal RBCs.

A low WBC count (leukopenia) indicates bone marrow depression, which may result from viral infections or toxic reactions, such as those following treatment with antineoplastics, ingestion of mercury or other heavy metals, or exposure to benzene or arsenicals. Leukopenia also accompanies influenza, typhoid fever, measles, infectious hepatitis, mononucleosis, and rubella. (See *WBC count interference.*)

What needs to be done
• Tell the patient that he should avoid strenuous exercise for 24 hours before the test to avoid altered readings and that he should also avoid ingesting a large meal before the test.
• Perform a venipuncture and collect the sample in a 7-ml tube containing EDTA.
• Completely fill the sample collection tube, and invert it gently several times to adequately mix the sample and anticoagulant.

White blood cell differential

A WBC differential can provide more specific information about a patient's immune system. In a WBC differential, the laboratory classifies 100 or more WBCs in a stained film of blood according to five major types of leukocytes — neutrophils, eosinophils, basophils, lymphocytes, and monocytes — and determines the percentage of each type.

Relatively speaking

The differential count is the relative number of each type of WBC in the blood. Multiply the percentage value of each type by the total WBC count to obtain the absolute number of each type of WBC.

What results mean
Here are the normal percentages of each WBC type in adults:
• *neutrophils* — 54% to 75% (SI, 0.54 to 0.75)
• *eosinophils* — 1% to 4% (SI, 0.01 to 0.04)
• *basophils* — 0% to 1% (SI, 0 to 0.01)
• *monocytes* — 2% to 8% (SI, 0.02 to 0.08)
• *lymphocytes* — 25% to 40% (SI, 0.25 to 0.40).

It depends

Abnormally high WBC levels are associated with allergic reactions and parasitic infections. When the normal values for the patient have been determined, an assessment can be made.

WBC count interference

Exercise, stress, or digestion may interfere with test results, making them inaccurate.

Most antineoplastics, anti-infectives (such as metronidazole and flucytosine), anticonvulsants (such as phenytoin derivatives), thyroid hormone antagonists, and nonsteroidal anti-inflammatory drugs (such as indomethacin) can decrease levels.

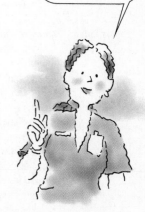

WBC differential counts must always be considered in relation to the patient's total WBC count.

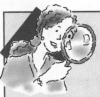

A closer look

How disease affects WBC differential values

White blood cell (WBC) differential aids diagnosis because some disorders affect only one WBC type. Below, each cell type is listed with its corresponding effect and causes.

Cell type	How affected
Neutrophils	**Increases count** • Infections: osteomyelitis, otitis media, septicemia, gonorrhea, endocarditis, chickenpox, herpes • Ischemic necrosis caused by myocardial infarction, burns, cancer • Metabolic disorders: diabetic acidosis, eclampsia, uremia, thyrotoxicosis • Stress response • Inflammatory diseases: rheumatic fever, rheumatoid arthritis, acute gout, vasculitis, myositis **Decreases count** • Bone marrow depression caused by radiation or cytotoxic drugs • Infections: typhoid, hepatitis, influenza, measles, mumps, rubella, infectious mononucleosis • Hypersplenism: hepatic disease and storage diseases • Collagen vascular diseases such as systemic lupus erythematosus • Deficiency of folic acid or vitamin B_{12}
Eosinophils	**Increases count** • Allergic disorders: asthma, hay fever, food or drug sensitivity, serum sickness, angioneurotic edema • Parasitic infections: trichinosis, hookworm, roundworm, amebiasis • Skin diseases: eczema, pemphigus, psoriasis, dermatitis, herpes simplex • Neoplastic diseases: chronic myelocytic leukemia, Hodgkin's disease, metastasis **Decreases count** • Stress response • Cushing's syndrome

Cell type	How affected
Basophils	**Increases count** • Chronic myelocytic leukemia, Hodgkin's disease, ulcerative colitis, chronic hypersensitivity states **Decreases count** • Hyperthyroidism, ovulation, pregnancy, stress
Lymphocytes	**Increases count** • Infections: tuberculosis, hepatitis, infectious mononucleosis, mumps, rubella, cytomegalovirus • Thyrotoxicosis, hypoadrenalism, ulcerative colitis, immune diseases, lymphocytic leukemia **Decreases count** • Severe debilitating illnesses: heart failure, renal failure, advanced tuberculosis • Defective lymphatic circulation, high levels of adrenal corticosteroids, immunodeficiency
Monocytes	**Increases count** • Infections: subacute bacterial endocarditis, tuberculosis, hepatitis, malaria • Collagen vascular diseases: systemic lupus erythematosus, rheumatoid arthritis • Carcinomas, monocytic leukemia, lymphomas

Looking at the big picture

Keep in mind that, to achieve an accurate diagnosis, differential test results must always be interpreted in relation to the total WBC count. Abnormal differential patterns suggest a range of disease states and other conditions. (See *How disease affects WBC differential values*.)

Action!

Some WBC differential findings indicate that immediate action is required. For instance, an absolute neutrophil count of 1,000/μl (SI, 1×10^9/L) or less requires neutropenic precautions, including protective isolation. (See *WBC differential interference*.)

What needs to be done

- Tell the patient to avoid strenuous exercise before a WBC count to ensure accurate results.
- Perform a venipuncture and collect the sample in a 7-ml tube containing EDTA.
- Completely fill the collection tube, and invert it gently several times to adequately mix the sample and anticoagulant.

> **WBC differential interference**
>
> Some drugs increase the eosinophil count in the WBC differential, including:
> - anticonvulsants
> - gold compounds
> - isoniazid
> - penicillins
> - phenothiazines
> - rifampin
> - streptomycin
> - sulfonamides
> - tetracyclines.
>
>   Other drugs decrease the eosinophil count, for example:
> - indomethacin
> - procainamide.

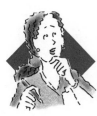

Quick quiz

1. Your patient's blood studies have returned and the serum ALT level is very high—up to 50 times the normal level. Which of the following conditions may cause this?

    A.   Hepatitis
    B.   Urinary tract infection
    C.   MI
    D.   Prostate cancer

Answer: A. Normally, serum ALT levels range from 8 to 50 IU/L (SI, 0.14 to 0.85 μkat/L). Very high ALT levels (up to 50 times the normal level) suggest viral or severe drug-induced hepatitis or another hepatic disease with extensive necrosis.

2. Your patient with cirrhosis and hepatic coma is being treated with lactulose. Which diagnostic test result indicates an improvement in the patient's condition?

    A.   Increased plasma rennin
    B.   Decreased plasma ammonia
    C.   Increased ALT
    D.   Decreased alkaline phosphatase

Answer: B. Lactulose depresses ammonia levels, thereby improving the patient's condition.

3. What condition results in an increased anion gap?
   A. Respiratory acidosis
   B. Respiratory alkalosis
   C. Metabolic acidosis
   D. Metabolic alkalosis

Answer: C. When acidosis results from accumulation of metabolic acids, as with lactic acidosis, the anion gap increases above 14 mEq/L (SI, 14 mmol/L) with the increase being in unmeasured anions. Metabolic acidosis caused by such accumulation is known as *high anion gap acidosis.*

4. Which drug may depress BUN levels?
   A. Chloramphenicol
   B. Diphenhydramine
   C. Digoxin
   D. Rifampin

Answer: A. Chloramphenicol can depress BUN levels. Nephrotoxic drugs, such as aminoglycosides, amphotericin B, and methicillin, can elevate BUN levels.

5. What C-reactive protein level is considered within normal limits?
   A. Less than 0.8 mg/dl
   B. 1 to 1.5 mg/dl
   C. 1.6 to 2 mg/dl
   D. Greater than 2 mg/dl

Answer: A. C-reactive protein isn't normally present in an adult. Normal results may be reported as less than 0.8 mg/dl (SI, less than 8 mg/L).

Scoring

☆☆☆ If you answered all five questions correctly, super! Your knowledge is coagulating nicely.

☆☆ If you answered four questions correctly, keep up the good work! You have a high "level" of understanding.

☆ If you answered fewer than four questions correctly, our diagnosis is test stress. Relax! You'll ace the next test on tests.

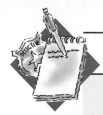

4

Nursing procedures

Just the facts

In this chapter, you'll learn:

♦ equipment needed for common nursing procedures

♦ required preparation for common procedures

♦ techniques for carrying out common procedures

♦ special documentation instructions for each procedure.

A look at nursing procedures

Performing nursing procedures requires skill and confidence. Before you perform a nursing procedure, review the procedure to refresh your memory. Next, explain the procedure to the patient to allay his anxiety and promote cooperation. Make sure that consent for the procedure was obtained, if required. Then gather all of the necessary equipment. Always wash your hands before and after patient contact and follow standard precautions. This chapter discusses more than 30 commonly used nursing procedures.

Arterial pressure monitoring

Direct arterial pressure monitoring permits continuous measurement of systolic, diastolic, and mean pressures and allows arterial blood sampling. It's generally more accurate than indirect methods (such as palpation and auscultation of audible pulse sounds).

Direct indication

Direct monitoring is indicated when highly accurate or frequent blood pressure measurements are required — for example, in patients receiving titrated doses of vasoactive drugs.

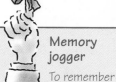

Memory jogger

To remember the steps you should take before performing every nursing procedure, think, "Remembering Every Component Guarantees Wonderfully Satisfied Patients."

*R*eview

*E*xplain

*C*heck consent (if required)

*G*ather equipment

*W*ash hands

*S*tandard Precautions

What you need

For catheter insertion

Gown ✳ mask ✳ protective eyewear ✳ sterile gloves ✳ 16G to 20G catheter (type and length depend on the insertion site, the patient's size, and other anticipated uses of the line) ✳ preassembled preparation kit (if available) ✳ sterile drapes for maximum barrier precautions ✳ linen-saver pad ✳ prepared pressure transducer system ✳ ordered local anesthetic ✳ chlorhexidine swabs ✳ sutures ✳ syringe and needle (21G to 25G, 1″) ✳ I.V. pole ✳ tubing and medication labels ✳ site care kit (containing sterile transparent semipermeable dressing and hypoallergenic tape) ✳ arm board and soft wrist restraint (ankle restraint for a femoral site) ✳ optional: shaving kit (for femoral artery insertion)

For blood sample collection

If an open system is in place

Gloves ✳ gown ✳ mask ✳ protective eyewear ✳ sterile 4″ × 4″ gauze pads ✳ linen-saver pad ✳ 5- or 10-ml syringe for discard sample ✳ syringes of appropriate size and number for ordered laboratory tests ✳ needleless blood transfer device ✳ laboratory request forms and labels ✳ Vacutainers

If a closed system is in place

Gloves ✳ gown ✳ mask ✳ protective eyewear ✳ syringes of appropriate size and number for ordered laboratory tests ✳ laboratory request forms and labels ✳ alcohol pad ✳ blood transfer unit ✳ Vacutainers

For arterial line tubing changes

Gloves ✳ gown ✳ mask ✳ protective eyewear ✳ linen-saver pad ✳ preassembled arterial pressure tubing with flush device and disposable pressure transducer ✳ I.V. pole ✳ 500-ml bag of I.V. flush solution (such as dextrose 5% in water or normal saline solution) ✳ 500 or 1,000 units of heparin (according to facility policy) ✳ alcohol pads ✳ medication label ✳ pressure bag ✳ site care kit ✳ tubing labels

For arterial catheter removal

Gloves ✳ gown ✳ mask ✳ protective eyewear ✳ two sterile 4″ × 4″ gauze pads ✳ linen-saver pad ✳ sterile suture removal set ✳ dressing ✳ alcohol pads ✳ hypoallergenic tape

I'll just relax while you gather all of that equipment.

For femoral line removal

Gloves * gown * mask * protective eyewear * six or more sterile 4″ × 4″ gauze pads * small sandbag (which you may wrap in a towel or place in a pillowcase) * adhesive bandage

For a catheter-tip culture

Sterile scissors * sterile container or agar plate * label

Getting ready

Set up the transducer system. Then set the alarms on the bedside monitor according to your facility's policy.

How you do it

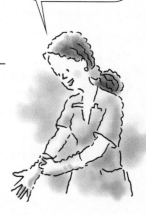

Gloves are an important piece of equipment for almost every aspect of arterial pressure monitoring.

• Make sure that an informed consent form has been signed. Check the patient's history for an allergy or a hypersensitivity to povidone-iodine ointment, chlorhexidine, heparin, or the ordered local anesthetic.
• Maintain asepsis and wear personal protective equipment throughout all procedures described.
• Position the patient for easy access to the catheter insertion site. Place a linen-saver pad under the site.
• If the catheter will be inserted into the radial artery, perform Allen's test on the ulnar artery *to assess collateral circulation in the hand.* To perform Allen's test, apply digital compression to the ulnar artery while the patient forms a tight fist. If blood fails to return to the palm and fingers when the patient opens his hand, blood flow in the artery is obstructed and the catheter shouldn't be inserted into the radial artery.

Inserting an arterial catheter

• Using a preassembled preparation kit, the doctor prepares and anesthetizes the insertion site. He covers the surrounding area with sterile drapes and then cleans the area with chlorhexadine using a vigorous side-to-side motion. He anesthetizes the area and inserts the catheter attached to the fluid-filled pressure tubing into the artery.
• While the doctor holds the catheter in place, activate the fast-flush release. After each fast-flush operation, observe the drip chamber *to verify that the continuous flush rate is at the desired level.* A waveform should appear on the bedside monitor.

• The doctor may suture the catheter in place, or you may secure it with hypoallergenic tape. Cover the insertion site with a dressing, as specified by facility policy.

No movement allowed

• Immobilize the insertion site. With a radial or brachial site, use an arm board. With a femoral site, maintain the patient on bed rest, with the head of the bed elevated no more than 15 to 30 degrees. Then zero the system to atmospheric pressure.
• Activate monitor alarms, as appropriate.

Obtaining a blood sample from an open system

• Assemble the equipment. Turn off or temporarily silence the monitor alarms, depending on your facility's policy. (However, some facilities require that alarms be left on.)
• Locate the stopcock nearest the patient. Open a sterile $4'' \times 4''$ gauze pad. Remove the dead-end cap from the stopcock, and place it on the gauze pad.

Just practicing

• Place the syringe for the discard sample into the stopcock. (This sample is discarded because it's diluted with flush solution.) Follow your facility's policy on how much discarded blood to collect. In most cases, you'll withdraw 5 to 10 ml through a 5- or 10-ml syringe.
• Next, turn the stopcock off to the flush solution. Allow the syringe to fill with blood until you obtain an adequate amount for your discard sample. If you feel resistance, reposition the affected extremity and check the insertion site for obvious problems (such as catheter kinking). After correcting the problem, resume blood withdrawal. Then turn the stopcock halfway back to the open position *to close the system in all directions.*
• Remove the discard syringe, and dispose of the syringe containing the blood, observing standard precautions.

Now for real

• Place a syringe for the laboratory sample in the stopcock, turn the stopcock off to the flush solution, and allow the syringe to fill with the required amount of blood. For each additional sample required, repeat this procedure. If the doctor has ordered coagulation tests, obtain blood for this sample from the final syringe *to prevent dilution from the flush device.*
• After you've obtained blood for the final sample, turn the stopcock off to the syringe and remove the syringe. Activate the fast-flush release. Then turn the stopcock off to the patient, and repeat the fast flush.

• Turn the stopcock off to the stopcock port, and replace the dead-end cap. Then turn the stopcock on to the flush solution. Reactivate the monitor alarms. Attach needleless devices to the filled syringes, and transfer the blood samples to the appropriate specimen collection tubes or Vacutainer, labeling them according to facility policy. Send all samples to the laboratory with appropriate documentation.

• Check the monitor for return of the arterial waveform and pressure reading. (See *Understanding the arterial waveform*, page 208.)

Obtaining a blood sample from a closed system

• Assemble the equipment, maintaining sterile technique. Locate the closed-system reservoir and blood sampling site. Deactivate or temporarily silence monitor alarms. (Some facilities require that alarms be left on.)

• Clean the sampling site with an alcohol pad.

• Holding the reservoir upright, grasp the flexures and slowly fill the reservoir with blood over 3 to 5 seconds. (This blood serves as discard blood.) If you feel resistance, reposition the affected extremity, and check the catheter for obvious problems (such as kinking). Then resume blood withdrawal.

• Turn the one-way valve off to the reservoir by turning the handle perpendicular to the tubing. Using a syringe with an attached cannula, insert the cannula into the sampling site. (Make sure that the plunger is depressed to the bottom of the syringe barrel.) Slowly fill the syringe. Then grasp the cannula near the sampling site, and remove the syringe and cannula as one unit. Repeat the procedure as needed *to fill the required number of syringes*. If the doctor has ordered coagulation tests, obtain blood for those tests from the final syringe.

• After filling the syringes, turn the one-way valve to its original position, parallel to the tubing. Then smoothly and evenly push down on the plunger until the flexures lock in place in the fully closed position and all fluid has been reinfused. The fluid should be reinfused over 3 to 5 seconds. Then activate the fast-flush release *to clear blood from the tubing and reservoir*.

• Clean the sampling site with an alcohol pad. Reactivate the monitor alarms. Using the blood transfer unit, transfer blood samples to the appropriate specimen collection tubes, labeling them according to facility policy. Send all samples to the laboratory with appropriate documentation.

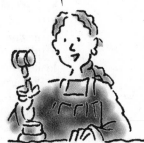

Open or closed case? Just remember that the procedure differs depending on this important detail.

Understanding the arterial waveform

Normal arterial blood pressure produces a characteristic waveform, representing ventricular systole and diastole. The waveform has five distinct components, which are shown below.

Going up...

The *anacrotic limb* marks the waveform's initial upstroke, which results as blood is rapidly ejected from the ventricle through the open aortic valve into the aorta. Rapid ejection causes a sharp rise in arterial pressure, which appears as the waveform's highest point, called the *systolic peak.*

...and coming down

As blood continues into the peripheral vessels, arterial pressure falls and the waveform begins a downward trend, called the *dicrotic limb.* Arterial pressure usually continues to fall until pressure in the ventricle is less than pressure in the aortic root. When this pressure change occurs, the aortic valve closes. This event appears as a small notch (the *dicrotic notch*) on the waveform's downside. When the aortic valve closes, diastole begins, progressing until aortic root pressure gradually descends to its lowest point. On the waveform, this lowest point appears as end diastolic pressure, which represents *end diastole.*

Normal arterial waveform

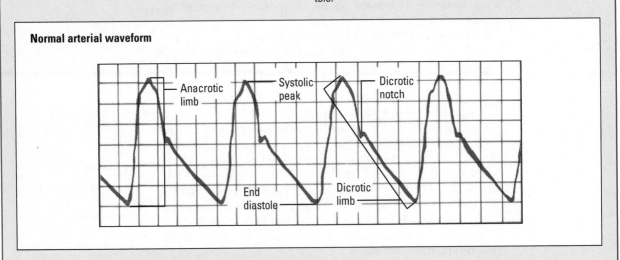

Changing arterial line tubing

- Assemble the new pressure monitoring system.
- Consult your facility's policy and procedure manual *to determine how much tubing length to change.*
- Inflate the pressure bag to 300 mm Hg, and check it for air leaks. Then release the pressure.
- Prepare the I.V. flush solution by adding heparin, if ordered, and prime the pressure tubing and transducer system. At this time, add the medication label and tubing label. Apply 300 mm Hg of pressure to the system. Then hang the I.V. bag on a pole.

Sound off

• Place the linen-saver pad under the affected extremity. Remove the dressing from the catheter insertion site, taking care not to dislodge the catheter or cause vessel trauma. Turn off or temporarily silence the monitor alarms. (Some facilities require that alarms be left on.)
• Turn off the flow clamp of the tubing segment that you'll change. Disconnect the tubing from the catheter hub, taking care not to dislodge the catheter. Immediately insert new tubing into the catheter hub. Secure the tubing and then activate the fast-flush release *to clear it.*

Sound on

• Reactivate the monitor alarms. Clean the site using a site care kit (if available) or a chlorhexidine swab. Apply an appropriate dressing.
• Zero the system to atmospheric pressure.

Removing an arterial line

• Consult facility policy *to determine whether you're permitted to perform this procedure.*
• Assemble all equipment. Follow standard precautions, including wearing personal protective equipment, for this procedure.
• Turn off the monitor alarms. Then turn off the flow clamp to the flush solution for the time predetermined by your facility.
• Carefully remove the dressing over the insertion site. Remove any sutures using the suture removal kit, and then carefully check that all sutures have been removed.

Steady withdrawal

• Withdraw the catheter using a gentle, steady motion. Keep the catheter parallel to the artery during withdrawal *to reduce the risk of traumatic injury.*
• Immediately after withdrawing the catheter, apply pressure to the site with a sterile gauze pad. Maintain pressure for at least 10 minutes (longer if bleeding or oozing persists). Apply additional pressure to a femoral site or if the patient has a coagulopathy or is receiving anticoagulants.
• Cover the site with an appropriate dressing and secure the dressing with tape. If stipulated by facility policy, make a pressure dressing for a femoral site by folding four sterile 4″ × 4″ gauze pads in half, and apply the dressing. Cover the dressing with a tight adhesive bandage, and then cover the bandage with a sandbag. Maintain the patient on bed rest for 6 hours with the sandbag in place.

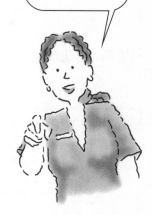

Be in the know! Know your facility's policy before removing an arterial line.

• Observe the site for bleeding. Assess circulation in the extremity distal to the site by evaluating color, pulses, and sensation. Repeat this assessment every 15 minutes for the first 4 hours, every 30 minutes for the next 2 hours, then hourly for the next 6 hours.

Culturing the catheter tip

• If the doctor has ordered a culture of the catheter tip (to diagnose a suspected infection), gently place the catheter tip on a sterile gauze pad. When the bleeding is under control, hold the catheter over the sterile container. Using sterile scissors, cut the tip so it falls into the sterile container. Some facilities prefer that the catheter tip be swabbed across an agar plate. Label the specimen or agar plate and send it to the laboratory.

Automated external defibrillation

Automated external defibrillators (AEDs) are commonly used to meet the need for early defibrillation, which is considered the most effective treatment for ventricular fibrillation. The AED is equipped with a microcomputer that senses and analyzes a patient's heart rhythm at the push of a button. Then it audibly or visually prompts you to deliver a shock. Some facilities now require an AED in every noncritical care unit.

What you need

AED ✳ two prepackaged electrodes

Getting ready

After discovering that your patient is unresponsive to your questions, pulseless, and apneic, follow basic life support and advanced cardiac life support (ACLS) protocols. Then ask a colleague to bring the AED into the patient's room and set it up before the code team arrives.

How you do it

• Open the foil packets containing the two electrode pads. Attach the electrode cable connector to the AED.

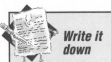

Write it down

Documenting arterial pressure monitoring

In your notes, document:
• date of system setup
• systolic, diastolic, and mean pressure readings
• circulation in the extremity distal to the site
• amount of flush solution infused
• patient positioning during each blood pressure reading.

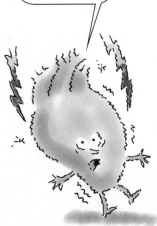

Automated external defibrillation can be quite shocking!

White to the right, red to the ribs

- Expose the patient's chest. Remove the plastic backing film from the electrode pads. Place one electrode pad on the right upper portion of the patient's chest, just beneath his clavicle.
- Place the second pad to the left of the heart's apex. (Placement for both electrode pads is the same as for manual defibrillation or cardioversion.)

Ghost in the machine

- Firmly press the device's ON button, and wait while the machine performs a brief self-test. Most AEDs signal their readiness by a computerized voice that says "Stand clear" or by emitting a series of loud beeps. (If the AED isn't functioning properly, it will convey the message: "Don't use the AED. Remove and continue CPR.") Report AED malfunctions according to facility policy.
- When the machine is ready, analyze the patient's heart rhythm. Have everyone stand clear, and press the ANALYZE button when the machine prompts you. Don't touch or move the patient while the AED is in analysis mode. (If the message "Check electrodes" appears, verify correct electrode placement and a secure patient cable attachment; then press the ANALYZE button again.)
- In 15 to 30 seconds, the AED will analyze the patient's rhythm. When the patient needs a shock, the AED displays a "Stand clear" message and emits a beep that changes to a steady tone as it charges.

Button down

- When fully charged and ready to deliver a shock, the AED will prompt you to press the SHOCK button. (Some fully automatic AED models automatically deliver a shock within 15 seconds after analyzing the patient's rhythm. If a shock isn't needed, the AED displays "No shock indicated" and prompts you to "Check patient.")
- Make sure that no one is touching the patient or his bed, and call out "Stand clear." Then, if necessary, press the SHOCK button on the AED. Most AEDs are ready to deliver a shock within 15 seconds.
- After the first shock, the AED automatically reanalyzes the patient's heart rhythm. If no additional shock is needed, the machine will prompt you to check the patient. If the patient is still in ventricular fibrillation, the AED will automatically begin recharging at a higher joule level to prepare for a second shock. Repeat the steps you performed before shocking the patient. According to the AED algorithm, the patient can be shocked up to three times at increasing joule levels (200, 200 to 300, and 360 joules).

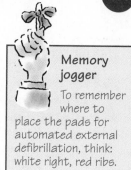

Memory jogger

To remember where to place the pads for automated external defibrillation, think: white right, red ribs.

Shock three, then start over

• If ventricular fibrillation persists after three shocks, resume CPR for 1 minute. Then press the ANALYZE button to identify the heart rhythm. If the patient is still in ventricular fibrillation, continue the algorithm sequence until the code team leader arrives.
• After the code, remove and transcribe the AED's computer memory module or tape, or prompt the AED to print a rhythm strip with code data. Follow your facility's policy for analyzing and storing code data.

Bladder irrigation, continuous

Continuous bladder irrigation can help prevent urinary tract obstruction by flushing out small blood clots that form after prostate or bladder surgery. It may also be used to treat an irritated, inflamed, or infected bladder lining.

Triple threat

This procedure requires placement of a triple-lumen catheter. One lumen controls balloon inflation, one allows irrigant inflow, and one allows irrigant outflow. The continuous flow of irrigating solution through the bladder also creates a mild tamponade that may help prevent venous hemorrhage. (See *Setup for continuous bladder irrigation.*)

What you need

One 4-L container or two 2-L containers of irrigating solution (usually normal saline solution) or the prescribed amount of medicated solution ✳ Y-type tubing made specifically for bladder irrigation ✳ alcohol pad or povidone-iodine pad ✳ I.V. pole

Getting ready

Before starting continuous bladder irrigation, double-check the irrigating solution against the doctor's order. If the solution contains an antibiotic, check the patient's chart *to make sure that he isn't allergic to the drug.*

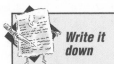

Write it down

Documenting AED use

After using an automated external defibrillator (AED), give a synopsis to the code team leader. Remember to report:
• patient's name, age, medical history, and reason for seeking care
• time you found the patient in cardiac arrest
• time you started cardiopulmonary resuscitation
• time you applied the AED
• number of shocks the patient received
• time the patient regained a pulse at any point
• postarrest care that was given, if any
• physical assessment findings.
    Later, be sure to document the code on the appropriate form.

How you do it

- Insert the spike of the Y-type tubing into the container of irrigating solution. (If you have a two-container system, insert one spike into each container.)
- Squeeze the drip chamber on the spike of the tubing.
- Open the flow clamp and flush the tubing; then close the clamp.

Hanging out

- To begin, hang the bag of irrigating solution on the I.V. pole.
- Clean the opening to the inflow lumen of the catheter with the alcohol or povidone-iodine pad.
- Insert the distal end of the Y-type tubing securely into the inflow lumen (third port) of the catheter.

Setup for continuous bladder irrigation

In continuous bladder irrigation, a triple-lumen catheter allows irrigating solution to flow into the bladder through one lumen and flow out through another, as shown in the inset. The third lumen is used to inflate the balloon that holds the catheter in place.

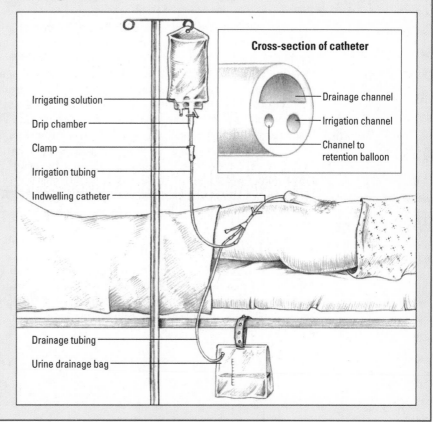

Cross-section of catheter

- Drainage channel
- Irrigation channel
- Channel to retention balloon

- Irrigating solution
- Drip chamber
- Clamp
- Irrigation tubing
- Indwelling catheter

- Drainage tubing
- Urine drainage bag

• Make sure that the catheter's outflow lumen is securely attached to the drainage bag tubing.
• Open the flow clamp under the container of irrigating solution, and set the drip rate as ordered.
• *To prevent air from entering the system*, don't let the primary container empty completely before replacing it.

Close this, open that

• If you have a two-container system, simultaneously close the flow clamp under the nearly empty container and open the flow clamp under the reserve container. *Doing so prevents reflux of irrigating solution from the reserve container into the nearly empty one.* Hang a new reserve container on the I.V. pole and insert the tubing, maintaining asepsis.
• Empty the drainage bag about every 4 hours, or as often as needed.

Central venous pressure monitoring

In central venous pressure (CVP) monitoring, the doctor inserts a catheter through a vein, such as the subclavian or jugular, and advances it until its tip lies in or near the right atrium. When connected to pressurized tubing, the catheter measures CVP, an index of right ventricular function. Normal CVP ranges from 5 to 10 cm H_2O or 2 to 8 mm Hg depending on the monitoring system. Any condition that alters venous return, circulating blood volume, or cardiac performance may affect CVP. If circulating volume increases , such as with enhanced venous return to the heart, CVP rises. If circulating volume decreases, such as with reduced venous return, CVP drops.

What you need

For continuous CVP monitoring

Appropriate protective clothing ✳ pressure monitoring kit with disposable pressure transducer ✳ leveling device ✳ bedside pressure module ✳ 500 ml of continuous I.V. flush solution ✳ 500 or 1,000 units of heparin (according to facility policy) ✳ pressure bag

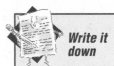

Write it down

Documenting continuous bladder irrigation

Each time you finish a container of irrigating solution, record the date, time, and amount of fluid given on the patient's intake and output record.

Each time you empty the drainage bag, record the time and amount of drainage, appearance of the drainage, and any patient complaints.

CVP monitoring is serious business. It can tell you about cardiovascular functioning.

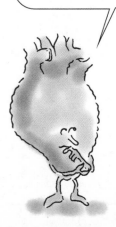

For withdrawing blood samples through the CV line

Appropriate protective clothing ✳ appropriate number of syringes for the ordered tests ✳ 5- or 10-ml syringe for the discard sample (size depends on the tests ordered)

For removing a CV catheter

Sterile gloves ✳ suture removal set ✳ sterile gauze pads ✳ povidone-iodine ointment ✳ dressing ✳ tape

Getting ready

Gather the equipment necessary for insertion of a CV catheter, and be ready to assist the doctor as necessary.

How you do it

Obtaining continuous CVP readings with a pressure monitoring system

• Make sure that the CV line or the proximal lumen of a pulmonary artery catheter is attached to the system. (If the patient has a CV line with multiple lumens, one lumen may be dedicated to continuous CVP monitoring and the other lumens may be used for fluid administration.)

• Set up a pressure transducer system. Connect the pressure tubing from the CVP catheter hub to the transducer. Then connect the flush solution container to a flush device.

• To obtain values, position the patient flat. If he can't tolerate this position, use semi-Fowler's position. Locate the level of the right atrium by identifying the phlebostatic axis. Zero the transducer, leveling the transducer air-fluid interface stopcock with the right atrium. Read the CVP value from the digital display on the monitor, and compare it to the value elicited by the waveform. Make sure that the patient is still when the reading is taken *to prevent artifact.* Be sure to use this position for all subsequent readings.

Removing a CV line

• You may assist the doctor in removing a CV line. (In some states, a nurse is permitted to remove the catheter with a doctor's order or when acting under advanced collaborative standards of practice.)

- Minimize the risk of air embolism during catheter removal—for instance, by placing the patient in Trendelenburg's position if the line was inserted using a superior approach. If he can't tolerate this position, have him lie flat.
- Turn the patient's head to the side opposite the catheter insertion site. The doctor removes the dressing and exposes the insertion site. If sutures are in place, he removes them carefully.
- Turn off the I.V. solution.
- The doctor pulls the catheter out in a slow, smooth motion and immediately applies pressure to the insertion site for several minutes or until all bleeding has stopped.
- Clean the insertion site, apply povidone-iodine ointment, and cover it with a dressing as ordered.
- Assess the patient for signs of respiratory distress, *which may indicate an air embolism.*

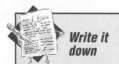

Write it down

Documenting CVP monitoring

Be sure to document all dressing, tubing, and solution changes. Also document:
- patient's tolerance of the procedure
- date and time of catheter removal
- type of dressing applied.

In addition, note the condition of the catheter insertion site and whether a culture specimen was collected. Note any complications and actions taken.

Chest physiotherapy

Chest physiotherapy includes postural drainage, chest percussion and vibration, and coughing and deep-breathing exercises. Together, these techniques mobilize and eliminate secretions, reexpand lung tissue, and promote efficient use of respiratory muscles.

What you need

Stethoscope ✳ pillows ✳ hospital bed ✳ emesis basin ✳ facial tissues ✳ suction equipment as needed ✳ equipment for oral care ✳ towel ✳ trash bag ✳ optional: sterile specimen container, supplemental oxygen

Getting ready

Gather the equipment at the patient's bedside. Set up suction equipment, if needed, and test its function.

How you do it

- Auscultate the patient's lungs *to determine baseline respiratory status.*
- Position the patient as ordered. *The lung's lower lobes commonly require drainage because the upper lobes drain during normal activity.*

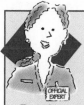

Advice from the experts

Performing percussion and vibration

To perform *percussion,* hold your hands in a cupped shape, with fingers flexed and thumbs pressed tightly against your index fingers. Percuss each segment for 1 to 2 minutes by alternating your hands against the patient in a rhythmic manner. Listen for a hollow sound on percussion to verify correct technique.

To perform *vibration,* ask the patient to inhale deeply and then exhale slowly through pursed lips. During exhalation, firmly press your fingers and the palms of your hands against his chest wall. Tense your arm and shoulder muscles in an isometric contraction to send fine vibrations through the chest wall. Vibrate during five exhalations over each chest segment.

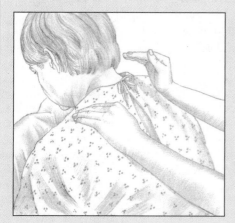
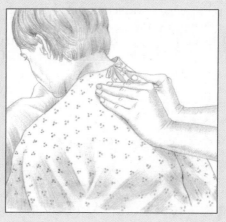

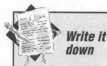

Write it down

Documenting chest PT

In your notes, record:
• date and time of chest physiotherapy (PT)
• positions used for secretion drainage and the duration each position is maintained
• chest segments percussed or vibrated
• color, amount, odor, and viscosity of secretions produced
• presence of blood
• complications and nursing actions taken
• patient's tolerance of the procedure.

Wanted: Drum players

• Instruct the patient to remain in each position for 10 to 15 minutes. During this time, perform percussion and vibration as ordered. (See *Performing percussion and vibration.*)
• After postural drainage, percussion, or vibration, instruct the patient to cough *to remove loosened secretions.* Give him an emesis basin and facial tissues *to dispose of secretions.* Have the patient perform exercises for about 1 minute and then rest for 2 minutes. Gradually progress to a 10-minute exercise period four times daily.
• Provide oral hygiene.
• Auscultate the patient's lungs *to evaluate the effectiveness of therapy.*

Colostomy and ileostomy care

A patient with an ascending or a transverse colostomy or an ileostomy must wear an external pouch to collect emerging fecal matter, which will be watery or pasty. In addition to collecting waste matter, the pouch helps control odor and protect the stoma and peristomal skin. Most disposable pouching systems can be used for 2 to 7 days; some models last longer.

What you need

Pouching system ✳ stoma measuring guide ✳ stoma paste (if drainage is watery to pasty or stoma secretes excess mucus) ✳ plastic bag ✳ water ✳ washcloth and towel ✳ closure clamp ✳ toilet or bedpan ✳ water or pouch cleaning solution ✳ gloves ✳ facial tissues ✳ optional: ostomy belt, paper tape, mild non-moisturizing soap, skin shaving equipment, liquid skin sealant, pouch deodorant

Getting ready

Provide privacy and emotional support.

How you do it

Fitting the pouch and skin barrier

• For a pouch with an attached skin barrier, measure the stoma with the stoma measuring guide. Select the opening size that matches the stoma.
• For an adhesive-backed pouch with a separate skin barrier, measure the stoma with the measuring guide and select the opening that matches the stoma. Trace the selected size opening onto the paper back of the skin barrier's adhesive side. Cut out the opening. (If the pouch has precut openings, which can be handy for a round stoma, select an opening that is ⅛″ [0.3 cm] larger than the stoma. If the pouch comes without an opening, cut the hole ⅛″ wider than the measured tracing.) The cut-to-fit system works best for an irregularly shaped stoma.
• For a two-piece pouching system with flanges, see *Applying a skin barrier and pouch.*

Can't feel a thing

• Avoid fitting the pouch too tightly *because the stoma has no pain receptors. A constrictive opening could injure the stoma or*

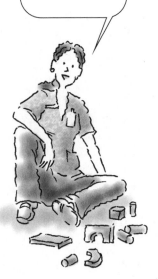

Ostomy pouching systems come in many shapes and sizes, so your patient can find a comfortable fit.

skin tissue without the patient feeling warning discomfort. Also, avoid cutting the opening too big because an opening that's too large may expose the skin to fecal matter and moisture.

Applying or changing the pouch
• Collect all equipment.
• Put on gloves.

Out with the old
• Remove and discard the old pouch. Wipe the stoma and peristomal skin gently with a facial tissue.
• Carefully wash with warm water and dry the peristomal skin by patting gently. Allow the skin to dry thoroughly. Inspect the peristomal skin and stoma. If necessary, clip surrounding hair (in a direction away from the stoma).
• If applying a separate skin barrier, peel off the paper backing of the prepared skin barrier, center the barrier over the stoma, and press gently *to ensure adhesion.*
• You may want to outline the stoma on the back of the skin barrier (depending on the product) with a thin ring of stoma paste *to provide extra skin protection.* (Skip this step if the patient has a sigmoid or descending colostomy, formed stools, and little mucus.)

Peel and press
• Remove the paper backing from the adhesive side of the pouching system and center the pouch opening over the stoma. Press gently *to secure it.*
• For a pouching system with flanges, align the lip of the pouch flange with the bottom edge of the skin barrier flange. Gently press around the circumference of the pouch flange, beginning at the bottom, until the pouch securely adheres to the barrier flange. (The pouch will click into its secured position.) Holding the barrier against the skin, gently pull on the pouch *to confirm the seal between flanges.*

Warm to the task
• Encourage the patient to stay quietly in position for about 5 minutes *to improve adherence.* The patient's body warmth also helps to improve adherence and soften a rigid skin barrier.
• Attach an ostomy belt to further secure the pouch, if desired. (Some pouches have belt loops, and others have plastic adapters for belts.)
• Leave a bit of air in the pouch *to allow drainage to fall to the bottom.*
• Apply the closure clamp if necessary.

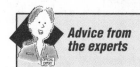

Advice from the experts

Applying a skin barrier and pouch

Fitting a skin barrier and ostomy pouch properly can be done in a few steps:
• Measure the stoma using a measuring guide.
• Trace the appropriate circle carefully on the back of the skin barrier.
• Cut the circular opening in the skin barrier. Bevel the edges to keep them from irritating the patient.
• Remove the backing from the skin barrier, and moisten it or apply barrier paste as needed along the edge of the circular opening.
• Center the skin barrier over the stoma, adhesive side down, and gently press it to the skin.
• Gently press the pouch opening onto the ring until it snaps into place.

- If desired, apply paper tape in a picture-frame fashion to the pouch edges *for additional security.*

Emptying the pouch

- Empty the pouch when it's one-third to one-half full. Tilt the bottom of the pouch upward and remove the closure clamp.
- Turn up a cuff on the lower end of the pouch and allow it to drain into the toilet or bedpan.
- Wipe the bottom of the pouch, fold the bottom of the pouch over once, and reapply the closure clamp.
- If desired, the bottom portion of the pouch can be rinsed with cool tap water. Don't aim water up near the top of the pouch *because this may loosen the seal on the skin.*
- A two-piece flanged system can also be emptied by unsnapping the pouch. Let the drainage flow into the toilet.
- Release flatus through the gas release valve if the pouch has one. Otherwise, release flatus by tilting the pouch bottom upward, releasing the clamp, and expelling the flatus. To release flatus from a flanged system, loosen the seal between the flanges. (Some pouches have gas release valves.)

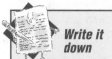

Write it down

Documenting colostomy and ileostomy care

In your notes, record:
- date and time of the pouching system change
- character of drainage, including color, amount, type, and consistency
- appearance of the stoma and peristomal skin
- patient teaching
- patient's response to self-care and evaluation of his learning progress.

Continuous ambulatory peritoneal dialysis

Continuous ambulatory peritoneal dialysis (CAPD) requires insertion of a permanent peritoneal catheter (such as a Tenckhoff catheter) to circulate dialysate in the peritoneal cavity. Inserted under local anesthetic, the catheter is sutured in place and its distal portion tunneled subcutaneously to the skin surface. There it serves as a port for the dialysate, which flows in and out of the peritoneal cavity by gravity. All equipment for infusing the dialysate and discontinuing the procedure must be sterile. Commercially prepared sterile CAPD kits are available.

CAPD gives dialysis patients more freedom.

What you need

To infuse dialysate

Prescribed amount of dialysate (usually in 2-L bags) ✳ heating pad or commercial warmer ✳ three face masks ✳ 42″ (106.7-cm) connective tubing with drain clamp ✳ six to eight packages of sterile 4″ × 4″ gauze pads ✳ medication, if ordered ✳ povidone-iodine pads ✳ hypoallergenic tape ✳

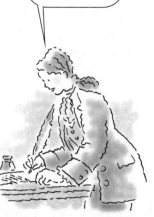

plastic snap-top container ✳ povidone-iodine solution ✳ sterile basin ✳ container of alcohol ✳ sterile gloves ✳ belt or fabric pouch ✳ two sterile waterproof paper drapes (one fenestrated) ✳ optional: syringes, labeled specimen container

To discontinue dialysis temporarily

Three sterile waterproof paper barriers (two fenestrated) ✳ eight or more 4″ × 4″ gauze pads (for cleaning and dressing the catheter) ✳ two face masks ✳ sterile basin ✳ hypoallergenic tape ✳ povidone-iodine solution ✳ sterile gloves ✳ sterile rubber catheter cap

Getting ready

Check the concentration of the dialysate against the doctor's order. Also check the expiration date and appearance of the solution. Warm the solution to body temperature with a heating pad or a commercial warmer if one is available. Don't warm the solution in a microwave oven because the temperature is unpredictable.

To minimize the risk of contaminating the bag's port, leave the dialysate container's wrapper in place. Wash your hands and put on a surgical mask. Remove the dialysate container from the warming setup, and remove its protective wrapper. Squeeze the bag firmly to check for leaks.

Insert the connective tubing into the dialysate container. Open the drain clamp to prime the tube. Then close the clamp.

Place a povidone-iodine pad on the dialysate container's port. Cover the port with a dry gauze pad, and secure the pad with tape. Remove and discard the surgical mask. Tear the tape so it will be ready to secure the new dressing. Commercial devices with povidone-iodine pads are available for covering the dialysate container and tubing connection.

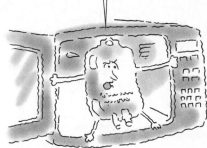

Warm the dialysate before infusion, but don't microwave it.

How you do it

• Weigh the patient at the same time and on the same scale every day *to help monitor fluid balance.*

Infusing dialysate

• Assemble all equipment at the patient's bedside. Prepare the sterile field by placing a waterproof, sterile paper drape on a dry surface near the patient. Take care to maintain the drape's sterility.

• Fill the snap-top container with povidone-iodine solution, and place it on the sterile field. Place the basin on the sterile field. Then place four pairs of sterile gauze pads in the sterile basin, and saturate them with the povidone-iodine solution. Drop the remaining gauze pads on the sterile field. Loosen the cap on the alcohol container, and place it next to the sterile field.

• Put on a clean surgical mask and provide one for the patient.

• Carefully remove the dressing covering the peritoneal catheter and discard it. Be careful not to touch the catheter or skin. Check skin integrity at the catheter site, and look for signs of infection. If drainage is present, obtain a swab specimen, and notify the doctor.

• Put on the sterile gloves and palpate the insertion site and subcutaneous tunnel route for tenderness or pain. If present, notify the doctor.

Catheter cleaning

• Wrap one gauze pad saturated with povidone-iodine solution around the distal end of the catheter, and leave it in place for 5 minutes. Clean the catheter and insertion site with the rest of the gauze pads, moving in concentric circles away from the insertion site. Use straight strokes to clean the catheter, beginning at the insertion site and moving outward. Use a clean area of the pad for each stroke. Loosen the catheter cap one notch and clean the exposed area. Place each used pad at the base of the catheter *to help support it.* After using the third pair of pads, place the fenestrated paper drape around the base of the catheter. Continue cleaning the catheter for another minute with one of the remaining pads soaked with povidone-iodine.

• Remove the povidone-iodine pad on the catheter cap, remove the cap, and use the remaining povidone-iodine pad *to clean the end of the catheter hub.* Attach the connective tubing from the dialysate container to the catheter. Be sure to secure the luer-lock connector tightly.

• Open the drain clamp on the dialysate container *to allow the solution to enter the peritoneal cavity by gravity over a period of 5 to 10 minutes.* Leave a small amount of fluid in the bag *to make folding it easier.* Close the drain clamp.

• Fold the bag and secure it with a belt, or tuck it in the patient's clothing or a small fabric pouch.

• After the prescribed dwell time (usually 4 to 10 hours), unfold the bag, open the clamp, and allow peritoneal fluid to drain back into the bag by gravity.

• When drainage is complete, attach a new bag of dialysate and repeat the infusion.

• Discard used supplies appropriately.

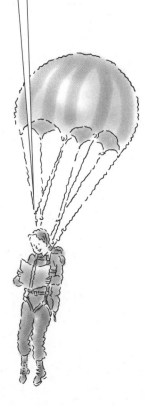

What goes up must come down. Gravity allows the solution to enter the peritoneal cavity.

Discontinuing dialysis temporarily

- Put on a surgical mask, and provide one for the patient.
- Using sterile gloves, remove and discard the dressing over the peritoneal catheter.
- Set up a sterile field next to the patient by covering a clean, dry surface with a waterproof drape. Be sure to maintain the drape's sterility. Place all equipment on the sterile field, and place the gauze pads in the basin. Saturate them with the povidone-iodine solution. Open the gauze pads to be used as the dressing, and drop them onto the sterile field. Tear pieces of tape as needed.
- Tape the dialysate tubing to the side rail of the bed.

Get more gloves

- Change to another pair of sterile gloves. Then place one of the fenestrated drapes around the base of the catheter.
- Use a pair of povidone-iodine pads to clean about 6″ (15.2 cm) of the dialysis tubing. Clean for 1 minute, moving in one direction only, away from the catheter. Then clean the catheter, moving from the insertion site to the junction of the catheter and dialysis tubing. Place used pads at the base of the catheter *to prop it up*. Use two more pairs of pads to clean the junction for a total of 3 minutes.
- Place the second fenestrated paper drape over the first at the base of the catheter. With the fourth pair of pads, clean the junction of the catheter and 6″ of the dialysate tubing for another minute.

Break in the line

- Disconnect the dialysate tubing from the catheter. Pick up the catheter cap and fasten it to the catheter, making sure that it fits securely over both notches of the hard plastic catheter tip.
- Clean the insertion site and a 2″ (5-cm) radius around it with povidone-iodine pads, working from the insertion site outward. Let the skin air-dry before applying the dressing.
- Discard used supplies appropriately.

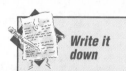

Write it down

Documenting continuous ambulatory peritoneal dialysis

In your notes, record:
- type and amount of fluid instilled and returned for each exchange
- time and duration of the exchange
- medications added to the dialysate
- color and clarity of the returned exchange fluid
- whether the returned fluid contains mucus, pus, or blood
- fluid intake and output balance
- signs of fluid imbalance, such as weight change, decreased breath sounds, peripheral edema, ascites, or skin turgor change
- patient's weight, blood pressure, and pulse rate after the day's last fluid exchange.

Defibrillation

The standard treatment for ventricular fibrillation and ventricular tachycardia that doesn't produce a pulse, defibrillation involves using electrode paddles to direct an electric current through the patient's heart. The current causes the myocardium to depolarize, which in turn encourages the sinoatrial node to resume control of the heart's electrical activity. The electrode paddles delivering the current may be placed on the patient's chest or, during cardiac surgery, directly on the myocardium.

For other types of arrhythmias, synchronized cardioversion may be used. (See *In sync with synchronized cardioversion.*)

OK for ICD?

Patients with a history of ventricular fibrillation may be candidates for an implantable cardioverter-defibrillator (ICD), a sophisticated device that automatically discharges an electric current when it senses a ventricular tachyarrhythmia.

What you need

Defibrillator ✳ external paddles ✳ conductive medium pads or gel ✳ electrocardiogram (ECG) monitor with recorder ✳ oxygen therapy equipment ✳ handheld resuscitation bag ✳ endotracheal (ET) tube ✳ emergency pacing equipment ✳ emergency cardiac medications

Getting ready

Assess the patient to determine if he lacks a pulse. Call for help and perform CPR until the defibrillator and other emergency equipment arrive.

How you do it

- If the defibrillator has "quick-look" capability, place the paddles on the patient's chest *to quickly view his cardiac rhythm.* Otherwise, connect the monitoring leads of the defibrillator to the patient, and assess his cardiac rhythm in two leads.

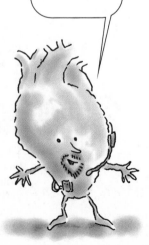

Defibrillation helps keep me *NSYNC.

In sync with synchronized cardioversion

Used to treat tachyarrhythmias, synchronized cardioversion delivers an electric charge to the myocardium at the peak of the R wave. This charge causes immediate depolarization, interrupting reentry circuits and allowing the sinoatrial node to resume control. Synchronizing the electric charge with the R wave ensures that the current won't be delivered on the vulnerable T wave and disrupt repolarization.

It's all about options

Synchronized cardioversion may be elective or urgent. It's the treatment of choice for arrhythmias that don't respond to drug therapy, such as atrial tachycardia, atrial flutter, atrial fibrillation, and symptomatic ventricular tachycardia.

Places, everyone!

• Expose the patient's chest, and apply conductive pads at the paddle placement positions or apply gel to the paddles. For anterolateral placement, place one paddle to the right of the upper sternum, just below the right clavicle, and the other over the fifth or sixth intercostal space at the left anterior axillary line. For anteroposterior placement, place the anterior paddle directly over the heart at the precordium, to the left of the lower sternal border. Place the flat posterior paddle under the patient's body beneath the heart and immediately below the scapulae (but not under the vertebral column).
• Turn on the defibrillator and, if performing external defibrillation, set the energy level for 200 joules for an adult patient.
• Charge the paddles by pressing the charge buttons, which are located either on the machine or on the paddles themselves.
• Place the paddles over the conductive pads (if used) and press firmly against the patient's chest, using 25 lb (11 kg) of pressure.

I'm clear, you're clear, we're all clear

• Reassess the patient's cardiac rhythm. If the patient remains in ventricular fibrillation or pulseless ventricular tachycardia, instruct all personnel to stand clear of the patient and the bed. Make sure that you're clear of the bed as well.
• Discharge the current by pressing both paddle discharge buttons simultaneously.
• Leaving the paddles in position on the patient's chest, reassess the patient's cardiac rhythm and have someone else assess the pulse.

Encore

• If necessary, prepare to defibrillate a second time. Instruct someone to reset the energy level on the defibrillator to 200 to 300 joules. Announce that you're preparing to defibrillate, and follow the procedure described above.
• Reassess the patient. If defibrillation is again necessary, instruct someone to reset the energy level to 360 joules. Then follow the same procedure as before.

If no success, start ACLS

• If the patient still has no pulse after three initial defibrillations, resume CPR and begin other ACLS measures.
• If defibrillation restores a normal rhythm, assess the patient. Obtain baseline arterial blood gas (ABG) levels and a 12-lead ECG. Provide supplemental oxygen, ventilation, and medications, as needed. (ET tube insertion may be necessary *to ensure ventilation*.) Check the patient's chest for electrical burns and treat them as ordered. Also prepare the defibrillator for immediate reuse. A temporary pacemaker may be inserted.

Write it down

Documenting defibrillation

In your notes, document:
• that the procedure was performed
• patient's electrocardiogram rhythms before and after defibrillation
• number of times defibrillation was performed
• voltage used during each attempt
• whether a pulse returned
• dosage, route, and time of drug administration
• whether cardiopulmonary resuscitation was used
• means of airway maintenance
• patient's outcome.

Doppler use

More sensitive than palpation in determining a pulse rate, the Doppler ultrasound blood flow detector is especially useful when a pulse is faint or weak. Unlike palpation, which detects arterial wall expansion and retraction, this instrument detects the movement of red blood cells.

What you need

Doppler ultrasound machine ✳ gel

Getting ready

Tell the patient what you're going to do and provide privacy.

How you do it

• Apply a small amount of transmission gel to the ultrasound probe.
• Position the probe on the skin directly over the selected artery.
• When using a Doppler probe with an amplifier, turn on the instrument and, moving counterclockwise, set the volume control to the lowest setting. If your model doesn't have a speaker, plug in the earphones and slowly raise the volume.

Centering in

• *To obtain the best signals,* put gel between the skin and the probe, and tilt the probe 45 degrees from the artery. Slowly move the probe in a circular motion to locate the center of the artery and the Doppler signal—a hissing noise at the heartbeat. Avoid moving the probe rapidly *because doing so distorts the signal.*
• Count the signals for 60 seconds *to determine the pulse rate.*

Feeding tube insertion and removal

Inserting a feeding tube into the stomach or duodenum allows a patient who can't or won't eat to receive nourishment. The feeding tube also permits administration of supplemental feedings to a patient who has high nutritional requirements, such as an uncon-

> RBCs like me may be on the move, but the Doppler can detect us.

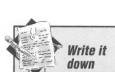

Write it down

Documenting Doppler use

Document the location, rate, and quality of the pulse and that it was detected with the Doppler ultrasound; record the setting of the Doppler device.

scious patient or one with extensive burns. The preferred feeding tube route is nasal, but the oral route may be used for patients with such conditions as a deviated septum or a head or nose injury.

What you need

For insertion

Feeding tube (#6 to #18 French, with or without guide) ✳ linen-saver pad ✳ gloves ✳ hypoallergenic tape ✳ water-soluble lubricant ✳ cotton-tipped applicators ✳ skin preparation (such as tincture of benzoin) ✳ facial tissues ✳ penlight ✳ small cup of water with straw or ice chips ✳ emesis basin ✳ 60-ml syringe ✳ pH test strip

During use

Mouthwash or saltwater solution ✳ toothbrush

For removal

Gloves ✳ linen-saver pad ✳ tube clamp ✳ bulb syringe

Getting ready

Have the proper size tube available. Usually, the doctor orders the smallest-bore tube that will allow free passage of the liquid feeding formula. Read the instructions on the tubing package carefully because tube characteristics vary according to the manufacturer.

Defect-free

Examine the tube to make sure that it's free from defects, such as cracks or rough or sharp edges. Next, run water through the tube. Doing so checks for patency, activates the coating, and facilitates guide removal.

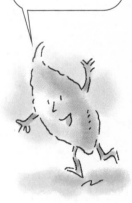

Running water through the tube checks the tube's patency and activates the coating.

How you do it

- Put on gloves.
- Assist the patient into semi-Fowler's or high Fowler's position *to prevent aspiration.*
- Place a linen-saver pad across the patient's chest.

Inner tube

- *To determine the tube length needed to reach the stomach,* first extend the distal end of the tube from the tip of the patient's nose to his earlobe. Coil this portion of the tube around your fingers *so the end will remain curved until you insert it.* Then extend the uncoiled portion from the earlobe to the xiphoid process. Use a small piece of hypoallergenic tape to mark the total length of the two portions.

Inserting the tube nasally

• Using the penlight, assess nasal patency. Occlude one nostril and then the other *to determine which has the better airflow.*
• Lubricate the curved tip of the tube (and the feeding tube guide, if appropriate) with a small amount of water-soluble lubricant *to ease insertion and prevent tissue injury.*
• Ask the patient to hold the emesis basin and facial tissues.
• To advance the tube, insert the curved, lubricated tip into the more patent nostril and direct it along the nasal passage toward the ear on the same side. Don't force the tube. When it passes the nasopharyngeal junction, turn the tube 180 degrees *to aim it downward into the esophagus.* Tell the patient to lower his chin to his chest *to close the trachea.* Then give him a small cup of water with a straw or ice chips. Direct him to sip the water or suck on the ice and swallow frequently *to ease the tube's passage.* Advance the tube as he swallows. If resistance is met, stop advancing the tube. Monitor the patient for cyanosis or choking. If either occurs, withdraw the tube and delay the procedure.

Inserting the tube orally

• Have the patient lower his chin *to close his trachea,* and ask him to open his mouth.
• Place the tip of the tube at the back of the patient's tongue, give water, and instruct the patient to swallow, as described above. Advance the tube as he swallows.

Positioning the tube

• Continue passing the tube until the tape marking the appropriate length reaches the patient's nostril or lips.

Your placement or mine?

• *To check tube placement,* attach the syringe to the end of the tube. Gently try to aspirate gastric secretions. If no gastric secretions return, the tube may be in the esophagus. You'll need to advance the tube or reinsert it before proceeding.
• Examine the aspirate and place a small amount on the pH test strip. Gastric placement is likely if aspirate has the typical gastric fluid appearance (green with clear, colorless mucus or brown) and the pH is less than or equal to 5.

Tale of the tape

- After confirming proper tube placement, remove the tape marking the tube length.
- Tape the tube to the patient's nose and remove the guide wire. *Note:* X-rays should always be ordered to verify tube placement before instilling anything into the tube.

Gravitational force

- *To advance the tube to the duodenum,* position the patient on his right side. *Doing so lets gravity assist tube passage through the pylorus.* Move the tube forward 2″ to 3″ (5 to 7.6 cm) hourly until X-rays confirm duodenal placement. (An X-ray must confirm placement before feeding begins *because duodenal feeding can cause nausea and vomiting if accidentally delivered to the stomach.*)
- Apply a skin preparation to the patient's cheek before securing the tube with tape. *This preparation helps the tube adhere to the skin and also prevents irritation.*
- Tape the tube securely to the patient's cheek *to avoid excessive pressure on his nostrils.*

Removing the tube

- Put on gloves.
- Protect the patient's chest with a linen-saver pad.
- Flush the tube with air, clamp or pinch it *to prevent fluid aspiration during withdrawal,* and withdraw it gently but quickly.
- Promptly cover and discard the used tube.

Femoral compression device use

Femoral compression is used to maintain hemostasis at the puncture site following a procedure involving an arterial access site (such as cardiac catheterization or angiography). A femoral compression device is used to apply direct pressure to the arterial access site. A nylon strap is placed under the patient's buttocks and attached to the device with an inflatable plastic dome. After the dome is positioned correctly over the puncture site, it's inflated to the recommended pressure, according the manufacturer. A doctor or a specially trained nurse may apply the device.

What you need

Femoral compression device strap ✳ compression arch with dome and three-way stopcock ✳ pressure inflation device

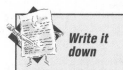

Write it down

Documenting feeding tube insertion and removal

Be sure to document details of tube insertion and removal.

Ins
For tube insertion, record:
- insertion date and time
- tube type and size
- insertion site
- placement area
- confirmation of proper placement
- name of the person who performed the procedure.

Outs
For tube removal, record:
- removal date and time
- patient's tolerance of the procedure.

✳ sterile transparent dressing ✳ gloves (nonsterile and sterile) ✳ protective eyewear

Getting ready

Obtain a doctor's order for the femoral compression device, including the amount of pressure to be applied and the length of time the device should remain in place. Position the patient on the stretcher or bed; don't flex the involved extremity. Assess the condition of the puncture site, obtain the patient's vital signs, perform neurovascular checks, and assess pain, according to your facility's policy for arterial access procedures.

How you do it

Applying a femoral compression device

• Put on nonsterile gloves and protective eyewear, and place the device strap under the patient's hips before sheath removal (in cases that warrant the use of a sheath).
• After achieving hemostasis, put on sterile gloves and apply a sterile transparent dressing over the puncture site using sterile technique.
• With the assistance of another nurse, position the compression arch over the puncture site. Apply manual pressure over the dome area while the straps are secured to the arch.
• When the dome is properly positioned over the puncture site, connect the pressure inflation device to the stopcock that's attached to the device. Turn the stopcock to the open position and inflate the dome with the pressure inflation device to the ordered pressure. Turn off the stopcock and remove the pressure-inflation device.
• Assess the puncture site for proper placement of the device and for signs of bleeding or hematoma. Assess distal pulses and perform neurovascular assessments according to your facility's policy. Confirm distal pulses after adjustments to the device.

Maintaining the device

• When the patient is transferred to the nursing unit, assess the distal pulses, the puncture site, and placement of the device and confirm the ordered amount of pressure.
• Check device placement, assess the patient's vital signs and the puncture site, and perform neurovascular checks according to your facility's policy.
• Deflate the device hourly and assess the puncture site for bleeding or a hematoma. Assess for proper placement of the dome over

the puncture site. Put on gloves and protective eyewear and reposition the compression arch and dome as necessary. Reinflate the device to the ordered pressure using the pressure inflation device.

Removing the device

• Put on nonsterile gloves and protective eyewear, remove the air from the dome, loosen the straps, and remove the device. Assess the puncture site for bleeding or a hematoma. Change the sterile transparent dressing according to your facility's policy.
• Check the puncture site and distal pulses, and perform neurovascular assessments every 15 minutes for the first half hour and every 30 minutes for the next 2 hours. Your facility may require more frequent monitoring. Observe for signs of bleeding, hematoma, or infection.
• Dispose of the device according to your facility's policy.

Gastrostomy feeding button use

A gastrostomy feeding button serves as an alternative feeding device for an ambulatory patient who's receiving long-term enteral feedings. The feeding button has a mushroom dome at one end and two wing tabs and a flexible safety plug at the other. When inserted into an established stoma, the button lies almost flush with the skin, with only the top of the safety plug visible.

What you need

Gastrostomy feeding button of the correct size (all three sizes, if the correct one isn't known) ✳ obturator ✳ water-soluble lubricant ✳ gloves ✳ feeding accessories, including adapter, feeding catheter, food syringe or bag, and formula ✳ catheter clamp ✳ cleaning equipment, including water, a syringe, a cotton-tipped applicator, a pipe cleaner, and mild soap or povidone-iodine solution ✳ optional: pump to provide continuous infusion over several hours

Getting ready

Explain that the doctor will perform the initial insertion. Put on gloves. (See *How to reinsert a gastrostomy feeding button*, page 232.)

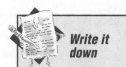

Write it down

Documenting femoral compression device use

When documenting femoral compression device use, record:
• initial application of the device
• sheath removal
• patient's tolerance of the procedure
• vital signs
• puncture site checks
• distal pulses
• neurovascular assessments
• hourly deflation
• repositioning of the device
• time the device was in place
• removal of the device
• patient and family teaching
• complications
• interventions.

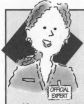

Advice from the experts

How to reinsert a gastrostomy feeding button

If your patient's gastrostomy feeding button pops out (with coughing, for instance), you or he will need to reinsert the device. Here are some steps to follow.

Prepare the equipment
Collect the feeding button, an obturator, and water-soluble lubricant. If the button will be reinserted, wash it with soap and water and rinse it thoroughly.

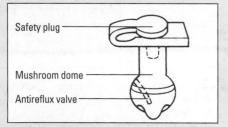

Insert the button
• Check the depth of the patient's stoma to make sure that you have the correct size feeding button. Then clean around the stoma.
• Lubricate the obturator with a water-soluble lubricant, and distend the button several times *to ensure the patency of the antireflux valve within the button.*

• Lubricate the mushroom dome and the stoma. Gently push the button through the stoma into the stomach.

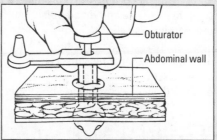

• Remove the obturator by gently rotating it as you withdraw it *to keep the antireflux valve from adhering to it.* If the valve still sticks, gently push the obturator back into the button until the valve closes.
• After removing the obturator, make sure that the valve is closed. Then close the flexible safety plug, which should be relatively flush with the skin surface.
• If you need to administer a feeding right away, open the safety plug and attach the feeding adapter and feeding tube. Deliver the feeding as ordered.

How you do it

• Attach the adapter and feeding catheter to the syringe or feeding bag. Clamp the catheter and fill the syringe or bag and catheter with formula. Refill the syringe before it's empty. *These steps prevent air from entering the stomach and distending the abdomen.*
• Open the safety plug and attach the adapter and feeding catheter to the button. Elevate the syringe or feeding bag above stomach level, and gravity-feed the formula for 15 to 30 minutes, varying the height as needed *to alter the flow rate.* Use a pump for continuous infusion or for feedings lasting several hours.

• After the feeding, flush the button with 10 ml of water, and clean the inside of the feeding catheter with a cotton-tipped applicator and water *to preserve patency and to dislodge formula or food particles.* Then lower the syringe or bag below stomach level *to allow burping.* Remove the adapter and feeding catheter. The antireflux valve should prevent gastric reflux. Then snap the safety plug in place *to keep the lumen clean and prevent leakage if the antireflux valve fails.* If the patient feels nauseated or vomits after the feeding, vent the button with the adapter and feeding catheter *to control emesis.*

• Wash the catheter and syringe or feeding bag in warm soapy water and rinse thoroughly. Clean the catheter and adapter with a pipe cleaner. Rinse well before using for the next feeding. Soak the equipment once per week according to the manufacturer's recommendations.

Write it down

Documenting gastrostomy feeding button use

Record feeding time and duration, amount and type of feeding formula used, and patient tolerance. Maintain intake and output records as necessary. Note the appearance of the stoma and surrounding skin.

Incentive spirometry

Incentive spirometry involves using a breathing device to help promote lung expansion after prolonged bed rest or surgery. The device requires that the patient take a deep breath and hold it for several seconds.

What you need

Flow or volume incentive spirometer, as indicated, with sterile disposable tube and mouthpiece (the tube and mouthpiece are sterile on first use and clean on subsequent uses) ✳ stethoscope ✳ watch

Getting ready

Assemble the ordered equipment at the patient's bedside. Read the manufacturer's instructions for spirometer setup and operation.

Remove the sterile flow tube and mouthpiece from the package and attach them to the device. Set the flow rate or volume goal as determined by the doctor or respiratory therapist and based on the patient's preoperative performance.

What a relief! Incentive spirometry promotes lung expansion after prolonged bed rest or surgery.

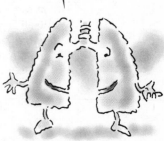

How you do it

- Assess the patient's condition.
- Help the patient into a comfortable sitting or semi-Fowler's position *to promote optimal lung expansion.* If you're using a flow incentive spirometer and the patient can't assume or maintain this position, he can perform the procedure in any position as long as the device remains upright. *Tilting a flow incentive spirometer decreases the required patient effort and reduces the exercise's effectiveness.*

Listen up!

- Auscultate the patient's lungs *to provide a baseline for comparison with posttreatment auscultation.*
- Instruct the patient to insert the mouthpiece and close his lips tightly around it *because a weak seal may alter flow or volume readings.*
- Instruct the patient to exhale normally and then inhale as slowly and as deeply as possible. If he has difficulty with this step, tell him to suck as he would through a straw but more slowly. Ask the patient to retain the entire volume of air he inhaled for 3 seconds.

Breathe easy

- Tell the patient to remove the mouthpiece and exhale normally. Allow him to relax and take several normal breaths before attempting another breath with the spirometer. Repeat this sequence 5 to 10 times during every waking hour. Note tidal volumes.
- Evaluate the patient's ability to cough effectively, and encourage him to cough after each effort *because deep lung inflation may loosen secretions and facilitate their removal.* Observe expectorated secretions.
- Auscultate the patient's lungs and compare findings with the first auscultation.

Over and out

- Instruct the patient to remove the mouthpiece. Wash the device in warm water and shake it dry. Avoid immersing the spirometer itself *because immersion enhances bacterial growth and impairs the internal filter's effectiveness in preventing inhalation of extraneous material.*
- Place the mouthpiece in a plastic storage bag between exercises, and label it and the spirometer, if applicable, with the patient's name *to avoid inadvertent use by another patient.*

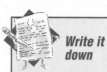
Write it down

Documenting incentive spirometry

In your notes, record:
- preoperative flow or volume levels
- preoperative teaching provided
- date and time of the procedure
- type of spirometer used
- flow or volume levels achieved
- number of breaths taken
- patient's condition before and after the procedure
- patient's tolerance of the procedure
- results of auscultation before and after use.

Indwelling urinary catheter insertion

> A urinary catheter drains urine from the bladder when a patient is unable to void or when urine output must be measured accurately.

An indwelling urinary catheter, also called a *Foley* or *retention catheter*, provides the patient with continuous urine drainage. The catheter is inserted into the bladder and a balloon is inflated at the catheter's distal end to prevent it from slipping out. Insert the catheter with extreme care to prevent injury and infection.

What you need

Sterile indwelling catheter (latex or silicone #10 to #22 French [average adult sizes are #16 to #18 French]) ✳ syringe filled with 5 to 8 ml of sterile water ✳ washcloth ✳ towel ✳ soap and water ✳ two linen-saver pads ✳ sterile gloves ✳ gloves ✳ sterile drape ✳ sterile fenestrated drape ✳ sterile cotton-tipped applicators (or cotton balls and plastic forceps) ✳ povidone-iodine or other antiseptic cleaning agent ✳ urine receptacle ✳ sterile water-soluble lubricant ✳ sterile drainage collection bag ✳ intake and output sheet ✳ optional: urine specimen container and laboratory request form, leg band with Velcro closure, gooseneck lamp or flashlight, pillows or rolled blankets or towels

At your disposal

Prepackaged sterile disposable kits that usually contain all the necessary equipment are available. The syringes in these kits are prefilled with 10 ml of sterile water.

In case of contamination

In addition, gather an extra pair of sterile gloves and two catheters of an appropriate size to be readily available at the bedside in case of contamination during insertion.

Getting ready

Check the order on the patient's chart to determine if a catheter size or type has been specified. Select the appropriate equipment, and assemble it at the patient's bedside.

How you do it

• Check the patient's chart and ask when he voided last. Percuss and palpate the bladder *to establish baseline data*. Ask if the patient feels the urge to void. Make sure that he isn't allergic to iodine solution or latex. If he's allergic to iodine solution, obtain another antiseptic cleaning agent; if he's allergic to latex, obtain a silicone catheter.

• Have a coworker hold a flashlight or place a gooseneck lamp next to the patient's bed *so that you can see the urinary meatus clearly, even in poor lighting.*

Assume the position

• Place the female patient in the supine position, with her knees flexed and separated and her feet flat on the bed, about 2′ (61 cm) apart. If she finds this position uncomfortable, have her flex one knee and keep the other leg flat on the bed. (See *Positioning an elderly female.*)

• Place the male patient in the supine position with his legs extended and flat on the bed. Ask the patient to hold the position *to give you a clear view of the urinary meatus and prevent contamination of the sterile field.*

Sterile fieldwork

• Put on gloves. Clean the patient's genital area and perineum thoroughly with soap and water. Dry the area with the towel. Then remove the gloves and wash your hands.

• Place the linen-saver pads on the bed between the patient's legs and under the hips. To create the sterile field, open the prepackaged kit or equipment tray and place it between the female patient's legs or next to the male patient's hip. If the sterile gloves are the first item on the top of the tray, put them on. Place the sterile drape under the patient's hips. Then drape the patient's lower abdomen with the sterile fenestrated drape *so that only the genital area remains exposed.* Take care not to contaminate your gloves.

• Open the rest of the kit or tray. Put on the sterile gloves if you haven't already done so.

• Tear open the packet of povidone-iodine or other antiseptic cleaning agent, and use it to saturate the sterile cotton balls or applicators.

• Open the packet of water-soluble lubricant and apply it to the catheter tip; attach the drainage bag to the other end of the catheter. (If you're using a commercial kit, the drainage bag may be attached.) Make sure that all tubing ends remain sterile and that the clamp at the emptying port of the drainage bag is closed *to prevent urine leakage from the bag.*

• Before inserting the catheter, inflate the balloon with sterile water *to inspect it for leaks.* To inflate the balloon, attach the prefilled syringe to the luer-lock, then push the plunger and check for seepage as the balloon expands. Aspirate the sterile water *to deflate the balloon.*

Ages and stages

Positioning an elderly female

The elderly female patient may need pillows or rolled towels or blankets for positioning support. If necessary, ask her to lie on her side with one knee drawn up to her chest during catheterization (as shown below). This position may also be helpful for disabled patients.

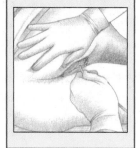

Female facts

• For the female patient, separate the labia majora and labia minora as widely as possible with the thumb, middle, and index fingers of your nondominant hand *so you have a full view of the urinary meatus.* Keep the labia well separated throughout the procedure *so they don't obscure the urinary meatus or contaminate the area when it's cleaned.*

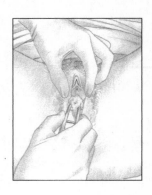

• With your dominant hand, use a sterile, cotton-tipped applicator (or pick up a sterile cotton ball with the plastic forceps) and wipe one side of the urinary meatus with a single downward motion. Wipe the other side with another sterile applicator or cotton ball in the same way. Then wipe directly over the meatus with still another sterile applicator or cotton ball (as shown in the top illustration at right). Take care not to contaminate your sterile glove.

• For the female patient, advance the catheter 2″ to 3″ (5 to 7.6 cm) while continuing to hold the labia apart until urine begins to flow (as shown in the middle illustration at right). If the catheter is inadvertently inserted into the vagina, leave it there as a landmark. Then begin the procedure again using new supplies.

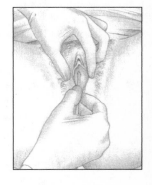

Male matters

• For the male patient, hold the penis with your nondominant hand. If he's uncircumcised, retract the foreskin. Then gently lift and stretch the penis to a 60- to 90-degree angle. Hold the penis this way throughout the procedure *to straighten the urethra and maintain a sterile field.*

• Use your dominant hand to clean the glans with a sterile cotton-tipped applicator or a sterile cotton ball held in the forceps. Clean in a circular motion, starting at the urinary meatus and working outward.

• Repeat the procedure, using another sterile applicator or cotton ball and taking care not to contaminate your sterile glove.

• Pick up the catheter with your dominant hand and prepare to insert the lubricated tip into the urinary meatus. *To facilitate insertion by relaxing the sphincter,* ask the patient to cough as you insert the catheter. Tell him to breathe deeply and slowly *to further relax the sphincter and spasms.* Hold the catheter close to its tip *to ease insertion and control its direction.* (See *Preventing indwelling catheter problems,* page 238.)

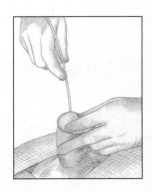

• For the male patient, advance the catheter to the bifurcation (7″ to 9″ [17.8 to 22.8 cm] and check for urine flow (as shown in the bottom illustration at right). If the foreskin was retracted, replace it *to prevent compromised circulation and painful swelling.*

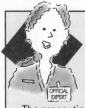

Advice from the experts

Preventing indwelling catheter problems

The precautions below can help prevent problems with an indwelling urinary catheter:
• Never force the catheter during insertion. Instead, maneuver it gently as the patient bears down or coughs. If you still meet resistance, stop and notify the doctor. Sphincter spasms, strictures, misplacement in the vagina (in females), or an enlarged prostate (in males) may cause resistance.
• Establish urine flow, then inflate the balloon. Doing so ensures that the catheter is in the bladder.

More helpful hints
Observe the patient carefully for hypovolemic shock and other adverse reactions caused by removing excessive volumes of residual urine. Check your facility's policy in advance to determine the maximum amount of urine that may be drained at one time. Some facilities limit the amount to between 700 and 1,000 ml. (However, controversy exists over limiting the amount of urine drainage.) Clamp the catheter at the first sign of an adverse reaction, and notify the doctor.

Inflate, hang, and secure

• When urine stops flowing, attach the sterile water-filled syringe to the luer-lock.
• Push the plunger and inflate the balloon *to keep the catheter in place in the bladder.*
• Hang the collection bag below bladder level *to prevent urine reflux into the bladder, which can cause infection, and to promote gravity drainage of the bladder.* Make sure that the tubing doesn't get tangled in the bed's side rails.
• Secure the catheter to the patient's thigh using a leg band with a Velcro closure (as shown at right). *Doing so decreases skin irritation, especially in patients with long-term indwelling catheters.*
• Alternatively, in male patients, secure the catheter to the abdomen *to avoid tension on the bladder neck and prevent accidental dislodgement.*
• Dispose of all used supplies properly.

Latex allergy protocol

Although latex is commonly used to make all sorts of products, many people are allergic to it. Those at increased risk include people who have had or will undergo multiple surgical procedures, health care workers (especially those in the critical care unit, emergency department, and operating room), workers who manufacture latex

Write it down

Documenting indwelling catheter insertion, care, and removal

Catheter insertion

When documenting catheter insertion, record:
- date and time of insertion
- size of the catheter
- volume and appearance of urine
- patient's tolerance of the procedure
- associated problems and interventions.

Catheter care

When documenting catheter care, record:
- care you performed
- care modifications required
- patient complaints
- condition of the perineum and urinary meatus

- characteristics of urine in the drainage bag
- whether a specimen was sent for laboratory analysis
- fluid intake and output. (Usually, an hourly record is required for critically ill patients and hemodynamically unstable patients with renal insufficiency.)

Catheter removal

When documenting catheter removal, record:
- date and time of catheter removal
- patient's tolerance of the procedure
- when and how much the patient voided after removal (usually for first 24 hours)
- associated problems and interventions.

and latex-containing products, and people with a genetic predisposition to latex allergy. (See *Choosing the right glove*, page 240.)

Telltale foods

People who are allergic to certain cross-reactive foods — including apricots, cherries, grapes, kiwis, passion fruit, bananas, avocados, chestnuts, tomatoes, and peaches — may also be allergic to latex. Exposure to latex produces an allergic response similar to the one that these foods produce.

Itching, sneezing, coughing

Latex allergy can cause various signs and symptoms, including generalized itching (on the hands and arms, for example); itchy, watery, burning eyes; sneezing and coughing (hay fever–type signs); rash; hives; bronchial asthma, scratchy throat, and difficulty breathing; edema of the face, hands, and neck; and anaphylaxis.

Letting history speak for itself

To help identify people at risk for latex allergy, ask latex allergy–specific questions during the health history. (See *Latex allergy screening*, page 241.)

Health care workers are at increased risk for latex allergy.

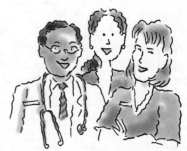

What you need

Latex allergy patient identification wristband ✳ latex-free equipment, including room contents ✳ anaphylaxis kit

Getting ready

After you've determined that the patient has a latex allergy or is sensitive to latex, arrange for him to be placed in a private room. If that isn't possible, make the room latex-free to prevent the

---

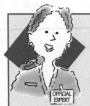

Advice from the experts

Choosing the right glove

Health care workers may develop allergic reactions as a result of their exposure to latex gloves and other products containing natural rubber latex. Patients may also have latex sensitivity.

General precautions
Take the following steps to protect yourself and your patient from allergic reactions to latex:
• Use nonlatex (for example, vinyl or synthetic) gloves for activities that aren't likely to involve contact with infectious materials (food preparation, routine cleaning, and so forth).
• Use appropriate barrier protection when handling infectious materials. If you choose latex gloves, use powder-free gloves with reduced protein content.
• After wearing and removing gloves, wash your hands with soap and dry them thoroughly.
• When wearing latex gloves, don't use oil-based hand creams or lotions (which can cause gloves to deteriorate) unless they've been shown to maintain glove barrier protection.

• Refer to the material safety data sheet for the appropriate glove to wear when handling chemicals.
• Learn procedures for preventing latex allergy, and learn how to recognize the signs and symptoms of latex allergy, including skin rashes; hives; flushing; itching; nasal, eye, or sinus symptoms; asthma; and shock.
• If you have (or suspect you have) a latex sensitivity, use nonlatex gloves, avoid contact with latex gloves and other latex-containing products, and consult a doctor experienced in treating latex allergy.

If you know you're allergic
If you have latex allergy, consider these precautions:
• Avoid contact with latex gloves and other products that contain latex.
• Avoid areas where you might inhale the powder from latex gloves worn by other workers.
• Inform your employers and your health care providers (doctors, nurses, dentists, and others).
• Wear a medical identification bracelet.
• Follow your doctor's instructions for dealing with allergic reactions to latex.

spread of airborne particles from latex products used on the other patient.

How you do it

- Check for latex allergy in all patients being admitted to the delivery room or short procedure unit or having a surgical procedure.
- If a patient has a latex allergy, bring a cart with latex-free supplies into his room.
- Document the allergy on the patient's chart, according to facility policy. If policy requires the patient to wear a latex allergy identification wristband, place it on him.

Write big

- If the patient will be receiving anesthesia, make sure that "LATEX ALLERGY" is clearly visible on the front of his chart. Notify the circulating nurse in the surgical unit, the postanesthesia care unit nurses, and other team members that the patient has a latex allergy.
- If the patient must be transported to another area of the facility, make certain that the latex-free cart accompanies him and that all health care workers who come in contact with him are wearing nonlatex gloves. The patient should wear a mask with cloth ties when leaving his room *to protect him from inhaling airborne latex particles.*

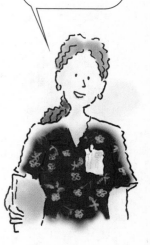

If your patient has a latex allergy, all health care team members involved in his care should be notified.

Latex allergy screening

To determine if your patient has a latex sensitivity or allergy, ask these screening questions:
- Do you have a history of allergies, dermatitis, or asthma? If so, what type of reaction do you have?
- Do you have any congenital abnormalities? If yes, explain.
- Do you have any food allergies? If so, what specific allergies do you have? Describe your reaction.
- Do you experience shortness of breath or wheezing when blowing up latex balloons? If so, describe your reaction.
- Have you had previous surgical procedures? Did you experience associated complications? If so, describe them.
- Have you had previous dental procedures? Did complications result? If so, describe them.
- Are you exposed to latex in your work? Have you experienced a reaction to latex products at work? If so, describe your reaction.

• If the patient is to have an I.V. line, make sure that it's inserted using latex-free products. Post a LATEX ALLERGY sign on the I.V. tubing *to prevent access of the line with latex products.*

First flush

• Flush I.V. tubing with 50 ml of I.V. solution because of latex ports in the I.V. tubing.
• Place a warning label on I.V. bags that says "Don't use latex injection ports."
• Use a nonlatex tourniquet. If none are available, use a latex tourniquet over clothing.
• Remove the vial stopper to mix and draw medications.
• Use latex-free oxygen administration equipment. Remove the elastic, and tie equipment on with gauze.
• Wrap your stethoscope with a nonlatex product *to protect the patient from latex contact.*
• Wrap Tegaderm over the patient's finger before using pulse oximetry.
• Use latex-free syringes when administering medication through a syringe.
• Keep an anaphylaxis kit nearby. If the patient has an allergic reaction to latex, treat him immediately.

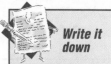

Write it down

Documenting latex allergy protocol

Document actions taken to protect the patient from latex exposure.

Lumbar puncture

Lumbar puncture involves the insertion of a sterile needle into the subarachnoid space of the spinal canal, usually between the third and fourth lumbar vertebrae. This procedure is used to detect blood in cerebrospinal fluid (CSF), to obtain CSF specimens for laboratory analysis, and to inject dyes or gases for contrast in radiologic studies. It's also used to administer drugs or anesthetics.

What you need

Overbed table ✳ one or two pairs of sterile gloves for the doctor ✳ sterile gloves for the nurse ✳ povidone-iodine solution ✳ sterile gauze pads ✳ alcohol pads ✳ sterile fenestrated drape ✳ 3-ml syringe for local anesthetic ✳ 25G ¾″ sterile needle for injecting anesthetic ✳ local anesthetic (usually 1% lidocaine) ✳ 18G or 20G 3½″ spinal needle with stylet (22G needle for a child) ✳ three-way stopcock ✳ manometer ✳ small adhesive bandage ✳ three sterile collection tubes with stoppers ✳ laboratory request forms ✳ labels ✳ light source such as a gooseneck lamp ✳ optional: patient-care reminder

The nurse's role during lumbar puncture is to help the patient maintain the proper position.

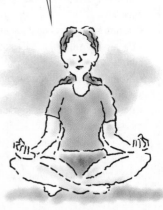

Disposable lumbar puncture trays contain most of the needed sterile equipment.

Getting ready

Gather the equipment and take it to the patient's bedside.

How you do it

- Make sure an informed consent form has been signed.
- Inform the patient that he may experience headache after lumbar puncture, but reassure him that his cooperation during the procedure minimizes such an effect.
- Immediately before the procedure, provide privacy, and instruct the patient to void.
- Wash your hands thoroughly.
- Open the equipment tray on an overbed table, being careful not to contaminate the sterile field when you open the wrapper.

Model behavior

- Provide adequate lighting at the puncture site, and adjust the height of the patient's bed *to allow the doctor to perform the procedure comfortably.*
- Position the patient, and reemphasize the importance of remaining as still as possible *to minimize discomfort and trauma.* (See *Positioning for lumbar puncture.*)

Positioning for lumbar puncture

To position the patient correctly for lumbar puncture, have him lie on his side at the edge of the bed, with his chin tucked to his chest and his knees drawn up to his abdomen. Make sure that the patient's spine is curved and his back is at the edge of the bed (as shown at right). This position widens the spaces between the vertebrae, easing needle insertion.

To help the patient maintain this position, place one of your hands behind his neck and the other hand behind his knees, and pull gently. Hold the patient firmly in this position throughout the procedure to prevent accidental needle displacement.

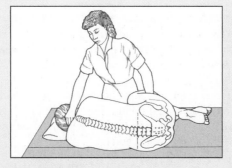

Needle insertion site
Typically, the doctor inserts the needle between the third and fourth lumbar vertebrae.

Careful preparation

- The doctor cleans the puncture site with sterile gauze pads soaked in povidone-iodine solution, wiping in a circular motion away from the puncture site; he uses three different pads *to avoid contaminating spinal tissues with the body's normal skin flora.* Next, he drapes the area with the fenestrated drape *to provide a sterile field.* (If the doctor uses povidone-iodine pads instead of sterile gauze pads, he may remove his sterile gloves and put on another pair *to avoid introducing povidone-iodine into the subarachnoid space with the lumbar puncture needle.*)
- If no ampule of anesthetic is included on the equipment tray, clean the injection port of a multidose vial of anesthetic with an alcohol pad. Then invert the vial 45 degrees so that the doctor can insert a 25G needle and syringe and withdraw the anesthetic for injection.
- Before the doctor injects the anesthetic, tell the patient he'll experience a transient burning sensation and local pain. Ask him to report other persistent pain or sensations *because they may indicate irritation or puncture of a nerve root, requiring repositioning of the needle.*

Still and steady

- When the doctor inserts the sterile spinal needle into the subarachnoid space between the third and fourth lumbar vertebrae, instruct the patient to remain still and breathe normally. If necessary, hold the patient firmly in position *to prevent sudden movement that may displace the needle.*
- If the lumbar puncture is being performed to administer contrast media for radiologic studies or spinal anesthetic, the doctor injects the dye or anesthetic at this time.

Meter reader

- When the needle is in place, the doctor attaches a manometer with a three-way stopcock to the needle hub to read CSF pressure. If ordered, help the patient extend his legs *to provide a more accurate pressure reading.*
- The doctor then detaches the manometer and allows CSF to drain from the needle hub into the collection tubes. When he has collected 2 to 3 ml in each tube, mark the tubes in sequence, insert a stopper *to secure them,* and label them.

Stop sign

- If the doctor suspects an obstruction in the spinal subarachnoid space, he may check for Queckenstedt's sign after he takes an initial CSF pressure reading. He checks for this sign by compressing

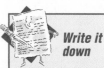

Write it down

Documenting lumbar puncture

In your notes, record:
- initiation and completion times of the procedure
- patient's response
- administration of drugs
- number of specimen tubes collected
- time of transport to the laboratory
- color, consistency, and other characteristics of the collected specimens
- complications and interventions taken.

the patient's jugular vein for 10 seconds. This compression increases intracranial pressure (ICP) and, if no subarachnoid block exists, causes CSF pressure to rise as well. The doctor then takes pressure readings every 10 seconds until the pressure stabilizes. If a block occurs, pressure isn't affected.

Finishing touches

- After the doctor collects the specimens and removes the spinal needle, put on sterile gloves, clean the puncture site with povidone-iodine, and apply a small adhesive bandage. Remove gloves and wash your hands.
- Send the CSF specimens with completed laboratory request forms to the laboratory immediately.

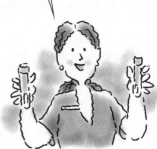

Send the CSF specimens to the lab immediately.

Manual ventilation

A handheld resuscitation bag is an inflatable device that can be attached to a face mask or directly to an ET tube or a tracheostomy tube. It allows manual delivery of oxygen or room air to the lungs of a patient who can't breathe by himself.

Hey! We've been disconnected

Usually used in an emergency, manual ventilation can also be performed while the patient is disconnected temporarily from a mechanical ventilator, such as during a tubing change, during transport, or before suctioning. In such instances, use of the handheld resuscitation bag maintains ventilation. Oxygen administration with a resuscitation bag can help improve a compromised cardiorespiratory system.

What you need

Handheld resuscitation bag ✳ mask ✳ oxygen source (wall unit or tank) ✳ oxygen tubing ✳ nipple adapter attached to oxygen flowmeter ✳ suction equipment ✳ optional: oxygen accumulator, positive end-expiratory pressure (PEEP) valve

Getting ready

Unless the patient is intubated or has a tracheostomy, select a mask that fits snugly over the mouth and nose. (See *Pediatric manual ventilation*.) Attach the mask to the resuscitation bag.

If oxygen is readily available, connect the handheld resuscitation bag to the oxygen. Attach one end of the tubing to the bottom

Ages and stages

Pediatric manual ventilation

When manually ventilating a pediatric patient, make sure that you have the proper bag and mask size. For a child, deliver 15 breaths/minute, or one compression of the bag every 4 seconds; for an infant, 20 breaths/minute, or one compression every 3 seconds. Infants and children should receive 250 to 500 cc of air with each bag compression.

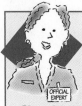

Advice from the experts

How to apply a handheld resuscitation bag and mask

Place the mask over the patient's face so that the apex of the triangle covers the bridge of his nose and the base lies between his lower lip and chin (as shown below left). Hold the mask on, taking care to avoid soft tissue by keeping your fingers on the bony part of the jaw.

Make sure that the patient's mouth remains open beneath the mask. Attach the bag to the mask and to the tubing leading to the oxygen source.

Alternatively, if the patient has a tracheostomy tube or an endotracheal tube in place, remove the mask from the bag and attach the handheld resuscitation bag directly to the tube (as shown below right).

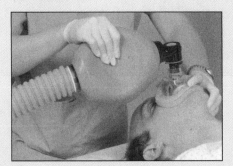
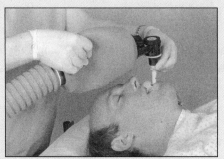

of the bag and the other end to the nipple adapter on the flowmeter of the oxygen source.

Turn on the oxygen, and adjust the flow rate according to the patient's condition. If time allows, set up suction equipment.

How you do it

- Before using the handheld resuscitation bag, check the patient's upper airway for foreign objects. If present, remove them. Suction the patient to remove secretions that may obstruct the airway. If necessary, insert an oropharyngeal or nasopharyngeal airway *to maintain airway patency*. If the patient has a tracheostomy tube or an ET tube in place, suction the tube.
- If appropriate, remove the bed's headboard and stand at the head of the bed *to help keep the patient's neck extended and to free space at the side of the bed for other activities such as CPR.*

Head back, jaw forward

- Tilt the patient's head backward, if not contraindicated, and pull his jaw forward *to move the tongue away from the base of the pharynx and prevent airway obstruction.* (See *How to apply a handheld resuscitation bag and mask.*)
- Keeping your nondominant hand on the patient's mask, exert downward pressure *to seal the mask against his face.* For an adult patient, use your dominant hand to compress the bag every 5 seconds to deliver approximately 1 L of air.
- Deliver breaths with the patient's own inspiratory effort, if present. Don't attempt to deliver a breath as the patient exhales.

Rise and fall

- Observe the patient's chest *to ensure that it rises and falls with each compression.* If ventilation fails to occur, check the fit of the mask and the patency of the patient's airway. If necessary, reposition his head and ensure patency with an oral airway.

Mechanical ventilation

A mechanical ventilator moves air in and out of a patient's lungs. Although the equipment serves to ventilate a patient, it doesn't ensure adequate gas exchange. Mechanical ventilators may use either positive or negative pressure to ventilate patients.

What you need

Oxygen source ✳ air source that can supply 50 psi ✳ mechanical ventilator ✳ humidifier ✳ ventilator circuit tubing, connectors, and adapters ✳ condensation collection trap ✳ spirometer, respirometer, or electronic device to measure flow and volume ✳ in-line thermometer ✳ probe for gas sampling and measuring airway pressure ✳ gloves ✳ handheld resuscitation bag with reservoir ✳ suction equipment ✳ sterile distilled water ✳ equipment for ABG analysis ✳ soft restraints, if indicated ✳ optional: oximeter, ordered sedative, ordered neuromuscular blocking agent

Getting ready

In most facilities, respiratory therapists assume responsibility for setting up the ventilator. If necessary, check the manufacturer's instructions for setting it up.

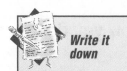

Write it down

Documenting manual ventilation

In your notes, record:
- date and time of manual ventilation efforts
- reason for the procedure
- length of time the patient received manual ventilation
- patient's response
- complications and nursing actions taken.

Hey! I think I'm in trouble. Can you help me out?

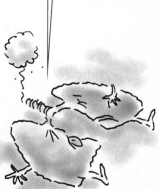

How you do it

• Verify the doctor's order for ventilator support. If the patient isn't already intubated, prepare him for intubation.
• Perform a complete physical assessment, and draw blood for ABG analysis *to establish a baseline.*

Adjust as necessary

• Plug the ventilator into the electrical outlet, and turn it on. Adjust the settings on the ventilator as ordered.
• Make sure that the ventilator's alarms are set as ordered and that the humidifier is filled with sterile distilled water.
• Ensure that suction equipment is readily available and functioning properly.

Is it working?

• Put on gloves if you haven't already. Connect the ET tube to the ventilator. Observe for chest expansion, and auscultate for bilateral breath sounds *to verify that the patient is being ventilated.*
• Monitor the patient's ABG values after the initial ventilator setup (usually 20 to 30 minutes), after changes in ventilator settings, and as the patient's clinical condition indicates *to determine whether the patient is being adequately ventilated and to avoid oxygen toxicity.* Be prepared to adjust ventilator settings based on ABG analysis.
• Keep the head of the patient's bed elevated to at least 30 degrees *to prevent nosocomial pneumonia.*
• Monitor pulse oximetry values.

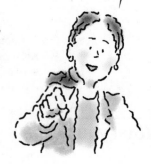

Here's something you should know. The head of the bed should be elevated to at least 30 degrees to prevent nosocomial pneumonia.

Water, temperature, breathing

• Check the ventilator tubing frequently for condensation, *which can cause resistance to airflow and may also be aspirated by the patient.* As needed, drain the condensate into a collection trap or briefly disconnect the patient from the ventilator (ventilating him with a handheld resuscitation bag if necessary), and empty the water into a receptacle. Don't drain the condensate into the humidifier *because the condensate may be contaminated with the patient's secretions.*
• Check the ventilator alarms and in-line thermometer *to make sure that the temperature of the air delivered to the patient is close to body temperature and alarms are activated.* (See *Responding to ventilator alarms.*)
• When monitoring the patient's vital signs, count spontaneous breaths as well as ventilator-delivered breaths.

Running smoothly

Responding to ventilator alarms

The chart below lists two possible ventilator alarm signals along with their possible causes and interventions.

Possible cause	Interventions	Possible cause	Interventions
Low-pressure alarm		*High-pressure alarm*	
• Tube disconnected from ventilator	• Reconnect the tube to the ventilator.	• Increased airway pressure or decreased lung compliance caused by worsening disease	• Auscultate the lungs for evidence of increasing lung consolidation, barotrauma, or wheezing. Call the doctor if indicated.
• Endotracheal (ET) tube displaced above vocal cords or tracheostomy tube extubated	• Check tube placement and reposition if needed. If extubation or displacement has occurred, ventilate the patient manually and call the doctor immediately.	• Patient biting on oral ET tube	• Insert a bite block if needed.
• Leaking tidal volume from low cuff pressure (from an underinflated or ruptured cuff or a leak in the cuff or one-way valve)	• Listen for a whooshing sound around the tube, indicating an air leak. If you hear one, check cuff pressure. If you can't maintain pressure, call the doctor; he may need to insert a new tube.	• Secretions in airway	• Look for secretions in the airway. To remove them, suction the patient or have him cough.
		• Condensate in large-bore tubing	• Check the tubing for condensate and remove fluid if found.
		• Patient coughing, gagging, or attempting to talk	• If the patient fights the ventilator, the doctor may order a sedative or neuromuscular blocker.

Time for a change

• Make sure that the respiratory therapist changes, cleans, or disposes of the ventilator tubing and equipment according to your facility's policy *to reduce the risk of bacterial contamination*. Typically, ventilator tubing should be changed every 48 to 72 hours and sometimes more often.

• When ordered, begin to wean the patient from the ventilator.

Write it down

Documenting mechanical ventilation

In your notes, document:
• date and time that mechanical ventilation was initiated
• type of ventilator used
• ventilator settings
• patient's subjective and objective response to ventilation, including vital signs, breath sounds, and accessory muscle use
• fluid intake and output
• body weight
• complications and nursing actions taken
• pertinent laboratory data, including arterial blood gas (ABG) analysis results and oxygen saturation levels.
   During weaning from the ventilator, record:
• date and time of each weaning session
• weaning method used

• baseline and subsequent vital signs, oxygen saturation levels, and ABG values
• patient's subjective and objective responses, including level of consciousness, respiratory effort, arrhythmias, skin color, and need for suctioning
• complications and nursing actions taken.

What else?
If the patient has been receiving pressure support ventilation (PSV) or using a T-piece or tracheostomy collar, note the duration of spontaneous breathing and the patient's ability to maintain the weaning schedule. If he has been using intermittent mandatory ventilation (with or without PSV), record the control breath rate and the rate of spontaneous respirations.

Nasogastric tube insertion and removal

Usually inserted to decompress the stomach, a nasogastric (NG) tube prevents vomiting after major surgery. An NG tube typically is in place for 48 to 72 hours after surgery, by which time peristalsis usually resumes.

And that isn't all

The NG tube can also be used to assess and treat upper GI bleeding, collect gastric contents for analysis, perform gastric lavage, aspirate gastric secretions, and administer medications and nutrients.

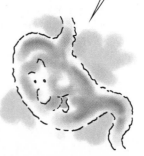

Postsurgery plans commonly include inserting an NG tube.

What you need

For NG tube insertion

Tube (usually #12, #14, #16, or #18 French for a normal adult) ✳ towel or linen-saver pad ✳ penlight ✳ 1″ or 2″ hypoallergenic tape or Opsite ✳ liquid skin barrier ✳ gloves ✳ water-soluble lubricant ✳ cup or glass of water with straw (if appropriate) ✳ tongue blade ✳ catheter-tip or bulb syringe or irrigation set ✳ pH test strip ✳ safety pin ✳ ordered suction equipment ✳ optional: metal clamp, ice, alcohol pad, warm water, large basin or plastic container, rubber band

For NG tube removal

Stethoscope ✳ gloves ✳ catheter-tip syringe ✳ normal saline solution ✳ towel or linen-saver pad ✳ adhesive remover ✳ optional: clamp

Getting ready

Check the patient's history for nasal surgery or a deviated septum. To ease insertion, increase a stiff tube's flexibility by coiling it around your gloved fingers for a few seconds or by dipping it into warm water. Stiffen a limp rubber tube by briefly chilling it in ice.

How you do it

• Provide privacy, wash your hands, and put on gloves.

Inserting an NG tube

• Tell the patient that she may experience some discomfort and that swallowing will ease the tube's advancement.
• Help the patient into high Fowler's position unless contraindicated.
• Stand at the patient's right side if you're right-handed or at her left side if you're left-handed *to ease insertion.*
• Drape the towel or linen-saver pad over the patient's chest.
• Put on gloves.

Measure for measure

• *To determine how long the NG tube must be to reach the stomach,* hold the end of the tube at the tip of the patient's nose. Extend the tube to the patient's earlobe and then down to the xiphoid process.
• Mark this distance on the tubing with the tape.

• To determine which nostril will allow easier access, use a penlight and inspect for a deviated septum or other abnormalities.
• Lubricate the first 3″ (7.6 cm) of the tube with a water-soluble gel.
• Instruct the patient to hold her head straight and upright.

Down the hatch

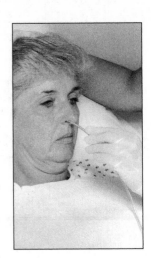

• Grasp the tube with the end pointing downward, curve it if necessary, and carefully insert it into the more patent nostril (as shown at right).
• Aim the tube downward and toward the ear closest to the chosen nostril. Advance it slowly *to avoid pressure on the turbinates and resultant pain and bleeding.*
• When the tube reaches the nasopharynx, you'll feel resistance. Instruct the patient to lower her head slightly *to close the trachea and open the esophagus.* Then rotate the tube 180 degrees toward the opposite nostril *to redirect it so that the tube won't enter the patient's mouth.*

Take a sip

• Unless contraindicated, offer the patient a cup of water with a straw. Direct her to sip and swallow as you slowly advance the tube *to help the tube pass to the esophagus.* (If you aren't using water, ask the patient to swallow.)
• Use a tongue blade and penlight to examine the patient's mouth and throat for signs of a coiled section of tubing.
• As you carefully advance the tube and the patient swallows, watch for respiratory distress signs, *which may mean the tube is in the bronchus and must be removed immediately.*
• Stop advancing the tube when the tape mark reaches the patient's nostril.
• Attach a catheter-tip or bulb syringe to the tube and try to aspirate stomach contents. If you don't obtain stomach contents, position the patient on her left side *to move the contents into the stomach's greater curvature,* and aspirate again.
• If you still can't aspirate stomach contents, advance the tube 1″ to 2″ (2.5 to 5 cm). Then gently attempt to aspirate stomach contents. Examine the aspirate and place a small amount on the pH test strip. Gastric placement is likely if aspirate has the typical gastric fluid appearance (green with clear, colorless mucus or brown) and the pH is less than or equal to 5.
• If this test doesn't confirm proper tube placement, you'll need X-ray verification.

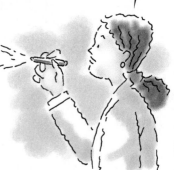

A penlight may help to reveal a coiled section of tubing.

Nobody move

• Secure the NG tube to the patient's nose with hypoallergenic tape (or other designated tube holder). If the patient's skin is oily, wipe the bridge of her nose with an alcohol pad and allow it to dry. Apply liquid skin barrier *to make the tape more adherent to the skin.* You'll need about 4″ (10 cm) of tape. Split one end of the tape up the center about 1½″ (3.8 cm). Make tabs on the split ends (by folding sticky sides together). Stick the uncut tape end on the patient's nose so that the split in the tape starts about ½″ (1.3 cm) to 1½″ from the tip of her nose. Crisscross the tabbed ends around the tube. Then apply another piece of tape over the bridge of the nose *to secure the tube.*

• Alternatively, stabilize the tube with Opsite or a prepackaged product that secures and cushions it at the nose.

• *To reduce discomfort from the weight of the tube,* tie a slipknot around the tube with a rubber band, and then secure the rubber band to the patient's gown with a safety pin, or wrap another piece of tape around the end of the tube and leave a tab. Then fasten the tape tab to the patient's gown.

• Attach the tube to suction equipment, if ordered, and set the designated suction pressure.

Removing an NG tube

• Explain the procedure to the patient and tell her that it may cause some discomfort.

• Assess bowel function by auscultating for peristalsis or flatus.

• Help the patient into semi-Fowler's position. Then drape a towel or linen-saver pad across her chest *to protect her from spills.*

• Put on gloves. Using a catheter-tip syringe, flush the tube with 10 ml of normal saline solution *to ensure that the tube doesn't contain stomach contents that could irritate tissues during tube removal.*

• Untape the tube from the patient's nose and then unpin it from her gown.

• Clamp the tube by folding it in your hand.

Pull slowly, then quickly

• Ask the patient to hold her breath *to close the epiglottis.* Then withdraw the tube gently and steadily. (When the distal end of the tube reaches the nasopharynx, you can pull it quickly.)

• Assist the patient with thorough mouth care, and clean the tape residue from her nose with adhesive remover.

• Monitor the patient for signs of GI dysfunction.

Pressure ulcer care

Most pressure ulcers develop over bony prominences, where friction and shearing force combine with pressure to break down skin

Write it down

Documenting NG tube insertion and removal

After inserting the tube, record:

• type and size of the nasogastric (NG) tube

• insertion date and time

• type and amount of suction, if used

• drainage characteristics, including amount, color, character, consistency, and odor

• patient's tolerance of the procedure.

When you remove the tube, record:

• removal date and time

• color, consistency, and amount of gastric drainage

• patient's tolerance of the procedure.

and underlying tissues. Common sites include the sacrum, coccyx, ischial tuberosities, and greater trochanters. Other common sites include the skin over the vertebrae, scapulae, elbows, knees, and heels in bedridden and relatively immobile patients. (See *Assessing pressure ulcers*.)

What you need

Hypoallergenic tape or elastic netting ✳ overbed table ✳ piston-type irrigating system ✳ two pairs of gloves ✳ normal saline solution as ordered ✳ sterile 4″ × 4″ gauze pads ✳ selected topical dressing ✳ linen-saver pads ✳ impervious plastic trash bag ✳ disposable wound-measuring device ✳ 21G needle and syringe ✳ optional: alcohol pad

Getting ready

Assemble the equipment at the patient's bedside. Cut tape into strips for securing dressings. Loosen lids on cleaning solutions and medications for easy removal. Loosen existing dressing edges and tapes before putting on gloves. Attach an impervious plastic trash bag to the overbed table to hold used dressings and refuse.

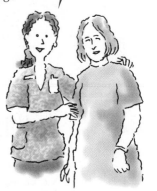

Keeping patients mobile is the key to preventing pressure ulcers.

How you do it

• Before any dressing change, wash your hands and review the principles of standard precautions.

Cleaning the pressure ulcer

• Provide privacy and explain the procedure to the patient.
• Position the patient in a way that maximizes his comfort while allowing easy access to the pressure ulcer site.
• Cover bed linens with a linen-saver pad.

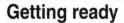

No splashing

• Open the normal saline solution container and the piston syringe. Carefully pour normal saline solution into an irrigation container. (The container may be clean or sterile, depending on facility policy.) Put the piston syringe into the opening provided in the irrigation container.
• Open the packages of supplies.
• Put on gloves to remove the old dressing and expose the pressure ulcer. Discard the soiled dressing in the impervious plastic trash bag.

Assessing pressure ulcers

To choose the most effective treatment for a pressure ulcer, you must first assess its characteristics. The pressure ulcer staging system described below, used by the National Pressure Ulcer Advisory Panel and the Agency for Health Care Research and Quality, reflects the anatomic depth of exposed tissue. Keep in mind that if the wound contains necrotic tissue, you won't be able to determine the stage until you can see the wound base.

Stage I
In stage I, the heralding lesion of a pressure ulcer is persistent redness in lightly pigmented skin, and persistent red, blue, or purple hues on darker skin. Other indicators include changes in temperature, consistency, or sensation.

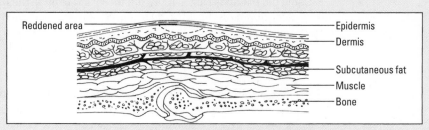

Stage II
Stage II is marked by partial-thickness skin loss involving the epidermis, dermis, or both. The ulcer is superficial and appears as an abrasion, a blister, or a shallow crater.

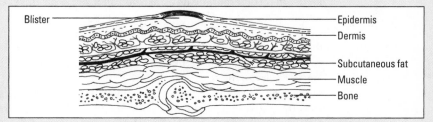

Stage III
In stage III, the ulcer constitutes a full-thickness wound penetrating the subcutaneous tissue, which may extend to — but not through — underlying fascia. The ulcer resembles a deep crater and may undermine adjacent tissue.

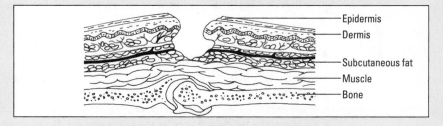

Stage IV
In stage IV, the ulcer extends through the skin, accompanied by extensive destruction, tissue necrosis, or damage to muscle, bone, or supporting structures (such as tendons and joint capsules).

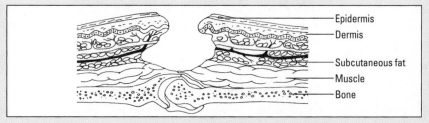

Tale of the tape

• Inspect the wound. Note the color, amount, and odor of drainage and necrotic debris. Measure the wound perimeter with the disposable wound-measuring device (a square, transparent card with concentric circles arranged in bull's-eye fashion and bordered with a straight-edge ruler).
• Using the piston syringe, apply full force and irrigate the pressure ulcer *to remove necrotic debris and help decrease bacteria in the wound.*
• Remove and discard your soiled gloves and put on a fresh pair.

Tunnel test

• Insert a gloved finger or sterile cotton-tipped applicator into the wound *to assess wound tunneling or undermining.* Tunneling usually signals wound extension along fascial planes. Gauge tunnel depth by determining how far you can insert your finger or the cotton swab.
• Next, reassess the condition of the skin and ulcer. Note the character of the clean wound bed and surrounding skin.
• If you observe adherent necrotic material, notify a wound care specialist or doctor.
• Prepare to apply the appropriate topical dressing. (See instructions for applying typical moist saline gauze, hydrocolloid, transparent, alginate, foam, and hydrogel dressings below.) For other dressings or topical agents, follow your facility's policy or the supplier's instructions.

Applying a moist saline gauze dressing

• Irrigate the pressure ulcer with normal saline solution. Blot the surrounding skin dry.
• Moisten the gauze dressing with normal saline solution.
• Gently place the dressing over the ulcer surface. To separate surfaces within the wound, gently place a dressing between opposing wound surfaces. To avoid damage to tissues, don't pack the gauze tightly.
• Change the dressing often enough to keep the wound moist.

Applying a hydrocolloid dressing

• Irrigate the pressure ulcer with normal saline solution. Blot the surrounding skin dry.

Smooth operator

• Choose a clean, dry, presized dressing, or cut one to overlap the pressure ulcer by about 1″ (2.5 cm). Remove the dressing from its package, pull the release paper from the adherent side of the dressing, and apply the dressing to the wound. *To minimize irritation,* carefully smooth out wrinkles as you apply the dressing.

• If the dressing's edges need to be secured with tape, apply a skin sealant to the intact skin around the ulcer. After the area dries, tape the dressing to the skin. The sealant protects the skin and promotes tape adherence. Avoid using tension or pressure when applying the tape.

• Remove your gloves and discard them in the impervious plastic trash bag. Dispose of refuse according to facility policy and wash your hands.

• Change a hydrocolloid dressing every 2 to 7 days as necessary—for example, if the patient complains of pain, the dressing no longer adheres, or leakage occurs.

Applying a transparent dressing

• Irrigate the pressure ulcer with normal saline solution. Blot the surrounding skin dry.

• Clean and dry the wound as described above.

• Select a dressing to overlap the ulcer by 2″ (5 cm). If the edges of the dressing begin to curl, straighten them.

Straighten the curls

• Gently lay the dressing over the ulcer. *To prevent shearing force,* don't stretch the dressing. Press firmly on the edges of the dressing *to promote adherence.* Although this type of dressing is self-adhesive, you may have to tape the edges *to prevent them from curling.*

• If necessary, aspirate accumulated fluid with a 21G needle and syringe. After aspirating the pocket of fluid, clean the aspiration site with an alcohol pad and cover it with another strip of transparent dressing.

• Change the dressing every 3 to 7 days, depending on the amount of drainage.

Applying an alginate dressing

• Irrigate the pressure ulcer with normal saline solution. Blot the surrounding skin dry.

• Apply the alginate dressing to the ulcer surface. Cover the area with a secondary dressing, such as gauze pads, as ordered. Secure the dressing with tape or elastic netting.

• If the wound is draining heavily, change the dressing once or twice daily for the first 3 to 5 days. As drainage decreases, change the dressing less frequently—every 2 to 4 days or as ordered. When the drainage stops or the wound bed looks dry, stop using alginate dressing.

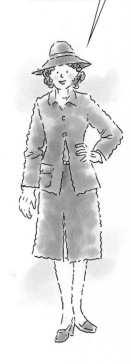

Choosing the appropriate wound dressing is important. Your dressing? Not so much.

Applying a foam dressing

• Irrigate the pressure ulcer with normal saline solution. Blot the surrounding skin dry.
• Gently lay the foam dressing over the ulcer.
• Use tape, elastic netting, or gauze to hold the dressing in place.
• Change the dressing when the foam no longer absorbs the exudate.

Applying a hydrogel dressing

• Irrigate the pressure ulcer with normal saline solution. Blot the surrounding skin dry.
• Apply gel to the wound bed.
• Cover the area with a secondary dressing.
• Change the dressing daily or as needed *to keep the wound bed moist.*
• If the dressing you select comes in sheet form, cut the dressing to match the wound base; *otherwise, the intact surrounding skin can become macerated.*
• Hydrogel dressings also come in a prepackaged, saturated gauze for wounds that require "dead space" to be filled. Follow the manufacturer's directions.

Preventing pressure ulcers

• Turn and reposition the patient every 1 to 2 hours unless contraindicated. For a patient who can't turn himself or who's turned on a schedule, use a pressure-reducing device, such as air, gel, or a 4″ foam mattress overlay. Low- or high-air-loss therapy may be indicated *to reduce excessive pressure and promote evaporation of excess moisture.* As appropriate, implement active or passive range-of-motion (ROM) exercises to relieve pressure and promote circulation. To save time, combine these exercises with bathing if applicable.

D'oh! No doughnut here.

• Direct the patient confined to a chair or wheelchair to shift his weight every 15 minutes *to promote blood flow to compressed tissues.* Show a paraplegic patient how to shift his weight by doing push-ups in the wheelchair. If the patient needs your help, sit next to him and help him shift his weight to one buttock for 60 seconds; then repeat the procedure on the other side. Provide pressure-relieving cushions as appropriate. However, avoid seating the patient on a rubber or plastic doughnut, *which can increase localized pressure at vulnerable points.*
• Apply lotion after bathing *to help keep the patient's skin moist.*

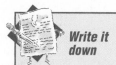

Write it down

Documenting pressure ulcer care

In your notes, record:
• date and time of initial and subsequent treatments
• specific treatment given
• preventive strategies performed
• pressure ulcer location and size (length, width, and depth)
• color and appearance of the wound bed
• amount, odor, color, and consistency of drainage
• condition of the surrounding skin.

  Reassess pressure ulcers at least weekly. Update the care plan as required, noting changes in ulcer condition or size and skin temperature elevation on the clinical record. Record when the doctor was notified of abnormal observations. Record daily temperature readings on the graphic sheet to allow easy assessment of body temperature patterns.

Minimize moisture

• If diarrhea develops or if the patient is incontinent, clean and dry soiled skin. Then apply a protective moisture barrier *to prevent skin maceration.*

Pulse oximetry

Pulse oximetry is a relatively simple, noninvasive procedure used to monitor arterial oxygen saturation (SpO_2). It can be performed continuously or intermittently.

Light reading

In this procedure, two diodes send red and infrared light through a pulsating arterial vascular bed such as the one in the fingertip. A photodetector slipped over the finger measures the transmitted light as it passes through the vascular bed, detects the relative amount of color absorbed by arterial blood, and calculates the exact mixed venous oxygen saturation without interference from surrounding venous blood, skin, connective tissue, or bone.

What you need

Oximeter ✳ finger or ear probe ✳ alcohol pads ✳ nail polish remover, if necessary

Getting ready

Review the manufacturer's instructions for assembling the oximeter.

How you do it

For pulse oximetry

• Select a finger for the test (or bridge of the nose if circulation in the extremities is compromised). Although the index finger is commonly used, a smaller finger may be selected if the patient's fingers are too large for the equipment. (See *Pediatric pulse oximetry.*) Make sure that the patient isn't wearing false fingernails, and remove any nail polish from the test finger. Place the transducer (photodetector) probe over the patient's finger so that light beams and sensors oppose each other. If the patient has long fingernails, position the probe perpendicular to the finger, if possible, or clip the fingernail. Always position the patient's hand at

Ages and stages

Pediatric pulse oximetry

If you must monitor arterial oxygen saturation in a neonate or small infant, wrap the oximeter's probe around the infant's foot so that light beams and detectors oppose each other. For a large infant, use a probe that fits on the great toe and secure it to the foot.

heart level *to eliminate venous pulsations and promote accurate readings.*

• Turn on the power switch. If the device is working properly, a beep will sound, a display will light momentarily, and the pulse searchlight will flash. The SpO_2 and pulse rate displays will show stationary zeros. After four to six heartbeats, the SpO_2 and pulse rate displays will supply information with each beat, and the pulse amplitude indicator will begin tracking the pulse.

Restraint application

Restraints are used only when other, less restrictive measures prove ineffective in protecting the patient and others from harm. *Soft restraints* limit movement to prevent the confused, disoriented, or combative patient from injuring himself or others. *Vest* and *belt restraints*, which permit full movement of arms and legs, are used to prevent falls from a bed or chair. *Limb restraints*, which allow only slight limb motion, are used to prevent the patient from removing supportive equipment (such as I.V. lines, indwelling catheters, and NG tubes). *Mitts* prevent the patient from removing supportive equipment, scratching rashes or sores, and injuring himself or others. *Body restraints*, which immobilize all or most of the body, are used to control the combative or hysterical patient. *Leather restraints* should be used only as a last resort for the combative patient who's at risk for injuring himself or others.

What you need

For soft restraints

Vest, belt, limb, or body restraints or mitts as needed ✳ gauze pads or washcloth if needed

For leather restraints

Two wrist and two ankle leather restraints ✳ four straps ✳ key ✳ large gauze pads to cushion each extremity

Getting ready

Before entering the patient's room, make sure that the restraints are the correct size, using the patient's build and weight as a guide. If you use leather restraints, make sure that the straps are unlocked and the key fits the locks.

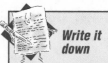

Write it down

Documenting pulse oximetry

In your notes, document the procedure, including the date, time, procedure type, oximetric measurement, and actions taken. Record the readings on appropriate flowcharts, if indicated.

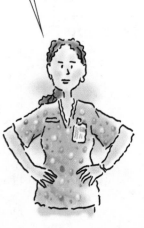

Restrain yourself from using restraints on a patient unless all other measures prove ineffective.

How you do it

• Obtain a doctor's order for the restraint. Keep in mind that the doctor's order must be time limited—4 hours for adults, 2 hours for children and adolescents ages 9 to 17, and 1 hour for patients younger than age 9 when used for behavioral purposes. When used for medical-surgical purposes, the order is limited to 24 hours. After the original order expires, the doctor must see and evaluate the patient before a new order can be written.

Team play

• If necessary, enlist the help of several coworkers and organize their effort before entering the patient's room, giving each person a specific task — for example, one person explains the procedure to the patient and applies the restraints while the others immobilize his arms and legs.
• Tell the patient what you're about to do, and describe the restraints to him. Assure him that they're being used to protect him from injury, rather than to punish him.

Applying a vest restraint

• Assist the patient to a sitting position if his condition permits.

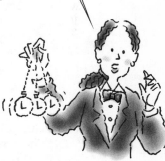

Remember, a restraint order must have a time limit.

Cross your heart

• Slip the vest over the patient's gown. Crisscross the cloth flaps at the front, placing the V-shaped opening at his throat. Never crisscross the flaps in the back, *which may cause him to choke if he tries to squirm out of the vest.*

Keep it a little loose

• Pass the tab on one flap through the slot on the opposite flap, and adjust the vest for the patient's comfort. You should be able to slip your fist between the vest and the patient. Avoid wrapping the vest too tightly *because doing so may restrict his breathing.*

Knot too tight

• Tie all restraints securely to the frame of the bed, chair, or wheelchair, out of the patient's reach, using a bow or a knot that can be released quickly and easily in an emergency. Never tie a regular knot to secure the straps.
• Leave 1″ to 2″ (2.5 to 5 cm) of slack in the straps.

Breathing behavior

• After applying the vest, check the patient's respiratory rate and breath sounds regularly. Watch for signs of respiratory distress.

• Make sure that the vest hasn't tightened with the patient's movement. Loosen the vest frequently, if possible, *so the patient can stretch, turn, and breathe deeply.*

Applying a limb restraint

• Wrap the patient's wrist or ankle with gauze pads *to reduce friction between the patient's skin and the restraint, which will help prevent irritation and skin breakdown.* Then wrap the restraint around the gauze pads.

Snug as a bug

• Pass the strap on the narrow end of the restraint through the slot in the broad end, and adjust for a snug fit. Alternatively, fasten the buckle or Velcro cuffs to fit the restraint. You should be able to slip one or two fingers between the restraint and the patient's skin. Avoid applying the restraint too tightly.
• Tie the restraint as you would a vest restraint, using a bow or a knot that can be released quickly and easily in an emergency.

Keep on movin'

• After applying limb restraints, watch for signs of impaired circulation in the extremity distal to the restraint. If the skin appears blue or feels cold or if the patient complains of a tingling sensation or numbness, loosen the restraint.
• Perform ROM exercises regularly *to stimulate circulation and prevent contractures and loss of mobility.*

Applying a mitt restraint

• Wash and dry the patient's hands.

Give 'em something to hold on to

• Roll up a washcloth or gauze pad, and place it in the patient's palm. Have him form a loose fist, if possible, and then pull the mitt over it and secure the closure.
• *To restrict the patient's arm movement,* attach the strap to the mitt, and tie it securely, using a bow or a knot that can be released quickly and easily in an emergency.
• When using mitts made of transparent mesh, check hand movement and skin color frequently *to assess circulation.*
• Remove the mitts regularly *to stimulate circulation* and perform passive ROM exercises *to prevent contractures.*

Applying a belt restraint

• Center the flannel pad of the belt on the bed. Then wrap the short strap of the belt around the bed frame, and fasten it under the bed.
• Position the patient on the pad. Then have him roll slightly to one side while you guide the long strap around his waist and through the slot in the pad.
• Wrap the long strap around the bed frame and fasten it under the bed.

Getting the right fit

• After applying the belt, slip your hand between the patient and the belt *to ensure a secure but comfortable fit*. A loose belt can be raised to chest level; a tight one can cause abdominal discomfort.

Applying a body (Posey net) restraint

• Place the restraint flat on the bed, with arm and wrist cuffs facing down and the V at the head of the bed.
• Place the patient in the prone position on top of the restraint.
• Lift the V over the patient's head. Thread the chest belt through one of the loops in the V to ensure a snug fit.
• Secure the straps around the patient's chest, thighs, and legs. Then turn the patient on his back.
• Secure the straps to the bed frame *to anchor the restraint*. Then secure the straps around the patient's arms and wrists.

Applying leather restraints

• Place the patient in a supine position on the bed, with each arm and leg securely held down *to minimize combative behavior and prevent injury*.
• Immobilize the patient's arms and legs at the knees, ankles, shoulders, and wrists.
• Apply gauze pads to the patient's wrists and ankles *to reduce friction between his skin and the leather and prevent skin irritation and breakdown*.

Not too tight; not too loose

• Wrap the restraint around the gauze pads, and insert the metal loop through the hole that gives the best fit.
• Apply the restraints securely but not too tightly. You should be able to slip one or two fingers between the restraint and the patient's skin.
• Thread the strap through the metal loop on the restraint, close the metal loop, and secure the strap to the bed frame, out of the patient's reach.

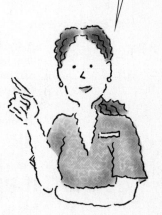

For all types of restraints, ensure a secure but comfortable fit.

Flex, lock, and release

• Flex the patient's arm or leg slightly before locking the strap *to allow room for movement and prevent joints from locking in place or dislocating.*
• Lock the restraint by pushing in the button on the side of the metal loop, and tug it gently to make sure that it's secure. After it's secure, a coworker can release the arm or leg.
• Place the key in an accessible location at the nurses' station.
• Check the patient's pulse rate and vital signs at least every 2 hours.

Give 'em a break

• Remove or loosen the restraints one at a time, every 2 hours, and perform passive ROM exercises if possible. To unlock the restraint, insert the key into the metal loop, opposite the locking button. This key releases the lock so you can open the metal loop.
• Watch for signs of impaired peripheral circulation such as cool, cyanotic skin.
• Observe the patient regularly and offer emotional support.

Write it down

Documenting restraint use

Document restraint use on a restraint flow sheet according to facility policy. Record:
• behavior that necessitated restraints
• when the restraints were applied and removed
• type of restraints used
• patient's vital signs, skin condition, respiratory status, peripheral circulation, and mental status.

Seizure management

Seizures are paroxysmal events associated with abnormal electrical discharges of neurons in the brain. Partial seizures are usually unilateral, involving a localized or focal area of the brain. Generalized seizures involve the entire brain.

Protect and observe

When a patient has a generalized seizure, nursing care aims to protect him from injury and prevent serious complications. Appropriate care also includes observation of seizure characteristics to help determine the area of the brain involved.

A step ahead

Patients considered at risk for seizures are those with a history of seizures and those with conditions, such as traumatic brain injury, that predispose them to seizures. These patients require precautionary measures to help prevent injury if a seizure occurs. (See *Seizure precautions.*)

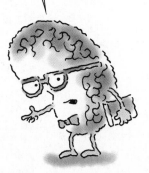

I hate to generalize, really, but generalized seizures involve the entire brain.

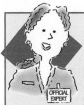

Advice from the experts

Seizure precautions

By taking appropriate precautions, you can help protect the patient from injury, aspiration, and airway obstruction in the event of a seizure.

Gathering equipment

Based on the patient's history, tailor your precautions to his needs. Start by gathering the appropriate equipment, including a hospital bed with full-length side rails, commercial side rail pads, or six bath blankets (four for a crib). Also gather adhesive tape, an oral airway, and oral or nasal suction equipment.

Preparing the bedside

• Explain to the patient why the precautions are necessary.
• To protect the patient from injury caused by a seizure while he's in bed, cover the side rails, headboard, and footboard with side rail pads or bath blankets. If you use blankets, secure them with adhesive tape. To prevent falls, always keep three side rails raised while the patient is in bed. Keep the bed in a low position.
• Place an airway at the bedside according to your facility's protocol. Keep suction equipment nearby in case you need to establish a patent airway. Explain to the patient how the airway will be used.
• If the patient has a history of frequent or prolonged seizures, insert an I.V. saline lock to administer emergency medications.
• After a seizure, place the patient in a side-lying position to prevent aspiration.

What you need

Oral airway ✳ oxygen and supplies (mask, tubing, source) ✳ suction equipment ✳ side rail pads ✳ seizure activity record

Getting ready

If you're with a patient when he experiences an aura, help him into bed, raise the side rails, and adjust the bed flat. If he's away from his room, lower him to the floor and place a pillow, blanket, or other soft material under his head to keep it from hitting the floor.

How you do it

• Stay with the patient during the seizure, and be ready to intervene if complications, such as airway obstruction, develop. If necessary, have another staff member obtain the appropriate equipment and notify the doctor of the obstruction.

• Move hard or sharp objects out of the patient's way, and loosen his clothing.

• Don't forcibly restrain the patient or restrict his movements during the seizure *because the force of the patient's movements against restraints could cause muscle strain or even joint dislocation.*

Take note

• Continually assess the patient during the seizure. Observe the earliest symptom, such as head or eye deviation, as well as how the seizure progresses, what form it takes, and how long it lasts. *Your description may help determine the seizure's type and cause.*

• If this is the patient's first seizure, notify the doctor immediately. If the patient has had seizures before, notify the doctor only if the seizure activity is prolonged or if the patient fails to regain consciousness. (See *Understanding status epilepticus.*)

When it's done

• If ordered, establish an I.V. line and infuse normal saline solution at a keep-vein-open rate.

• If the seizure is prolonged and the patient becomes hypoxemic, administer oxygen as ordered. He may require ET intubation.

• For a patient with diabetes, administer 50 ml of dextrose 50% in water by I.V. push as ordered. For an alcoholic patient, a 100-mg bolus of thiamine may be ordered *to stop the seizure.*

• After the seizure, turn the patient on his side and apply suction if necessary *to facilitate drainage of secretions and maintain a patent airway.* Insert an oral airway if needed.

• Check for injuries.

• Reorient and reassure the patient as necessary.

• When the patient is comfortable and safe, document what happened during the seizure.

• After the seizure, monitor the patient's vital signs and mental status every 15 to 20 minutes for 2 hours.

• Ask the patient about his aura and activities preceding the seizure. The type of aura (auditory, visual, olfactory, gustatory, or somatic) helps pinpoint the site in the brain where the seizure originated.

Understanding status epilepticus

Status epilepticus is a state of continuous seizure without intervening periods of consciousness. It can occur in any seizure type. The most life-threatening form of status epilepticus is generalized tonic-clonic status epilepticus.

Name the causes

Always an emergency, status epilepticus is accompanied by respiratory distress. It can result from abrupt withdrawal of anticonvulsant medications, hypoxic or metabolic encephalopathy, acute head trauma, or septicemia secondary to encephalitis or meningitis.

Stop the seizure

Emergency treatment usually consists of lorazepam or diazepam followed by phenytoin and, possibly, dextrose 50% I.V. (when seizures result from hypoglycemia).

Write it down

Documenting seizure management

When documenting seizure management, record:
- patient's need for seizure precautions
- seizure precautions taken
- date and time the seizure began
- seizure duration
- precipitating factors
- sensations the patient reported or experienced before the seizure (possibly an aura)
- involuntary behavior at seizure onset, such as lip smacking, chewing movements, or hand and eye movements
- where body movements began and body parts involved
- progression or pattern to body movements

- deviation of the eyes to one side
- change in pupil size, shape, equality, or reaction to light
- whether the patient's teeth were clenched or open
- incontinence, vomiting, or salivation during the seizure
- patient's response to the seizure (for instance, whether he was aware of what happened, fell into a deep sleep afterward, or was upset or ashamed)
- medications given
- complications during the seizure and nursing actions
- patient's postseizure mental status.

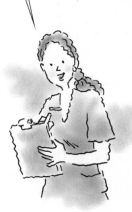

Remember that documentation is an important step for every nursing procedure.

Sequential compression therapy

Sequential compression therapy massages the legs in a wavelike, milking motion that promotes blood flow and deters thrombosis. It may be used with other measures to prevent deep vein thrombosis, such as antiembolism stockings and anticoagulant medications. Antiembolism stockings and sequential compression sleeves are commonly used preoperatively, intraoperatively, and postoperatively because blood clots tend to form during surgery.

What you need

Measuring tape ✳ sizing chart for the brand of sleeves you're using ✳ pair of compression sleeves in correct size ✳ connecting tubing ✳ compression controller

Getting ready

Wash your hands, explain the procedure to the patient, and have the patient rest in bed so that you can measure the circumference of the upper thigh at the gluteal fold. Find the patient's thigh measurement on the sizing chart, and locate the corresponding size of the compression sleeve.

Remove the compression sleeves from the package and unfold them, laying them down with the cotton lining facing up.

How you do it

- Place the patient's leg on the cotton sleeve lining, positioning the back of the knee over the popliteal opening and the back of the ankle over the ankle marking.
- Starting at the side opposite the clear plastic tubing, wrap the sleeve snugly around the patient's leg, beginning with the ankle and calf and then the thigh, and secure it with Velcro fasteners.
- Using the same procedure, apply the second sleeve.

Connect with a click

- Connect each sleeve to the tubing leading to the controller, making sure that the tubing isn't kinked. Line up the blue arrows on the connectors and push the ends together firmly. Listen for a click, signaling a firm connection.
- Plug the compression controller into the wall outlet and turn on the power. The controller automatically sets the compression sleeve pressure at 45 mm Hg, which is the midpoint of the normal range (35 to 55 mm Hg).
- Check the AUDIBLE ALARM key. The green light should be lit, indicating that the alarm is working.
- When discontinuing therapy, dispose of the sleeves, but store the tubing and compression controller according to your facility's policy.

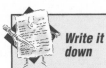

Write it down

Documenting sequential compression therapy

In your notes, record:
- procedure
- patient's response to and understanding of the procedure
- status of the alarm and cooling settings.

Surgical site verification

Wrong-site surgery is a general term referring to a surgical procedure performed on the wrong body part or side of the body — or even the wrong patient. This error may occur in the operating room or in other settings, such as ambulatory care or interventional radiology. Because serious consequences may result from wrong-site surgery, the nurse must confirm that the correct site has been identified before surgery begins.

What you need

Surgical consent ✳ medical record ✳ procedure schedule ✳ hypoallergenic, nonlatex permanent marker

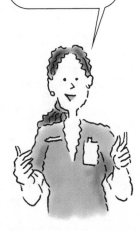

It's a nurse's responsibility to verify that the correct site has been identified before surgery.

Getting ready

Before the procedure, check the patient's chart for documentation and compare the information using the history and physical examination form, nursing assessment, preprocedure checklist, signed informed consent with the exact procedure site identified, procedure schedule, and the patient's verbal confirmation of the correct site.

How you do it

- The doctor performing the surgery should mark the correct site with a permanent marker after verbally confirming the site with the patient or a family member.
- Ensure that the surgical team (surgeon, operating room or procedure staff, and anesthesia personnel) takes a "time out" to identify the patient and verify the correct procedure and correct site before beginning the surgery.
- The nurse should verify that the surgeon confirms the site with the patient or family member.

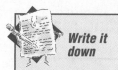

Write it down

Documenting surgical site verification

Complete the preprocedure checklist used by your facility, record that the correct site was verified, and note that the surgeon has marked the correct site with a permanent marker.

Thoracic drainage

Thoracic drainage uses gravity (and occasionally suction) to restore negative pressure, remove material that collects in the pleural cavity, or reexpand a partially or totally collapsed lung. An underwater seal in the drainage system allows air and fluid to escape from the pleural cavity but doesn't allow air to reenter.

Multi-tasker

The system is a self-contained, disposable system that collects drainage, creates a water seal, and controls suction.

What you need

Thoracic drainage system (Pleur-evac, Argyle, Ohio, or Thora-Klex system, which can function as gravity drainage systems or be connected to suction to enhance chest drainage) ✳ sterile distilled water (usually 1 L) ✳ adhesive tape ✳ sterile clear plastic tubing ✳ bottle or system rack ✳ two rubber-tipped Kelly clamps ✳ sterile 50-ml catheter-tip syringe ✳ suction source, if ordered ✳ pain medication, if ordered

Getting ready

Check the doctor's order to determine the type of drainage system to be used and specific procedure details. If appropriate, request the drainage system and suction system from the central supply department. Collect the appropriate equipment, and take it to the patient's bedside.

How you do it

• Maintain sterile technique throughout the entire procedure and whenever you make changes in the system or alter any of the connections *to avoid introducing pathogens into the pleural space.*

Setting up a commercially prepared disposable system

• Open the packaged system, and place it on the floor in the rack supplied by the manufacturer *to avoid accidentally knocking it over or dislodging the components.* After the system is prepared, it may be hung from the side of the patient's bed.

Just add water

• Remove the plastic connector from the short tube attached to the water-seal chamber. Using a 50-ml catheter-tip syringe, instill sterile distilled water into the water-seal chamber until it reaches the 2-cm mark or the mark specified by the manufacturer. (The Ohio and Thora-Klex systems are ready to use; however, with the Thora-Klex system, 15 ml of sterile water may be added *to help detect air leaks.*) Replace the plastic connector.
• If suction is ordered, remove the cap (also called the *muffler* or *atmosphere vent cover*) on the suction-control chamber to open the vent. Next, instill sterile distilled water until it reaches the 20-cm mark or the ordered level, and recap the suction-control chamber.
• Using the long tube, connect the patient's chest tube to the closed drainage collection chamber. Secure the connection with tape.
• Connect the short tube on the drainage system to the suction source, and turn on the suction. Gentle bubbling should begin in the suction chamber, indicating that the correct suction level has been reached.

Managing closed-chest underwater seal drainage

• Repeatedly note the character, consistency, and amount of drainage in the drainage collection chamber.

• Mark the drainage level in the drainage collection chamber by noting the time and date at the drainage level on the chamber every 8 hours (or more often if there's a large amount of drainage).

Look for the level

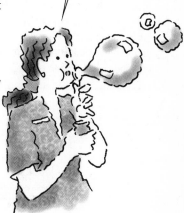

What can I say? One nursing responsibility associated with thoracic drainage is checking for bubbles.

• Check the water level in the water-seal chamber every 8 hours. If necessary, carefully add sterile distilled water until the level reaches the 2-cm mark indicated on the water-seal chamber of the commercial system.
• Check for fluctuation in the water-seal chamber as the patient breathes. Normal fluctuations of 2″ to 4″ (5 to 10 cm) reflect pressure changes in the pleural space during respiration. To check for fluctuation when a suction system is being used, momentarily disconnect the suction system so the air vent is open, and observe for fluctuation.
• Check for intermittent bubbling in the water-seal chamber. *This bubbling occurs normally when the system is removing air from the pleural space.* If bubbling isn't readily apparent during quiet breathing, have the patient take a deep breath or cough. *Absence of bubbling indicates that the pleural space has sealed.*
• Check the water level in the suction-control chamber. Detach the chamber from the suction source; when bubbling ceases, observe the water level. If necessary, add sterile distilled water to bring the level to the –20-cm line or as ordered.
• Check for gentle bubbling in the suction-control chamber because it indicates that the proper suction level has been reached. *Vigorous bubbling in this chamber increases the rate of water evaporation.*
• Periodically check that the air vent in the system is working properly. *Occlusion of the air vent results in a buildup of pressure in the system that could cause the patient to develop tension pneumothorax.*

Always ready to clamp down

• Be sure to keep two rubber-tipped clamps at the bedside *to clamp the chest tube if the system cracks or to locate an air leak in the system.*
• Encourage the patient to cough frequently and breathe deeply *to help drain the pleural space and expand the lungs.*
• Tell him to sit upright *for optimal lung expansion* and splint the insertion site while coughing *to minimize pain.*
• Check the rate and quality of the patient's respirations, and auscultate his lungs periodically *to assess air exchange in the affected lung.* Diminished or absent breath sounds may indicate that the lung hasn't reexpanded.

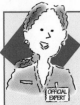

To strip or not to strip

When clots are visible, you may be able to strip (or milk) the tubing, depending on your facility's policy. This procedure is controversial because it creates high negative pressure that could suck viable lung tissue into the tube's drainage ports, with subsequent ruptured alveoli and pleural air leaks.

If you're ready for the challenge…
Strip the tubing only when clots are visible. Use an alcohol pad or lotion as a lubricant on the tube, and pinch it between your thumb and index finger about 2″ (5 cm) from the insertion site. Using the other thumb and index finger, compress the tubing as you slide your fingers down the tube or use a mechanical stripper. After stripping, release the thumb and index finger that are pinching the tube near the insertion site.

Cause for alarm

- Tell the patient to report breathing difficulty immediately. Notify the doctor immediately if the patient develops cyanosis, rapid or shallow breathing, subcutaneous emphysema, chest pain, or excessive bleeding.
- Check the chest tube dressing at least every 8 hours. Palpate the area surrounding the dressing for crepitus or subcutaneous emphysema, which indicates that air is leaking into the subcutaneous tissue surrounding the insertion site. Change the dressing if necessary or according to facility policy. (See *To strip or not to strip.*)
- Give ordered pain medication as needed *for comfort and to help with deep breathing and coughing.*

Tracheal suction

Tracheal suction involves the removal of secretions from the trachea or bronchi by means of a catheter inserted through the mouth or nose, a tracheal stoma, a tracheostomy tube, or an ET tube. Performed as frequently as the patient's condition warrants, tracheal suction calls for strict sterile technique.

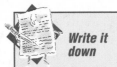

Documenting thoracic drainage

In your notes, record:
- date and time thoracic drainage began
- type of system used
- amount of suction applied to the pleural cavity
- presence or absence of bubbling or fluctuation in the water-seal chamber
- initial amount and type of drainage
- patient's respiratory status.

At the end of each shift, record:
- frequency of system inspection
- amount, color, and consistency of drainage
- presence or absence of bubbling or fluctuation in the water-seal chamber
- patient's respiratory status
- condition of chest dressings
- administration of pain medication
- complications and nursing actions taken.

What you need

Oxygen source (wall or portable unit and handheld resuscitation bag with a mask, 15-mm adapter, or a PEEP valve, if indicated) ✳ wall or portable suction apparatus ✳ collection container ✳ connecting tube ✳ suction catheter kit or a sterile suction catheter, one sterile glove, one clean glove, and a disposable sterile solution container ✳ 1 L bottle of sterile water or normal saline solution ✳ sterile water-soluble lubricant (for nasal insertion) ✳ syringe for deflating the cuff of the ET or tracheostomy tube ✳ waterproof trash bag ✳ optional: sterile towel

Tracheal suctioning helps maintain a patent airway.

Getting ready

Choose a suction catheter of the appropriate size. The diameter should be no larger than half of the inside diameter of the tracheostomy or ET tube to minimize hypoxia during suctioning. (A #12 or #14 French catheter may be used for an 8 mm or larger tube.) Place the suction apparatus on the patient's overbed table or bedside stand. Position the table or stand on your preferred side of the bed to facilitate suctioning.

Attach the collection container to the suction unit and the connecting tube to the collection container. Label and date the normal saline solution or sterile water. Open the waterproof trash bag.

How you do it

• Before suctioning, determine whether your facility requires a doctor's order and obtain one, if necessary.
• Assess the patient's vital signs, breath sounds, and general appearance *to establish a baseline for comparison after suctioning.* Review the patient's ABG values and oxygen saturation levels if they're available. If you'll be performing nasotracheal suctioning, check the patient's history for a deviated septum, nasal polyps, nasal obstruction, nasal trauma, epistaxis, or mucosal swelling.
• Wash your hands. Explain the procedure to the patient even if he's unresponsive.

Positioned to cough

• Unless contraindicated, place the patient in semi-Fowler's or high Fowler's position *to promote lung expansion and productive coughing.*
• Remove the top from the normal saline solution or water bottle.
• Open the package containing the sterile solution container.
• Using strict sterile technique, open the suction catheter kit, and put on gloves. If using individual supplies, open the suction

catheter and gloves, placing the nonsterile glove on your nondominant hand and then the sterile glove on your dominant hand.
• Using your nondominant (nonsterile) hand, pour the normal
saline solution or sterile water into the solution container.
• Place a small amount of water-soluble lubricant on the sterile
area. Lubricant may be used *to facilitate passage of the catheter
during nasotracheal suctioning.*
• Place a sterile towel over the patient's chest, if desired, *to provide an additional sterile area.* Using your dominant (sterile)
hand, remove the catheter from its wrapper. Keep it coiled so it
can't touch a nonsterile object. Using your other hand to manipulate the connecting tubing, attach the catheter to the tubing.
• Using your nondominant hand, set the suction pressure according to facility policy. Typically, pressure may be set between 80
and 120 mm Hg or lower for pediatric patients. Higher pressures
don't enhance secretion removal and may cause traumatic injury.
Occlude the suction port *to assess suction pressure.*
• Dip the catheter tip in the saline solution *to lubricate the outside of the catheter and reduce tissue trauma during insertion.*
• With the catheter tip in the sterile solution, occlude the control
valve with the thumb of your nondominant hand. Suction a small
amount of solution through the catheter *to lubricate the inside of
the catheter, thus facilitating passage of secretions through it.*
• For nasal insertion of the catheter, lubricate the tip of the
catheter with the sterile, water-soluble lubricant *to reduce tissue
trauma during insertion.*
• If the patient isn't intubated or is intubated but isn't receiving
supplemental oxygen or aerosol, instruct him to take three to six
deep breaths *to help minimize or prevent hypoxia during suctioning.*

Add oxygen

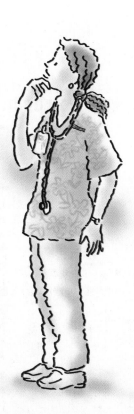

• If the patient isn't intubated but is receiving oxygen, evaluate
his need for preoxygenation. If indicated, instruct him to take
three to six deep breaths while using his supplemental oxygen. (If
needed, the patient may continue to receive supplemental oxygen
during suctioning by leaving his nasal cannula in one nostril or
keeping the oxygen mask over his mouth.)
• If the patient is being mechanically ventilated, preoxygenate
him by using a handheld resuscitation bag, adjusting the sigh
mode on the ventilator, or adjusting the fraction of inspired oxygen (FIO_2) to 0.1. To use the resuscitation bag, set the oxygen
flowmeter at 15 L/minute, disconnect the patient from the ventilator, and deliver three to six breaths with the resuscitation bag.
• If the patient is being maintained on PEEP, evaluate the need to
use a resuscitation bag with a PEEP valve.

Nasotracheal insertion in a nonintubated patient

- Disconnect the oxygen from the patient, if applicable.
- Using your nondominant hand, raise the tip of the patient's nose *to straighten the passageway and facilitate catheter insertion.*
- Gently roll the catheter between your fingers while inserting it into the patient's nostril *to help it advance through the turbinates.*
- As the patient inhales, quickly but gently advance the catheter as far as possible. *To avoid oxygen loss and tissue trauma,* don't apply suction during insertion.
- If the patient coughs as the catheter passes through the larynx, briefly hold the catheter still, and then resume advancement when the patient inhales.

Insertion in an intubated patient

- If you're using a closed system, see *Closed tracheal suctioning,* page 276.
- Using your nondominant hand, disconnect the patient from the ventilator.
- Using your dominant hand, gently insert the suction catheter into the artificial airway. Gently advance the catheter, without applying suction, until you meet resistance. If the patient coughs, pause briefly and then resume advancement.

Suctioning the patient

- After inserting the catheter, apply suction intermittently by removing and replacing the thumb of your nondominant hand over the control valve. Simultaneously use your dominant hand to withdraw the catheter as you roll it between your thumb and forefinger. *This rotating motion prevents the catheter from pulling tissue into the tube as it exits, avoiding tissue trauma.* Never suction more than 10 seconds at a time *to prevent hypoxia.*
- If the patient is intubated, use your nondominant hand to stabilize the tip of the ET tube as you withdraw the catheter *to prevent mucous membrane irritation or accidental extubation.*

Use the source, Luke

- If applicable, resume oxygen delivery by reconnecting the source of oxygen or ventilation and hyperoxygenating the patient's lungs before continuing *to prevent or relieve hypoxia.*
- Observe the patient, and allow him to rest for a few minutes before the next suctioning.

Closed tracheal suctioning

A closed tracheal suctioning system can ease removal of secretions and reduce patient complications. The system, which consists of a sterile suction catheter in a clear plastic sleeve, permits the patient to remain connected to the ventilator during suctioning. As a result, the patient can maintain the tidal volume, oxygen concentration, and positive end-expiratory pressure delivered by the ventilator while being suctioned and, in turn, reduce the occurrence of suction-induced hypoxemia.

Another advantage of this system is a reduced risk of infection, even when the same catheter is used many times. Because the catheter stays in a protective sleeve, gloves aren't required. The caregiver doesn't need to touch the catheter and the ventilator circuit remains closed.

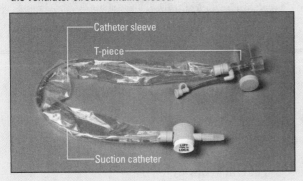

Catheter sleeve

T-piece

Suction catheter

How you do it

To perform the procedure, gather a closed suction control valve, a T-piece to connect the artificial airway to the ventilator breathing circuit, and a catheter sleeve that encloses the catheter and has connections at each end for the control valve and the T-piece. Then follow these steps:

• Remove the closed suction system from its wrapping. Attach the control valve to the connecting tubing.

• Depress the thumb suction control valve and keep it depressed while setting the suction pressure to the desired level.

• Connect the T-piece to the ventilator breathing circuit, making sure that the irrigation port is closed; then connect the T-piece to the patient's endotracheal or tracheostomy tube (as shown above right).

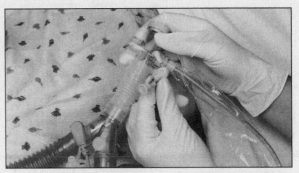

• With one hand keeping the T-piece parallel to the chin, use the thumb and index finger of the other hand to advance the catheter through the tube (as shown below). You may need to gently retract the catheter sleeve as you advance the catheter.

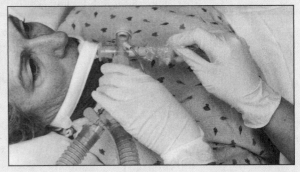

• While continuing to hold the T-piece and control valve, apply intermittent suction and withdraw the catheter until it reaches its fully extended length in the sleeve. Repeat the procedure as necessary.

• After you've finished suctioning, flush the catheter by maintaining suction while slowly introducing normal saline solution or sterile water into the irrigation port.

• Place the thumb control valve in the off position.

• Dispose of and replace the suction equipment and supplies according to your facility's policy.

• Change the closed suction system every 24 hours to minimize the risk of infection.

Taking the secret out of secretions

• Observe the secretions. If they're thick, clear the catheter periodically by dipping the tip in the saline solution and applying suction. If the patient's heart rate and rhythm are being monitored, observe for arrhythmias. If they occur, stop suctioning and ventilate the patient.
• Patients who can't mobilize secretions effectively may need to perform tracheal suctioning after discharge.

After suctioning

• After suctioning, hyperoxygenate the patient being maintained on a ventilator with the handheld resuscitation bag by adjusting the FiO_2 to 0.1 or using the ventilator's sigh mode.
• Readjust the FiO_2 and, for ventilated patients, the tidal volume to the ordered settings.
• After suctioning the lower airway, assess the patient's need for upper airway suctioning. If the cuff of the ET or tracheostomy tube is inflated, suction the upper airway before deflating the cuff with a syringe. Always change the catheter and sterile glove before resuctioning the lower airway *to avoid introducing microorganisms into the lower airway.*
• Discard the gloves and catheter in the waterproof trash bag. Clear the connecting tubing by aspirating the remaining saline solution or water. Discard and replace suction equipment and supplies according to your facility's policy. Wash your hands.
• Auscultate the lungs bilaterally and take the patient's vital signs, if indicated, *to assess the procedure's effectiveness.*

> *Write it down*
>
> ### Documenting tracheal suctioning
>
> In your notes, document:
> • date and time of the procedure
> • suctioning technique used
> • reason for suctioning
> • amount, color, consistency, and odor of secretions
> • complications and nursing actions taken
> • patient's tolerance of the procedure.

Transcutaneous pacemaker use

A temporary pacemaker consists of an external, battery-powered pulse generator and a lead or electrode system. In a life-threatening situation, when time is critical, a transcutaneous pacemaker is the best choice. This device works by sending an electrical impulse from the pulse generator to the patient's heart by way of two electrodes, which are placed on the front and back of the patient's chest. Transcutaneous pacing is quick and effective, but it's used only until the doctor can institute transvenous pacing.

What you need

Transcutaneous pacing generator ✳ transcutaneous pacing electrodes ✳ cardiac monitor

Getting ready

If necessary, clip the hair over the areas of electrode placement. However, don't shave the area. If you nick the skin, the current from the pulse generator could cause discomfort.

How you do it

• Attach monitoring electrodes to the patient in the lead I, II, or III position. Do so even if the patient is already on telemetry monitoring because you'll need to connect the electrodes to the pacemaker. If you select the lead II position, adjust the LL (left leg) electrode placement to accommodate the anterior pacing electrode and the patient's anatomy.

Get plugged in

• Plug the patient cable into the ECG input connection on the front of the pacing generator. Set the selector switch to the MONITOR ON position.
• You should see the ECG waveform on the monitor. Adjust the R-wave beeper volume to a suitable level and activate the alarm by pressing the ALARM ON button. Set the alarm for 10 to 20 beats lower and 20 to 30 beats higher than the intrinsic rate.
• Press the START/STOP button for a printout of the waveform.
• Now you're ready to apply the two pacing electrodes. First, make sure that the patient's skin is clean and dry *to ensure good skin contact*.

One for the back...

• Pull off the protective strip from the posterior electrode (marked BACK) and apply the electrode on the left side of the back, just below the scapula and to the left of the spine.

...one for the front

• The anterior pacing electrode (marked FRONT) has two protective strips — one covering the gelled area and one covering the outer rim. Expose the gelled area and apply it to the skin in the anterior position — to the left side of the precordium in the usual lead V_2 to V_5 position. Move this electrode around to get the best waveform. Then expose the electrode's outer rim and firmly press it to the skin. (See *Proper electrode placement*.)
• Now you're ready to pace the heart. After making sure that the energy output in milliamperes (mA) is on 0, connect the electrode cable to the monitor output cable.
• Check the waveform for a tall QRS complex in lead II.

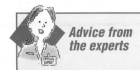

Advice from the experts

Proper electrode placement

Place the two pacing electrodes for a noninvasive temporary pacemaker at heart level on the patient's chest and back (as shown). This placement ensures that the electrical stimulus must travel only a short distance to the heart.

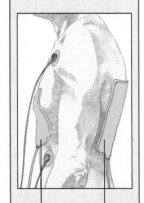

Anterior pacing electrode   Posterior pacing electrode

• Next, turn the selector switch to PACER ON. Tell the patient that he may feel a thumping or twitching sensation. Reassure him that you'll give him medication if he can't tolerate the discomfort.

But you still can't get FM

• Then set the rate dial to 10 to 20 beats higher than the patient's intrinsic rhythm. Look for pacer artifact or spikes, which will appear as you increase the rate. If the patient doesn't have an intrinsic rhythm, set the rate at 60.

• Slowly increase the amount of energy delivered to the heart by adjusting the OUTPUT mA dial. Continue adjusting until capture is achieved. You'll see a pacer spike followed by a widened QRS complex that resembles a premature ventricular contraction (PVC), which indicates that the appropriate pacing threshold has been reached. To ensure consistent capture, increase output by 10%. Don't go higher because you could cause the patient needless discomfort.

• With full capture, the patient's heart rate should be approximately the same as the pacemaker rate set on the machine. The usual pacing threshold is between 40 and 80 mA.

Transvenous pacemaker insertion and care

In addition to being more comfortable for the patient, a transvenous pacemaker is more reliable than a transcutaneous pacemaker. Transvenous pacing involves threading an electrode catheter through a vein into the patient's right atrium or right ventricle. The electrode then attaches to an external pulse generator. As a result, the pulse generator can provide an electrical stimulus directly to the endocardium.

What you need

Temporary pacemaker generator with new battery ✳ guide wire or introducer ✳ electrode catheter ✳ sterile gloves ✳ sterile dressings ✳ adhesive tape ✳ povidone-iodine solution ✳ nonconducting tape or rubber surgical glove ✳ pouch for external pulse generator ✳ emergency cardiac drugs ✳ intubation equipment ✳ defibrillator ✳ cardiac monitor with strip-chart recorder ✳ equipment to start a peripheral I.V. line, if appropriate ✳ I.V. fluids ✳ sedative ✳ bridging cable ✳ percutaneous introducer tray or venous cutdown tray ✳ sterile gowns ✳ linen-saver pad ✳ antimicrobial soap ✳ alcohol pads ✳ vial of 1% lidocaine ✳ 5-ml syringe ✳ fluoroscopy

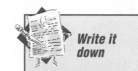

Write it down

Documenting transcutaneous pacemaker use

In your notes, record:
• reason for pacemaker use
• time that pacing began
• electrode locations
• pacemaker settings
• patient's response to the procedure and to temporary pacing
• complications and nursing actions taken.

If possible, obtain rhythm strips before, during, and after pacemaker placement; when pacemaker settings are changed; and when the patient receives treatment for a complication caused by the pacemaker.

equipment, if necessary ✳ fenestrated drape ✳ prepackaged cut-down tray (for antecubital vein placement only) ✳ sutures ✳ receptacle for infectious wastes ✳ optional: elastic bandage or gauze strips, restraints

Getting ready

Check the patient's history for hypersensitivity to local anesthetics.

How you do it

- If applicable, explain the procedure to the patient.
- Attach the cardiac monitor to the patient and obtain a baseline assessment, including the patient's vital signs, skin color, level of consciousness, heart rate and rhythm, and emotional state. Next, insert a peripheral I.V. line if the patient doesn't already have one. Begin an I.V. infusion of the specified I.V. fluid at a keep-vein-open rate.
- Insert a new battery into the external pacemaker generator, and test it to make sure that it has a strong charge. Connect the bridging cable to the generator, and align the positive and negative poles. *This cable allows slack between the electrode catheter and the generator, reducing the risk of accidental catheter displacement.*

Clean entry

- Place the patient in the supine position. If necessary, clip the hair around the insertion site. Next, open the supply tray while maintaining a sterile field. Using sterile technique, the doctor will clean the insertion site with antimicrobial soap and then wipe the area with povidone-iodine solution. He'll cover the insertion site with a fenestrated drape. Because fluoroscopy may be used during the placement of leadwires, put on a protective apron.
- Provide the doctor with the local anesthetic.
- After anesthetizing the insertion site, the doctor will puncture the brachial, femoral, subclavian, or jugular vein. Then he'll insert a guide wire or an introducer and advance the electrode catheter.

Map to the heart

- As the catheter advances, watch the cardiac monitor. When the electrode catheter reaches the right atrium, you'll notice large P waves and small QRS complexes. Then, as the catheter reaches the right ventricle, the P waves become smaller while the QRS complexes enlarge. When the catheter touches the right ventricular endocardium, expect to see elevated ST segments, PVCs, or both.

• When the electrode catheter is in the right ventricle, it will send an impulse to the myocardium, causing depolarization. If the patient needs atrial pacing (alone or with ventricular pacing), the doctor may place an electrode in the right atrium.

• When the electrode catheter is in place, attach the catheter leads to the bridging cable, lining up the positive and negative poles.

• Check the battery's charge by pressing the BATTERY TEST button.

• Set the pacemaker as ordered. (See *When a temporary pacemaker malfunctions.*)

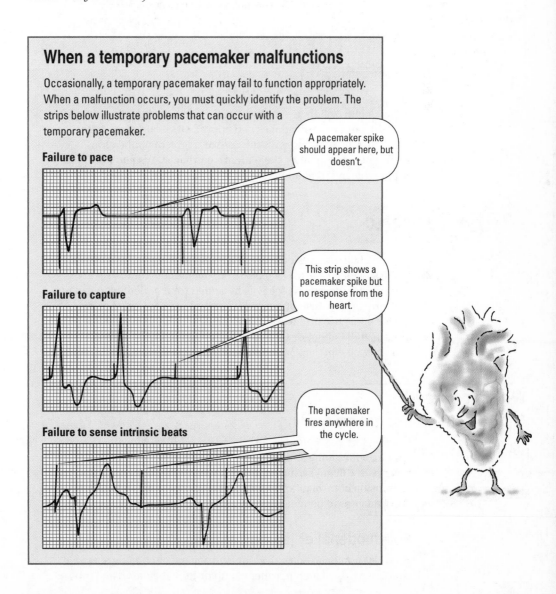

When a temporary pacemaker malfunctions

Occasionally, a temporary pacemaker may fail to function appropriately. When a malfunction occurs, you must quickly identify the problem. The strips below illustrate problems that can occur with a temporary pacemaker.

Failure to pace

A pacemaker spike should appear here, but doesn't.

Failure to capture

This strip shows a pacemaker spike but no response from the heart.

Failure to sense intrinsic beats

The pacemaker fires anywhere in the cycle.

Write it down

Documenting transvenous pacemaker insertion

In your notes, record:
- reason for pacemaker use
- time that pacing began
- electrode locations
- pacemaker settings
- patient's response to the insertion procedure and to temporary pacing
- complications and nursing actions taken.

If possible, obtain rhythm strips before, during, and after pacemaker placement, record when pacemaker settings are changed, and record when the patient receives treatment for a complication caused by the pacemaker.

• The doctor will then suture the catheter to the insertion site. Afterward, put on sterile gloves and apply a sterile dressing to the site. Label the dressing with the date and time of application.

• Continuously monitor the patient's cardiac status and pacemaker function and treat arrhythmias, as appropriate.

Tube feeding

Tube feeding involves delivery of a liquid feeding formula directly to the stomach (known as *gastric gavage*), duodenum, or jejunum. Gastric gavage typically is indicated for a patient who can't eat normally because of dysphagia or oral or esophageal obstruction or injury. Gastric feeding also may be given to an unconscious or intubated patient or to a patient recovering from GI tract surgery who can't ingest food orally.

What you need

For gastric feeding

Feeding formula ✳ graduated container ✳ 120 ml of water ✳ gavage bag with tubing and flow regulator clamp ✳ towel or linen-saver pad ✳ 60-ml syringe ✳ pH test strip ✳ stethoscope ✳ optional: infusion controller and tubing set (for continuous administration), adapter to connect gavage tubing to feeding tube

For duodenal or jejunal feeding

Feeding formula ✳ enteral administration set containing a gavage container, drip chamber, roller clamp or flow regulator, and tube connector ✳ I.V. pole ✳ 60-ml syringe with adapter tip ✳ water ✳ optional: pump administration set (for an enteral infusion pump), Y-connector

For nasal and oral care

Cotton-tipped applicators ✳ water-soluble lubricant ✳ petroleum jelly ✳ sponge-tipped applicators

Getting ready

Be sure to refrigerate formulas prepared in the dietary department or pharmacy. Refrigerate commercial formulas only after opening them. Check the date on all formula containers. Discard expired commercial formula. Use powdered formula within 24 hours of mixing. Always shake the container well to mix the solution thoroughly.

Warm, not hot

Let the formula warm to room temperature before administration. Cold formula can increase the chance of diarrhea. Pour 60 ml of water into the graduated container. After closing the flow clamp on the administration set, pour the appropriate amount of formula into the gavage bag.

Letting the air out

Open the flow clamp on the administration set to remove air from the lines.

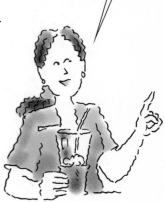

The only feeding that I prefer through a tube is drinking a milkshake. Waitress, another please!

How you do it

• Cover the patient's chest with a towel or linen-saver pad.
• Assess the patient's abdomen for bowel sounds and distention.

For gastric feeding

• Elevate the bed to semi-Fowler's or high Fowler's position *to promote digestion and prevent aspiration from gastroesophageal reflux.*

Tube check

• Check placement of the feeding tube *to make sure that it hasn't slipped out since the last feeding.*
• *To check tube patency and position,* remove the cap or plug from the feeding tube, and use the syringe to aspirate stomach contents (should be green with clear mucus or brown). Place a small amount of aspirate on a pH test strip; the pH of aspirate should be less than or equal to 5.

- To assess gastric emptying, aspirate and measure residual gastric contents. Withhold feedings if residual volume is greater than the predetermined amount specified in the doctor's order (usually 50 to 100 ml). Reinstill any aspirate obtained.
- Connect the gavage bag tubing to the feeding tube. Depending on the type of tube used, you may need to use an adapter to connect the two.
- If you're using a bulb or catheter-tip syringe, remove the bulb or plunger and attach the syringe to the pinched-off feeding tube *to prevent excess air from entering the patient's stomach and causing distention*. If you're using an infusion controller, thread the tube from the formula container through the controller according to the manufacturer's directions.
- Open the regulator clamp on the gavage bag tubing, and adjust the flow rate appropriately. When using a bulb syringe, fill the syringe with formula and release the feeding tube *to allow formula to flow through it*. The height at which you hold the syringe will determine the flow rate. When the syringe is three-quarters empty, pour more formula into it.

No air allowed

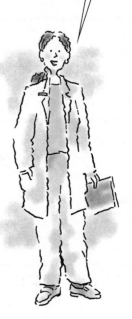

Always administer a tube feeding slowly.

- *To prevent air from entering the tube and the patient's stomach,* never allow the syringe to empty completely. Always administer a tube feeding slowly—typically 200 to 350 ml over 15 to 30 minutes, depending on the patient's tolerance and the doctor's order—*to prevent sudden stomach distention, which can cause nausea, vomiting, cramps, or diarrhea.* If you're using an infusion controller, set the flow rate according to the manufacturer's directions. (See *Managing tube feeding problems.*)
- After administering the appropriate amount of formula, flush the tubing by adding about 60 ml of water to the gavage bag or bulb syringe, or manually flush it using a barrel syringe. *Flushing the tube maintains its patency by removing excess formula, which could occlude the tube.*
- If you're administering a continuous feeding, flush the feeding tube every 4 hours *to help prevent tube occlusion.* Monitor gastric emptying every 4 hours.

When dinner is done

- To discontinue gastric feeding, close the regulator clamp on the gavage bag tubing, disconnect the syringe from the feeding tube, or turn off the infusion controller.
- Cover the end of the feeding tube with its plug or cap *to prevent leakage and contamination of the tube.*
- Leave the patient in semi-Fowler's or high Fowler's position for at least 30 minutes.

Running smoothly

Managing tube feeding problems

Administering a tube feeding isn't always problem-free. If your patient develops complications, you'll need to intervene quickly to avoid serious problems.

Complication	Interventions
Aspiration of gastric secretions	• Discontinue feeding immediately. • Perform tracheal suction of aspirated contents, if possible. • Notify the doctor. Prophylactic antibiotics and chest physiotherapy may be ordered. • Check tube placement before feeding to prevent complications.
Tube obstruction	• Flush the tube with warm water. If necessary, replace the tube. • Flush the tube with 50 ml of water after each feeding to remove excess sticky formula, which could occlude the tube.
Oral, nasal, or pharyngeal irritation or necrosis	• Provide frequent oral hygiene using mouthwash or moist sponge-tipped swabs. Use petroleum jelly on cracked lips. • Change the tube's position. If necessary, replace the tube.

• Rinse all reusable equipment. Dry it and store it in a convenient place. Change equipment every 24 hours or according to your facility's policy.

For duodenal or jejunal feeding

• Elevate the head of the bed and place the patient in low Fowler's position.
• Open the enteral administration set and hang the gavage container on the I.V. pole.
• If you're using a nasoduodenal tube, measure its exposed length to check tube placement. Remember that you may not get residual gastric contents when you aspirate the tube.
• Open the flow clamp and regulate the flow to the desired rate. To regulate the rate using a volumetric infusion pump, follow the manufacturer's directions for setting up the equipment. Most patients receive small amounts initially, with volumes increasing gradually when tolerance is established.
• Flush the tube every 4 hours with water *to maintain patency and provide hydration.*

Write it down

Documenting tube feedings

In your notes, document:
• amount, type, and time of feeding
• abdominal assessment findings (including tube exit site, if appropriate)
• amount of residual gastric contents
• tube placement verification
• tube patency
• patient's tolerance of the feeding, recording such problems as nausea, vomiting, cramping, diarrhea, and distention
• patient's hydration status
• drugs given through the tube
• date and time of administration set changes
• oral and nasal hygiene performed
• results of specimen collections
• blood and urine test results.
   On the patient's intake and output sheet, record the date, volume of formula administered, and volume of water administered.

Venipuncture

Venipuncture involves piercing a vein with a needle and collecting a blood sample in a syringe or evacuated tube. You'll typically use a vein in the antecubital fossa (the triangular area that lies anterior to and below the elbow). However, a vein in the wrist, on the back of the hand or foot, or in another accessible location can be used if necessary.

What you need

Tourniquet ✳ gloves ✳ syringe or evacuated tubes and needle holder ✳ alcohol or povidone-iodine pads ✳ 20G or 21G needle for the forearm or 25G needle for the wrist, hand, ankle, and children ✳ color-coded collection tubes containing appropriate additives ✳ labels ✳ laboratory request form ✳ 2″ × 2″ gauze pads ✳ adhesive bandage

Getting ready

If you're using evacuated tubes, open the needle packet, attach the needle to its holder, and select the appropriate tubes. If you're using a syringe, choose one large enough to hold all the blood required for the test, and then attach the appropriate needle to it. Label all collection tubes clearly with the patient's name and room number, the doctor's name, and the date and time of collection.

How you do it

• Wash your hands thoroughly and put on gloves.
• Tell the patient that you're about to collect a blood sample, and explain the procedure.
• If the patient is on bed rest, ask him to lie in a supine position with his head slightly elevated and his arms at his sides; if he's ambulatory, ask him to sit in a chair and support his arm securely on an armrest or a table.

Scouting sites

• Assess the patient's veins *to determine the best puncture site.* (See *Common venipuncture sites.*)
• Observe the skin for the vein's blue color, or palpate the vein for a firm rebound sensation.
• Tie a tourniquet 2″ (5 cm) proximal to the area chosen. *By impeding venous return to the heart while still allowing arterial*

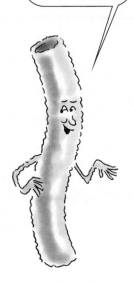

I'm not trying to be vain, but the veins in the antecubital fossa are usually best for venipuncture.

flow, a tourniquet produces venous dilation. (If the tourniquet fails to dilate the vein, have the patient open and close his fist repeatedly. Then ask him to close his fist as you insert the needle and open it again when the needle is in place.)

Don't cancel

• Clean the venipuncture site with an alcohol or a povidone-iodine pad. Don't wipe off the povidone-iodine solution with alcohol *because alcohol cancels the effect of povidone-iodine.* Wipe in a circular motion, spiraling outward from the site *to avoid introducing potentially infectious skin flora into the vessel during the procedure.* If you use alcohol, apply it with friction for 30 seconds or until the final pad comes away clean. Allow the skin to dry before performing the venipuncture.

• Immobilize the vein by pressing just below the venipuncture site with your thumb and drawing the skin taut.

Hold that position

• Position the needle holder or syringe with the needle bevel up and the shaft parallel to the path of the vein and at a 30-degree angle to the arm. Insert the needle into the vein. If you're using a syringe, venous blood will appear in the hub; withdraw the blood slowly, pulling the plunger of the syringe gently to create steady suction until you obtain the required sample. *Pulling the plunger too forcibly may collapse the vein.* If you're using a needle holder and an evacuated tube, grasp the holder securely to stabilize it in the vein, and push down on the collection tube until the needle

Common venipuncture sites

These illustrations show the most common sites for venipuncture. The best sites are the veins in the forearm, followed by those on the hand.

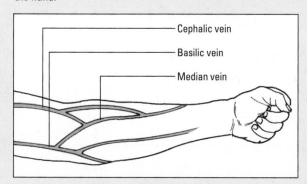

Cephalic vein
Basilic vein
Median vein

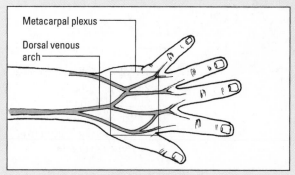

Metacarpal plexus
Dorsal venous arch

punctures the rubber stopper. Blood will flow into the tube automatically.

• Remove the tourniquet as soon as blood flows adequately *to prevent stasis and hemoconcentration, which can impair test results.* If the flow is sluggish, leave the tourniquet in place longer but always remove it before withdrawing the needle.

Gentle rotation

• Continue to fill the required tubes, removing one and inserting another. Gently rotate each tube as you remove it *to help mix the additive with the sample.*

• After you have drawn the sample, place a gauze pad over the puncture site and slowly and gently remove the needle from the vein. When using an evacuated tube, remove it from the needle holder to release the vacuum before withdrawing the needle from the vein.

Gentle pressure

• Apply gentle pressure to the puncture site for 2 to 3 minutes or until bleeding stops. *This pressure prevents extravasation into the surrounding tissue, which can cause a hematoma.*

• After bleeding stops, apply an adhesive bandage.

• If you've used a syringe, transfer the sample to a collection tube. Detach the needle from the syringe, open the collection tube, and gently empty the sample into the tube, being careful to avoid foaming, which can cause hemolysis.

• Finally, check the venipuncture site to see if a hematoma has developed. If it has, apply warm soaks to the site.

• Discard syringes, needles, and used gloves in the appropriate containers.

• Label the specimen and send it to the laboratory with the appropriate request form.

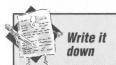

Write it down

Documenting venipuncture

In your notes, record:
• date, time, and site of the venipuncture
• name of the test
• time the sample was sent to the laboratory
• amount of blood collected
• patient's temperature
• adverse reactions to the procedure.

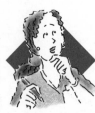

Quick quiz

1. Which of the following complications can be caused by arterial pressure monitoring?

   A.   Arterial spasm
   B.   Thrombophlebitis
   C.   Urinary tract infection
   D.   Hyperglycemia

Answer: A. Direct arterial pressure monitoring can cause such complications as arterial spasm, arterial bleeding, infection, air embolism, and thrombosis.

2. You're assessing the patient with a CV catheter, who's being treated for hypovolemia. A normal CVP reading is:
- A. 1 cm water.
- B. 3 cm water.
- C. 7 cm water.
- D. 14 cm water.

Answer: C. Normal CVP ranges from 5 to 10 cm H_2O or 2 to 8 mm Hg. Any condition that alters venous return, circulating blood volume, or cardiac performance may affect CVP.

3. If a patient with CAPD is experiencing slowed inflow and out-flow, you should:
- A. connect a new bag of dialysate.
- B. take the patient's blood pressure and pulse.
- C. check the tubing for kinks.
- D. call the doctor.

Answer: C. If inflow and outflow are slow or absent, check the tubing for kinks. You can also try raising the solution or reposi-tioning the patient to increase the inflow rate. Repositioning the patient or applying manual pressure to the lateral aspects of the patient's abdomen may also help increase drainage.

4. The initial defibrillation setting for an adult patient is:
- A. 200 joules.
- B. 250 joules.
- C. 300 joules.
- D. 350 joules.

Answer: A. After turning on the defibrillator, set the energy level to 200 joules for an adult patient.

5. In a patient with a femoral compression device, assess the patient's:
- A. respiratory rate.
- B. cardiac rate.
- C. distal pulses.
- D. history.

Answer: C. Assess the puncture site for proper placement of the device and for signs of bleeding or hematoma. Assess distal pulses and perform neurovascular assessments according to your facili-ty's policy. Confirm distal pulses after adjustments to the device.

Scoring

☆☆☆   If you answered all five questions correctly, super! You're a pro at nursing procedures.

☆☆   If you answered four questions correctly, good job! You followed the recommended procedure and documented your success.

☆   If you answered fewer than four questions correctly, don't fret— gather the necessary equipment (perhaps a sandwich and a glass of water) and review this chapter.

Ready to proceed to the next chapter?

⑤

I.V. therapy

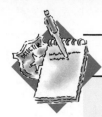

Just the facts

In this chapter, you'll learn:

♦ methods of initiating and maintaining peripheral I.V. therapy

♦ ways to assist with and maintain central venous access

♦ proper administration of blood products.

A look at I.V. therapy

Although you may not be responsible for insertion of all types of I.V. lines, you are responsible for maintaining these lines and preventing complications throughout therapy. You're also responsible for helping the doctor perform I.V.-related procedures, such as central and arterial line insertion. This chapter explains the essentials for assisting with these types of procedures as well as calculating I.V. flow rates and administering blood products.

Peripheral I.V. therapy

Peripheral I.V. therapy is ordered whenever venous access is needed — for example, when a patient requires surgery, transfusion therapy, or emergency care. You may also use peripheral I.V. therapy to maintain hydration, restore fluid and electrolyte balance, provide fluids for resuscitation, or administer I.V. drugs and nutrients for metabolic support.

Quick and easy

Peripheral I.V. therapy offers easy access to veins and rapid administration of solutions, blood, and drugs. It allows continuous administration of drugs to produce rapid systemic changes. It's also easy to monitor.

> Peripheral I.V. therapy can be used to maintain hydration and restore fluid and electrolyte balance, among other things.

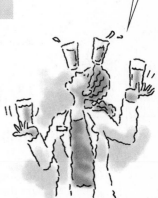

Peripheral concerns — and cost

Peripheral I.V. therapy is an invasive vascular procedure that carries such associated risks as bleeding, infiltration, and infection. Rapid infusion of some drugs can produce hearing loss, bone marrow depression, kidney or heart damage, and other irreversible adverse effects. Finally, peripheral I.V. therapy can't be used indefinitely and costs more than oral, subcutaneous, or I.M. drug therapy.

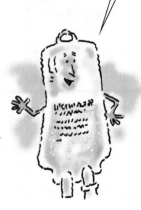

Face it. Any invasive procedure carries certain risks.

Focusing on the good

Despite its risks, peripheral I.V. therapy remains a mainstay of modern medicine and a crucial contribution that nurses make to their patients' well being. The key is to do it well, and that starts with preparation.

Preparing the equipment

After you select and gather the infusion equipment, you'll need to prepare it for use. Preparation involves inspecting the I.V. container and solution, preparing the solution, attaching and priming the administration set, and setting up the infusion pump.

Inspecting the container and solution

Check that the container size is appropriate for the volume to be infused and that the type of I.V. solution is correct. Note the expiration date and discard any outdated solutions.

Preparing the solution

Make sure that the container is labeled with the following information: your name; the patient's name, identification number, and room number; the date and time the container was hung; any additives; and the container number (if such information is required by your facility). For pediatric patients, you may label the volume-control set instead of the container.

Keep it clean

After the container is labeled, use sterile technique to remove the cap or the pull tab. Be careful not to contaminate the port.

Attaching the administration set

Make sure that the administration set is correct for the patient and the type of I.V. container and solution you're using. Also make sure that the set has no cracks, holes, or missing clamps. If the solution container is glass, check whether it's vented or nonvented to determine how to prepare it before attaching it to the administration set. (Plastic containers are prepared differently.)

Nonvented bottle

When attaching a nonvented bottle to an administration set, take these steps:
- Remove the metal cap and inner disk, if necessary.
- Place the bottle on a stable surface, and wipe the rubber stopper with an alcohol swab.
- Close the flow clamp on the administration set.
- Remove the protective cap from the spike.
- Push the spike through the center of the rubber stopper. Avoid twisting or angling the spike to prevent pieces of the stopper from breaking off and falling into the solution. If the vacuum is intact, you should hear a "swoosh" sound, indicating that the solution hasn't been contaminated. (You may not hear this sound if a medication has been added to the bottle.)
- Invert the bottle. If the vacuum isn't intact, discard the bottle. If it's intact, hang the bottle on the I.V. pole, about 36″ (91 cm) above the venipuncture site.

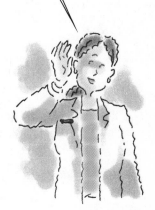

Listen for that swoosh. It lets you know the infusate hasn't been contaminated.

Vented bottle

When attaching a vented bottle to an administration set, take these steps:
- Remove the metal cap and latex diaphragm to release the vacuum. If the vacuum isn't intact, discard the bottle (unless a medication has been added).
- Place the bottle on a stable surface, and wipe the rubber stopper with an alcohol swab.
- Close the flow clamp on the administration set.
- Remove the protective cap from the spike.
- Push the spike through the insertion port, which is located next to the air vent.
- Hang the bottle on the I.V. pole about 36″ above the venipuncture site.

Plastic bag

When attaching a plastic bag to an administration set, take these steps:
- Place the bag on a flat, stable surface or hang it on an I.V. pole.
- Remove the protective cap or tear the tab from the tubing insertion port.
- Slide the flow clamp up close to the drip chamber, and close the clamp.
- Remove the protective cap from the spike.

• Hold the port carefully and firmly with one hand, and then quickly insert the spike with your other hand.
• Hang the bag about 36″ (91 cm) above the venipuncture site.

Priming the administration set

Before you prime any administration set, label it with the date and time you opened it. Make sure that you have also labeled the container. When priming a set for an electronic infusion device, the procedure is similar to priming other infusion sets. (See *Electronic infusion devices*.)

Basic training

When priming a basic set, take these steps:
• Close the roller clamp below the drip chamber.
• Squeeze the drip chamber until it's half full.
• Aim the distal end of the tubing at a receptacle.
• Open the roller clamp, and allow the solution to flow through the tubing to remove the air. (Most distal tube coverings allow the solution to flow without having to remove the protective end.)
• Close the clamp after the solution has run through the line and all the air has been purged from the system.

Taking control

To prime a volume-control set, take these steps:
• Attach the set to the solution container, and close the lower clamp on the I.V. tubing below the drip chamber.
• Open the clamp between the solution container and the fluid chamber, and allow about 50 ml of the solution to flow into the chamber.
• Close the upper clamp.
• Open the lower clamp, and allow the solution in the chamber to flow through the remainder of the tubing. Make sure that some fluid remains in the chamber so that air won't fill the tubing below it.
• Close the lower clamp.
• Fill the chamber with the desired amount of solution.

What about a filter?

If you're using a filter on any of these sets and it isn't an integral part of the infusion path, attach it to the primed distal end of the I.V. tubing, and follow the manufacturer's instructions for filling and priming it. Most filters are positioned with the distal end of the tubing facing upward so the solution will wet the filter membrane completely and the line will be purged of all air bubbles.

Electronic infusion devices

Electronic infusion devices help regulate the rate and volume of infusions. This regulation improves the safety and accuracy of drug and fluid administration.

Priming the set
Follow these steps to prime an infusion set with an electronic infusion device:
1. Fill the drip chamber to the halfway mark.
2. Slowly open the roller clamp.
3. As gravity assists the flow, invert chambered sections of the tubing to expel the air and fill them with the I.V. fluid or infusate. The chambered sections fit into the pump of the electronic infusion device. They must be filled exactly so they won't activate the air-in-line alarm during use.
4. Reinvert the pump chamber, continuing to purge the air along the fluid path and out of the tubing.

Setting up and monitoring an infusion pump

Infusion pumps help maintain a steady flow of liquid at a set rate over a specified period of time. After gathering your equipment, follow these steps:

• Attach the infusion pump to the I.V. pole. Insert the administration spike into the I.V. container.

• Fill the drip chamber completely to prevent air bubbles from entering the tubing. To avoid fluid overload, clamp the tubing whenever the pump door is open.

• Follow the manufacturer's instructions for priming and placing the I.V. tubing.

• Be sure to flush all the air out of the tubing before connecting it to the patient to lower the risk of an air embolism.

• Place the infusion pump on the same side of the bed as the I.V. setup and the intended venipuncture site.

• Set the appropriate controls to the desired infusion rate or volume.

• Check the patency of the venous access device, watch for infiltration, and monitor the accuracy of the infusion rate.

You may hear an alarm when the infusion rate changes. Don't be alarmed.

Don't alarm the patient

Be sure to explain the alarm system to the patient, so he isn't frightened when a change in the infusion rate triggers the alarm. Also, be prepared to disengage the device if infiltration occurs; otherwise the pump will continue to infuse medication into the infiltrated area.

Frequently check the infusion pump to make sure that it's working properly — specifically, note the flow rate. Monitor the patient for signs of infiltration and other complications such as infection.

Going tubing

After the equipment is up and running, you'll also need to change the tubing according to the manufacturer's instructions and your facility's policy.

Selecting a venipuncture site

The metacarpal, cephalic, and basilic veins, along with the branches or accessory branches that merge with them, are commonly used for placement of venipuncture devices. When selecting an I.V. site, choose distal veins first, unless the solution is very irritating (for example, potassium chloride). Generally, your best choice is a peripheral vein that's full and pliable and appears long enough to accommodate the length of the intended catheter. It should be large enough to allow blood flow around the catheter to minimize venous lumen irritation. If the patient has an area that's bruised, tender, or phlebitic, choose a vein proximal to it. Avoid flexion areas, such as the wrist and antecubital fossa.

Refrain from these veins

Some veins are best to avoid, including those in the:
- legs (circulation can be easily compromised)
- inner wrist and arm (they're small and inserting an I.V. into them can cause discomfort)
- affected arm of a mastectomy patient
- arm with an arteriovenous shunt or fistula
- arm being treated for thrombosis or cellulitis
- arm that has experienced trauma (such as burns or scarring from surgery).

Performing the venipuncture

To perform a venipuncture, you need to dilate the vein, prepare the access site, and insert the device. After the infusion starts, you can complete the I.V. placement by securing the device with tape or a transparent semipermeable dressing.

Dilating the vein

To dilate or distend a vein effectively, you need to use a tourniquet, which traps blood in the veins by applying enough pressure to impede venous flow. A properly distended vein should appear and feel round, firm, and fully filled with blood and should rebound when gently compressed. Because the amount of trapped blood depends on circulation, a patient who is hypotensive, very cold, or experiencing vasomotor changes (such as septic shock) may have inadequate filling of the peripheral blood vessels.

Pretourniquet prep

Before applying the tourniquet, place the patient's arm in a dependent position to increase capillary flow to the lower arm and hand. If his skin is cold, warm it by rubbing and stroking his arm or by covering the entire arm with warm moist towels for 5 to 10 minutes. As soon as you remove the warm towels, apply the tourniquet and continue to perform the insertion procedure.

Applying a tourniquet

The ideal tourniquet is one that can be secured easily, doesn't roll into a thin band, stays relatively flat, and releases easily. (To review the steps for applying a tourniquet, see *Applying a tourniquet*.)

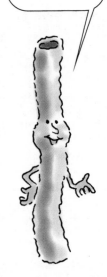

A properly distended vein should appear and feel round, firm, and full.

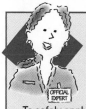

Advice from the experts

Applying a tourniquet

To safely apply a tourniquet, follow these steps:

1. Place the tourniquet under the patient's arm, about 6″ (15 cm) above the venipuncture site. Position the arm on the middle of the tourniquet.
2. Bring the ends of the tourniquet together, placing one on top of the other.
3. Holding one end on top of the other, lift and stretch the tourniquet, and tuck the top tail under the bottom tail. Don't allow the tourniquet to loosen.
4. Tie the tourniquet smoothly and snugly; be careful not to pinch the patient's skin or pull his arm hair.

No more than 2 minutes

Leave the tourniquet in place for no more than 2 minutes. If you can't find a suitable vein and prepare the venipuncture site in this amount of time, release the tourniquet for a few minutes. Then reapply it and continue the procedure. You may need to apply the tourniquet, find the vein, remove the tourniquet, prepare the site, and then reapply the tourniquet for the venipuncture.

As flat as possible

Keep the tourniquet as flat as possible. It should be snug but not uncomfortably tight. If it's too tight, it will impede arterial and venous blood flow. Check the patient's radial pulse. If you can't feel it, the tourniquet is too tight and must be loosened. Also loosen and reapply the tourniquet if the patient complains of severe tightness.

Intend to distend

After you've applied the tourniquet about 6″ (15 cm) above the intended site, have the patient open and close his fist tightly four to six times to distend the vein. If necessary, gently flick the skin over the vein with one or two short taps of your forefinger. This tapping is less traumatic than slapping the skin, but it achieves the same result. If the vein still feels small and uniform, release the tourniquet, reapply it, and reassess the intended access site. If the vein still isn't well distended, remove the tourniquet; apply a warm, moist towel for 5 minutes; then reapply the tourniquet. This step is especially helpful if the patient's skin feels cool.

Preparing the access site

Before performing the venipuncture, you'll need to clean the site and stabilize the vein. You may also need to administer a local anesthetic.

Cleaning the venipuncture site

Wash your hands, then put on gloves. If necessary, clip the hair over the insertion site to make the veins and the site easier to see and reduce pain when the tape is removed. Avoid shaving the patient because it can cause microabrasion of the skin, which increases the risk of infection.

Have a hairy patient? Clip hair at the insertion site. Shaving may cause microabrasion of the skin.

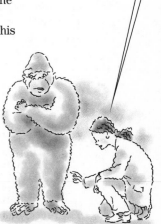

Check with the patient to see if he has an allergy to iodine or other antimicrobial solutions. Clean the skin with 2% chlorhexidine solution. (Other antimicrobial solutions include tincture of iodine 2% and 70% alcohol solution.) Using a swab stick or swab, start at the center of the insertion site and move outward in a side-to-side motion. Allow the solution 30 to 60 seconds to dry thoroughly.

Using a local anesthetic

If an anesthetic is ordered, first check with the patient and review his record for an allergy to lidocaine or other drugs. Then describe the procedure to him and explain that it will reduce the discomfort of the venipuncture.

Next, administer the local anesthetic, as ordered. The anesthetic will begin to work in 2 to 3 seconds. Lidocaine anesthetizes the site to pain but allows the patient to feel touch and pressure. Also, 0.9% sodium chloride solution has proven effective.

Stabilizing the vein

Stabilizing the vein helps ensure a successful venipuncture the first time and decreases the chances of bruising. If the tip of the venipuncture device repeatedly probes a moving vein wall, it can nick the vein and cause it to leak blood. When a vein gets nicked, it can't be reused immediately. Finding a new venipuncture site will cause the patient the discomfort of another needle puncture.

Hold still, vein

To stabilize the vein, stretch the skin and hold it taut, and then lightly press it with your fingertips about 1½ ″ (3.5 cm) from the insertion site. (Never touch the prepared site or you'll recontaminate it.) The vein should feel round, firm, fully engorged, and resilient. Remove your fingertips. If the vein returns to its original position and appears larger than it did before you applied the tourniquet, then it's adequately distended.

To help prevent the vein from "rolling," apply adequate traction with your nondominant hand to hold the skin and vein in place. This traction is particularly helpful in those with poor skin turgor or loosely anchored veins.

Insertion

When you have prepared the venipuncture site, you're ready to insert the venous access device. The process involves three steps: positioning, inserting, and advancing. You might also need to add an intermittent infusion device, use deep veins rather than superficial, or collect a blood sample.

Positioning the venous access device

While still wearing gloves, use the appropriate method for the type of venous access device being used.

Going "over"-board

When using an over-the-needle catheter, grasp the plastic hub with your dominant hand, remove the cover, and examine the device. If the edge isn't smooth, discard the device and obtain another. Position the device bevel up for insertion.

Don't wing it; follow these steps

When using a winged catheter, hold the edges of the wings between your thumb and forefinger, with the bevel facing upward. Then squeeze the wings together. Remove the protective cover from the needle, being careful not to contaminate the steel needle or the catheter.

Inserting the venous access device

Tell the patient that you're about to insert the device. Ask him to remain still and refrain from pulling away. Explain that the initial needle stick will hurt but that the pain will quickly subside. Then insert the device, using the direct approach. Place the bevel up and enter the skin directly over the vein at a 5- to 15-degree angle (deeper veins require a wider angle).

Steady...steady...

When you insert the device, use a steady, smooth motion while keeping the skin taut. You'll know the device is in the vein because you'll see blood return in the flashback chamber. (You may not see a rapid blood return with a small vein.)

Don't always expect to feel a "pop" or a sense of release when the device enters the vein. This "pop" usually occurs only when a venous access device enters a large, thick-walled vein or when the patient has good tissue tone.

As soon as the device enters the vein, lower the distal portion of the adapter until it's almost parallel with the skin. Doing so lifts the tip of the needle so it doesn't penetrate the opposite wall of the vein.

Advancing the venous access device

To advance the catheter before starting the infusion, first release the tourniquet. While stabilizing the vein with one hand, use the other to advance the catheter up to the hub. Make sure to advance only the catheter to avoid puncturing the vein with the needle. Next, remove the inner needle. Apply digital pressure to the catheter (to minimize blood exposure) and, using aseptic tech-

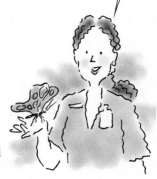

An over-the-needle catheter or a winged catheter may be used as a venous access device.

nique, attach the primed I.V. tubing or flush the inserted device with saline solution. The advantage of this method is that it commonly results in less blood being spilled.

In mid-infusion

To advance the catheter while infusing the I.V. solution, release the tourniquet and remove the inner needle. Using aseptic technique, attach the I.V. tubing and begin the infusion. While stabilizing the vein with one hand, use the other to advance the catheter into the vein. When the catheter is advanced, slow the I.V. flow rate. Using this method to advance the catheter reduces the risk of vein wall puncture because the catheter is advanced without the steel needle and the rapid flow dilates the vein. However, this method increases the risk of infection.

Needles of steel

If you're using a steel needle winged infusion set, advance the needle fully, if possible, and hold it in place. Release the tourniquet, slightly open the administration set clamp, and check for free flow or infiltration. Next, tape the infusion set in place, using the wings as an anchor to prevent catheter movement (which could cause irritation and phlebitis). When using an over-the-needle winged infusion set, you can advance the catheter using either of the methods described above.

Wrapping it up

After the venous access device has been successfully inserted and securely taped, clean the skin if necessary. Cover the access site with a transparent semipermeable dressing or the dressing used by your facility. If your facility's policy and procedures require doing so, further stabilize the device. Dispose of the inner needle in a nonpermeable receptacle. Finally, regulate the flow rate and then remove your gloves and wash your hands.

Intermittent infusion device

Also called a *saline lock*, an intermittent infusion device may be used when venous access must be maintained for intermittent use and a continuous infusion isn't necessary. This device keeps the access device sterile and prevents blood and other fluids from leaking from an open end. Much like the administration set injection port, the intermittent injection cap is self-sealing after the needle or needleless injector is removed. The ends of these devices are universal in size and fit the female end of any catheter or tubing designed for infusion therapy. Caps should have a luer-lock design to prevent disconnections.

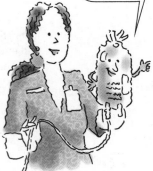

Advancing the catheter while infusing I.V. fluids reduces the risk of puncturing the vein wall...

...but increases the risk of infection.

Continuous infusion not required

The intermittent infusion device can be filled with diluted saline solution to expel air from the equipment. Doing so makes it possible to maintain venous access in patients who must receive I.V. medications regularly or intermittently but don't require continuous infusion.

Less means more

The intermittent infusion device has many benefits. It minimizes the risks of fluid overload and electrolyte imbalance that may be associated with a keep-vein-open infusion. By eliminating the continuous use of I.V. solution containers and administration sets, it reduces the risk of contamination and lowers costs. Finally, it allows for patient mobility, which helps reduce anxiety.

Do you accept tips?

Here are two tips related to intermittent infusion devices:
• If the patient feels a burning sensation as you inject the saline solution, stop the injection and check the catheter placement. If it's in the vein, inject the solution at a slower rate to minimize irritation.
• If the doctor orders discontinuation of an I.V. infusion, you can convert the existing line from a continuous to an intermittent venous access device. Just disconnect the I.V. tubing and insert an adapter plug into the device that's already in place. In addition, occlusion is possible if the device isn't flushed to ensure patency before and after medication is infused.

Insertion into deep veins

If a superficial vein isn't available, you may have to insert the venous access device into a deep vein that isn't visible. Here's how:
• Put on gloves.
• Palpate the area with your fingertips until you feel the vein.
• Clean the skin over the vein with an approved cleaning solution, such as chlorhexidine, swiping in a side-to-side motion.
• Aim the device directly over the intended vein, stretch the skin with your gloved fingertips, and insert the venous access device at a 15-degree angle to the skin.

> Don't be afraid to delve deeper. If a superficial vein isn't available, you may have to go fishing for a deep vein.

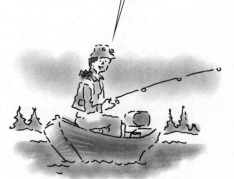

Making sure

Expect to insert the device one-half to two-thirds its length; that way you'll make sure that the needle and the catheter are in the vein lumen. When you see blood in the flashback chamber, remove the tourniquet and inner steel needle, and advance the catheter with or without infusing fluid.

Collecting a blood sample

If a blood sample is ordered, you can collect it while performing the venipuncture. First, gather the necessary equipment: one or more evacuated tubes, a 19G needle or needleless system, an appropriate-size syringe without a needle, and a protective pad. Then follow the steps outlined in *Collecting a blood sample*.

Securing the venous access device

After the infusion begins, you need to secure the venous access device at the insertion site. You can do this with tape and a transparent semipermeable dressing.

Applying tape
Stabilize the device and keep the hub from moving by using a standard taping method, such as the chevron, U, or H method. (See *Taping techniques*.)

Applying a transparent dressing
To prevent infection, nurses in many health care facilities cover the insertion site with a transparent, semipermeable dressing. (See *How to apply a transparent semipermeable dressing*, page 304.) This dressing allows air to pass through but is impervious to microorganisms.

Using an arm board
An arm board is an immobilization device that helps secure correct venous access device positioning and prevent unnecessary motion that could cause infiltration or inflammation. This immobilization device is sometimes necessary when the insertion site is near a joint or in the dorsum of the hand. An arm board may be used with a restraint in certain situations (for example, if the patient is confused or disoriented).

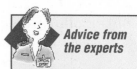

Advice from the experts

Collecting a blood sample

To smoothly and safely collect a blood sample, follow this step-by-step technique after assembling your equipment and making the venipuncture:

1. Place a pad underneath the site to protect the bed linens.
2. When the venous access device is correctly placed, remove the inner needle if you're using an over-the-needle device.
3. Leave the tourniquet tied.
4. Attach the syringe to the venous access device's hub, and withdraw the appropriate amount of blood.
5. Release the tourniquet and disconnect the syringe.
6. Quickly attach the saline lock or I.V. tubing, regulate the flow rate, and stabilize the device.
7. Attach a 19G needle or needleless device to the syringe, and insert the blood into the evacuated tubes.
8. Properly dispose of the needle and syringe; then complete I.V. line placement.

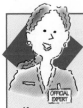

Advice from the experts

Taping techniques

If you use tape to secure the venous access device to the insertion site, use one of the methods described below. Use as little tape as possible, and remove hair from around the access area. In addition to improving visibility and reducing pain when the tape is removed, removing hair helps decrease colonization by bacteria present on the hair.

Chevron method
1. Cut a long strip of ½″ tape. Place it sticky side up under the hub.
2. Cross the ends of the tape over the hub and secure the tape to the patient's skin on the opposite sides of the hub, as shown below.
3. Apply a piece of 1″ tape across the two wings of the chevron. Loop the tubing and secure it with another piece of 1″ tape. Once a dressing is secured, apply a label. On the label, write the date and time of insertion, type and gauge of the needle, and your initials.

U method
1. Cut a strip of ½″ tape. With the sticky side up, place it under the hub of the catheter.
2. Bring each side of the tape up, folding it over the wings of the catheter, as shown below. Press it down, parallel to the hub.
3. Next, apply tape to stabilize the catheter. After a dressing is secured, apply a label. On the label, write the date and time of insertion, type and gauge of the catheter, and your initials.

H method
1. Cut three strips of ½″ tape.
2. Place one strip of tape over each wing, keeping the tape parallel to the catheter.
3. Place the third strip of tape perpendicular to the first two, as shown below. Put the tape directly on top of the wings. Make sure that the catheter is secure, then apply a dressing and label. On the label, write the date and time of insertion, type and gauge of the catheter, and your initials.

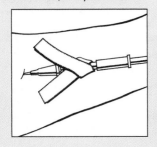
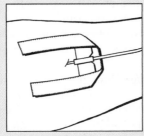
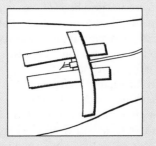

Board of regulations

Because it's an immobilization device, the use of an arm board may be restricted by state or facility policies—so check first. Better yet, don't place the tip of the infusion device in a flexion area; then you won't need an arm board.

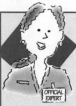

Advice from the experts

How to apply a transparent semipermeable dressing

Here's how to apply a transparent semipermeable dressing, which allows for visual assessment of the catheter insertion site:

• Make sure the insertion site is clean and dry.

• Remove the dressing from the package and, using aseptic technique, remove the protective seal. Avoid touching the sterile surface.

• Place the dressing directly over the insertion site and the hub, as shown at right. Don't cover the tubing. Also, don't stretch the dressing; doing so may cause itching.

• Tuck the dressing around and under the catheter hub to make the site occlusive to microorganisms.

• To remove the dressing, grasp one corner; then lift and stretch.

If this dressing remains intact, daily changes aren't necessary.

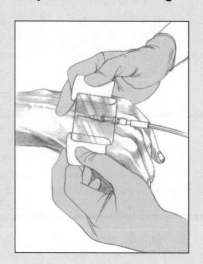

If the flow doesn't go

To determine whether an arm board is needed, move your patient's arm through its full range of motion (ROM) while watching the I.V. flow rate. If the flow stops during movement, you may need to use the arm board to prevent flexion of the extremity. Choose one that's long enough to prevent flexion and extension at the tip of the device. If necessary, cover it with a soft material before you secure it to the patient's arm. Make sure that you can still observe the insertion site.

Keep in mind that an arm board applied too tightly can cause nerve and tendon damage. If you need to use an arm board, remove it periodically according to facility policy so the patient can perform ROM activities, and you can better observe for complications from restricted activity and infusion therapy.

Maintaining peripheral I.V. therapy

Routine care measures help prevent complications. They also give you an opportunity to observe the I.V. site for signs of inflammation or infection — two of the most common complications. Perform these measures according to your facility's policy and procedures. Wash your hands and wear gloves whenever you work near the venipuncture site.

Changing the dressing

The insertion site should be inspected and palpated for tenderness daily, through the intact dressing. Depending on your facility's policy, gauze dressings should be changed routinely every 48 hours. A transparent semipermeable dressing should be changed whenever its integrity is compromised because it has become soiled, wet, or loose.

Getting ready

Before performing a dressing change, gather this equipment:
• alcohol swab or other approved solution
• sterile gauze pad, or transparent semipermeable dressing
• clean adhesive tape
• sterile gloves.
    To change a dressing, follow the steps outlined in *Changing a peripheral I.V. dressing*. Of course, use aseptic technique.

Changing the I.V. solution

To avoid microbial growth, don't allow an I.V. container to hang for more than 24 hours. Before changing the I.V. container, check the new one for cracks, leaks, and other damage. Also check the

> I can't stand those microbes, so please don't leave me hanging for more than 24 hours.

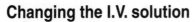

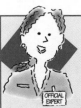

Advice from the experts

Changing a peripheral I.V. dressing

To change a peripheral I.V. dressing, follow these steps.
• Wash your hands and put on sterile gloves.
• Hold the needle or catheter in place with your nondominant hand to prevent movement or dislodgment that could lead to infiltration; then gently remove the tape and the dressing.
• Assess the venipuncture site for signs of infection (redness and tenderness), infiltration (coolness, blanching, edema), and thrombophlebitis (redness, firmness, pain along the path of the vein, edema).
• If you detect these signs, apply pressure to the area with a sterile gauze pad and remove the catheter or needle. Maintain

pressure on the area until the bleeding stops; then apply an adhesive bandage. Using new equipment, insert the I.V. access device at another site.
• If you don't detect complications, hold the needle or catheter at the hub and carefully clean around the site with an alcohol swab or other approved solution. Work in a swiping motion to avoid introducing pathogens into the cleaned area. Allow the area to dry completely.
• Retape the device and apply a transparent semipermeable dressing, if available, or apply gauze and secure it.

solution for discoloration, turbidity, and particulates. Note the date and time the solution was mixed and the expiration date.

Cleanliness is key

After washing your hands, clamp the line, remove the spike from the old container, and quickly insert the spike into the new one. Then hang the new container and adjust the flow rate as prescribed.

Changing the administration set

Change the administration set according to your facility's policy (usually every 72 hours if it's a primary infusion line), and whenever you note or suspect contamination. If possible, change the set when you start a new venous access device during routine site rotation.

Getting equipped again

Before changing the set, gather:
- I.V. administration set
- sterile 2″ × 2″ gauze pads
- adhesive tape for labeling or appropriate labeling tapes supplied by the facility
- gloves.

Then follow the guidelines set out in *A change in administration.*

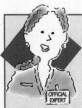

Advice from the experts

A change in administration

To quickly change the administration set for a peripheral infusion, follow these steps:
- Wash your hands and put on gloves.
- Reduce the I.V. flow rate. Then remove the old spike from the container and place the cover of the new spike over it loosely.
- Keeping the old spike upright and above the patient's heart level, insert the new spike into the I.V. container and prime the system.
- Place a sterile gauze pad under the needle or hub of the plastic catheter to create a sterile field.
- Disconnect the old tubing from the venous access device, being careful not to dislodge or move the device. If you have trou-

ble disconnecting the old tubing, try using a pair of hemostats to hold the hub securely while twisting and removing the end of the tubing. Alternatively, try grasping the venous access device with one pair of hemostats and the hard plastic of the luer-lock end of the administration set with another pair and pull the hemostats in opposite directions. *Don't clamp the hemostats shut; this may crack the tubing adapter or the venous access device.*
- Using aseptic technique, quickly attach the new primed tubing to the device.
- Adjust the flow to the prescribed rate.
- Label the new tubing with the date and time of the change and your initials.

Changing the I.V. site

As a standard of care, rotate the I.V. site every 48 to 72 hours, according to facility policy. Sometimes, limited venous access will prevent you from changing sites this often. If that's the case, notify the doctor of the situation and discuss alternatives for long-term insertion.

A complete change may be in order

Be prepared to change the entire system, including the venous access device, if you detect signs of thrombophlebitis, cellulitis, or I.V. therapy-related bacteremia.

Patients with special needs

I.V. therapy for pediatric and elderly patients poses special nursing challenges, especially regarding the effects of age-related differences in the skin and veins on I.V. line insertion and maintenance.

Pediatric patients

Inserting a venous access device in an infant or toddler can prove difficult because their veins are imbedded in fat, making them hard to isolate. (A premature infant has less subcutaneous fat, making the veins more prominent.)

The scalp is the top site

In infants, the best sites for I.V. insertion include the hands, feet, antecubital fossa, dorsum of the hand and, especially, the scalp (in infants under age 6 months), which has an abundant supply of veins. The head veins most commonly used are the bilateral superficial temporal veins above the ear and the metopic vein running down the middle of the forehead. (See *Identifying scalp veins*.)

Feel first

Before performing a venipuncture on a scalp vein, palpate to ensure you have a vein—not an artery. In the scalp, arteries and veins may look similar. Remember, you'll feel a pulse with an artery. However, in hypotensive or premature infants, the pulse may be more difficult to detect.

Consider using a topical or transdermal anesthetic to decrease discomfort. If necessary, use clove-hitch and mummy restraints. Also, engage the parents to help keep the infant calm. If you need a tourniquet effect, tip the infant's head down to facilitate filling of the superficial veins—don't use a tourniquet or rubber band. Insert the venous access device caudally to make stabilizing easier.

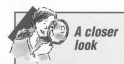

A closer look

Identifying scalp veins

This illustration shows the scalp veins most commonly used for venipuncture in infants.

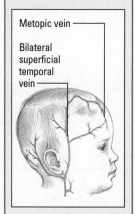

Metopic vein

Bilateral superficial temporal vein

When you see blood return (usually it will be slight), tip the child back to a horizontal or vertical position.

Device advice

The preferred venous access device for infants and young children, no matter which vein you're using, is a small-diameter, winged over-the-needle catheter (commonly called a *scalp vein catheter*). This device is less likely to cause traumatic injury to the vein. Over-the-needle catheters are also recommended for long-term therapy and antibiotic therapy when venous access is poor.

Perfect site

Stabilizing the I.V. site can be challenging with pediatric patients. Tape the site as you would for an adult so the skin over the access site is easily visible. Avoid overtaping the I.V. site; it makes inspecting the site and the surrounding tissues more difficult, and practically guarantees trauma when the device is removed. Instead, cover the site with a stretch net, which can be rolled back easily for inspection. Some clinicians protect the insertion site by taping a plastic medicine cup or commercial protective cover over it, especially when a scalp vein is used.

The scalp, with its abundant supply of veins, is one of the best sites for I.V. line insertion in an infant.

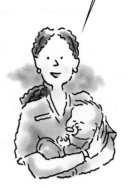

Elderly patients

Because elderly patients' veins are usually more prominent and their skin is less resistant, you may find venipuncture easier in this population than in pediatric patients. Even so, the normal aging process also presents drawbacks. Because the tissues are looser, you may have more difficulty stabilizing the vein. Also, because the thickness and amount of connective tissue in the outer layer of the veins decreases, the veins become more fragile due to the thickness of the tunica adventitia. You'll need to perform the venipuncture quickly and efficiently to avoid excessive bruising. Thus, a smaller gauge needle, such as a 24G ¾″ needle, may be more appropriate and easier to insert. You'll also need to remove the tourniquet promptly to prevent bleeding through the vein wall around the infusion device from increased vascular pressure.

Go smaller and shorter

To help stabilize the vein for insertion, stretch the skin proximal to the insertion site and anchor it firmly with your nondominant hand. Smaller, shorter venous access devices usually work best with elderly patients' fragile veins.

Complications of therapy

Complications of peripheral I.V. therapy can arise from the venous access device, the infusion, or the medication being administered and can be local or systemic. (For a description of local and systemic complications, see *Risks of peripheral I.V. therapy*, pages 310 to 312.)

It's in your hands

Fortunately, you can minimize or prevent most complications by using proper insertion techniques and carefully monitoring the patient. I.V. sites should be checked by a nurse every 2 to 4 hours, or according to facility policy.

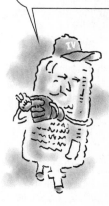

Proper technique and careful monitoring are a winning team.

Discontinuing the infusion

To discontinue the infusion, first clamp the infusion line. Then remove the venous access device using aseptic technique. Here's how to proceed:

• After putting on gloves, lift the tape from the skin to expose the insertion site. You don't need to remove the tape or dressing as long as you can peel it back to expose the venous access device and the patient's skin.

• Be careful to avoid manipulating the device in the skin to prevent skin organisms from entering the bloodstream. Moving the device may also cause discomfort, especially if the insertion site has become phlebitic.

• Apply a sterile dressing directly over the insertion site, then quickly remove the device. (Never use an alcohol pad to clean the site when discontinuing an infusion; this may cause bleeding and a burning sensation.)

• Maintain direct pressure on the I.V. site for several minutes, then tape a dressing over it, being careful not to encircle the limb. If possible, hold the limb upright for about 5 minutes to decrease venous pressure.

• Tell the patient to restrict his activity for about 10 minutes and to leave the site dressing in place for at least 8 hours. If he feels lingering tenderness at the I.V. site, apply warm, moist packs.

• Dispose of the used venipuncture equipment, tubing, and solution containers in a receptacle designated by your facility.

• Document the time of removal, the catheter length and integrity, and the condition of the site. Also, record how the patient tolerated the procedure and any nursing interventions.

(Text continues on page 312.)

Risks of peripheral I.V. therapy

Complications of peripheral I.V. therapy may be local or systemic. This chart lists some common complications along with their signs and symptoms, possible causes, and nursing interventions, including preventive measures.

Signs and symptoms	Possible causes	Nursing interventions
Local complications		
Phlebitis • Tenderness at tip of device and above • Redness at tip of catheter and along vein • Puffy area over vein • Vein hard on palpation • Elevated temperature	• Poor blood flow around device • Friction from catheter movement in vein • Device left in vein too long • Clotting at catheter tip (thrombophlebitis) • Solution with high or low pH or high osmolarity	• Remove device. • Apply warm pack. • Notify doctor. • Document patient's condition and your interventions. *Prevention* • Restart infusion using larger vein for irritating infusate, or restart with a smaller-gauge device to ensure adequate blood flow. • Use filter to reduce risk of phlebitis as indicated. • Tape device securely to prevent motion.
Infiltration • Swelling at and around I.V. site (may extend along entire limb) • Discomfort, burning, or pain at site • Feeling of tightness at site • Decreased skin temperature around site • Blanching at site • Continuing fluid infusion even when vein is occluded, although rate may decrease • Absent backflow of blood • Slower flow rate	• Device dislodged from vein or perforated vein	• Remove device. • Apply warm soaks to aid absorption. • Elevate limb. • Notify doctor if severe. • Periodically assess circulation by checking for pulse, capillary refill, and numbness or tingling. • Restart infusion preferably in another limb or above infiltration site. • Document patient's condition and your interventions. *Prevention* • Check I.V. site frequently (especially when using I.V. pump). • Don't obscure area above site with tape. • Teach patient to report discomfort, pain, or swelling.
Occlusion • No increase in flow rate when I.V. container is raised • Blood backup in line • Discomfort at insertion site	• I.V. flow interrupted • Intermittent device not flushed • Blood backup in line when patient walks • Hypercoagulable patient • Line clamped too long	• Use a low flush pressure syringe, such as a 5cc syringe, during injection. Don't use force. If resistance is met, stop immediately. If unsuccessful, reinsert I.V. device. *Prevention* • Maintain I.V. flow rate. • Flush promptly after intermittent piggyback administration. • Have patient walk with his arm below heart level to reduce risk of blood backup.

Risks of peripheral I.V. therapy *(continued)*

Signs and symptoms	Possible causes	Nursing interventions
Local complications (continued)		
Vein irritation or pain at I.V. site • Pain during infusion • Possible blanching if vasospasm occurs • Red skin over vein during infusion • Rapidly developing signs of phlebitis	• Solution with high or low pH or high osmolarity, such as potassium chloride, phenytoin, and some antibiotics (vancomycin and nafcillin)	• Slow the flow rate. • Try using an electronic flow device to achieve a steady regulated flow. ***Prevention*** • Dilute solutions before administration. For example, give antibiotics in 250-ml rather than 100-ml solution. If drug has low pH, ask pharmacist if drug can be buffered with sodium bicarbonate. (Refer to facility policy.) • If long-term therapy of irritating drug is planned, ask doctor to use central I.V. line.
Systemic complications		
Circulatory overload • Neck vein engorgement • Respiratory distress • Increased blood pressure • Crackles • Large positive fluid balance (intake is greater than output)	• Roller clamp loosened to allow run-on infusion • Flow rate too rapid • Miscalculation of fluid requirements	• Raise the head of the bed. • Slow infusion rate (but don't remove the venous access device). • Administer oxygen as needed. • Notify doctor. • Administer medications (probably furosemide) as ordered. ***Prevention*** • Use pump or volume control set for elderly or compromised patients. • Recheck calculations of fluid requirements. • Monitor infusion frequently.
Systemic infection (septicemia or bacteremia) • Fever, chills, and malaise for no apparent reason • Contaminated I.V. site, usually with no visible signs of infection at site	• Failure to maintain aseptic technique during insertion or site care • Severe phlebitis, which can set up ideal conditions for organism growth • Poor taping that permits venous access device to move, which can introduce organisms into bloodstream • Prolonged indwelling time of device • Immunocompromised patient	• Notify doctor. • Administer medications as prescribed. • Culture site and device. • Monitor vital signs. ***Prevention*** • Use scrupulous aseptic technique when handling solutions and tubings, inserting venous access device, and discontinuing infusion. • Secure all connections. • Change I.V. solutions, tubing, and venous access device at recommended times. • Use I.V. filters. *(continued)*

Risks of peripheral I.V. therapy *(continued)*

Signs and symptoms	Possible causes	Nursing interventions

Systemic complications (continued)

Air embolism
- Respiratory distress
- Unequal breath sounds
- Weak pulse
- Increased central venous pressure
- Decreased blood pressure
- Confusion, disorientation, loss of consciousness

- Empty solution container
- Solution container empties; next container pushes air down line
- Tubing disconnected from venous access device or I.V. bag

- Discontinue infusion.
- Place patient in Trendelenburg's position and on his left side to allow air to enter right atrium and disperse through the pulmonary artery.
- Administer oxygen.
- Notify doctor.
- Document patient's condition and your interventions.

Prevention
- Purge tubing of air completely before infusion.
- Use air-detection device on pump or air-eliminating filter proximal to I.V. site.
- Secure connections.

Central venous therapy

In central venous (CV) therapy, drugs or fluids are infused directly into a major vein. CV therapy is used in various situations, including emergencies or when a patient's peripheral veins are inaccessible.

Patients must be physically and mentally prepared for CV therapy.

On the upside

CV therapy offers many benefits, such as:
- access to the central veins
- rapid infusion of medications or large amounts of fluids
- a way to draw blood samples and measure CV pressure, an important indicator of circulatory function
- reduced need for repeated venipunctures, which decreases the patient's anxiety and preserves (or restores) the peripheral veins
- reduced risk of vein irritation from infusing irritating or caustic substances.

Preparing for CV therapy

The first step in preparing for CV therapy is selecting an insertion site for the catheter. You also need to prepare the patient physically and mentally. The doctor must also obtain informed consent.

You can then gather and prepare the appropriate equipment, which will vary depending on which procedure is used.

Selecting the insertion site

With the exception of a peripherally inserted central catheter (PICC), CV devices are usually inserted by a doctor. If inserting a central line is an elective rather than an emergency procedure, you may collaborate with the patient and doctor in selecting a site.

Commonly used insertion sites include the subclavian, internal and external jugular, and brachiocephalic veins. Although uncommon, the femoral and brachial veins may be used.

Subclavian vein

The subclavian vein is one of the most common insertion sites for CV therapy. It affords easy access and a short, direct route to the superior vena cava and CV circulation.

The subclavian vein is a large vein with high-volume blood flow, making clot formation and vessel irritation less likely. The subclavian site also allows the greatest patient mobility after insertion.

Meet me in the angle of Louis

When using the subclavian site, the doctor inserts the catheter into the vein percutaneously (through the skin and into the vessel with one puncture), threading it into the superior vena cava. This technique requires a venipuncture close to the apex of the lung and major vessels of the thorax. As the catheter enters the skin between the clavicle and first rib, the doctor directs the needle toward the angle of Louis, under the clavicle. The procedure may be difficult if the patient moves during insertion, has a chest deformity, or displays poor posture.

Internal jugular vein

The internal jugular vein provides easy access. In many cases, it's the preferred site. This insertion site is commonly used in children but not in infants.

Too close for comfort

The right internal jugular vein provides a more direct route to the superior vena cava than does the left internal jugular vein. This site is also used for vascular access port insertion. However, its proximity to the common carotid artery can lead to serious complications, such as uncontrolled hemorrhage, emboli, or impeded flow, especially if the carotid artery is punctured during catheter insertion (which can cause irreversible brain damage).

Using the internal jugular vein has other drawbacks. For example, it limits the patient's movement and may be a poor choice for home therapy because it's difficult to immobilize the catheter. Because of the location of the internal jugular vein, it's also difficult to keep a dressing in place.

Femoral veins

Femoral veins may be used if other sites aren't suitable. Although the femoral veins are large vessels, using them for catheter insertion entails some complications. Insertion may be difficult, especially in larger individuals, and carries the risk of puncturing the local lymph nodes.

Dress code

Dressing adherence is a big concern when selecting an insertion site. The femoral site inherently carries a greater risk of local infection because of the difficulty of keeping a dressing clean and intact in the groin area.

Straighten it out

When a femoral vein is used in CV therapy, the patient's leg needs to be kept straight and movement limited. Doing so prevents bleeding and keeps the catheter from becoming kinked internally or dislodged. Infection can also occur at the insertion site from catheter movement into and out of the incision.

Peripheral veins

The peripheral veins most commonly used as insertion sites include basilic, cephalic, external jugular, and median cubital of the antecubital fossa.

Far from internal organs

Because they're located far from major internal organs and vessels, peripheral veins cause fewer traumatic complications on insertion. However, accessing peripheral veins may cause phlebitis. The tight fit of the catheter in the smaller vessel allows only minimal blood flow around the catheter. Catheter movement may irritate the inner lumen or block it, causing blood pooling (stasis) and thrombus formation.

Vein pursuits

Although the cephalic vein is more accessible than the basilic vein, its sharp angle and location below the shoulder make it more difficult to thread a catheter through it. The larger, straighter basilic vein is usually the preferred insertion site. Bedside ultra-

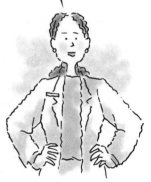

When using the femoral vein for CV therapy, keep the patient's leg straight and limit his movement.

sound may be used to locate the basilic vein and determine if the vein's condition is appropriate for catheter insertion.

The external jugular vein may provide a CV insertion site. Using the external jugular vein this way presents few complications. However, threading a catheter into the superior vena cava may be difficult because of the sharp angle encountered on entering the subclavian vein from the external jugular vein. For this reason, the catheter tip may remain in the external jugular vein. This position allows high-volume infusions but makes CV pressure measurements less accurate.

Accessing peripheral sites in the antecubital space may limit the patient's mobility because the device exits the skin at the bend of the elbow. Inserting the catheter above the antecubital space increases patient mobility and prevents kinking but makes it difficult to palpate the veins.

Dilution dilemma

External jugular veins shouldn't be used to administer highly caustic medications because blood flow around the tip of the catheter may not be strong enough to sufficiently dilute the solutions as they enter the vein.

Let's look alive men! One of us is about to be chosen for a big chore.

Preparing the patient

Accurate and thorough patient teaching increases the success of CV therapy. Before therapy begins, make sure that the patient understands the procedure and its benefits. Be sure to let him know what to expect during and after catheter insertion. Also, cover all self-care measures.

The primary responsibility for explaining the procedure and its goals rests with the doctor. Your role may include allaying the patient's fears and answering questions about movement restrictions, cosmetic concerns, and management regimens.

Explaining the procedure

Ask the patient if he has ever received I.V. therapy before, particularly CV therapy. Evaluate the patient's learning capabilities and adjust your teaching technique accordingly. For example, when describing the procedure to a child, use appropriate language and ask the parents to help you phrase the procedure in terms their child understands. If time and resources permit, use pictures and physical models to enhance your teaching.

All dressed up

If catheter insertion is to take place at the bedside, explain that sterile procedures require the staff to wear gowns, masks, and gloves. Tell your patient that he may need to wear a mask as well.

If time allows, let the patient, especially if he is a child, try on the mask.

An important position

To minimize the patient's anxiety, explain how he'll be positioned during the procedure. If the subclavian or jugular vein will be used, he'll be in Trendelenburg's position for at least a short period, and a towel may be placed under his back between the scapulae. (In Trendelenburg's position, the head is low and the body and legs are on an inclined plane.)

Reassure the patient that he won't be in this position longer than necessary. Stress the position's importance for dilating the veins, which aids insertion and helps prevent insertion-related complications.

The sting

Warn the patient to expect a stinging sensation from the local anesthetic and a feeling of pressure during catheter insertion.

Testing, testing

Explain any other tests that may be done. For example, the doctor may obtain a venogram before the catheter insertion to check the status of the vessels, especially if the catheter is intended for long-term use. After CV catheter insertion, blood samples are commonly drawn to establish baseline coagulation profiles, and a chest X-ray is always done to confirm catheter placement.

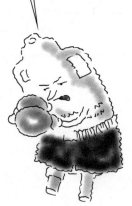

What's that saying? Float like a butterfly; sting like an anesthetic.

Explaining self-care measures

In explaining self-care measures to your patient, make sure that you cover these topics:

• Teach the patient Valsalva's maneuver, and have him demonstrate it to you at least twice. This maneuver helps prevent air embolism. The patient may need to perform it in the future whenever the catheter is open to the air. This training is especially important when the patient is taking care of his catheter at home.

• If the catheter is to be in place long-term or will be managed at home, thoroughly explain all care procedures, such as how to change the dressing and how to flush the device. Ask the patient to demonstrate the various techniques and procedures, and include other family members, as appropriate. A home-therapy coordinator or discharge planner should coordinate teaching and follow-up assessments before and after catheter insertion.

Preparing the equipment

In addition to the I.V. solution, infusion equipment typically includes an administration set with tubing containing an air-eliminating in-line filter if total parenteral nutrition is being infused and an infusion pump. Some facilities use drip controllers for CV therapy, which permit infusion at a lower pressure. Drip controllers are used most commonly with infants and children, who could suffer serious complications from high-pressure infusion.

Gather 'round

When you're assisting with an insertion at the patient's bedside, first collect the necessary equipment. Most facilities use pre-assembled disposable trays that include the CV catheter. Although most trays include the necessary equipment, be sure to check. If you don't have a preassembled tray, gather the following items:
- linen-saver pad
- scissors
- povidone-iodine solution
- sterile gauze pads
- chlorhexidine
- local anesthetic
- 3-ml syringe with 25G needle for introduction of anesthetic
- sterile syringe for blood samples
- sterile towels or drapes
- suture material
- sterile dressing
- CV catheter.

You also need to obtain extra syringes and blood sample containers if the doctor wants venous blood samples to be drawn during the procedure.

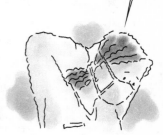

Gowns, masks, and gloves are required for bedside catheter insertion.

Proper precautions

Make sure that everyone participating in the insertion has a mask, a gown, and gloves. You may also need such protection for the patient, especially if there's a risk of site contamination from oral secretions or if the patient is unable to cooperate.

Some assembly required

To set up the equipment, follow these steps:
- Attach the tubing to the solution container.
- Prime the tubing with the solution.
- Fill the syringes with saline or heparin flush solutions, based on policy and procedures at your facility.
- Prime and calibrate pressure monitoring setups.

Aseptic, air-free, secure, and sealed

In addition, take the following precautions:
- All priming must be done using strict aseptic technique.
- All tubing must be free from air.
- After you have primed the tubing, recheck all the connections to make sure that they're secure.
- Make sure that all open ends are covered with sealed caps.

Performing central venous therapy

Although specific steps may vary, the same basic procedure is used whether catheter insertion is done at the bedside or in the operating room. Before the doctor inserts the catheter, you need to position the patient and prepare the insertion site. Some patients may require sedation for the catheter to be placed. Such patients must be carefully monitored by staff trained in this procedure.

Positioning the patient

After you have assembled the equipment, position the patient to make him as comfortable as possible. For insertion in the subclavian or internal jugular veins, position the patient in Trendelenburg's position. This position distends neck and thoracic veins, making them more visible and accessible. Filling the veins also lessens the chance of air emboli because the venous pressure is higher than atmospheric pressure.

On a roll

If the subclavian vein is to be used, you may need to place a rolled towel or blanket between the patient's scapulae. Doing so allows for more direct access and may prevent puncture of the lung apex or adjacent vessels. If a jugular vein is to be used, place a rolled blanket under the opposite shoulder to extend the neck and make anatomic landmarks more visible.

Preparing the insertion site

To prepare the insertion site, place a linen-saver pad under the site to prevent soiling the bed. Make sure that the skin is free from hair because the follicles can harbor microorganisms. (See *Removing hair from a CV insertion site.*)

Wipe the site

Prepare the intended venipuncture site with chlorhexidine. Use a side-to-side motion to prepare the skin. Don't wipe the same area

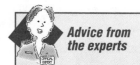
Advice from the experts

Removing hair from a CV insertion site

Infection-control practitioners and the Infusion Nurses Society recommend clipping the hair close to the skin rather than shaving.

Irritation, open wounds, infection
Shaving may cause skin irritation and create multiple, small, open wounds, increasing the risk of infection. To avoid irritation, clip the patient's hair with single-patient-use clipper blades.

Rinse, wash, and remove
After you remove the hair, rinse the skin with saline solution to remove hair clippings. You may also need to wash the skin with soap and water before the actual skin prep to remove surface dirt and body oils.

twice, and be sure to discard each gauze pad or swab stick after each complete cycle. Be sure to let the solution dry completely before proceeding with vascular access device insertion.

Drape in place

After the site is prepared, the doctor places sterile drapes around it and, possibly, around the patient's face. (The drapes make the patient's mask unnecessary.) If the patient's face is draped, you can help ease anxiety by uncovering his eyes. The drapes should provide a work area at least as large as the length of the catheter or guide wire.

Inserting the catheter

During catheter insertion, you may be responsible for monitoring the patient's tolerance of the procedure and providing emotional support. The doctor usually prepares the equipment, which comes with a CV access kit and requires aseptic technique.

After inserting the catheter

You may obtain venous blood samples after the catheter is inserted. You'll need a sterile syringe that's large enough to hold all of the needed blood such as a 10-ml syringe. Place the blood in the proper sample container or, using a needle or needleless system, access a saline lock at the end of the port with a Vacutainer. This device draws blood directly into the appropriate tube.

Patient participation

Each time the catheter hub is open to air — such as when the syringe is changed — tell the patient to perform Valsalva's maneuver or clamp the port to decrease the risk of air embolism.

After the fact

After the catheter is inserted, your primary responsibilities are monitoring the patient and administering therapy. You'll also need to apply a dressing to the insertion site and document your interventions and all information related to the catheter insertion.

Monitoring the patient

Monitor the patient for complications. Make sure that you tailor your assessment and interventions to the particular catheter insertion site. For example, if the site is close to major thoracic organs, as with a subclavian or internal jugular vein site, you should closely monitor the patient's respiratory status, watching for dyspnea, shortness of breath, and sudden chest pain.

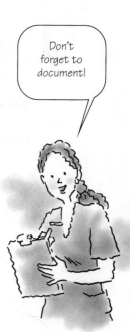

Don't forget to document!

Arrhythmia alert

Inserting the catheter can cause arrhythmias if the catheter enters the right atrium (irritating the node) or right ventricle (irritating the cardiac muscle). For this reason, make sure that you monitor the patient's cardiac status. (Arrhythmias usually abate as the catheter is withdrawn.) If the patient isn't attached to a cardiac monitor, palpate the radial pulse to detect rhythm irregularities.

Some patients have sutures in their futures

When the proximal end of the catheter rests on the sterile drape, the doctor will use one or two sutures to secure the catheter to the skin. Most short-term catheters have preset tabs to hold the sutures.

X-ray vision

Finally, a chest X-ray is ordered to confirm the location of the catheter tip before starting infusions. The line should be capped and flushed with normal saline solution until an X-ray confirms placement. After confirmation, begin the infusion by connecting the I.V. tubing or intermittent cap to the catheter hub. Adjust the flow rate as prescribed.

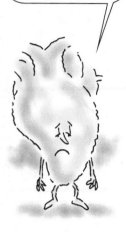

Make sure you monitor how I'm doing. Catheter insertion can cause arrhythmias.

Applying a dressing

Maintain sterile technique and place a sterile dressing over the insertion site of a short-term catheter or exit site of the PICC or tunneled catheter. To apply the dressing, follow these steps:
• Clean the site with chlorhexidine using the same method as the initial skin preparation. Allow the skin to dry; then cover the site with a transparent semipermeable dressing.
• Seal the dressing with nonporous tape, checking that all edges are well secured. Label the dressing with the date and time, your initials, and the catheter length.
• After you apply the dressing, place the patient in a comfortable position and reassess his status. Elevate the head of the bed 45 degrees to help the patient breathe more easily. Remember to keep the site clean and dry to prevent infection. Also remember to keep the dressing occlusive to prevent contamination.

Maintaining central venous therapy

One of your primary responsibilities is maintaining CV infusions. Doing so includes meticulous care of the CV catheter insertion site as well as the catheter and tubing. Expect to perform the following care measures:
• Change the transparent semipermeable dressing weekly or whenever it becomes moist, loose, or soiled.

- Change the I.V. tubing and solution.
- Flush the catheter.
- Change the catheter cap.
- Administer a secondary infusion or obtain blood samples, if needed.
- Record your assessment findings and interventions according to your facility's policy.

Changing dressings

To reduce the risk of infection, always wear gloves and a mask when changing a dressing. The patient should also wear a mask. If the patient can't tolerate a facial mask, have him turn his head away from the catheter during the dressing change.

Well equipped

Many facilities use a preassembled dressing-change tray that contains all the necessary equipment. If your facility doesn't use this type of tray, gather the necessary equipment, including:
- chlorhexidine swabs
- transparent semipermeable dressing
- sterile drape
- sterile gloves and masks
- clean gloves
- bag to dispose of old dressing.

Dress for success

Change the patient's dressing according to the type of dressing and your facility's policy and procedures. Some CV dressings are changed every 48 hours, but other dressings can remain in place for as long as 7 days. Change dressings immediately if they become soiled or loose. (See *Changing a CV dressing*, page 322.)

Changing solutions and tubing

Change the I.V. solution every 24 hours and tubing every 72 hours or as directed by your facility's policy, maintaining strict aseptic technique. You don't need to wear a mask unless there's a contamination risk — for example, if you have an upper respiratory tract infection.

To prevent air embolism, have the patient perform Valsalva's maneuver and clamp the port each time the catheter hub is open to air. Many facilities eliminate the need for this by using a connecting tubing with a slide clamp between the catheter hub and the I.V. tubing, which allows the I.V. tubing to be clamped during changes.

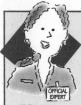

Advice from the experts

Changing a CV dressing

After you assemble all needed equipment, follow the step-by-step technique below to safely change a central venous (CV) dressing.

Getting ready
• Wash your hands. Then place the patient in a comfortable position.
• Prepare a sterile field. Open the bag, placing it away from the sterile field but still within reach.

Out with the old
• Put on clean gloves and remove the old dressing.
• Inspect the old dressing for signs of infection. You may want to culture any discharge at the site or on the old dressing. If not, discard the dressing and gloves in the bag. Be sure to report an infection to the doctor immediately and to document it in the nurses' notes.
• Check the position of the catheter and the insertion site for signs of infiltration or infection, such as redness, swelling, tenderness, or drainage.

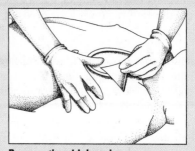

Remove the old dressing.

In with the new
• Put on sterile gloves and clean the skin around the catheter with chlorhexidine using a side-to-side motion. Don't wipe the same area twice.
• Don't use solutions containing acetone; they may cause some catheters to disintegrate.
• Redress the site with a transparent semipermeable dressing.
• If the catheter is taped (not sutured) to the skin, carefully replace the soiled tape with sterile tape, using the chevron method. To do so, first cut a strip of tape about ½″ (1.3 cm) wide and slide it under the catheter, sticky side up. Then crisscross the tape over the top of the catheter. Finally, place a second strip of tape over the first strip. Make sure the catheter is secure.

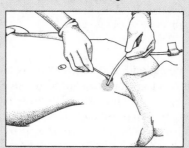

Clean the insertion site.

Write it down
• Label the dressing with the date, time, and your initials.
• Discard all used items properly; reposition the patient comfortably.

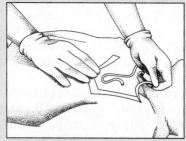

Redress the site.

Switching solutions

To change the solution, follow these steps:
- Gather a solution container and an alcohol swab.
- Wash your hands.
- Put on gloves.
- Remove the cap and seal from the solution container.
- Clamp the CV line.
- Remove the spike quickly from the solution container, and reinsert it into the new container.
- Hang the new container and adjust the flow rate.

Turning over the tubing

To change the tubing, gather an I.V. administration set, an extension set, an alcohol wipe, and gloves. For instructions on what to do next, see *Changing CV tubing*.

Two things at once

If possible, change the solution and tubing at the same time. You may not be able to do this if, for example, the tubing is damaged or the solution runs out before it's time to change the tubing. To change the tubing and solution simultaneously, follow these steps:
- Wash your hands.
- Hang the new I.V. bag and primed tubing on the I.V. pole.
- Stop the flow in the old tubing.

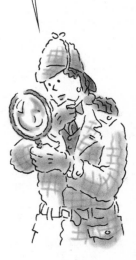

Perhaps the best solution is to change the I.V. solution and the tubing at the same time.

Advice from the experts

Changing CV tubing

After assembling the needed equipment, follow these guidelines to safely and quickly change central venous (CV) tubing:

1. Wash your hands.
2. Reduce the I.V. flow rate, and remove the old spike from the bag. Loosely spread the cover from the new spike over the old spike.
3. Keep the old spike in an upright position above the patient's heart, and insert the new spike into the I.V. container. Prime the system.
4. Instruct the patient to perform Valsalva's maneuver. Quickly disconnect the old tubing from the needle or catheter hub, being careful not to dislodge the venipuncture device. If it's difficult to disconnect, use a hemostat to hold the hub securely while the end of the tubing is twisted and removed. Don't clamp the hemostat shut because the tubing adapter, needle, or catheter hub may crack, requiring a change of equipment and I.V. site.
5. Quickly attach the new primed tubing to the venipuncture device, using aseptic technique.
6. Adjust the flow to the prescribed rate.
7. Label the new tubing with the date and time of the change.

• Quickly disconnect the old tubing and connect the new tubing, as described in *Changing CV tubing*.

Flushing the catheter

Flush the CV catheter with saline solution routinely, according to your facility's policy, to maintain patency. When the system is maintained as an intermittent infusion device, the flushing procedure varies, depending on facility policy, type of catheter used, and medication administration schedule.

How often? How much?

Flushing recommendations vary from once every 8 hours to once per day. The recommended amount of flushing solution also varies. (See *How much flushing solution?*) Some facilities use positive pressure (alone or with saline solution) to flush the CV catheter.

Don't overdo the heparin

Some facilities use a heparinized saline flush solution, available in premixed, 10-ml multidose vials. Recommended concentration strengths vary from 10 to 1,000 units of heparin/ml. Be sure to use the lowest possible effective heparin concentration because higher concentrations can interfere with the patient's clotting factors.

Know your catheter needs

Different catheters require not only different amounts of solution but different flushing schedules as well. Generally, a CV catheter with a two-way valve (Groshong tip) is flushed with saline solution once per day when not in use. All lumens of a multilumen catheter (unless it's a valved catheter) must be flushed regularly with a heparin or saline solution, depending on your facility's policy and practice. (No flushing is needed with a continuous infusion through a single-lumen catheter.) It's also recommended that you obtain a blood return of 3 to 5 ml of free-flowing blood from the catheter before each use.

Mismatched medications

A heparin or normal saline solution flush should also be performed before and after the administration of incompatible medications.

Flushing made simple

To flush the catheter, follow these steps:
• Put on gloves.
• Clean the cap with an alcohol swab (using a 70% alcohol solution).
• Allow the cap to dry.
• Inject the recommended or prescribed type and amount of flush solution.

How much flushing solution?

The recommended amount of flushing solution varies. The Infusion Nurses Society states to flush with at least two times the volume capacity of the catheter and add-on devices. Facility policies recommend using 3 to 5 ml of solution to flush the catheter, although some policies allow for as much as 10 ml of solution.

To prevent blood backflow and possible clotting in the line, continue with these steps:
• Maintain positive pressure by keeping your thumb on the plunger of the syringe (usually 10 ml).
• Engage the clamping mechanism on the central line.
• Withdraw the syringe.

Changing caps

CV catheters used for infrequent infusions have intermittent injection caps similar to saline lock adapters used for peripheral I.V. infusion therapy. The frequency of cap changes varies according to facility policy and the number of times that the cap is used. However, the cap should be changed at least every 7 days. Needleless caps should be used whenever possible.

Don't say we didn't warn you

Use strict aseptic technique when changing the cap. Repeated puncturing of the injection port increases the risk of infection. Also, pieces may break off after repeated punctures, placing the patient at risk for embolism. Many needleless caps don't have a rubber port.

Caps off

To change the cap, follow these steps:
• Close the clamping mechanism on the line.
• Clean the connection site with an alcohol swab.
• Instruct the patient to perform Valsalva's maneuver while you quickly disconnect the old cap and connect the new cap, using aseptic technique. If the patient can't perform Valsalva's maneuver, time the disconnect maneuver with the patient's respiratory cycle and remove the cap during the expiratory phase. Make sure that the new cap is purged of air and ready to be applied.

Infusing secondary fluids and drawing blood

To add other fluids to the patient's CV infusion, make sure that solutions running in the same line are compatible and connections are luer-locked or well secured with tape. Secondary I.V. lines may be piggybacked into a side port or Y-port of a primary infusion line instead of being connected directly to the catheter lumen. However, if there's no primary infusion prescribed, the medication may be infused through the CV line.

You may use the CV catheter to obtain ordered blood samples, especially if the patient requires frequent laboratory work. (See *Drawing blood from a CV catheter*, page 326.)

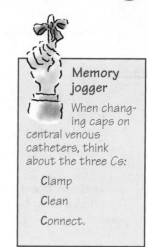

Memory jogger

When changing caps on central venous catheters, think about the three Cs:

Clamp

Clean

Connect.

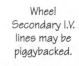

Whee! Secondary I.V. lines may be piggybacked.

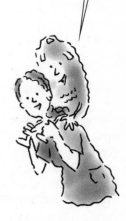

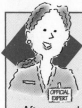

Advice from the experts

Drawing blood from a CV catheter

After assembling your equipment, use these step-by-step instructions to safely draw blood from a central venous (CV) catheter.

Collecting with an evacuated tube
To draw blood using an evacuated tube, follow the steps listed below.

Get ready
• Wash your hands and put on sterile gloves.
• Stop the I.V. infusion and place an injection cap on the lumen of the catheter.
• If multiple infusions are running, stop them and wait 1 minute before drawing blood from the catheter to allow I.V. fluids and medications to be carried away from the catheter, preventing them from becoming mixed with the blood sample you'll be drawing.
• Clean the end of the injection cap with antiseptic swabs (such as with alcohol).

Draw the blood
• Place a 5-ml lavender-top evacuated tube into its plastic sleeve. Use this tube to collect and discard the filling volume of the catheter, plus an extra 2 to 3 ml. Most studies indicate that about 5 ml is enough blood to discard. (At some health care facilities, the first 5 ml of blood isn't discarded if the patient is scheduled for multiple blood studies. Instead, the blood is infused back into the patient after the sample is drawn.)
• Insert the needleless device into the injection cap of the catheter. The first milliliter may be clear until the blood flows through the catheter.
• When blood stops flowing into the tube, remove and discard the tube, if appropriate.
• Use the appropriate evacuated tubes for the ordered blood tests. After you've drawn the necessary blood, flush the catheter with saline solution and a 10-ml syringe and resume the infusion. If you're not going to use the lumen immediately, heparinize the catheter.
• If you can't get blood flowing from the catheter, the tip of the catheter could be against the vessel wall. To correct this problem, ask the patient to raise his arms over his head, turn on his side, cough, or perform Valsalva's maneuver. You can also try flushing the catheter with saline solution before making another attempt to draw blood.

Collecting with a syringe
If evacuated tubes for collecting blood aren't available, obtain the blood sample with a syringe. To do so, collect syringes, evacuated tubes for the sample, gloves, and saline or heparin flush solution. Then follow the steps listed below.

Get ready
• First, stop all infusions.
• Select the port from which to withdraw the blood. The port should be 16G to 20G.
• Put on gloves.
• Using aseptic technique, disconnect the tubing or saline lock cap. (If the catheter has a clamp, use it before disconnecting. If the catheter doesn't have a clamp, have the patient perform Valsalva's maneuver.)

Draw the blood
• Insert the syringe and draw back 5 ml of blood.
• Discard the syringe.
• Connect a second syringe, and draw the amount of blood you need.
• Flush the catheter with the recommended amount of saline solution or heparin. (The amount depends on the type of catheter and the frequency and type of infusions. Check the manufacturer's recommendations and your facility's policy.)
• Place the blood in the evacuated tubes.
• Label the evacuated tubes, and send them to the laboratory.

Common infusion problems

During CV infusions, you may encounter such problems as catheter tears or kinking and clots. Follow the recommendations below to deal with these common infusion problems.

Tears to bear

A serrated hemostat will eventually break down silicone rubber and tear the catheter, causing blood to back up and fluid to leak from the device. If air enters the catheter through the tear, an air embolism could result. Prevent catheter tears by using nonserrated clamps. If the catheter or part of the catheter breaks, cracks, or becomes nonfunctional, the doctor may replace the entire CV line with a new one or use a repair kit if available.

Working out the kinks

The catheter can become kinked or pinched above or beneath the skin. Kinks beneath the skin are detected by X-ray and are usually located between the clavicle and the first rib. The catheter may need to be unsutured and repositioned or replaced.

Never attempt to straighten kinks in stiff catheters such as those made from polyvinyl chloride. These catheters fracture easily. Fractured particles may enter the circulation and act as an embolus. The doctor may try to unkink a long-term catheter, which is made of pliable silicone rubber. The unkinking is done under guided fluoroscopy using aseptic technique.

You may be able to prevent external catheter kinks by taping and positioning the catheter properly. For example, looping the extension tubing once and securing it with tape adjacent to the dressing prevents the catheter from being pulled if the tubing gets entangled. Doing so also helps prevent the catheter from moving or telescoping at the insertion site, a major cause of catheter-related infections and site irritations.

Lots and lots about clots

If you have difficulty withdrawing blood or infusing fluid, there may be a fibrin sheath at the tip of the catheter. This type of sheath impedes the flow of blood and provides a protein-rich environment for bacterial growth.

Occasionally, this sheath forms so that fluids infuse easily while blood aspiration is difficult or impossible. The fibrin sheath may be removed surgically or dissolved by instilling a thrombolytic agent. The agent may be instilled by a doctor or registered nurse trained in the procedure.

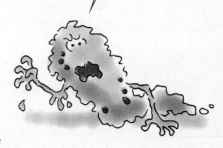

A fibrin sheath at the catheter tip provides a protein-rich environment for bacterial growth.

This procedure is usually recommended for long-term CV catheters because they're difficult and costly to replace. However, attempting to salvage a device isn't always appropriate or possible.

Patients with special needs

There are a few additional considerations involved in caring for pediatric, elderly, and home therapy patients.

Across the generation gap

Essentially the same catheters are used in both pediatric and elderly patients. However, four possible differences include catheter length, lumen size, insertion sites, and amount of fluid infused.

In infants, for example, the jugular vein is the preferred insertion site, even though it's much more difficult to maintain than are other sites. Usually, the doctor and the patient's family select a mutually acceptable site if the catheter will be used for long-term therapy. Furthermore, because pediatric patients are smaller, they require shorter catheters with smaller lumens than those needed for adults. As pediatric patients grow, larger catheters are required.

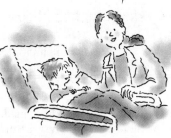

Pediatric patients require short catheters with small lumens.

Homework

Long-term CV catheters allow patients to receive fluids, medications, and blood infusions at home. These catheters have a much longer life because they're less thrombogenic and less prone to infection than are short-term devices.

The care procedures used in the home are the same as those used in the hospital, including aseptic technique. A candidate for home CV therapy must have:
• a family member or friend who can assist in safe and competent administration of I.V. fluids
• a suitable home environment
• a telephone
• transportation
• the ability to prepare, handle, store, and dispose of the equipment.

To ensure your patient's safety, patient teaching begins before he's discharged. After discharge, a home-therapy coordinator provides follow-up care. This care helps ensure compliance until the patient or caregiver can independently provide catheter care and infusion therapy at home. The home therapy patient can learn to care for the catheter himself and to infuse his own medications and solutions.

Traumatic and systemic complications

Complications can occur at any time during CV therapy. Traumatic complications, such as pneumothorax, typically occur on insertion but may not be noticed until after the procedure is completed. Systemic complications, such as sepsis, typically occur later in therapy.

Traumatic topic: Pneumothorax

Pneumothorax, the most common traumatic complication of catheter insertion, is associated with the insertion of a CV catheter into the subclavian or internal jugular vein. It's usually discovered on the chest X-ray that confirms catheter placement if the patient doesn't have symptoms immediately.

Pneumothorax may be minimal and may not require intervention (unless the patient is on positive-pressure ventilation). A thoracotomy is performed and a chest tube inserted if pneumothorax is severe enough to cause signs and symptoms, such as chest pain, dyspnea, cyanosis, and decreased or absent breath sounds on the affected side.

Sneaky signs and symptoms

Initially, the patient may be asymptomatic; signs of distress gradually show up as pneumothorax gets larger. For this reason, you need to monitor the patient closely and auscultate for breath sounds for at least 8 hours after catheter insertion. If unchecked, pneumothorax may progress to tension pneumothorax, a medical emergency. The patient exhibits such signs as:
- acute respiratory distress
- asymmetrical chest wall movement
- possibly, a tracheal shift away from the affected side.

A chest tube must be inserted immediately before respiratory and cardiac decompensation occur.

Let's talk puncture at this juncture

The second most common life-threatening complication is arterial puncture. Arterial puncture may lead to hemothorax and internal bleeding, which may not be detected immediately. A hemothorax is treated like pneumothorax, except that the chest tube is inserted lower in the chest to help evacuate the blood.

Left untreated, internal bleeding caused by arterial puncture leads to hypovolemic shock. Signs and symptoms include:
- increased heart rate
- decreased blood pressure
- cool, clammy skin
- obvious swelling in the neck or chest

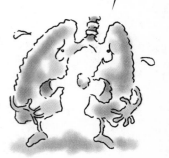

Yikes! Insertion of a catheter into subclavian or internal jugular veins may cause pneumothorax.

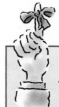

Memory jogger

Use the mnemonic ACT to remember the signs and symptoms of tension pneumothorax so that you can "act" fast to protect your patient:

Acute respiratory distress

Chest wall motion that's asymmetrical

Tracheal shifting.

• mental confusion (especially if the common carotid arteries are involved)
• formation of a hematoma (a large, blood-filled sac), which causes pressure on the trachea and adjacent vessels.

Rare but risky

There are a few additional, but rare, complications of CV therapy:
• Tracheal puncture is associated with insertion of a catheter into the subclavian vein.
• Development of a fistula between the brachiocephalic vein and the subclavian artery may result from perforation by the guide wire on insertion into the vessel.
• Chylothorax results when a lymph node is punctured and lymph fluid leaks into the pleural cavity.
• Hydrothorax (or infusion of solution into the chest), thrombosis, and local infection are also potential complications of CV therapy.

Serious business: Sepsis

Catheter-related sepsis is the most serious systemic complication. It may lead to septic shock, multisystem organ failure, and death. Most sepsis attributed to CV catheters is caused by skin surface organisms, such as *Staphylococcus epidermidis*, *S. aureus*, and *Candida albicans*.

Strict aseptic technique and close observation are the best defense against sepsis. Regularly check the catheter insertion site for signs of localized infection, such as redness, drainage, and tenderness along the catheter path. If the patient shows signs of generalized infection, such as unexplained fever, draw blood cultures from a peripheral site as well as from the device itself, according to facility protocol.

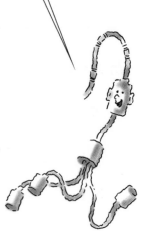

If sepsis is suspected, I may need to be replaced by a new catheter in a different site.

Out with the old, in with the new

If catheter-related sepsis is suspected, the catheter may be removed and a new one inserted in a different site. Culture the catheter tip after removal. Administer antibiotics, as ordered, and draw blood for repeat cultures after the antibiotic course is complete.

PICC-specific complications

PICC therapy causes fewer and less severe complications than does therapy using other CV lines. Pneumothorax is extremely rare because the insertion site is peripheral. Catheter-related sepsis is usually related to site contamination.

Phlebitis — mechanical or bacterial

Mechanical phlebitis—painful inflammation of a vein—may be the most common PICC complication. It may occur during the first 72 hours after PICC insertion and is more common in left-sided insertions and when a large-gauge catheter is used. If the patient develops mechanical phlebitis, apply warm, moist compresses to his upper arm; elevate the extremity; and restrict activity to mild exercise. If the phlebitis continues or worsens, remove the catheter, as ordered.

Bacterial phlebitis can occur with PICCs; however, it usually occurs later in the infusion therapy. If drainage occurs at the insertion site and the patient's temperature increases, notify the doctor. The catheter may have to be removed.

Quick PICC info

Expect minimal bleeding from the PICC insertion site for the first 24 hours. Bleeding that persists needs additional evaluation. A pressure dressing should be left in place over the insertion site for at least 24 hours. After that, if there's no bleeding, the dressing can be changed and a new transparent dressing applied without a gauze pressure dressing.

Some patients complain of pain at the PICC insertion site, usually because the device is located in an area of frequent flexion. Pain may be treated by applying warm compresses and restricting activities until the patient becomes adjusted to the presence of the PICC.

Air embolism in PICC therapy is less common than it is in traditional CV lines because the line is inserted below the level of the heart.

Discontinuing central venous therapy

You or the doctor may remove the catheter, depending on your state's nurse practice act, your facility's policy, and the type of catheter. Long-term catheters and implanted devices are always removed by the doctor. However, PICC lines may be removed by a qualified nurse.

Discontinue continuous; implement intermittent

You may receive an order to discontinue continuous infusion therapy and begin intermittent infusion therapy. If so, follow the same procedure used for peripheral I.V. therapy.

Removing the catheter

Begin catheter removal with a couple of precautions:

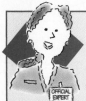

Advice from the experts

Removing a CV catheter

After assembling your equipment, follow the step-by-step guidelines listed below to safely remove a central venous (CV) catheter.

Getting ready
- Place the patient in a supine position to prevent emboli.
- Wash your hands and put on clean gloves.
- Turn off all infusions.
- Remove the old dressing.
- Inspect the site for signs of drainage or inflammation.

Removing the catheter
- Clip the sutures and remove the catheter in a slow, even motion. Have the patient perform Valsalva's maneuver as the catheter is withdrawn to prevent air emboli.
- Apply povidone-iodine or antibiotic ointment to the insertion site to seal it.
- Inspect the catheter to see if any portions broke off during the removal. If so, notify the doctor immediately and monitor the patient closely for signs of distress. If a culture is to be obtained, use sterile scissors to clip approximately 1" (2.5 cm) off the distal end of the catheter, letting it drop into the sterile specimen container.

- Place a transparent semipermeable dressing over the site. Label the dressing with the date and time of the removal and your initials.
- Properly dispose of the I.V. tubing and equipment you used.

Monitoring the patient
Insidious bleeding may develop after removing the catheter. Remember that some vessels, such as the subclavian vein, aren't easily compressed. By 72 hours, the site should be sealed and the risk of air emboli should be past; however, you may still need to apply a dry dressing to the site.

Make a notation on the nursing care plan to recheck the patient and insertion site frequently for the next few hours. Check for signs of respiratory decompensation, possibly indicating air emboli, and for signs of bleeding, such as blood on the dressing, decreased blood pressure, increased heart rate, paleness, or diaphoresis.

Noteworthy
Document the time and date of the catheter removal and any complications that occurred, such as catheter shearing, bleeding, or respiratory distress. Also be sure to record the length of the catheter and signs of blood, drainage, redness, or swelling of the site.

Check the patient's record or other documentation (such as the nurses' notes, physicians' notes, or the written X-ray report) for the most recent placement confirmed by an X-ray to trace the catheter's path as it exits the body (as directed by facility policy).

Make sure that backup assistance is available if a complication, such as uncontrolled bleeding, occurs during catheter removal. This complication is common in patients with coagulopathies.

Patient prep

Before you remove the catheter, explain the procedure to the patient. Tell him that he'll need to turn his face away from the site and perform Valsalva's maneuver when the catheter is withdrawn. If necessary, review the maneuver with him.

Get your gear

Before removing the catheter, gather the necessary equipment, including:
- sterile gauze
- clean gloves
- forceps
- sterile scissors
- povidone-iodine or antibiotic ointment
- alcohol swabs
- transparent semipermeable dressing
- tape.

If you're sending the catheter tip for culture, you also need a sterile specimen container. (See *Removing a CV catheter*.)

Note this

After removing the catheter, be sure to document:
- patient tolerance
- condition of the catheter, including its length
- time of discontinuation of therapy
- cultures ordered and sent
- dressings applied
- other pertinent information.

Calculating I.V. flow rates

A key aspect of administering I.V. therapy is maintaining accurate flow rates for the solutions. If an infusion runs too quickly or too slowly, your patient may suffer complications, such as phlebitis, infiltration, circulatory overload (possibly leading to heart failure and pulmonary edema), and adverse drug reactions.

Volume-control devices and the correct administration set help prevent such complications. You can help, too, by being familiar with all of the information in doctors' orders and being able to recognize incomplete or incorrectly written orders for I.V. therapy.

Calculating flow rates

Two basic types of flow rates are available with I.V. administration sets: macrodrip and microdrip. Each set delivers a specific number of drops per milliliter (gtt/ml). Macrodrip delivers 10, 15, or 20 gtt/ml; microdrip delivers 60 gtt/ml. Regardless of the type of set you

No matter what size administration set you use, the formula for calculating flow rates is the same.

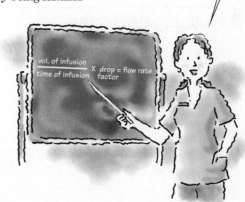

$$\frac{\text{vol. of infusion}}{\text{time of infusion}} \times \text{drop} = \text{flow rate factor}$$

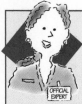

Advice from the experts

Calculating flow rates

When calculating the flow rate (drops per minute) of I.V. solutions, remember that the number of drops required to deliver 1 ml varies with the type of administration set used and its manufacturer:

• Administration sets are of two types— macrodrip (the standard type) and micro-drip. Macrodrip delivers 10, 15, or 20 drops per milliliter (gtt/ml); microdrip usually delivers 60 gtt/ml (see illustrations).

• Manufacturers calibrate their devices differently, so be sure to look for the "drop factor"—expressed in gtt/ml—in the packaging that accompanies the set you're using. (This packaging also has crucial information about such things as special infusions and blood transfusions.)

When you know your device's drop factor, use the following formula to calculate specific flow rates:

$$\frac{\text{volume of infusion (in milliliters)}}{\text{time of infusion (in minutes)}} \times \text{drop factor (in drops per milliliter)} = \text{flow rate (in drops per minute)}$$

After you calculate the flow rate for the set you're using, remove your watch or position your wrist so you can look at your watch and the drops at the same time. Next, adjust the clamp to achieve the ordered flow rate, and count the drops for 1 full minute. Readjust the clamp as necessary and count the drops for another minute. Keep adjusting the clamp and counting the drops until you have the correct rate.

Macrodrip

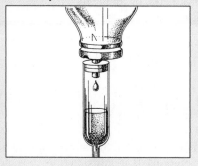

Microdrip

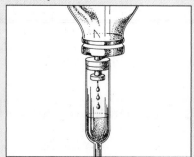

use, the formula for calculating flow rates is the same. (See *Calculating flow rates.*)

Regulating flow rates

When a patient's condition requires you to maintain precise I.V. flow rates, use an infusion control device such as clamps, volumetric pumps, and rate minders.

ml/hour or gtt/minute?

When you regulate I.V. flow rate with a clamp, the rate is usually measured in drops per minute (gtt/minute). If you use a pump, the flow rate is measured in milliliters per hour (ml/hour).

I.V. clamps

You can regulate the flow rate with two types of clamps: screw and roller. The screw clamp offers greater accuracy, but the roller clamp, used for standard fluid therapy, is faster and easier to manipulate. A third type, the slide clamp, can stop or start the flow but can't regulate the rate.

Pumps

New pumps are being developed all the time; be sure to attend instruction sessions to learn how to use them. On your unit, keep a file of instruction manuals (provided by the manufacturers) for each piece of equipment used.

Rate minder

Another type of flow control device is the rate minder, which resembles a roller clamp. This device is added to the I.V. tubing. By setting the rate minder to the desired flow rate, you adjust the clamp to deliver that rate. Be sure to label the infusion bag with the rate in milliliters per hour.

Mind these limitations

Rate minders have some limitations. Because the flow rate may vary by as much as 5%, the infusion must be checked frequently to prevent too-rapid infusion or nonflow situations. The other drawback is that the rate minders usually don't deliver infusions at rates lower than 5 to 10 ml/hour. For this reason, they're used mainly for adult patients and only with noncritical infusions.

Factor in these factors

When you're using a clamp for flow regulation, you must monitor the flow rate closely and adjust as needed. Such factors as vein spasm, vein pressure changes, patient movement, manipulations of the clamp, and bent or kinked tubing can cause the rate to vary markedly. For easy monitoring, use a time tape, which marks the prescribed solution level at hourly intervals.

Other factors that affect flow rate include the type of I.V. fluid and its viscosity, the height of the infusion container, the type of administration set, and the size and position of the venous access device.

Checking flow rates

Flow rates can be fickle; they should be checked and adjusted regularly. The frequency of flow rate check depends on the patient's condition and age and the solution or medication being administered.

I'll be back soon!

Many nurses check the I.V. flow rate every time they're in a patient's room and after each position change. The flow rate should be assessed more frequently for critically ill patients, patients with conditions that might be exacerbated by fluid overload, pediatric patients, elderly patients, and patients receiving a drug that can cause tissue damage if infiltration occurs.

When checking the flow rate, inspect and palpate the I.V. insertion site, and ask the patient how it feels.

Minor (not major) adjustments

If the infusion rate slows significantly, you can usually get it back on schedule by adjusting the rate slightly. Don't make a major adjustment, though. If the rate must be increased by more than 30%, check with the doctor.

You should also time an infusion control device or rate minder for 1 to 2 hours per shift. (These devices have an error rate ranging from 2% to 10%.) Before using any infusion control device, become thoroughly familiar with its features. Attend instruction sessions and perform return demonstrations until you learn the system.

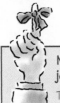

Memory jogger

To remind yourself of the need to check and adjust flow rates, remember the following tongue twister:

Fight fickle flow with frequent follow-up.

Administering blood products

Most states allow nurses with RN licenses (but not LPN or LVN licenses) to administer blood and blood components. In some states, nurses with LPN licenses may regulate transfusion flow rates, observe patients for reactions, discontinue transfusions, and document procedures. Know your state practice act before performing a transfusion or a transfusion-related procedure.

Safer but still risky

Because of careful screening and testing, the supply of blood is safer today than it has ever been. Even so, a patient who receives a transfusion is still at risk for life-threatening complications, such as a hemolytic reaction (which destroys red blood cells [RBCs]), and exposure to infectious diseases, such as human immunodeficiency virus (HIV) and hepatitis. Therefore, the doctor, the nurse, and the

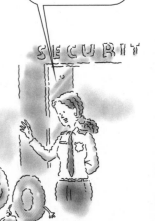

Although blood products are carefully screened, transfusions still expose patients to certain risks.

patient (when able) must weigh the benefits of a transfusion against the risks. Patients must be informed of the risks of transfusions. Many facilities have special consent forms for transfusions.

Transfusion methods

The two ways to administer blood and blood products are through a peripheral I.V. line and through a CV line.

Peripheral I.V. line

Blood products can be transfused through a peripheral I.V. line, but this set-up isn't the best method if large volumes must be transfused quickly. It's recommended that a 20G or larger peripheral I.V. catheter be used for rapid transfusions in acute situations. Peripheral veins are commonly used in nonacute transfusion situations. The small diameter of the vein and peripheral resistance (resistance to blood flow in the vein) can slow the transfusion.

CV line

Large volumes of blood products can be delivered quickly through a CV line because of the large size of the blood vessels and their decreased resistance to infusion.

Blood products

Generally, only a patient who has lost a massive amount of blood in a short time requires a whole blood transfusion. Most patients can be treated with individual blood products—the separate components that make up whole blood.

Partial components but full solutions

Current technology allows freshly donated whole blood to be separated into its component parts: RBCs, plasma, platelets, leukocytes, and plasma proteins, such as immune globulin, albumin, and clotting factors. Individual blood components can be used to correct specific blood deficiencies. The availability of blood components usually makes it unnecessary to transfuse whole blood.

Compatibility

Recipient blood is choosy about donor blood. Any incompatibility can cause serious adverse reactions. The most severe is a hemolytic reaction, which destroys RBCs and may become life-threatening. Before a transfusion, testing helps to detect incompatibilities between recipient and donor blood.

> It's important to make sure that donor blood and recipient blood match.

Making a match

Typing and crossmatching establish the compatibility of donor and recipient blood. This precaution minimizes the risk of a hemolytic reaction. The most important tests include ABO blood typing, Rh typing, crossmatching, direct antiglobulin test, antibody screening test, screening for such diseases as hepatitis B and C, HIV, human T-cell lymphotrophic virus type I (HTLV-1) and type II (HTLV-2, or hairy cell leukemia), syphilis and, for certain patients, cytomegalovirus (CMV).

ABO blood type

The four blood types in the ABO system are A, B, AB, and O. An antigen is a substance that can stimulate the formation of an antibody. Each blood group in the ABO system is named for antigens—A, B, both of these, or neither—that are carried on a person's RBCs. An antigen may induce the formation of a corresponding antibody if given to a person who doesn't normally carry the antigen.

An antibody is an immunoglobulin molecule synthesized in response to a specific antigen. The ABO system includes two naturally occurring antibodies: anti-A and anti-B. One, both, or neither of these antibodies may be found in the plasma. The interaction of corresponding antigens and antibodies of the ABO system can cause agglutination (clumping together).

The major antigens, such as those in the ABO system, are inherited. Blood transfusions can introduce other antigens and antibodies into the body. Most are harmless, but any could cause a transfusion reaction.

A mismatch is a hemolytic hazard

A hemolytic reaction occurs when donor and recipient blood types are mismatched. It could happen, for example, if blood containing anti-A antibodies is transfused to a recipient who has blood with A antigens.

A hemolytic reaction can be life-threatening. With as little as 10 ml infused, symptoms can occur quickly—including chest pain, dyspnea, facial flushing, fever, chills, hypotension, flank pain, burning sensation along the vein receiving blood, shock, and renal failure. Because this reaction is so fast, always adhere strictly to your facility's policy and procedures for assessing vital signs during transfusions.

Blood feud

When mismatching occurs, antigens and antibodies of the ABO system do battle. Antibodies attach to the surfaces of the recipient's RBCs, causing the cells to agglutinate (clump together).

Eventually, the clumped cells can plug small blood vessels. This antibody-antigen reaction activates the body's complement system, a group of enzymatic proteins that cause RBC destruction (hemolysis). RBC hemolysis releases free hemoglobin (an RBC component) into the bloodstream, which can damage renal tubules and lead to kidney failure.

O, you're everybody's type

Because group O blood lacks both A and B antigens, it can be transfused in limited amounts in an emergency to any patient — regardless of the recipient's blood type — with little risk of adverse reaction. That's why people with group O blood are called *universal donors.*

Any donor will do

A person with AB blood type has neither anti-A nor anti-B antibodies. This person may receive A, B, AB, or O blood, making him a universal recipient.

Rh blood group

Another major blood antigen system, the Rhesus (Rh) system, has two groups: Rh-positive and Rh-negative. The Rh system consists of different inherited antigens — D, C, E, c, or e. These antigens are highly immunogenic — they have a high capacity for initiating the body's immune response.

D is the difference

D, or D factor, is the most important Rh antigen. The presence or absence of D is one of the factors that determines whether a person has Rh-positive or Rh-negative blood.

Rh-positive blood contains a variant of the D antigen or D factor; Rh-negative blood doesn't have this antigen. A person with Rh-negative blood who receives Rh-positive blood will gradually develop anti-Rh antibodies. The first exposure won't cause a reaction because anti-Rh antibodies are slow to form. Subsequent exposures, however, may pose a risk of hemolysis and agglutination. A person with Rh-positive blood doesn't carry anti-Rh antibodies because they would destroy his own RBCs. (See *Ethnicity and Rh type.*)

Bridging the gap

Ethnicity and Rh type

Nearly 95% of Blacks, Native Americans, and Asians have Rh-positive blood. About 85% of Whites have Rh-positive blood. The rest of the population has Rh-negative blood.

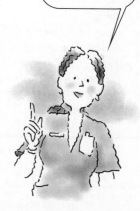

I'm positive that Rh-positive blood is a popular type.

Administering transfusions

There are two kinds of transfused blood: autologous (from the recipient himself) and homologous (from a donor). Autologous blood reduces the risks normally associated with transfusions, but it may not be available. Homologous blood undergoes rigorous screening and testing to ensure its quality. Part of this screening involves the donors themselves.

A big responsibility

Whatever the source of the blood or blood products, your primary responsibility is to prevent a potentially fatal hemolytic reaction by making sure the patient receives the correct product. Whether you transfuse whole blood, cellular products, or plasma, you'll follow the same basic procedure: Obtain baseline vital signs and then send for the ordered blood product. After receiving the blood product, always begin by checking, verifying, and inspecting. (See *Check, verify, and inspect.*)

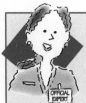

Advice from the experts

Check, verify, and inspect

The most common cause of a severe transfusion reaction is receiving the wrong blood. Before administering any blood or blood product, take the steps described here.

Check
Check to make sure an informed consent form was signed. Then double-check the patient's name, medical record number, ABO and Rh status (and other compatibility factors), and blood bank identification number against the label on the blood bag. Also check the expiration date on the bag.

Verify
Make sure to use two patient identifiers, such as the patient's name and medication record number. Ask another nurse or doctor to verify all information, according to facility policy. Make sure that you and the nurse or doctor who checked the blood or blood product have signed the blood confirmation slip. If even a slight discrepancy exists, don't administer the blood or blood product. Instead, immediately notify the blood bank and return the blood or blood product.

Inspect
Inspect the blood or blood product to detect abnormalities. Then confirm the patient's identity by checking the name, room number, and bed number on his wristband and, if possible, with the patient himself.

Whole blood and cellular products

Before a transfusion, you need to send for the blood or cellular products ordered. Then gather and set up the appropriate equipment. The patient's condition dictates which type of cellular product is needed in transfusion therapy. Transfused cellular products include whole blood, packed RBCs, leukocyte-poor RBCs, white blood cells (WBCs), and platelets.

Would you like that whole or packed?

To replenish decreased blood volume or to boost the oxygen-carrying capacity of blood, the doctor orders a transfusion of whole blood or packed RBCs (blood from which 80% of the plasma has been removed).

If your patient is receiving whole blood or packed RBCs, don't send for the blood until just before you gather the equipment because RBCs deteriorate after 4 hours at room temperature. Whole blood transfusions are used to increase blood volume. They're usually needed because of massive hemorrhage (loss of more than 25% of total blood) resulting from trauma or vascular or cardiac surgery.

Packed RBCs are transfused to maintain or restore oxygen-carrying capability. They can also replace RBCs lost because of GI bleeding, dysmenorrhea, surgery, trauma, or chemotherapy.

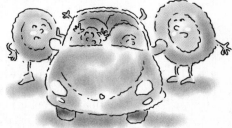

I know that looks like a tight squeeze, but packed RBCs maintain or restore oxygen-carrying capability.

Leaving out the leukocytes

Leukocyte-poor RBCs are transfused when a patient has had a febrile, nonhemolytic transfusion reaction, caused by WBC antigens reacting with the patient's WBC antibodies or platelets. Several methods are used to remove leukocytes from blood, including:
• centrifugal force along with filtration and the addition of sedimentary agents, such as dextran and hydroxyethyl starch
• leukocyte removal filters
• washing the cells in a special solution (the most expensive and the least effective method, which also removes about 99% of the plasma).

Granulocytes to go

Transfusion of granulocytes (leukocytes containing granules) may be ordered to fight antibiotic-resistant septicemia and other life-threatening infections or when granulocyte supply is severely low (granulocytopenia). This therapy is repeated for 4 to 5 days or longer, as ordered, unless the bone marrow recovers or severe reactions occur.

Because some RBCs normally remain in WBC concentrates, granulocytes are tested for compatibility (ABO, Rh, and HLA).

Platelets step to the plate

Platelets can be transfused to:
• control or prevent bleeding or correct an extremely low platelet count (20,000/µl or less) in a patient who doesn't have a disease that destroys platelets
• increase the number of platelets in a patient who's receiving a platelet-destroying therapy, such as chemotherapy, or who has a hematologic disease, such as aplastic anemia or leukemia.

Selecting equipment

Before beginning a transfusion, gather the following equipment:
• gloves, a gown, a mask, and goggles to wear when handling blood products
• in-line or add-on filters as specified by the doctor's order or as appropriate for the product being infused
• I.V. pole
• transfusion component, exactly as ordered
• venipuncture equipment, if necessary.

Normal saline solution only

No I.V. solution other than normal saline (0.9% sodium chloride) should be given with blood. If a primary line has been used to deliver any solution other than normal saline, a blood administration set shouldn't be affixed or "piggybacked" to it without first flushing the line.

Ready to filter through some advice?

Always use blood filters on blood products to avoid infusing fibrin clots or cellular debris that forms in the blood bag. There are many types of filters, each with unique features and indications. A standard blood administration set comes with a 170-micron filter, which traps particles that are 170 microns or larger. This filter doesn't remove smaller particles, called *microaggregates*, which form after only a few days of blood storage.

Microaggregates form from degenerating platelets and fibrin strands, and may contribute to formation of microemboli (small clots that obstruct circulation) in the lungs. To remove microaggregates, the doctor may order a 20- to 40-micron filter, called a *microaggregate filter*. This filter removes smaller particles but is costly and may slow the infusion rate — a particular problem when seeking to deliver a massive, rapid transfusion.

Filters may be used to screen out leukocytes during the transfusion of RBCs or platelets. Use new tubing and a new filter for every 1 to 2 units of blood you transfuse. Never use a microaggregate filter to transfuse WBC concentrates or platelets; the filter

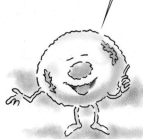

Only normal saline solution should be given with blood. Other isotonic solutions may cause cells to clump.

will trap them. Instead, use a leukocyte reduction filter made specifically for the component.

Heat it up

A blood warmer may be ordered to prevent hypothermia (for example, from large volumes of blood administered quickly) or to prevent arrhythmias from hypothermia (86° F [30° C]).

Let's jump to a pump

In some facilities, an infusion pump is used to regulate the administration of blood and blood products. Always check the manufacturer's instructions to find out whether a particular pump can be used to administer blood or blood products.

Starting the transfusion

So far, you have identified the patient, inspected and verified the blood product, obtained baseline vital signs, and assembled the necessary equipment and supplies. Now you're ready to begin the transfusion. (See *Transfusing blood*, page 344.)

After you begin the transfusion, assess the patient, and monitor vital signs according to the patient's transfusion history and your facility's policy—usually every 15 minutes for the first hour.

Stop the transfusion!

Watch for signs and symptoms of a transfusion reaction, including fever, chills, headache, nausea, and facial flushing. If you detect any of these signs or symptoms, quickly stop the transfusion, and reestablish the normal saline solution infusion. *Note:* If you're using a Y-set, don't restart the infusion by opening the clamp; you'll just deliver more of the blood that's causing the problem. Instead, use a new bag and tubing to restart the infusion.

Next, check and record the patient's vital signs. Notify the doctor immediately, and don't dispose of the blood. If no signs of a reaction appear within 15 minutes, adjust the flow clamp to achieve the ordered infusion rate. Monitor the patient throughout the entire transfusion according to your facility's policy and procedures. (See *Transfusion don'ts*, page 346.)

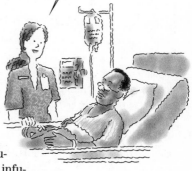

I'll need to monitor your status throughout the entire transfusion.

Terminating the transfusion

After a transfusion is complete, follow these steps:
• Flush the blood tubing with an adequate amount of normal saline solution according to the patient's condition.
• On a Y-type set, close the clamp on the blood line and open the clamp on the saline solution line.

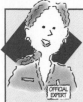

Advice from the experts

Transfusing blood

To begin transfusing blood, follow the steps described here.

Let's begin
• Explain the procedure to the patient. Obtain consent according to your facility policy.
• Wash your hands and put on gloves, a gown, goggles, and a mask.
• If you're using a straight-line set, insert the set's tubing spike into the bag of normal saline solution.
• Hang the bag on the I.V. pole, and prime the filter and tubing with saline solution to reduce the risk of microclots forming in the tubing. Leave the bag of normal saline solution attached to the tubing until you're ready to start the transfusion.

Check, recheck, and verify
When you're ready to start the transfusion, proceed with these steps:
• Check, recheck, and verify the type, Rh, and expiration date of the blood or cellular component. Also, double-check that you're giving the right blood or cellular component to the right patient using two patient identifiers, as shown below.
• Observe the blood or cellular component for abnormal color, clumping of red blood cells (RBCs), gas bubbles, and extraneous material that might indicate bacterial contamination. If you see any of these signs, return the bag to the blood bank.

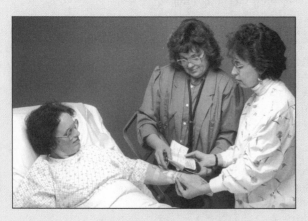

Ready to start
• When you're ready to start the transfusion, prepare the equipment. Use a Y-type blood administration set. Blood and saline are both connected and can be clamped without opening the system.
• Next, remove the clamp from the normal saline solution line. Insert the spike on the regular administration set into the bag of saline solution and prime the line.
• When using a Y-type set, close all the clamps on the set. Then insert the spike of the line you're using for the normal saline solution into the bag of normal saline solution. Next, open the port on the blood bag, and insert the spike of the line you're using to administer the blood or cellular component into the port. Close the clamps. Hang the bag of normal saline solution and blood or cellular component on the I.V. pole.
• Open the clamp on the line of normal saline solution, and squeeze the drip chamber until it's half full of normal saline solution. Then remove the adapter cover at the tip of the blood administration set, open the main flow clamp, and prime the tubing with normal saline solution. Close the clamp and recap the adapter.

The transfusion itself
To transfuse the blood or cellular component, follow these steps:
• Take the patient's vital signs to serve as baseline values. Recheck vital signs after 15 minutes (or according to facility policy).
• If the patient doesn't have an I.V. device in place, perform a venipuncture, using a 20G or larger catheter.
• Attach the prepared blood administration set to the venous access device using a needleless connection, and flush it with normal saline solution.

(continued)

Transfusing blood *(continued)*

• When using a Y-type set, close the clamp on the normal saline solution line and open the clamp on the blood side (as shown below left).

• When administering whole blood or white blood cells, gently invert the bag several times during the procedure to mix the cells. (During the transfusion, gently agitate the bag to prevent the viscous cells from settling.)

• After you've flushed the venous access device, begin to transfuse the blood.

• Adjust the flow clamp closest to the patient to deliver a slow rate (usually about 20 gtt/minute) for the first 10 to 30 minutes, as shown below right. The type of blood product given and the patient's clinical condition determine the rate of transfusion. A unit of RBCs may be given over a period of 1 to 4 hours. Platelets and coagulation factors can be given more quickly than can RBCs and granulocytes.

• A transfusion should be administered over 4 hours at room temperature because the risk of contamination and sepsis increases after that. Discard or return to the blood bank any blood or blood products not given within this time, as facility policy directs.

Hanging the bag

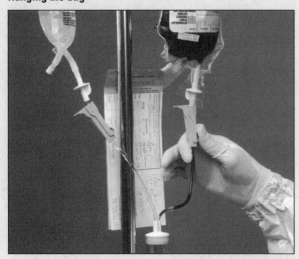

Adjusting the clamp

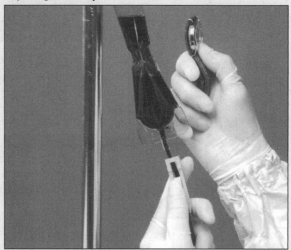

• Discard the tubing, filter, and blood bag according to your facility's policy.

• Reassess the patient's condition and vital signs.

Plasma and plasma fractions

Plasma and plasma fractions are the anticoagulated clear portion of blood that have been run through a centrifuge. They make up about 55% of the blood and are used in transfusion therapy to:

• correct blood deficiencies such as a low platelet count

• control bleeding tendencies that result from clotting factor deficiencies

• increase the patient's circulating blood volume.

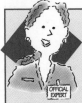

Advice from the experts

Transfusion don'ts

A blood transfusion requires extreme care. Here are some tips on what not to do when administering a transfusion:
• Don't add any medications to the blood bag.
• Never give blood products without checking the order against the blood bag label. Checking the
order is the only way to tell if the request form has been stamped with the wrong name. Most life-
threatening reactions occur when this step is omitted.
• Don't transfuse the blood product if you discover a discrepancy in the blood number, blood slip
type, or patient identification number.
• Don't piggyback blood into the port of an existing infusion set. Most solutions, including dextrose in water, are incompatible with blood. Administer blood only with normal saline solution.
• Don't hesitate to stop the transfusion if your patient shows changes in vital signs, is dyspneic or
restless, or develops chills, hematuria, or pain in the flank, chest, or back. Your patient could go
into shock, so don't remove the I.V. device that's in place. Keep it open with a slow infusion of normal saline solution; call the doctor and the laboratory.

Perusing plasma products

Before a transfusion, obtain the plasma or plasma fractions ordered. Commonly transfused plasma products include fresh frozen
plasma, albumin, cryoprecipitate, and prothrombin complex. The
patient's condition dictates which plasma product is needed.

Plasma proxies

Plasma substitutes may be used to maintain blood volume in
an emergency, such as acute hemorrhage and shock. Plasma
substitutes lack oxygen-carrying and coagulation properties,
but using them allows time to get the patient's blood typed
and crossmatched.

Depending on the circumstances, you may give:
• synthetic volume expander such as dextran in saline solution
• natural volume expander, such as plasma protein fraction
and albumin.

> Plasma and
> plasma fractions
> give a boost to
> the circulating
> blood volume.

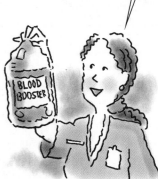

Selecting equipment

Gather the following infusion equipment:
• in-line or add-on filters or a filter system designated for the
ordered component (usually a 170-micron filter) (*Note:* Never
use a microaggregate filter to infuse platelets or plasma; it
could remove essential components from the transfusion.)

- normal saline solution
- I.V. pole
- clean gloves, a gown, a mask, and goggles
- ordered plasma or plasma fractions
- venipuncture equipment, if necessary.

Starting the transfusion

To transfuse plasma or plasma fractions, follow these steps:
- Obtain baseline vital signs.
- Make sure that the patient has a functional venous access device (20G or greater), or insert one as needed.
- Flush the patient's venous access device with normal saline solution.

   When you're ready to begin the transfusion, follow these steps:
- Put on clean gloves and other protective equipment that your facility requires.
- Verify that you have the correct blood product and verify the patient's identity with another nurse using two patient identifiers.
- Check the expiration date of the plasma or plasma fraction.
- Double-check that you're giving the right plasma or plasma fraction.
- Inspect the plasma or plasma fraction for cloudiness and turbidity, which could indicate possible contamination.
- Spike the bag with component-specific tubing (if the blood bank provided it) or with the blood tubing specified by your facility's policy and procedures.
- Prime the tubing.
- Explain the procedure to the patient.
- Obtain baseline vital signs, and continue to check vital signs frequently according to your facility's policy.
- Attach the plasma, fresh frozen plasma, albumin, factor VIII concentrate, prothrombin complex, platelets, or cryoprecipitate to the patient's flushed venous access device.
- Begin the transfusion, and adjust the flow rate as ordered.
- Take the patient's vital signs, and assess him frequently for signs or symptoms of a transfusion reaction, such as fever, chills, or nausea. If a reaction occurs, quickly stop the infusion and start a normal saline solution infusion at a keep-vein-open rate. Check and record the patient's vital signs. Notify the doctor.
- After the infusion, flush the line with saline solution, according to your facility's policy. Then disconnect the I.V. line. If therapy will continue, hang the original I.V. solution and adjust the flow rate as ordered.
- Record the type and amount of plasma or plasma fraction administered, duration of transfusion, baseline vital signs, adverse reactions, and how the patient tolerated the procedure.

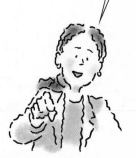

Don't forget to flush — the I.V. line, that is!

Patients with special needs

Pediatric and elderly patients require special care during transfusion therapy. For instance, transfusing blood into a neonate requires specialized skills because the neonate's physiologic requirements differ vastly from those of an older infant, child, adolescent, or adult.

Pediatric patients

Transfusions in children differ significantly from transfusions in adults.

Half-unit packs for half-pint patients

Blood units for pediatric patients are prepared in half-unit packs, and a 24G catheter is used to administer the blood.

Rating children differently

The rate of the infusion also differs. Usually, a child receives 5% to 10% of the total transfusion in the first 15 minutes of therapy. To maintain the correct flow rate, be sure to use an electronic infusion device.

Volume control

A child's normal circulating blood volume determines the amount of blood transfused. The average blood volume for children and infants older than 1 month is 75 ml/kg. The proportion of blood volume to body weight decreases with age.

Good communication

Whenever you transfuse blood in an infant or child, explain the procedure, its purpose, and its possible complications to the parents or legal guardian. If appropriate, also include the child in the explanation. Ask the parents for the child's transfusion history, and obtain their consent.

A watchful eye

Closely monitor the child, particularly during the first 15 minutes to detect early signs of a reaction. Use a blood warmer, if indicated, to prevent hypothermia and cardiac arrhythmias, especially if you're administering blood through a central line.

A child's problem with grown-up indications

In massive hemorrhage and shock, the indications for blood component transfusion in children remain similar to those for adults, although accurate assessment is difficult. Draw blood from a central vein to get more accurate hemoglobin and hematocrit measurements, or use blood pressure readings to assess blood volume.

Elderly patients

An elderly patient with preexisting heart disease may be unable to tolerate rapid transfusion of an entire unit of blood without exhibiting shortness of breath or other signs of heart failure. The patient may be better able to tolerate half-unit blood transfusions.

Delayed reaction

Age-related slowing of the immune system puts an older adult at risk for delayed transfusion reactions. Because greater quantities of blood products transfuse before signs or symptoms appear, the patient may experience a more severe reaction. Also, an elderly patient tends to be less resistant to infection.

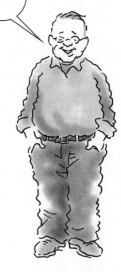

> At my age, rapid transfusion of an entire unit of blood may be too much.

Complications

Always take steps to prevent transfusion complications, and know how to manage them when they arise. (See *Correcting transfusion problems.*)

Correcting transfusion problems

A patient who receives excellent care can still encounter problems during a transfusion. Here's how to proceed when common transfusion problems occur.

It stopped!

If the transfusion stops, follow these steps.
- Check that the I.V. container is at least 3′ (1 m) above the level of the I.V. site.
- Make sure that the flow clamp is open.
- Make sure that the blood completely covers the filter. If it doesn't, squeeze the drip chamber until it does.
- Gently rock the bag back and forth, agitating any blood cells that may have settled on the bottom.
- If using a Y-type blood administration set, close the flow clamp to the patient and lower the blood bag. Next, open the normal saline solution line clamp, and allow the solution to flow into the blood bag. Rehang the blood bag, open the flow clamp to the patient, and reset the flow rate.

Hematoma

If a hematoma develops at the I.V. site, follow these steps:
- Immediately stop the infusion.
- Remove the needle or catheter, and then cap the tubing with a new, needleless connection.
- Notify the doctor and expect to place ice on the site for 24 hours; after that, apply warm compresses.
- Promote reabsorption of the hematoma by having the patient gently exercise the affected limb.
- Document your observations and actions.

An empty bag

If the blood bag empties before the next one arrives when using a Y-type set, follow these steps:
- Close the blood line clamp.
- Open the normal saline solution line clamp.
- Let the normal saline solution run slowly until the new blood arrives.
- Make sure that you decrease the flow rate or clamp the line before attaching the new unit of blood.

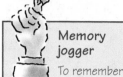

Memory jogger

To remember what to do in the event of a transfusion reaction, think of the acronym **SPIN**:

Stop the infusion.

Pulse and other vital signs (check 'em).

Infuse normal saline solution.

Notify the doctor.

Transfusion reactions

Usually attributed to major antigen-antibody reactions, transfusion reactions may occur up to 96 hours after the transfusion begins. Transfusion reactions occur more commonly with the administration of platelets, WBCs, and cryoprecipitate than they do with whole blood, RBCs, or plasma.

Stop immediately!

Whenever you detect signs or symptoms of an acute transfusion reaction, immediately stop the transfusion. Then follow these steps:
• Change the I.V. tubing to prevent infusing more blood. Save the blood tubing and bag for analysis.
• Administer normal saline solution to keep the vein patent (open).
• Take and record the patient's vital signs.
• Notify the doctor.
• Obtain a urine specimen and blood sample and send them to the laboratory.
• Prepare for further treatment.
• Complete a transfusion reaction report and an incident report according to your facility's policies and procedures.
    The doctor or blood bank may eliminate some of these steps if a patient has a history of frequent mild reactions.

The rundown on reactions

Transfusion of blood products that have been processed and preserved increases the patient's risk of complications, especially if the patient receives frequent transfusions of large amounts. Hemolytic, febrile, and allergic reactions can follow any transfusion. (See *Managing transfusion reactions.*)

Hemolytic reactions

An acute hemolytic reaction, which is life-threatening, occurs as a result of incompatible blood. This type of reaction can also occur as a result of improper storage of blood. It may progress to shock and renal failure.

Clean up clerical errors

A hemolytic reaction almost always results from a clerical error, such as mislabeling or failing to identify the patient properly.

Febrile reactions

Nonhemolytic febrile reactions are characterized by a temperature increase of 1.8° F (1° C). Such reactions are related to a transfusion and aren't caused by disease.

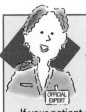

Advice from the experts

Managing transfusion reactions

If your patient experiences a transfusion reaction, stop the infusion and consult the chart below for further steps and tips for preventing future reactions.

Reaction	Nursing interventions	Prevention
Hemolytic	• Monitor blood pressure. • Treat shock as indicated by patient's condition, using I.V. fluids, oxygen, epinephrine, a diuretic, and a vasopressor. • Obtain posttransfusion reaction blood and urine samples for evaluation. • Observe for signs of hemorrhage resulting from disseminated intravascular coagulation.	• Before transfusion, check donor and recipient blood types to ensure blood compatibility. Also identify patient with another nurse or doctor present. • Transfuse blood slowly for the first 15 to 20 minutes. Closely observe patient for the first 30 minutes of the transfusion.
Febrile	• Relieve symptoms with an antipyretic or antihistamine.	• Premedicate with an antipyretic, an antihistamine and, possibly, a steroid. • Use leukocyte-poor or washed red blood cells (RBCs). Use a leukocyte removal filter specific to the component.
Allergic	• Administer antihistamines. • Monitor for anaphylactic reaction and administer epinephrine and steroids, if indicated.	• Premedicate with an antihistamine if the patient has a history of allergic reactions. • Observe the patient closely for the first 30 minutes of the transfusion.
Plasma protein incompatibility	• Treat for shock by administering oxygen, fluids, epinephrine and, possibly, a steroid as ordered.	• Transfuse only immunoglobulin A-deficient blood or well-washed RBCs.
Bacterial contamination	• Treat with a broad-spectrum antibiotic and a steroid.	• Inspect blood before the transfusion for gas, clots, and dark purple color. • Use air-free, touch-free methods to draw and deliver blood. • Maintain strict storage control. • Change the blood tubing and filter every 4 hours. • Infuse each unit of blood over 2 to 4 hours. Terminate the infusion if blood is at room temperature for 4 hours. • Maintain sterile technique when administering blood products.

(continued)

Managing transfusion reactions *(continued)*

Reaction	Nursing interventions	Prevention
Circulation overload	• Stop the transfusion. • Maintain the I.V. with normal saline solution. • Administer oxygen. • Elevate the patient's head. • Administer diuretics as ordered by the doctor.	• Transfuse blood slowly. • Don't exceed 2 units in 4 hours (less for elderly patients, infants, or patients with cardiac conditions).
Hemosiderosis	• Perform a phlebotomy to remove excess iron.	• Administer blood only when absolutely necessary.
Bleeding tendencies	• Administer platelets. • Monitor the platelet count.	• Use only fresh blood (less than 7 days old) when possible.
Elevated blood ammonia level	• Monitor the ammonia level. • Decrease the amount of protein in the diet. • If indicated, give neomycin sulfate or lactulose.	• Use only RBCs, fresh frozen plasma, or fresh blood, especially if the patient has hepatic disease.
Increased oxygen affinity for hemoglobin	• Monitor arterial blood gas levels, and give respiratory support as needed.	• Use only RBCs or fresh blood if possible.
Hypothermia	• Stop the transfusion. • Warm the patient with blankets. • Obtain an electrocardiogram (ECG).	• Warm the blood to 95° to 98° F (35° to 37° C), especially before massive transfusions.
Hypocalcemia	• Monitor potassium and calcium levels. • Use blood less than 2 days old if administering multiple units. • Slow or stop transfusion, depending on reaction. Expect a worse reaction in hypothermic patients or patients with elevated potassium levels. • Slowly administer calcium gluconate I.V.	• Infuse blood slowly.
Potassium intoxication	• Obtain an ECG. • Administer sodium polystyrene sulfonate (Kayexalate) orally or by enema.	• Use fresh blood when administering massive transfusions.

Antibodies battling antigens

Febrile reactions usually result from the patient's anti-HLA antibodies reacting against antigens on the donor's WBCs or platelets. Febrile reactions may occur in approximately 1% of transfusions. They can occur immediately or within 2 hours after completion of a transfusion. Signs and symptoms of febrile reactions include fever, chills, headache, nausea and vomiting, hypotension, chest pain, dyspnea, nonproductive cough, and malaise.

Allergic reactions

An allergic reaction is the second most common transfusion reaction. It occurs because of an allergen in the transfused blood. Signs of an allergic reaction may include itching, hives, fever, chills, facial swelling, wheezing, and throat swelling.

An anaphylactic advance

An allergic reaction may progress to an anaphylactic reaction. This reaction can occur immediately or within 1 hour after infusion. Severe anaphylactic reactions produce bronchospasm, dyspnea, pulmonary edema, and hypotension. Treatment includes immediate administration of epinephrine, corticosteroids, and antihistamines.

Plasma protein incompatibility

Plasma protein incompatibility usually results from blood that contains immunoglobulin A (IgA) proteins being infused into an IgA-deficient recipient who has developed anti-IgA antibodies. The reaction can be life-threatening and usually resembles anaphylaxis. Signs and symptoms include flushing and urticaria, abdominal pain, chills, fever, dyspnea and wheezing, hypotension, shock, and cardiac arrest.

Bacterial contamination

Blood and blood products may be contaminated during the collection process. As storage times and temperature increase, growth of microorganisms also increases. The resulting transfusion reaction is most commonly related to the endotoxins produced by gram-negative bacteria. Signs and symptoms of bacterial contamination include chills, fever, vomiting, abdominal cramping, diarrhea, shock, and kidney failure.

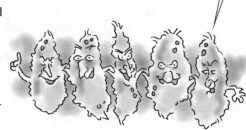

As storage time and temperature increase, growth of microorganisms like us also increases.

Reactions from multiple transfusions

Reactions from multiple transfusions include hemosiderosis, bleeding tendencies, elevated blood ammonia levels, increased oxygen affinity for hemoglobin, hypothermia, hypocalcemia, and potassium intoxication.

Hemosiderosis

Accumulation of an iron-containing pigment (hemosiderin) may be associated with RBC destruction in patients who receive many transfusions. In hemosiderosis, the patient's iron plasma level is greater than 200 mg/dl.

Bleeding tendencies

A low platelet count — which can develop in stored blood — can cause bleeding tendencies. Signs and symptoms may include abnormal bleeding, oozing from a cut or break in the skin surface, and abnormal clotting values.

Elevated blood ammonia level

Blood ammonia levels can increase in patients receiving transfusions of stored blood. Signs and symptoms of high blood ammonia levels include forgetfulness and confusion. The patient may also have a sweet mouth odor. High ammonia levels can cause behaviors that range from stuporlike to combative.

Increased oxygen affinity for hemoglobin

A blood transfusion can cause a decreased level of 2,3-diphosphoglycerate (2,3-DPG). Found on RBCs but scarce in stored blood, 2,3-DPG affects the oxyhemoglobin dissociation curve. This curve represents hemoglobin saturation and desaturation in graph form. Levels of 2,3-DPG (as well as other factors) cause the curve to shift to the right (causing a decrease in oxygen affinity) or the left (causing an increase in oxygen affinity).

A shift to the left

When 2,3-DPG levels are low, they produce a shift to the left. This shift causes an increase in oxygen affinity for hemoglobin, so the oxygen stays in the patient's bloodstream and isn't released into other tissues. Signs of this reaction include a depressed respiratory rate, especially in patients with chronic lung disease.

Hypothermia

A rapid infusion of large amounts of cold blood can cause hypothermia. The patient may experience shaking chills, hypotension, and cardiac arrhythmias, which may become life threatening. Cardiac arrest can occur if core temperature falls below 86° F (30° C).

Hypocalcemia

If blood is infused too rapidly, citrate toxicity can occur. (Citrate is used to preserve blood.) Because citrate binds with calcium, calcium deficiency results. Hypocalcemia can also occur if normal citrate metabolism is hindered by a liver disorder. Signs and symptoms of calcium deficiency include tingling in the fingers, muscle cramps, nausea, vomiting, hypotension, cardiac arrhythmias, and seizures.

Potassium intoxication

Some cells in stored RBCs may leak potassium into the plasma. Intoxication usually doesn't occur with transfusions of 1 to 2 units of blood. Larger volumes, however, may cause potassium toxicity. Signs and symptoms of potassium toxicity may include irritability; intestinal colic; diarrhea; muscle weakness; oliguria; renal failure; ECG changes with tall, peaked T waves; and bradycardia that may proceed to cardiac arrest.

Transmission of disease

Unlike a transfusion reaction, an infectious disease transmitted during a transfusion may go undetected until days, weeks, or months later, when signs and symptoms appear. Remember, all blood products are potential carriers of infectious disease, including hepatitis, HIV, and CMV.

Testing, testing, one, two

Steps to prevent disease transmission include laboratory testing of blood products and careful screening of potential donors. Neither of these precautions is foolproof.

Facilities also test blood for the presence of syphilis, although the routine practice of refrigerating blood kills the syphilis organism. These measures have virtually eliminated the risk of transfusion-related syphilis.

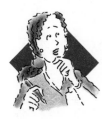

Quick quiz

1. The fluid located inside the cell is called:
   A. interstitial fluid.
   B. intracellular fluid.
   C. extracellular fluid.
   D. internal fluid.

Answer: B. The fluid inside the cells—about 55% of the total body fluid—is called *intracellular fluid*. The rest is called *extracellular fluid*.

2. The major extracellular electrolytes are:
   A. sodium and chloride.
   B. potassium and phosphorus.
   C. potassium and sodium.
   D. phosphorus and chloride.

Answer: A. The major extracellular electrolytes are sodium and chloride.

3. An example of a hypertonic solution is:
   A.   half-normal saline.
   B.   0.33% sodium chloride.
   C.   dextrose 2.5% in water.
   D.   dextrose 5% in half-normal saline.

Answer: D. Some examples of hypertonic solutions are dextrose 5% in half-normal saline (405 mOsm/L), dextrose 5% in normal saline (560 mOsm/L), and dextrose 5% in lactated Ringer's (527 mOsm/L).

4. When selecting a peripheral I.V. site, it's best to avoid:
   A.   an arm with a tattoo.
   B.   an arm with a sunburn.
   C.   an arm with an arteriovenous shunt.
   D.   an unaffected arm of a patient with a mastectomy.

Answer: C. Some veins are best to avoid, including those in the legs (circulation may be easily compromised); the inner wrist and arm (these veins are small and make I.V. therapy uncomfortable for the patient); the affected arm of a mastectomy patient; an arm with an arteriovenous shunt or fistula; an arm being treated for thrombosis or cellulitis; and an arm that has experienced trauma (such as burns or scarring from surgery).

5. How often should an I.V. solution be changed?
   A.   Every 8 hours
   B.   Every 12 hours
   C.   Every 16 hours
   D.   Every 24 hours

Answer: D. To avoid microbial growth, don't allow an I.V. container to hang for more than 24 hours.

Scoring

☆☆☆   If you answered all five questions correctly, right on! You took a central route to understanding this chapter.

☆☆   If you answered four questions correctly, congratulations! For the most part, you delivered the correct solutions.

☆   If you answered fewer than four questions correctly, don't worry! Check, verify, and inspect the material in this chapter again.

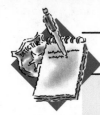

6

Pain management

Just the facts

In this chapter, you'll learn:

♦ the physiology behind pain

♦ methods to assess pain

♦ methods to adequately manage pain.

A look at pain

The process of pain involves complex physiologic and psychological responses that vary from person to person and even from day to day. Pain alerts us to injury or illness and serves as a protective mechanism. Reactions to pain vary among individuals. In fact, they even vary within the same person at different times.

Although pain may seem like a simple sensation, it's actually a complex experience influenced by:

• cultural background
• anticipation of pain
• previous experience with pain
• context in which pain occurs
• emotional and cognitive responses.

Nociception

To fully understand pain, you must be familiar with its physiologic aspects, called *nociception,* and its psychological aspects.

Nosing into nociception

Nociception simply means the sensation of pain. It results from the stimulation of nociceptors—special injury-sensing receptors embedded in the skin or in the walls of internal organs. Injury may come from a physical source (mechanical, thermal, or electrical) or a chemical source (such as a toxin).

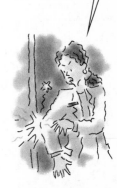

Ouch! Pain produces complex physiologic and psychological responses.

Millions of nociceptors

The body contains millions of nociceptors—roughly 1,300 for every square inch of skin. Some nociceptors detect burns while others detect cuts, chemical changes, pressure, infection, and other sensations. Nociceptors use nerve impulses to send messages to other nerves, which in turn forward the messages to the spinal cord and brain at lightning speed. This process activates involuntary (autonomic and reflexive) responses. Involuntary responses caused by painful stimuli include elevated blood pressure, an increasing pulse rate, an increased respiratory rate, or breath holding and muscle flexion (withdrawal) of the affected part of the body.

Making a distinction

Nociception and the pain experience aren't identical. Nociception refers to the neurologic events and reflex responses caused by an event that damages or threatens to damage tissue. Pain, on the other hand, is an unpleasant sensory and emotional experience associated with actual or potential tissue injury. Pain is subjective; nociception isn't. Nociception doesn't necessarily cause the perception of pain, and pain can occur without nociception, which explains why patients with certain pain syndromes may have no obvious pathology yet still experience debilitating pain.

Stages of nociception

Nociception has four stages:

transduction—mechanical, chemical, or thermal activity is converted into electrical activity in the nervous system

transmission— neurons transfer electrical impulses to the central nervous system, which processes nociceptive signals to extract relative information

perception—the patient actually perceives the pain; perception constantly changes according to the patient's developmental stage, environment, disease, or injury; pain perception can be brief (seconds to hours), prolonged (hours to weeks), or even permanent

modulation—internal and external controls reduce or increase pain (internal controls include pain control mechanisms in the midbrain; external controls include analgesics).

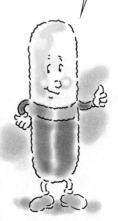

Analgesics are examples of external pain controls.

Types of pain

Pain falls into three broad categories—acute pain, chronic nonmalignant pain (also called *chronic persistent pain*), and cancer pain.

Acute pain

Acute pain comes on suddenly—for instance, after trauma, surgery, or an acute disease—and lasts from a few days to a few weeks. It causes a withdrawal reflex and may trigger involuntary bodily reactions, such as sweating, fast heart and respiratory rates, and elevated blood pressure. Acute pain may be constant (as in a burn), intermittent (as in a muscle strain that hurts only with activity), or both (as in an abdominal incision that hurts a little at rest and a lot with movement or coughing). The cause of acute pain can be diagnosed and treated, and the pain resolves when the cause is treated or analgesics are given.

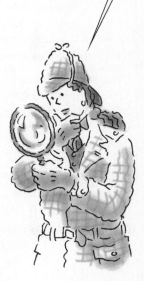

Unlike acute pain, the cause of chronic pain isn't always easily identifiable.

Chronic nonmalignant pain

Pain is considered chronic when it lasts beyond the normal time expected for an injury to heal or an illness to resolve. Many experts define chronic nonmalignant pain as pain lasting 6 months or longer that may continue during the patient's lifetime.

A world of pain

Chronic nonmalignant pain is unrelated to cancer. This type of pain affects more people—roughly 100 million Americans—than any other type. It can cause serious disability (as in arthritis or avascular necrosis), or it may be related to poorly understood disorders such as fibromyalgia and complex regional pain syndrome. Neuropathic pain is one type of chronic pain. (See *Understanding neuropathic pain*, page 360.)

Treatment. What a pain!

Medical treatment for chronic nonmalignant pain must be based on the patient's long-term benefit, not just the current complaint of pain. Drug therapy and surgery, which typically provide only partial and temporary relief, should be individualized. Drug treatment alone almost never effectively relieves chronic nonmalignant pain. The patient must receive a combination of treatments. These may include drugs, temporary or permanent invasive therapies (such as nerve blocks or surgery), cognitive-behavioral therapy, alternative and complementary therapies, and self-management techniques.

Understanding neuropathic pain

Commonly described as tingling, burning, or shooting, neuropathic pain is a puzzling type of chronic pain generated by the nerves. It commonly has no apparent cause and responds poorly to standard pain treatment.

We don't know the precise mechanism of neuropathic pain. Possibly, the peripheral nervous system has experienced damage that injures sensory neurons, causing continuous depolarization and pain transmission. Alternatively, perhaps repeated noxious stimuli cause hypersensitivity and excitement in the spinal cord, resulting in chronic neuropathy in which a normally harmless stimulus causes pain.

Phantom pain syndrome

Phantom pain syndrome is one example of neuropathic pain. This condition occurs when an arm or a leg has been removed but the brain still gets pain messages from the nerves that originally carried the limb's impulses. The nerves seem to misfire, causing pain.

Types of neuropathic pain

Neuropathic pain can involve either peripheral or central pain.

Peripheral pain

Peripheral neuropathic pain can occur as:
• polyneuropathy, which is pain felt along the peripheral nerves, as in diabetic neuropathy
• mononeuropathy, which is pain associated with an established injury and felt along the nerve, as in trigeminal neuralgia.

Central pain

Central neuropathic pain also comes in two varieties:
• sympathetic pain, which results from dysfunction of the autonomic nervous system
• deafferentation pain, which is marked by elimination of sensory (afferent) impulses, as from damage to the central or peripheral nervous system (as in phantom limb pain).

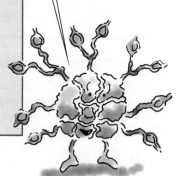

I'm puzzled because I don't know why I'm in pain.

It's painful to hear but...

Even with medical management, chronic nonmalignant pain can be lifelong. For this reason, treatments that carry significant risks or aren't likely to prove effective over the long term may be inappropriate. In many cases, treatment of chronic nonmalignant pain must focus on rehabilitation rather than a cure. Rehabilitation aims to:
• maximize physical and psychological functional abilities
• minimize pain experienced during rehabilitation and for the rest of the patient's life
• teach the patient how to manage residual pain and handle pain exacerbation caused by increased activity or unexplained reasons.

Cancer pain

Cancer pain is a complex problem. It may result from the disease itself or from its treatment. About 70% to 90% of patients with advanced cancer experience pain. Although cancer pain can be treated with oral medications, only one-third of patients with cancer pain achieve satisfactory relief. Whether pain results from cancer or its treatment, it may cause the patient to lose hope — especially if he thinks the pain means his illness is progressing. He's then likely to suffer additional feelings of helplessness, anxiety, and depression.

Sometimes pain results from the pressure of a tumor impinging on organs, bones, nerves, or blood vessels. In other cases, limitations in activities of daily living (ADLs) may lead to muscle aches.

A host of causes

These cancer treatments may cause pain:
• chemotherapy, radiation, or drugs used to offset the impact of these therapies
• surgery
• biopsies
• blood withdrawal
• lumbar punctures.

Under the radar

Most types of cancer pain can be managed effectively, diminishing physical and mental suffering. Unfortunately, cancer pain commonly goes undertreated because of:
• inadequate knowledge of — or attention to — pain control by health care professionals
• failure of health care professionals to properly assess pain
• reluctance of patients to report their pain
• reluctance of patients and doctors to use morphine and other opioids for fear of addiction.

Undertreated cancer pain diminishes the patient's activity level, appetite, and sleep. It may prevent the patient from working productively, enjoying leisure activities, or participating in family or social situations.

Assessing pain

To ensure that a patient receives effective pain relief, you must conduct a thorough and accurate pain assessment. That's a tall order because pain is so subjective. Pain is influenced not just by physical pathology but by cultural and social factors, expectations, mood, and perceptions of control. What's more, you and the patient may have dramatically different pain thresholds and tolerances, expectations about pain, and ways of expressing pain.

In some cases, you may even doubt the patient's complaints of pain — particularly if you think his behavior doesn't match his report of pain. For instance, he may tell you he has moderate pain yet continue to chat and laugh with visitors. If no pathologic cause for pain is found, you may even question the patient's report of its existence.

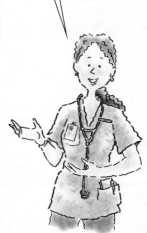

Pain can be a tricky symptom and, therefore, may be difficult for health care providers to assess.

While we're on the subject-ive

To keep your pain assessment on track, keep in mind the first principle of pain assessment: Pain is subjective. It is whatever the patient says it is, occurring whenever he says it does. The patient's self-report of the presence and severity of pain is the most accurate, reliable means of pain assessment. If the patient reports pain, respect what he says and act promptly to assess and control it.

On the threshold

Pain threshold refers to the intensity of the stimulus a person needs to sense pain. Pain tolerance is the duration and intensity of pain that a person tolerates before openly expressing pain. Tolerance has a strong psychological component. Identifying pain threshold and tolerance are crucial to pain assessment and the development of a pain management plan. But remember — pain threshold and tolerance vary widely among patients. They may even fluctuate in the same patient as circumstances change.

> A patient's actions may make you doubt her pain. Remember, however, that pain is subjective.

Team spirit

An interdisciplinary team approach promotes effective pain control. Team members typically include a doctor, a nurse, a pharmacist, a social worker, a spiritual advisor, a psychologist, physical and occupational therapists, an anesthesiologist or a certified registered nurse anesthetist, a pain management specialist and, of course, the patient and his family.

Thorough documentation and pain assessment tools communicate vital patient information to all team members. If the patient has chronic pain, periodic team meetings may also be crucial.

Differentiating acute and chronic pain

When you assess pain remember that it can be classified in several ways. One simple classification is based on its duration — acute or chronic.

Acute pain

Acute pain comes on abruptly after a sudden physical crisis. Typically, it's sharp, intense, and easily localized. Acute pain activates the sympathetic branch of the autonomic nervous system (ANS), causing such responses as heavy perspiration, increasing blood pressure, and rapid heart and respiratory rates.

Acute pain can be prolonged or recurrent. (See *Acute pain versus chronic pain.*)

Acute pain versus chronic pain

Acute pain may cause certain physiologic and behavioral changes that you won't observe in a patient with chronic pain. The chart below compares the physiologic and behavioral changes of each type of pain.

Type of pain	Physiologic evidence	Behavioral evidence
Acute	• Diaphoresis • Dilated pupils • Increased blood pressure • Increased pulse • Increased respirations	• Distraction • Distress • Restlessness • Worry
Chronic	• No diaphoresis • Normal respirations, pulse, blood pressure, and pupil size	• Despair, depression • Hopelessness • Reduced or absent physical activity

Prolonged acute pain

Prolonged acute pain can last days to weeks. Usually it results from tissue injury and inflammation (as from a sprain or surgery) and subsides gradually. At the injury site, release or synthesis of chemicals heightens sensitivity in nearby tissues. This hypersensitivity, called *hyperalgesia*, is normal. In fact, tenderness and tissue hypersensitivity help protect the injury site and prevent further damage.

Recurrent acute pain

Recurrent acute pain refers to brief painful episodes that recur at variable intervals. Examples include sickle cell vaso-occlusive crisis and migraine headache. In migraine and some other recurrent conditions, pain serves no apparent useful purpose—no protective action can be taken and tissue damage can't be prevented. However, in others, such as sickle cell disease, acute pain encourages the person to seek medical treatment.

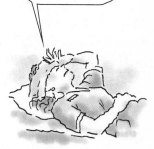

Migraine headaches are an example of recurrent acute pain.

Chronic pain

Remember, chronic pain is commonly defined as pain lasting 6 months or longer and may continue during the patient's lifetime. Although in some patients it begins as acute pain, more typically it starts slowly and builds gradually. Unlike acute pain, chronic pain isn't protective and doesn't warn of significant tissue damage.

Causes of chronic pain include nerve damage, such as in brain injury, tumor growth, or unexplained and abnormal responses to tissue injury by the central nervous system.

High cost of chronic pain

Chronic pain may be severe enough to limit a patient's ability and desire to participate in career, family life, and even ADLs. If it's severe or intractable, the patient may experience decreased function, pain behaviors, depression, opioid dependence, "doctor shopping," and suicide.

You may find pain assessment especially difficult in a patient with chronic pain. Over time, the ANS adapts to pain, so the patient may lack typical autonomic responses — dilated pupils, increased blood pressure, and fast heart and respiratory rates. Also, his facial expression may not suggest he's in pain. He may sleep periodically and shift his attention away from his pain. But don't let the lack of outward signs lead you to conclude that he isn't in pain.

JCAHO pain management standards

In 2000, the Joint Commission on Accreditation of Healthcare Organizations (JCAHO) issued new standards for pain assessment, management, and documentation. These standards require that patients be asked about pain when admitted to a JCAHO-accredited facility. Any patient who reports pain must be assessed further by licensed personnel. Facility policies must identify a standard pain screening tool to be used for all patients able to use it.

If you work in a JCAHO-accredited facility, check policies and procedures for information on which screening tool to use, how often to assess pain, and which pain level warrants further assessment and action. (In many facilities, this level is 4 or higher on a scale of 0 to 10.)

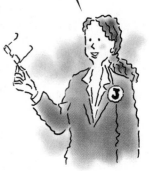

JCAHO requires that all patients be asked about pain on admission.

The fifth vital sign

Pain is commonly called the fifth vital sign because pain assessment scores must be monitored and recorded regularly — and at least as vigilantly as you monitor and record vital signs. To meet JCAHO standards, you must record pain assessment data in a way that promotes reassessment.

JCAHO standards also mandate that health care facilities plan and support activities and resources that assure pain recognition and use of appropriate interventions. These activities include:
• initial pain assessment using methods that are appropriate to the patient's age and abilities
• regular reassessment of pain
• patient education that includes understanding pain, the risk of pain, the importance of effective pain management, the pain assessment process, and methods for managing pain
• education of health care workers about pain assessment and management

• development of performance improvement plans that address pain assessment, reassessment, and the effectiveness of pain management.

Pain assessment tools

When a patient is admitted, ask him if he's currently in pain or has ongoing problems with pain. If he has ongoing pain, find out if he has an effective treatment plan. If so, continue with this plan if possible. If he doesn't have such a plan, use an assessment tool, such as a pain rating scale, to further assess his pain.

Pain rating scales

Pain rating scales quantify pain intensity — one of pain's most subjective aspects. These scales offer several advantages over semi-structured and unstructured patient interviews. They're easier to administer and take less time. They can uncover concerns that warrant a more thorough investigation. Also, when used before and after a pain control intervention, they can help determine if the intervention was effective.

Weighing pain rating scale options

Pain rating scales come in many varieties. When choosing an appropriate scale for your patient, consider his visual acuity, age, reading ability, and level of understanding. (See *Common pain rating scales*, page 366.)

Overall pain assessment tools

Overall pain assessment tools evaluate pain in multiple dimensions, providing a wider range of information. These tools are time-consuming and may be more practical for outpatient use. Still, you might want to use one for a hospitalized patient with hard-to-control chronic pain.

Pain assessment guide

Although lengthy, a pain assessment guide can help you collect important information about the patient's overall pain experience. These guides may vary from one facility to the next. (See *Pain assessment guide*, page 367.)

Brief pain inventory

The brief pain inventory (BPI) focuses on the patient's pain during the past 24 hours. The patient or health care provider can complete it in about 15 minutes. It comes in several languages besides English, including Chinese, French, and Vietnamese. To use the

Common pain rating scales

These scales are examples of the rating systems you can use to help a patient quantify pain levels.

Visual analog scale

To use a visual analog scale, ask the patient to place a line across the scale to indicate the current level of pain. The scale is a 10-cm line with "No pain" at one end and "Pain as bad as it can be" at the other end. The pain rating is determined by using a ruler to measure the distance, in millimeters, from "No pain" to the patient's mark.

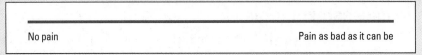

No pain   Pain as bad as it can be

Numeric rating scale

To use a numeric rating scale, ask the patient to choose a number from 0 (indicating no pain) to 10 (indicating the worst pain imaginable) to indicate the current pain level. The patient may circle the number on the scale or verbally state the number that best describes the pain.

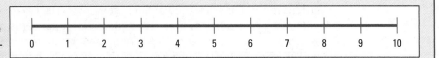

0 1 2 3 4 5 6 7 8 9 10

Faces scale

A pediatric or adult patient with language difficulty may not be able to describe the current pain level using the visual analog scale or the numeric rating scale. In that case, use a faces scale like the one shown at right. Ask your patient to choose the face on a scale from 1 to 6 that best represents the severity of his current pain.

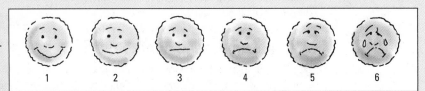

1   2   3   4   5   6

BPI, have the patient rate the least and worst pain he's experienced over the past 24 hours and at the present time. Have him point to the location of his pain on a body map.

The BPI also asks questions that focus on:
• whether the patient has had pain other than common types (such as a headache or toothache)
• whether pain has interfered with his activities (such as walking, work, and sleep) in the past 24 hours and, if so, to what extent
• whether the patient's current pain management plan is effective.

Pain assessment guide

A pain assessment guide like the one below can help you conduct a thorough assessment of the patient's pain status on admission. Although lengthy, this guide provides more information than does a simple rating scale. It may be especially appropriate for a patient with chronic pain.

Patient name: *Marie Kollar*

Patient goal: *Pain rating of 3 or less*

Past medical conditions: *Arthritis, cataracts*

Past surgeries and hospitalization: *None*

Past tests and results: *N/A*

Drug allergies and reactions: *NKA*

Do you drink alcohol?
(Specify substance and amount.) *No*

Do you smoke?
(Specify substance and amount.) *No*

Do you use drugs?
(Specify substance and amount.) *No*

When did your pain begin? *6 months ago*

Are you aware of something that started it? *No*

Where is your pain?

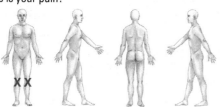

How severe is your pain right now?

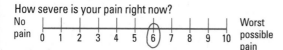

No pain 0 1 2 3 4 5 (6) 7 8 9 10 Worst possible pain

How would you describe your pain? (Circle all that apply.)
(Shooting) Stabbing Burning Numb (Sharp)
Dull Aching Gnawing Unbearable (Throbbing)
Radiating

Is your pain intermittent, occasional, or (continuous)?
(Circle one.)

What makes your pain better? *Rest and heat*

What makes your pain worse? *Activity*

To what extent does your pain affect the following aspects of your life? (Circle one each.)

Mood

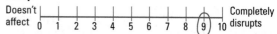

Doesn't affect 0 1 2 3 4 5 6 (7) 8 9 10 Completely disrupts

Sleep

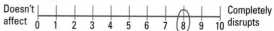

Doesn't affect 0 1 2 3 4 5 6 7 8 (9) 10 Completely disrupts

Daily activites

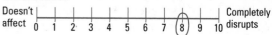

Doesn't affect 0 1 2 3 4 5 6 7 (8) 9 10 Completely disrupts

Concentration

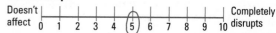

Doesn't affect 0 1 2 3 4 5 6 7 (8) 9 10 Completely disrupts

Relationships

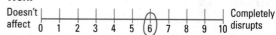

Doesn't affect 0 1 2 3 4 (5) 6 7 8 9 10 Completely disrupts

Work

Doesn't affect 0 1 2 3 4 5 (6) 7 8 9 10 Completely disrupts

Which medicines or therapies have you tried to relieve your pain? How effective is each one? (Circle one each.)

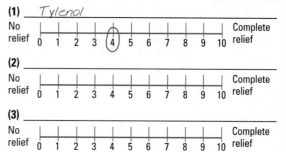

(1) *Tylenol*

No relief 0 1 2 3 (4) 5 6 7 8 9 10 Complete relief

(2) _____

No relief 0 1 2 3 4 5 6 7 8 9 10 Complete relief

(3) _____

No relief 0 1 2 3 4 5 6 7 8 9 10 Complete relief

McGill pain questionnaire

The McGill pain questionnaire assesses the multiple dimensions of neuropathic pain (a tingling, burning, or shooting pain generated by nerves). It provides word descriptors to measure sensory, affective, and evaluative pain domains. This tool is available in a short and long form. The short form has 15 word descriptors and takes less than 5 minutes. The long form consists of 78 word descriptors and takes about 20 minutes. The McGill questionnaire can be used for baseline and periodic assessments. However, it doesn't quantify the patient's pain and isn't useful for frequent assessments.

Minnesota Multiphasic Personality Inventory

Used particularly for patients with chronic pain, the Minnesota Multiphasic Personality Inventory consists of 566 true-or-false questions that help assess personality characteristics in patients. The main value of this test lies in predicting responses to pain interventions.

Self-monitoring record

If your patient has chronic or recurrent pain, consider giving him a self-monitoring record to help him accurately describe pain occurrence and severity. The patient can record the time symptoms occurred, how severe the pain was, what he was doing at the time, what he did for the pain and if it was effective.

Patient interview

Assessment begins with a patient interview. If the patient has acute pain from a traumatic injury, the interview may last for mere seconds. If he has chronic pain, it may be lengthy.

Shine a light

When interviewing a patient with chronic pain, try to elicit information that sheds light on his thoughts, feelings, behaviors, and physiologic responses to pain. Also find out about the environmental stimuli that can alter his response to pain.

Going for goals

During the interview, assess the cognitive, affective, and behavioral components of the patient's pain experience. Assessing these components can help you later when working with the patient to develop pain management goals. Also ask questions to determine how his pain affects his mental state, relationships, and work performance.

Pain characteristics

Question the patient about these characteristics of his pain:
• *onset and duration* — When did the pain begin? Did it come on suddenly or gradually? Is it intermittent or continuous? How often does it occur? How long does it last? Is it prolonged or recurrent?
• *location* — Ask the patient to point to the painful parts of his body or to mark these areas on a diagram. Be sure to assess each pain site separately.
• *intensity* — Using a pain rating scale, ask the patient to quantify the intensity of his pain at its worst and at its best.
• *quality* — Ask the patient what the pain feels like, in his own words. Does it have a burning quality? Is it knifelike? Does he feel pressure? Throbbing? Soreness?
• *relieving factors* — Does anything help relieve the pain, such as a certain position or heat or cold applications? Besides helping to pinpoint the cause of the pain, his answers may aid in developing a pain management plan.
• *aggravating factors* — What seems to trigger the pain? What makes it worse? Does it get worse when the patient moves or changes position?

You may find the PQRST technique valuable when assessing pain. Each letter stands for a crucial aspect of pain to explore. (See *PQRST: The alphabet of pain*, page 370.)

Medical and surgical history

The patient's medical history may offer clues to the source of pain or a condition that may exacerbate it. Ask him to list all of his past medical conditions, even those that have been resolved. Also question him about previous surgeries.

Past experiences with pain

Explore the patient's experiences with pain. If he experienced significant pain in the past, he may have anticipatory fear of future pain — especially if he received inadequate pain relief. Ask the patient which previous treatments — pharmacologic and otherwise — he tried, and find out which treatments helped and which didn't. Keep in mind that nonpharmacologic treatments include physical and occupational therapy, acupuncture, hypnosis, meditation, biofeedback, heat and cold therapy, transcutaneous electrical nerve stimulation (TENS), and psychological counseling.

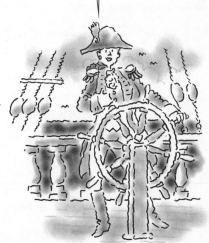

History is an important subject. The patient's med-surg history, that is!

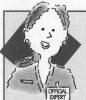

Advice from the experts

PQRST: The alphabet of pain

Use the PQRST mnemonic device to obtain more information about the patient's pain. Asking the questions below elicits important details about his pain.

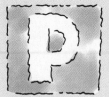 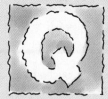 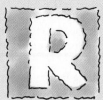 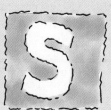 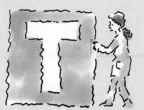

P: Provocative or palliative
Ask the patient:
• What provokes or worsens your pain?
• What relieves or causes the pain to subside?

Q: Quality or quantity
Ask the patient:
• What does the pain feel like? Is it aching, intense, knifelike, burning, or cramping?
• Are you having pain right now? If so, is it more or less severe than usual?
• To what degree does the pain affect your normal activities?
• Do you have other symptoms along with the pain, such as nausea or vomiting?

R: Region and radiation
Ask the patient:
• Where is your pain?
• Does the pain radiate to other parts of your body?

S: Severity
Ask the patient:
• How severe is your pain? How would you rate it on a 0-to-10 scale, with 0 being no pain and 10 being the worst pain imaginable?
• How would you describe the intensity of your pain at its best? At its worst? Right now?

T: Timing
Ask the patient:
• When did your pain begin?
• At what time of day is your pain least intense? What time is it worst?
• Is the onset sudden or gradual?
• Is the pain constant or intermittent?

Drug history

Obtain a complete list of the patient's medications. (Many medications can alter the effectiveness of analgesics.) Besides prescribed drugs, ask if he takes over-the-counter preparations, vitamins, nutritional supplements, or herbal or home remedies. Record the name, dose, frequency, administration route, and adverse effects of each drug he has used. Also ask him about drug allergies.

Find out if the patient currently takes or has previously taken medications to control pain and whether these were effective. If he currently receives analgesics, have him describe exactly how he takes them. If he hasn't been taking them according to instructions, he may need additional teaching on proper administration. If a particular analgesic drug or regimen didn't work for him in the past, you may be able to teach him how to use it effectively by tailoring the dosage or regimen to his needs.

Can't get no satisfaction?

Ask the patient if he's satisfied with the level of pain relief his current medications bring. Find out how long these drugs take to work and whether the pain returns before the next dose is due.

Examine effects

Question the patient about adverse effects, such as nausea, constipation, or drowsiness. If he's taking opioids for pain relief, note any worries he has about becoming drug dependent. Listen carefully for concerns he may have about any medication.

Social history

Thorough pain assessment includes a social history. Many social factors can influence the patient's perception and reports of pain and vice versa. This information helps guide interventions as well.

Social studies

Find out how the patient feels about himself, his place in society, and his relationships with others. Ask about his marital status, occupation, support systems, financial status, hobbies, exercise and sleep patterns, responsibilities, and religious, spiritual, and cultural beliefs. Determine his patterns of alcohol use, smoking, and illicit drug use.

Chronic pain can have wide-ranging effects on a person's life. If your patient has chronic pain, explore the impact it has on his moods, emotions, expectations, coping efforts, and resources. Also ask how his family responds to his condition. (See *Cultural influence on pain*.)

Physical examination

Start the physical examination by inspecting the patient. He may display a broad range of behaviors to convey pain, distress, and suffering. Some behaviors are controllable. Others, such as heavy perspiring or pupil dilation, are involuntary.

Conduct clues

As you observe the patient before or during the physical examination, note and document his behaviors. Use your observations to

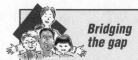

Bridging the gap

Cultural influence on pain

To provide culturally sensitive care, you must determine the meaning of pain for each patient, particularly in the context of his culture and religion. Determine how his cultural background and religious beliefs may affect his pain experience.

In some cultures, pain is openly expressed. Other cultures value stoicism and denial of pain. A patient who comes from a stoic culture may lead you to believe that he isn't in pain. Even so, be sure not to stereotype your patient. Keep in mind that, within each culture, the response to pain may vary from person to person.

Also, recognize your own cultural values and biases. Otherwise, you may end up evaluating a patient's response to pain according to your own beliefs instead of his.

help quantify his pain. These overt behaviors may indicate that the patient is experiencing pain:

- verbal reports of pain
- vocalizations, such as sighs and moans
- altered motor activities (frequent position changes, guarded positioning, slow movements, rigidity)
- limping
- grimacing and other expressions
- functional limitations, including reclining for long periods
- actions to reduce pain such as taking medication.

Autonomic indications

Next, measure the patient's blood pressure, heart and respiratory rates, and pupil size. Acute pain may raise blood pressure, speed the heart and respiratory rates, and dilate pupils. Remember, however, that these autonomic responses may be absent in a patient with chronic pain because the body gradually adapts to pain. Don't assume lack of autonomic responses means lack of pain.

You know the drill: Palpate, percuss, and auscultate

To complete the examination, use a systematic technique to perform palpation, percussion, and auscultation. If the patient is in severe pain, you may need to shorten the examination, completing it later when his pain has decreased.

Pain medications

Uncontrolled or poorly controlled pain diminishes a patient's physical and mental health. Because pain can be so difficult to treat, many drug and nondrug treatments have been developed for all types of pain. Ranging from mild to potent, many drugs are used to manage pain, including:

- nonopioid analgesics
- opioid agonists and opioid antagonists
- adjuvant analgesics (such as local anesthetics, anticonvulsants, antidepressants, and muscle relaxants).

A mix of opioid and nonopioid analgesics may pack the right punch.

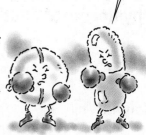

Nonopioid analgesics

Nonopioid (nonnarcotic) analgesics are used to treat pain that's either nociceptive (caused by stimulation of injury-sensing receptors) or neuropathic (arising from nerves). These drugs are particularly effective against the somatic component of nociceptive pain, such as with joint and muscle pain. Besides controlling pain, nonopioid analgesics reduce inflammation and fever.

Drug types in this category include:
- acetaminophen
- nonsteroidal anti-inflammatory drugs (NSAIDs)
- salicylates.

Team work

When used alone, acetaminophen and NSAIDs provide relief from mild pain. NSAIDs also can relieve moderate pain; in high doses, they may help relieve severe pain. Given in combination with opioids, nonopioid analgesics provide additional analgesia, allowing a lower opioid dose and thus a lower risk of adverse opioid effects.

Acetaminophen

Acetaminophen relieves mild pain and reduces fever. It's commonly the drug of choice for patients who need a mild analgesic, especially when aspirin and NSAIDs are contraindicated. Unlike those drugs, acetaminophen has no anti-inflammatory effects. Additionally, it doesn't alter platelet function and rarely causes GI problems.

What a relief!

Acetaminophen is used to relieve headache, muscle aches, and general pain as well as to reduce fever. It's the first-choice drug for treating fever and flulike symptoms in children. According to the American Arthritis Association, acetaminophen also effectively relieves pain in some forms of arthritis.

Adjusting the thermostat

Acetaminophen's pain control mechanism isn't well understood, but the drug is thought to inhibit prostaglandin synthesis in the central nervous system (CNS). Fever reduction comes from direct action on the body's "thermostat" — the temperature-regulating center in the brain's hypothalamus.

NSAIDs

NSAIDs provide temporary relief from mild to moderate pain. They're mainly used to treat inflammation, such as arthritis. Secondary uses include relief from menstrual cramps and mild to moderate pain after certain types of surgery. NSAIDs are also used adjunctively to manage cancer pain — especially in patients with bone metastasis. For long-term treatment, they may be prescribed for osteoarthritis or rheumatoid arthritis. They don't cause CNS or respiratory depression when used in therapeutic doses.

NSAIDs can be taken orally and are generally available without a prescription. Many types are available. Examples include celecoxib, diclofenac, fenoprofen, ibuprofen, indomethacin, nabumetone, naproxen, oxaprozin, piroxicam, sulindac, and tolmetin.

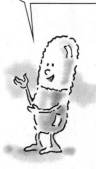

I don't want to brag, but acetaminophen has no anti-inflammatory effects.

Running prostaglandin interference

NSAIDs work by interfering with prostaglandin production. Prostaglandins are hormonelike substances. They're produced by the enzyme cyclooxygenase (COX). COX comes in two types—COX-1 and COX-2. Both types produce prostaglandins that promote inflammation, pain, and fever; however, only COX-1 produces prostaglandins that protect the stomach lining and support platelet function.

The downside

Traditional NSAIDs inhibit COX-1 and COX-2. By blocking COX-1, they may damage the stomach lining, causing GI distress, stomach bleeding and ulcers, and altered platelet function. A newer class of NSAIDs, COX-2 inhibitors, suppresses only COX-2. Because they spare COX-1, these agents reduce the risk of GI toxicity and altered platelet function.

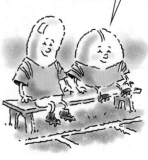

NSAIDs may be good blockers, but sometimes that's a bad thing.

Salicylates

Salicylates, such as aspirin, are among the most commonly used pain medications. A single salicylate dose of 650 mg brings maximum pain relief and fever-reducing effects. Doses of up to 5 g/day confer maximum anti-inflammatory effects.

Fewer prostaglandins, less pain

Salicylates relieve pain by inhibiting prostaglandin synthesis. They're used mainly to relieve pain and inflammation and reduce fever. They aren't effective against visceral pain (pain arising from the organs or smooth muscle) or severe pain related to trauma.

Opioids

Opioids (narcotics) include derivatives of the opium (poppy) plant and synthetic drugs that imitate natural narcotics. Unlike NSAIDs, which act peripherally, opioids produce their primary effects in the CNS. Opioids include opioid agonists, opioid antagonists, and mixed agonist-antagonists.

Opioid agonists

Opioid agonists are used to treat moderate to severe pain without causing loss of consciousness. They're also used to relieve severe pain in acute, chronic, and terminal conditions. Opioid agonists include codeine, fentanyl, hydromorphone, levorphanol tartrate, meperidine, methadone, morphine (including sustained-release tablets and intensified oral solution), and oxycodone.

Get more with morphine

Morphine is the gold standard against which the effectiveness and adverse reactions of other pain medications are measured. It's also used to relieve shortness of breath in patients with pulmonary edema and left-sided heart failure.

Agonist action

Opioid agonists reduce pain by binding to opiate receptor sites in the CNS. When these drugs stimulate opiate receptors, they mimic the effects of endorphins—naturally occurring opiates that are part of the body's pain relief system.

Adversity with agonists

Although this receptor-site binding produces an analgesic effect and cough suppression, it can also cause adverse reactions, such as respiratory depression and constipation. (See *How opioid agonists control pain*, page 376.)

Opioid antagonists

Opioid antagonists aren't actually pain medications; rather, they block the effects of opioid agonists. They're used to reverse adverse drug reactions, such as respiratory and CNS depression produced by opioid agonists. Examples of opioid antagonists include naloxone and naltrexone.

Naloxone to the rescue

Naloxone is the preferred drug for managing opioid overdose. It reverses respiratory depression and sedation and helps stabilize vital signs within seconds. Because naloxone reverses opioids' analgesic effects, a patient who receives an opioid for pain relief may complain of pain or even experience withdrawal symptoms after naloxone administration.

Naltrexone's opioid-free zone

Naltrexone is used to treat drug abuse—typically in combination with psychotherapy. It's given only to patients who've gone through a detoxification program to eliminate all opioids from the body. When naltrexone is given to someone who still has opioids in his body, acute withdrawal symptoms may occur.

It's back!

Opioid antagonists attach to opiate receptors but don't stimulate them. As a result, they prevent other opioids, enkephalins, and endorphins from producing their effects. Unfortunately, by reversing analgesic effects, opioid antagonists may cause the patient's pain to recur.

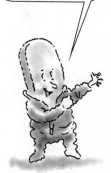

Looks like this is going to be a rescue mission. I'd better suit up!

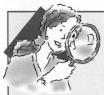

A closer look

How opioid agonists control pain

Opioid agonists, such as morphine, inhibit pain transmission by mimicking the body's natural pain-control mechanisms.

Where neurons meet
In the dorsal horn of the spinal cord, peripheral pain neurons meet central nervous system (CNS) neurons. At the synapse, the pain neuron releases substance P (a pain neurotransmitter). This agent helps transfer pain impulses to the CNS neurons that carry the impulses to the brain.

Taking up space
In theory, spinal interneurons respond to stimulation from descending CNS neurons by releasing endogenous opiates. These opiates bind to the peripheral pain neuron to inhibit release of substance P and retard the transmission of pain impulses.

Stopping substance P
Synthetic opiates supplement this pain-blocking effect by binding with free opiate receptors to inhibit the release of substance P. Opiates also alter consciousness of pain, but how this mechanism works remains unknown.

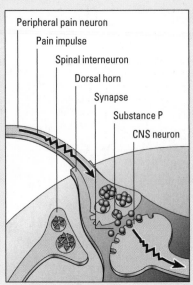

Peripheral pain neuron
Pain impulse
Spinal interneuron
Dorsal horn
Synapse
Substance P
CNS neuron

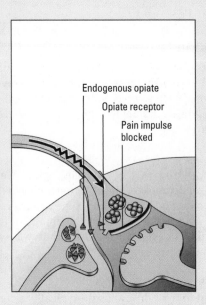

Endogenous opiate
Opiate receptor
Pain impulse blocked

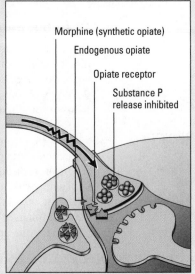

Morphine (synthetic opiate)
Endogenous opiate
Opiate receptor
Substance P release inhibited

Mixed opioid agonist-antagonists

Mixed opioid agonist-antagonists are used mainly to relieve moderate to severe pain, reduce preoperative anxiety and pain, and provide analgesia during childbirth. As their name implies, mixed opioid agonist-antagonists have agonist and antagonist properties. The agonist component relieves pain, while the antagonist component reduces the risk of toxicity and drug dependence. These drugs also decrease the risk of respiratory depression and drug abuse and include buprenorphine, butorphanol, dezocine, nalbuphine, and pentazocine (combined with pentazocine lactate, naloxone, aspirin, or acetaminophen).

Not so fast

Although mixed opioid agonist-antagonists generally seem to have less addiction potential than that of pure opioid agonists, as well as a lower risk of drug dependence, butorphanol and pentazocine have been known to cause dependence.

What's the action, Jackson?

The exact mechanism of action for mixed opioids isn't known. However, it's clear that buprenophine binds with CNS receptors, altering the perception of pain and the emotional response to it. The drug releases slowly from binding sites, producing a longer duration than that of other drugs in this class.

Some good, some bad

Because of their lower risks of drug dependence and respiratory depression, mixed opioids may be preferred over opioid agonists. However, they can produce other adverse reactions, such as bradycardia, nausea, and vomiting.

Adjuvant analgesics

Adjuvant analgesics are drugs that have other primary indications but are used as analgesics in some circumstances. Adjuvants may be given in combination with opioids or used alone to treat chronic pain. Patients receiving adjuvant analgesics should be reevaluated periodically to monitor their pain level and check for adverse reactions.

Drugs used as adjuvant analgesics include:
- anesthetics (local and topical)
- certain anticonvulsants
- benzodiazepines
- corticosteroids
- muscle relaxants
- psychostimulants
- selective serotonin reuptake inhibitors (SSRIs)
- serotonin 5-HT1 agonists
- tricyclic antidepressants (TCAs).

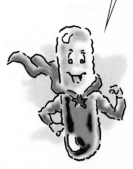

Adjuvant analgesics moonlight as pain control medications.

Local anesthetics

Local anesthetics are used to prevent and relieve pain from medical procedures, disease, or injury. They're also prescribed for severe pain not relieved by topical anesthetics or analgesics, to help

manage neuropathic pain, or as an alternative to general anesthesia. These drugs include:
- amides, such as bupivacaine, etidocaine, lidocaine, mepivacaine, prilocaine, and ropivacaine
- esters, such as benzocaine, cocaine, chloroprocaine, procaine, and tetracaine. (See *Pain-numbing cousins.*)

And... action!

Local anesthetics selectively block sodium channel permeability, thereby disrupting ectopic nerve impulses centrally and peripherally. They don't affect normal nerve conduction.

Topical anesthetics

Topical anesthetics are applied directly to the skin or mucous membranes. They're used to:
- relieve or prevent pain, especially from minor burns
- relieve itching and irritation
- numb a selected area before an injection
- numb mucosal surfaces before tube insertion
- relieve sore throat or mouth pain (when used as a spray or solution).

You're a friend amide

These drugs include amides (such as dibucaine and lidocaine) and esters (benzocaine, cocaine, dyclonine, pramoxine, and tetracaine) as well as topical combinations of local anesthetics, such as:
- aerocaine—a mixture of benzocaine and benzethonium
- cetacaine—a mixture of benzocaine, butamben, dyclonine, lidocaine, and tetracaine
- EMLA (eutetic mixture of local anesthetics), which contains lidocaine and prilocaine.

But can they act?

Topical anesthetics relieve pain by preventing nerve impulse transmission. These drugs accumulate in the nerve membrane, causing it to expand and lose its ability to depolarize, thus blocking impulse transmission.

Anticonvulsants

Anticonvulsants help prevent excessive nerve impulses, which may be perceived as pain, and can be used to treat neuropathic pain (pain generated by peripheral nerves). These drugs include carbamazepine, clonazepam, divalproex, gabapentin, lamotrigine, oxcarbazepine, phenytoin, tiagabine, topiramate, valproic acid, and zonisamide.

> ## Pain-numbing cousins
>
> Local anesthetics include two main groups. *Amides* (which include lidocaine and prilocaine) contain nitrogen in their molecular makeup.
>
> **Give them oxygen**
> In contrast, *esters* (such as cocaine and procaine) contain oxygen, not nitrogen.

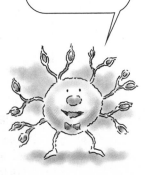

I can be a little impulsive sometimes, but anticonvulsants keep me in line.

The chosen ones

Carbamazepine and gabapentin are the anticonvulsants most commonly used as adjuvant analgesics. Both may be prescribed adjunctively to help relieve neuropathic pain in adults. In addition, carbamazepine is the drug of choice for treating trigeminal neuralgia (shooting pains of the facial area around one or more branches of the trigeminal nerve).

Anti action

Gabapentin and valproic acid suppress excessive nerve impulses by blocking the calcium channel and boosting production of gamma-aminobutyric acid (GABA), an inhibitory neurotransmitter. Carbamazepine and phenytoin act on the sodium channel.

Benzodiazepines

In pain management, benzodiazepines are used mainly for short-term relief of acute musculoskeletal pain characterized by muscle spasms. (When used for longer periods, these drugs have sedating affects that impede the patient's functional status.) Other uses for benzodiazepines include preoperative sedation and treatment of anxiety disorders. Benzodiazepines include alprazolam, diazepam, lorazepam, midazolam, and oxazepam.

Availability action

Benzodiazepines work by increasing the availability of the neurotransmitter GABA to brain neurons. At low doses, they ease anxiety by acting on the limbic system and related brain areas that help regulate emotional activity. At higher doses, they have sleep-inducing properties.

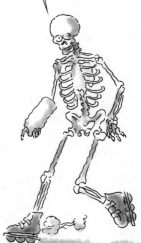

Benzodiazepines can help get pain in line. They're effective for short-term relief of musculoskeletal pain.

Corticosteroids

Corticosteroids are used to treat pain and inflammation. Based on their activity, they fall into two groups:
• mineralocorticoids, which regulate electrolyte and fluid homeostasis and include cortisone, fludrocortisone acetate, and hydrocortisone
• glucocorticoids, which regulate the body's reaction to inflammation, stimulate conversion of fat and protein into glucose by the liver, and regulate the immune response to diverse stimuli and include betamethasone, dexamethasone, methylprednisolone, prednisone, and triamcinolone.

Muscle relaxants

Muscle relaxants are used to relieve common musculoskeletal pain or acute traumatic sprains or strains. Drugs used for short-term relief of pain and muscle spasms are prescribed to relax skeletal muscles. Muscle relaxants can be classified as:

• neuromuscular drugs (such as metocurine and tubocurarine), used primarily as adjuncts to general anesthesia and secondarily to induce muscle relaxation and promote relaxation in patients on mechanical ventilation

• antispasmodic drugs, used to relieve spasticity associated with CNS disorders (baclofen, dantrolene, diazepam, and tizanidine)

• drugs for short-term pain relief and muscle spasms (carisoprodol, chlorzoxazone, cyclobenzaprine, methocarbamol, and tizanidine).

Antispasmodic exploits

Antispasmodic effects of baclofen and diazepam are similar. Baclofen suppresses release of excitatory neurotransmitters by binding to GABA-B receptors in the dorsal horn of the spinal cord, brain stem, and other CNS sites. Diazepam acts on GABA-A receptors.

Central activity

Although their precise mechanism of action is unknown, the centrally acting drugs don't relax skeletal muscles directly or depress neuronal conduction, neuromuscular transmission, or muscle excitability. Rather, centrally acting drugs are known to be CNS depressants. The skeletal muscle relaxant effects that they cause are most likely related to their sedative effects.

> Baclofen eases muscle spasms by binding to GABA receptors in the brain and spinal cord.

Psychostimulants

Psychostimulants are used mainly to treat such disorders as Parkinson's disease and attention deficit hyperactivity disorder. In pain management, they may be used adjunctively to manage acute or chronic pain disorders.

Psychostimulants include caffeine, dextroamphetamine, and methylphenidate. Dextroamphetamine has an analgesic affect in patients with postoperative pain. Methylphenidate helps ease pain associated with Parkinson's disease and cancer and also reduces opioid-induced sedation and cognitive impairments associated with opioid use.

Oh so stimulating

Psychostimulants appear to act on the cerebral cortex, stimulating the nervous system by promoting nerve impulse transmission.

SSRIs

A well-known class of antidepressants, SSRIs are being investigated as neuropathic pain relievers as well. These drugs have also shown potential in treating chronic nonmalignant pain syndromes. However, evidence doesn't support their role in managing acute pain. As analgesics, SSRIs perform best when used as adjuncts to opioids. SSRIs include fluoxetine, paroxetine, and sertraline.

SSRI endeavors

SSRIs block neuronal reuptake of the neurotransmitter serotonin, increasing the amount of serotonin available at the synapse of a neuron. Serotonin levels then increase, thereby relieving depression.

Serotonin 5-HT1 receptor agonists

Serotonin 5-HT1 receptor agonists (commonly called *triptans*) prevent or relieve migraine. These drugs include almotriptan, frovatriptan, naratriptan, rizatriptan, sumatriptan, and zolmitriptan.

The serotonin 5-HT1 receptor agonists are also known as the triptans.

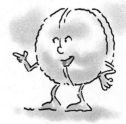

Active agonists bind beautifully

Serotonin 5-HT1 receptor agonists bind to serotonin receptors on the trigeminal nerve. This binding results in cranial vessel constriction and inhibition and reduction of the inflammatory process along the trigeminal nerve pathway. These actions may abort or provide symptomatic relief for a migraine.

Tricyclic antidepressants

Of the various types of antidepressants, TCAs have the longest history in managing pain—particularly neuropathic pain. TCAs include amitriptyline, amoxapine, clomipramine, desipramine, doxepin, imipramine, maprotiline, nortriptyline, and protriptyline.

Antidepressant action

Although the mechanism of action varies with the specific TCA, generally, TCAs inhibit reuptake of brain neurotransmitters (norepinephrine, serotonin, or dopamine) at nerve terminals. They may also block noradrenergic neuronal firing, providing analgesia to damaged nerve fibers.

Drug administration routes

Drugs can be delivered through many routes. Each route has advantages and drawbacks.

You can't get there from here

Keep in mind that administration routes aren't therapeutically interchangeable. The administration route influences a drug's absorption and distribution — in turn, affecting drug action and patient response. For instance, when given orally, the anxiolytic diazepam is readily absorbed. When given I.M., it's absorbed slowly and erratically.

> Liquid pain medications are absorbed faster than tablets and capsules.

Oral administration

For most patients, oral administration is the most convenient and easiest way to take analgesics. Oral pain medications generally are available in tablet, capsule, and liquid forms. After ingestion, tablets and capsules are absorbed by the GI system. How extensively and quickly absorption occurs depends on such factors as whether the drug is formulated for immediate or controlled release. Also, liquid preparations are absorbed faster.

Sublingual administration

Sublingual medications are placed under the tongue, providing rapid, convenient analgesia. Most sublingual medications are rapidly disintegrating tablets or soft gelatin capsules filled with a liquid drug. High drug concentration is achieved in the sublingual region before being absorbed by the mucosa.

Transdermal administration

Transdermal administration involves drugs that come as ointments or transdermal patches. Because they're lipid-soluble, transdermal drugs are absorbed through the skin, bypassing the GI tract. Many specially compounded creams, gels, and ointments can be applied to the skin for pain relief. Fentanyl, lidocaine, and clonidine are available in transdermal systems, or *patches*.

Buccal administration

Buccal medications are inserted between the cheek and mouth. The patient closes his mouth and holds the tablet against his cheek until it's absorbed. Because the buccal mucosa is less permeable than the sublingual area, absorption is slower and drug availability is somewhat decreased.

SubQ administration

Subcutaneous drugs are injected into the fatty tissue beneath the skin. Drug absorption and action depend on the specific drug and its properties. Subcutaneous administration usually provides rapid pain relief.

Patient at the pump

Subcutaneous medications can be given through single injections or through a patient-controlled analgesia (PCA) pump. With PCA, a catheter is implanted under the skin and attached to an external electronic pump. The patient self-administers basal (continuous) and bolus (additional) doses as needed. Disadvantages of PCA include possible discomfort and irritation at the injection or infusion site.

I.M. administration

Intramuscular (I.M.) injections deliver medication deep into muscle tissue. Typically, the I.M. route is used when subcutaneous, oral, or I.V. access isn't available or possible. Absorption and action of I.M. drugs depend on the specific drug and various patient factors. Drugs given I.M. have a faster onset than oral drugs, but a slower onset than that of I.V. drugs. Pain and irritation at the injection site are common.

I.V. administration

Delivering a drug directly into a vein allows rapid onset because the drug enters the bloodstream quickly. The I.V. route is a good choice if the patient can't swallow, has persistent nausea and vomiting, or needs rapid onset. On the downside, I.V. administration may cause drug infiltration and infection at the catheter site. I.V. drugs are absorbed rapidly but have a short duration of action. Almost all opioids can be given I.V. or through a PCA pump.

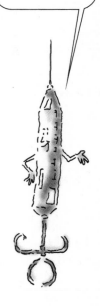

Unfortunately, just the sight of me has instilled fear in countless children — and some adults, too.

Intranasal administration

Intranasal administration (typically using a nasal spray) may be indicated for patients who can't tolerate the oral route. The vascular nasal mucosa absorbs medication rapidly. Intranasally administered pain medications include butorphanol, lidocaine, and sumatriptan succinate.

Epidural administration

A drug may be administered into the epidural space to provide local relief to irritated nerves in patients with chronic or acute pain. Epidurally administered pain medications include local anesthetics, opioids, and steroids. An epidural injection achieves pain relief within 2 to 10 days, on average. Duration of action ranges from days to months, depending on the patient's diagnosis and response. Drawbacks of epidural delivery include potential infection, local bleeding, and site tenderness.

Catheter control

Continuous and intermittent epidural medication delivery can be achieved by placing a catheter in the epidural space and attaching it to a pump. Catheters usually are placed temporarily for increased joint mobilization or intense physical therapy or to assess the patient's response to drug therapy. Pain relief occurs within minutes, although finding the dose that brings optimal relief may take a few days.

Intrathecal administration

Intrathecal administration refers to delivery of a drug into the subarachnoid space of the spinal canal. This method is used to administer drugs that don't readily cross the blood-brain barrier. Drugs that may be given intrathecally include morphine, baclofen, clonidine, and ziconotide.

    Some anesthetics may be given intrathecally to achieve regional anesthesia, as in spinal anesthesia or epidural block, or to treat patients with chronic pain by injecting a neurolytic agent into the cerebrospinal fluid (CSF).

Even more about pumps

Sometimes, intrathecal drugs are delivered through an implanted pump to allow precise delivery of continuous doses. The pump is embedded below the skin and a catheter is tunneled to the precise location of pain in the spine. The drug enters the CSF and then the spinal cord, where it acts on the targeted site.

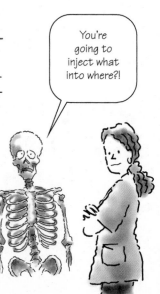

You're going to inject what into where?!

Intrathecal administration typically allows smaller doses of pain medication and causes fewer adverse reactions. When a pump is used, it must be refilled with medication every 1 to 3 months, depending on the delivery rate. Typically, the pump must be replaced every 5 years because of limited battery life.

Rectal administration

Medications given rectally (as a gelatin or waxy suppository capsule) have a slow onset and variable absorption. Because absorption varies, the degree of pain relief with this administration route also varies. Although cost-effective, rectal administration isn't widely accepted. Opioids, such as morphine, oxymorphone, and hydromorphone, are sometimes given rectally when other routes can't be tolerated.

Intra-articular administration

Intra-articular administration delivers drugs directly to the synovial joint cavity to relieve pain, reduce inflammation, and produce localized numbness. Drugs given by this route include corticosteroids, local anesthetics, and hyaluronic acid derivatives (used to treat osteoarthritis of the knee).

Intra-articular drugs absorb shock and lubricate the joint. Duration depends on the specific agent. For instance, hylan G-F 20 is given weekly for 3 weeks; hyaluronate is given weekly for 5 weeks.

Nonpharmacologic approaches

Managing pain doesn't necessarily involve capsules, syringes, I.V. lines, or medication pumps. Many nonpharmacologic therapies are available, too — and they're gaining popularity among the general public and health care professionals alike.

Self-help trends

What accounts for this trend? For one thing, many people are concerned about the overuse of drugs for conventional pain management. For another, some people simply prefer to self-manage their health problems.

Something for everyone

Collectively speaking, nonpharmacologic approaches offer something for nearly everyone. Many of them can be used either alone or combined with drug therapy. A combination approach may improve pain relief

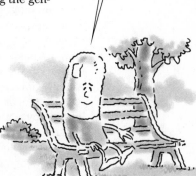

Looks like I'm going to be sitting out this section.

by enhancing drug effects and allow lower dosages. These therapies fall into three main categories:

- physical therapies
- alternative and complementary therapies
- cognitive and behavioral therapies.

And that's not all

Nonpharmacologic approaches have other benefits besides pain management. They help reduce stress, improve mood, promote sleep, and give the patient a sense of control over pain. By understanding how these techniques work and how best to use them, you can provide additional options for patients who experience pain.

License and occupation, please

Although the techniques discussed in this chapter can be effective for a wide range of patients, they're best administered, prescribed, or taught by licensed practitioners or experienced, credentialed lay people. A few require a doctor's order.

Physical therapies

Physical therapies involve the use of physical agents and methods to aid rehabilitation and restore normal functioning after illness or injury. They can also reduce inflammation, ease muscle spasms, and promote relaxation. These therapies are relatively cheap and easy to use. With appropriate teaching, patients and their families can use them on their own, which helps them participate in pain management.

Types of physical therapy include hydrotherapy, thermotherapy, cryotherapy, vibration, TENS, exercise, and range-of-motion (ROM) exercises.

Hydrotherapy

Hydrotherapy is the use of water to treat pain and disease. Sometimes considered the ultimate natural pain reliever, water comforts and soothes while providing support and buoyancy. It's most commonly prescribed for burns and relaxes muscles, raises or lowers tissue temperature (depending on water temperature), and eases joint stiffness (as in rheumatoid arthritis or osteoarthritis). In pain management, hydrotherapy is most commonly used to treat acute pain—for instance, from muscle sprains or strains. Depending on the patient's problem, the water can be hot or cold, and liquid, solid (ice), or steam. It can be applied externally or internally.

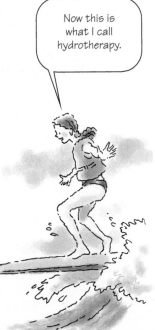

Now this is what I call hydrotherapy.

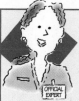

Advice from the experts

Pool rules

Hydrotherapy commonly takes the form of a whirlpool bath (shown at right), which uses water jets to help ease pain. Here are some tips to keep in mind while administering whirlpool therapy:

• Keep the water temperature between 56° and 109° F (13° and 43° C), depending on the body surface area being treated and the patient's physical condition.

• Use a hydraulic chair to help the patient get into and out of the whirlpool tub.

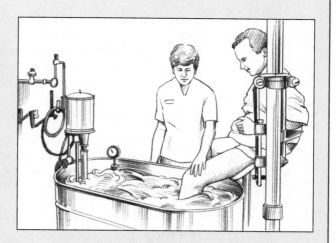

Jet set

Whirlpool baths—bathtubs with jets that force water to circulate—aid in rehabilitating injured muscles and joints. Depending on the desired effect, the water can be either hot or cold. The water jets act to massage and soothe muscles. (See *Pool rules*.)

Should I stay or should I go?

Whirlpools and certain other hydrotherapy treatments can be done at home. But the more intensive forms are best done in a supervised clinical setting, where the treatment and the patient's response can be monitored.

How it works

Hot-water hydrotherapy eases pain through a sequence of events triggered by increased skin temperature. As skin temperature rises, blood vessels widen and skin circulation increases. As resistance to blood flow through veins and capillaries drops, blood pressure decreases. The heart rate then rises to maintain blood pressure. The result is a significant drop in pain and greater comfort.

A hot bath eases pain as it lowers blood pressure and speeds the heart rate.

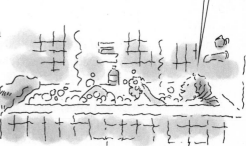

Special considerations

• Be aware that hydrotherapy may cause burns, falls, or light-headedness.
• Stop the treatment session if the patient feels lightheaded.
• Don't keep the patient in a heated whirlpool for more than 20 minutes.
• Instruct the patient to wipe his face frequently with a cool wash-cloth so he won't get overheated.
• Know that hydrotherapy isn't recommended for pregnant women, children, elderly patients, or patients with diabetes, hypertension, hypotension, or multiple sclerosis.

Thermotherapy

Thermotherapy refers to application of dry or moist heat to decrease pain, relieve stiff joints, ease muscle aches and spasms, improve circulation, and increase the pain threshold.

Dry heat and moist heat involve conductive heating (heat transfer that occurs when the skin directly contacts a warm object). Thermotherapy is used to treat pain caused by:
• headache
• muscle aches and spasms
• earache
• menstrual cramps
• temporomandibular joint (TMJ) disease
• fibromyalgia (a syndrome of chronic pain in the muscles and soft tissues surrounding joints).

Dry heat can be applied with a hot water bottle, a K-pad, or an electric heating pad. Moist heat can be applied with a hot pack, a warm compress, or a special heating pad. (See *Heaping on the hot packs.*)

How it works

Thermotherapy enhances blood flow, increases tissue metabolism, and decreases vasomotor tone. It produces analgesia by suppressing free nerve endings and also may reduce the perception of pain in the cerebral cortex.

Special considerations

• Before administering thermotherapy, determine the patient's awareness level and ability to communicate his response to the treatment.
• If the patient has a cognitive impairment, measure the temperature of the heating agent before applying it. It should be 104° to 113° F (40° to 45° C) when it contacts the skin.

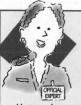

Advice from the experts

Heaping on the hot packs

Hot packs promote pain relief by delivering moist heat. Follow these tips to ensure safe, effective treatment:
• Make sure your patient can tolerate the weight of the hot pack on the affected body part.
• Wrap the pack with insulation and several layers of toweling so it won't burn the patient's skin.
• Position the pack and the patient carefully.
  The illustration at right shows a hot pack treatment for a patient with lower back pain.

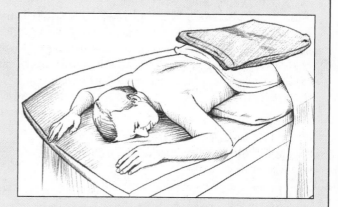

• Be aware that some patients may prefer a slightly lower (or higher) temperature. Keep the heating agent at a temperature that's comfortable for the patient.
• Wrap the heating agent so it doesn't directly contact the patient's skin.
• Regularly assess the skin at a heat application site for irritation and redness.
• Frequently evaluate the patient's response to treatment and his pain level.
• Stop the treatment if the patient's pain increases.
• Don't apply heat to an area that's infected, bleeding, or receiving radiation therapy or where oil or menthol has been applied.
• Know that thermotherapy is contraindicated in patients with vascular insufficiency, neuropathy, skin desensitization, or neoplasms.

Cryotherapy methods include cold packs, ice bags, and ice massage. Brrr.

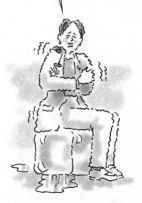

Cryotherapy

Cryotherapy involves applying cold to a specific body area. In addition to reducing fever, cryotherapy can provide immediate pain relief and help reduce or prevent edema and swelling. Cryotherapy methods include cold packs, ice bags, and ice massage. Ice massage has a temporary anesthetic effect and is used during brief painful procedures. (See *Reducing pain with ice massage*, page 390.)

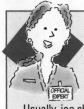
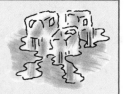

Advice from the experts

Reducing pain with ice massage

Usually, ice shouldn't be applied directly to the skin because it may damage the skin surface and underlying tissues. Even so, when carefully performed, this technique, called *ice massage,* may help patients tolerate brief, painful procedures, such as bone marrow aspiration, lumbar puncture, and chest tube or suture removal.

Get ready...
Prepare for ice massage by gathering the ice, a porous covering to hold it (if desired), and a cloth for wiping water off the patient's skin as the ice melts.

Get set...
Just before the procedure begins, rub the ice over the appropriate area to numb it. Assess the site frequently. Stop rubbing immediately if you detect signs of tissue intolerance.

Go!
To start the procedure, rub the ice over a point near—but not at—the affected site. This distracts the patient and gives him another stimulus on which to concentrate.

If the painful procedure lasts longer than 10 minutes or if you think tissue damage may occur, move the ice to a different site and continue the massage. If you know in advance that the procedure will last longer than 10 minutes, massage the site intermittently—2 minutes of massage alternating with a rest period until the skin regains normal color.

Alternatively, you can divide the area into several sites and apply ice to each one for several minutes at a time.

Putting a freeze on pain

Cryotherapy may be indicated for pain resulting from:
- acute trauma
- joint disorders such as rheumatoid arthritis
- headache such as migraine
- muscle aches and spasms
- incisions
- surgery.

Compare and contrast

In another cryotherapy technique, called *contrast therapy*, cold and heat application are applied alternately during the same session. Contrast therapy may benefit patients with rheumatoid arthritis and certain other conditions.

Typically, the session begins by immersing the patient's feet and hands in warm water for 10 minutes. Next come four cycles of cold soaks (each lasting 1 to 4 minutes) alternating with warm soaks (each lasting 4 to 6 minutes).

How it works
Cryotherapy constricts blood vessels at the injury site, reducing blood flow to the site. This flow reduction, in turn, thickens the

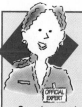

Advice from the experts

Applying cold to a muscle sprain

Cryotherapy helps reduce pain and edema when used during the first 24 to 72 hours after an injury. For best results, follow the guidelines below.

Method and materials
• Apply cold to the painful area four times daily for 20 to 30 minutes each time.
• Use enough crushed ice to cover the area.
• Place the ice in a plastic bag, and place the bag inside a pillowcase or a large piece of cloth, as shown below. Then apply the bag over the painful area for the specified treatment time.

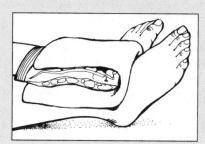

The old switcheroo
• After 24 to 72 hours, when swelling has subsided or when cold can no longer help, switch to thermotherapy.

Wise words
• Inform the patient that ice eases pain in a joint that has begun to stiffen, but caution him not to let the analgesic effect lull him into overusing the joint.

blood, resulting in decreased bleeding and increased blood clotting. Cryotherapy also slows edema development, prevents further tissue damage, and minimizes bruising. What's more, it decreases sensitivity to pain by cooling nerve endings and eases muscle spasms by cooling muscle spindles — the part of the muscle tissue responsible for the stretch reflex. (See *Applying cold to a muscle sprain.*)

Stimulating contrast

Contrast therapy is thought to stimulate endocrine function, reduce inflammation, decrease congestion, and improve organ function.

Special considerations

• As appropriate, encourage your patient to try cold application. Many patients aren't aware that cold relieves pain.
• Before applying cold, assess the pain or injury site and the patient's pain level. Evaluate for impaired circulation (such as from Raynaud's disease), inability to sense temperature (as from neuropathy), extreme skin sensitivity, and inability to report response to treatment (for instance, if he's a young child or a confused elderly patient).
• If the patient has a cognitive impairment, measure the temperature of the cooling agent. It should be no colder than 59° F (15° C).
• When administering moist cold, keep in mind that moisture intensifies cold.

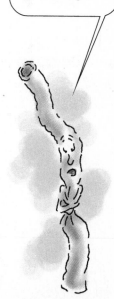

Brrr... Cryotherapy is so cold it constricts me at the injury site and reduces bleeding.

- Wrap cold packs so they don't directly contact the patient's skin.
- Stop the treatment if the patient's skin becomes numb.
- Use caution when applying ice to the elbow, wrist, or outer part of the knee. These sites are more susceptible to cold-induced nerve injury.
- Regularly assess the patient for adverse effects, such as skin irritation, joint stiffness, numbness, frostbite, and nerve injury.
- Don't apply cold to areas that have poor circulation or have received radiation.

Vibration

Vibration therapy eases pain by inducing numbness in the treated area. This technique, which works like an electric massage, may be effective in such disorders as muscle aches, headache, chronic nonmalignant pain, cancer pain, fractures, and neuropathic pain.

That's an order

Hospitalized patients need a doctor's order to use a vibrating device. Outpatients may choose from various devices available without a prescription. A vibrating device can be stationary or handheld. Stationary devices range from vibrating cushions to full beds and recliners. The patient lies or sits on the device and receives the treatment passively. Vibration therapy reduces pain by numbing the stimulated area. It also has a soothing effect.

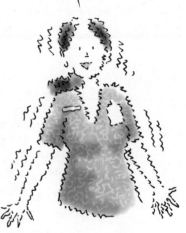

V-v-vibration th-therapy eases p-p-pain b-by inducing numb-n-ness.

Special considerations

- Before using vibration therapy, teach your patient about this method, including how it works and when it should and shouldn't be used.
- Tell the patient he may feel a warm sensation initially.
- Apply the vibrator to an area above or below the pain site.
- For more effective pain relief, use the highest vibration speed the patient can tolerate.
- Apply the vibrating device for 1 to 15 minutes at a time, two to four times daily, or as ordered.
- Determine the length of treatment needed to achieve adequate pain relief. Continue to assess the patient's response to treatment.
- Stop the treatment if the patient experiences discomfort, pain, or excessive skin redness or irritation.
- Don't use vibration therapy if the patient has thrombophlebitis or bruises easily.
- Don't apply the vibrator over burns, cuts, or incision sites.

TENS

In TENS therapy, a portable, battery-powered device transmits painless alternating electrical current to peripheral nerves or directly to a painful area. Used postoperatively and for patients with chronic pain, TENS reduces the need for analgesic drugs and helps the patient resume normal activities. TENS therapy must be prescribed by a doctor.

The patient usually wears the TENS unit on a belt. Units have several channels and lead placements. The settings allow adjustment of wave frequency, duration, and intensity. (See *Positioning TENS electrodes*.)

Top 10 TENS uses

Specific pain problems that have responded to TENS include:
- chronic nonmalignant pain
- cancer pain

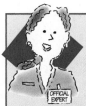

Advice from the experts

Positioning TENS electrodes

In transcutaneous electrical nerve stimulation (TENS), electrodes placed around peripheral nerves or an incision site transmit mild electrical impulses, which presumably block pain messages.

Perfect placement
Electrode placement usually varies, even for patients with similar complaints. Electrodes can be placed to:
- cover or surround the painful area, as for muscle tenderness or spasm or painful joints
- capture the painful area between electrodes, as for incisional pain.

The illustrations at right show combinations of electrode placement (dark squares) and areas of nerve stimulation (shaded strips) for low back and leg pain.

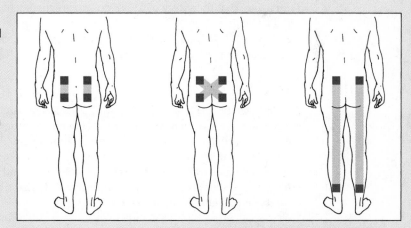

Placement tips
- If the patient has peripheral nerve injury, place electrodes proximal to the injury (between the brain and the injury site) to avoid increasing his pain.

- If a site lacks sensation, place electrodes on adjacent dermatomes (areas of skin innervated by sensory fibers from a single spinal nerve).
- Don't place electrodes in a hypersensitive area. Doing so can increase pain.

- bone fracture pain
- lower back pain
- sports injuries
- myofascial pain
- neurogenic pain (as in neuralgias and neuropathies)
- phantom limb pain
- arthritis
- menstrual pain.

A golden gate theory

Although TENS has existed for about 30 years, experts still aren't sure exactly how it relieves pain. Some believe that it works according to the *gate control theory,* which proposes that painful impulses pass through a "gate" in the brain. According to this theory, TENS alters the patient's perception of pain by closing the gate to painful stimuli.

Special considerations

- To ensure that your patient is a willing and active participant in TENS therapy, provide complete instructions on using and caring for the TENS unit.
- Before TENS therapy begins, assess the patient's pain level and evaluate for skin irritation at the sites where electrodes will be placed.
- Be aware that the safety of TENS during pregnancy hasn't been established.
- Don't use TENS if the patient has undiagnosed pain, uses a pacemaker, or has a history of heart arrhythmias.

Exercise

Exercise can be a valuable therapy for patients with acute or chronic pain. In most successful pain management programs, mobilization through exercise is an important component. Active exercise — muscle contraction entirely through the patient's own efforts — is the best way to achieve early mobilization and normal function. Exercise is commonly the treatment of choice in fibromyalgia and other chronic pain conditions.

How it works

Exercise may reduce pain by boosting the release of endorphins (the body's natural painkillers), which promotes a sense of comfort and alters the perception of pain. Moving about also increases the patient's self-esteem and gives him a sense of control.

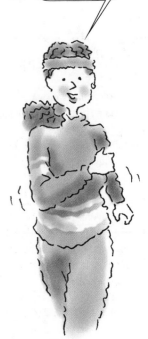

Exercise can ease pain and raise pain tolerance.

Special considerations
• Be sure to choose an exercise program that's appropriate for your patient. The program may range from simple stretching exercises to low-impact aerobic exercises such as walking.
• Teach the patient about the benefits of exercise in pain management.
• Consult an occupational or physical therapist, as appropriate, to develop an exercise program tailored to the patient's abilities and interests.
• Let the patient pace his activities according to his pain level.
• Before an exercise session, assess the patient's pain level and mobility limitations.
• Encourage a patient with chronic pain to set a daily exercise or activity goal and to record progress toward that goal. Advise him to rest only after completing the specified activity, instead of when pain occurs.
• Reassess the patient if exercise worsens his pain.

Range-of-motion exercises
ROM exercises are a simple yet encompassing technique for moving a body part through all the motions permitted by the involved joint. Each joint has a normal ROM. To maintain a normal ROM, the joint must be moved regularly. Limited ROM can lead to increased pain by impeding functional status (such as the ability to ambulate) and causing physical complications (such as skin breakdown).

> ROM exercises are even better than a lube job for keeping me limber.

Down with pain
Besides maintaining normal joint movement, ROM exercises decrease pain caused by stiffness and muscle spasms. Plus, they help the patient maintain or increase flexibility and preserve muscle strength (especially important if he can't exercise actively on his own).

It's only natural
ROM exercises take muscles and joints through all natural movements: extension, flexion, rotation, pronation, supination, abduction, adduction, eversion, and inversion. ROM exercises can be passive, active, or active-assistive.

Pass the passive ROM
Passive ROM refers to movement of a joint through its entire range without active muscle contraction. Another person moves the patient's limb (or other body part) for him. However, many patients can be trained to self-apply this technique. Also, passive

ROM can be done with an electrically powered continuous passive motion device.

Active and effective

In active ROM, the patient contracts his muscles through his own efforts. Compared to passive ROM, active ROM exercises more effectively return the body to normal functioning.

Exercise your judgment

In early healing stages, a patient may be unable to move the body part actively through the complete ROM and may benefit from an active-assistive routine. This type of ROM incorporates an additional passive force, applied by either a caregiver or the patient, along with the patient's own active efforts.

How it works

ROM exercises stretch the muscles, ligaments, and tendons surrounding a joint. They promote increased joint flexibility and movement and may reduce joint pain and stiffness from arthritis and other painful disorders.

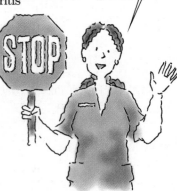

Stop passive ROM exercises if the patient's pain increases.

Special considerations

• During an episode of acute pain, limit the patient's exercise to self-administered ROM.
• Be aware that some patients benefit from heat or cold application before ROM exercises.
• Perform passive ROM exercises slowly, gently, and to the end of the normal ROM or to the point of pain — but no further.
• If a muscle spasm occurs, move the joint to the point of tightness and hold.
• Stop passive ROM exercises if the patient's pain increases.

Alternative and complementary therapies

Alternative and complementary therapies greatly expand the range of therapeutic choices for patients suffering pain. Today, patients are increasingly seeking these therapies, not just to treat pain but also to address many other common health conditions. Regardless of the problem for which they're used, alternative and complementary therapies address the whole person — body, mind, and spirit — rather than just signs and symptoms.

Together but different

Although alternative and complementary therapies are usually discussed together, they aren't exactly the same:

• *Alternative therapies* are those used instead of conventional or mainstream therapies—for example, the use of acupuncture rather than analgesics to relieve pain.

• *Complementary therapies* are those used in conjunction with conventional therapies—such as meditation used as an adjunct to analgesic drugs.

When conventional means ineffective

Alternative and complementary therapies commonly relieve some types of pain that don't respond to conventional techniques. They may prove especially valuable when a precise cause evades conventional medicine, as commonly occurs with chronic low back pain. These types of therapies include acupuncture, aromatherapy, chiropractic, massage, music therapy, Therapeutic Touch, and yoga.

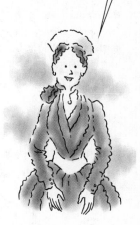

You know who was a big advocate of complementary and alternative therapies? I'll give you one guess.

Acupuncture

Acupuncture involves inserting thin metal needles just under the skin at specific points. Typically, the needles stay in place for 20 to 30 minutes. To enhance their intended benefits, they may be set in motion or connected to low-voltage electric generators.

The World Health Organization lists 100 conditions that can benefit from acupuncture. Pain-related conditions on the list include arthritis, back pain, carpal tunnel syndrome, dental pain, fibromyalgia, headache, menstrual cramps, postoperative pain, peripheral neuropathy, and trigeminal neuralgia.

How it works

Although acupuncture is one of the most thoroughly researched alternative therapies, Western scientists aren't sure how it works. Various theories have been proposed. (See *Insight into acupuncture*, page 398.)

Special considerations

• If your patient is considering acupuncture, advise him to get a practitioner referral from the National Commission for the Certification of Acupuncturists.

• Be aware that acupuncture has a lower incidence of adverse effects than many accepted medical procedures used for the same conditions. Nonetheless, some types of acupuncture carry a slight risk of life-threatening reactions, such as pneumothorax.

• Know that some third-party payers cover acupuncture treatments by a qualified practitioner. However, inability to pay continues to be a problem for many patients seeking acupuncture and other alternative treatments.

Insight into acupuncture

Various theories provide a possible explanation for how acupuncture works.

Endorphin stimulation

According to the endorphin stimulation theory, acupuncture needles stimulate peripheral nerves, triggering the release of endorphins and enkephalins (the body's natural painkilling chemicals). Researchers have found that during acupuncture analgesia, endorphin levels rise in the blood and cerebrospinal fluid and fall in specific brain regions.

Neurotransmitter effect

The neurotransmitter theory proposes that acupuncture affects levels of serotonin and norepinephrine, neurotransmitters that help relay nerve impulses across brain synapses.

Gate control

The popular gate control theory proposes that pain perception is controlled by a "gate"—a part of the nervous system that regulates pain impulses. When bombarded by too many impulses, as during acupuncture, the gate becomes overwhelmed and closes.

Inserting acupuncture needles is thought to "close the gate" on the nerve fibers that carry pain impulses to the brain.

Electrical conductance

The electrical conductance theory hinges on findings that acupuncture points (acupoints) have a higher level of electrical conductance than that of other sites. Some scientists theorize that acupoints amplify minute electrical signals as they travel through the body and that acupuncture needles interrupt that flow. This effect then blocks transmission of pain impulses.

Enhanced immunity

Some researchers suspect acupuncture may raise the white blood cell count and increase prostaglandin, gamma globulin, and overall antibody levels.

Circulation control

The circulation control theory proposes that acupuncture works by narrowing or widening blood vessels, possibly through control of vasodilators.

Aromatherapy

Used since ancient times to heal the body, mind, and spirit, aromatherapy refers to the inhalation or application of essential oils distilled from various plants. Health care providers say the technique reduces stress, prevents disease, and even treats certain illnesses.

Aromatherapy has been used for:
- headaches
- muscle disorders
- arthritis
- shingles
- premenstrual syndrome.

Tiptoe through the tulips

Aromatherapy oils come from many parts of the plant, including the leaf, stem, flower, seed, bark, and root. A transference of the life force of the plant is a crucial component of aromatherapy. Specific oils are thought to have either relaxing or stimulating effects. Oils that supposedly reduce pain include basil, eucalyptus, chamomile, geranium, lavender, rosemary, and tea tree.

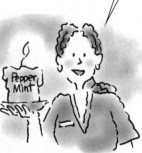

Choose wisely. Some scents are relaxing, whereas others are stimulating.

Aromatherapy may be self-administered or administered by a trained health care provider. Essential oils can be applied on the skin through gentle massage, added to bath water, or inhaled through an aerosol device.

How it works

When absorbed by body tissues, essential oils are thought to interact with hormones and enzymes to produce changes in blood pressure, pulse rate, and other physiologic functions.

Aromatherapists also believe smells can affect physiologic function through their effects on the limbic system—the part of the brain associated with emotion and memory. Odors stimulate receptors in the nose. These receptors convert the odors to nerve impulses that travel to the limbic system, where they may trigger memories associated with the odors.

Stop and smell the roses

According to aromatherapy researchers, the emotions evoked—joy, sadness, anger, anxiety—can affect heart rate, blood pressure, breathing, brain wave activity, and release of hormones that regulate insulin production, body temperature, stress, metabolism, and hunger. Odors also may stimulate release of neurotransmitters and endorphins in the brain, affecting emotional well-being and the perception of pain.

Special considerations

• Be aware that essential oils must be diluted carefully according to the distributor's instructions.
• Caution your patient never to massage essential oils into open or excoriated skin or to ingest the oils.
• Instruct the patient to wash essential oil off the skin before venturing into the sun because some oils are highly photosensitive.
• Warn the patient to keep essential oils away from the eyes and mucous membranes. If contact occurs, he should flush the eyes or mucous membranes copiously with water. If flushing doesn't relieve pain, he should get prompt medical attention.
• Many essential oils are toxic to children younger than age 5. Rose and eucalyptus oils have an especially high potential for toxicity.
• Know that aromatherapy is contraindicated in pregnancy because many essential oils pose a toxic risk to the mother and fetus.

Chiropractic

Chiropractic is a therapeutic system based on the belief that most medical problems result from vertebral

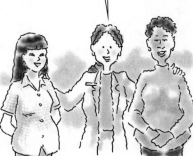

Sorry gals, but aromatherapy is contraindicated during pregnancy.

misalignments and can be corrected by spinal manipulation (called *adjustments*).

Two biggies

Health care providers believe chiropractic has two main benefits:
- It relieves musculoskeletal pain and disability.
- It reestablishes internal organ function.

Typically, chiropractors assess the source of pain and determine whether chiropractic treatment is an appropriate therapeutic choice. If the patient's problem requires medical care, the chiropractor makes referrals.

Chiropractic treatment may be useful in managing pain in patients of all ages, especially those with:
- neck and shoulder pain
- headaches
- sports injuries
- work-related injuries such as carpal tunnel syndrome.

How it works

Today, the most widely accepted theory of how chiropractic works centers on intervertebral motion and segmental dysfunction. (See *Understanding spinal manipulation*.)

Understanding spinal manipulation

Early theories of how chiropractic spinal adjustment worked relied on the anatomic understanding of the time. Misaligned vertebrae were thought to put pressure on spinal nerves, blocking the flow of nerve impulses. Spinal manipulation (adjustment) restored the free flow of neural impulses, relieving symptoms.

Because patients commonly reported significant relief of their complaints and increased function after an adjustment, this explanation was deemed satisfactory for many years. However, better understanding of anatomy and physiology over the years has made this explanation less acceptable.

No X-ray evidence
Another problem with the original explanation is that positive changes in health status aren't always reflected in vertebral alignment. That is, an adjustment may cause immediate and dramatic pain relief, but X-rays may show no detectable change in spinal alignment.

Also, no clearly demonstrated physiologic link exists between spinal manipulation and the organ responses they sup-

posedly cause. Because of these problems with the original explanation, alternative theories of how chiropractic achieves results have been proposed.

Fixating on a new theory
Currently, the most widely accepted theory is that of intervertebral motion and segmental dysfunction. This theory centers on loss of correct spinal joint mobility, not vertebral misalignment. Neighboring pairs of vertebrae and their surrounding tissues make up a motion segment. Loss of mobility within a segment is called a *fixation*. These fixations are most amenable to spinal manipulative therapy.

Recent neurophysiologic advances may explain how spinal manipulation can lead to visceral organ responses. Studies show that spinal adjustment initiates nerve signals that travel to internal organs through autonomic nervous system pathways. These signals provide a physiologic link between spinal manipulation and visceral organs.

Special considerations

• If your patient is seeking chiropractic care, explain the nature of chiropractic medicine and advise him on how to find a licensed practitioner.
• Tell your patient that chiropractic hasn't been proven effective in treating serious illnesses such as cancer.
• Know that chiropractic manipulation is contraindicated in patients with a condition that might worsen with spinal adjustment such as osteoporosis.

Massage

Massage involves rubbing and kneading of soft tissues for therapeutic purposes. As a therapy for pain relief and relaxation, massage has existed throughout history in almost all cultures. Different systems of therapeutic massage have been developed and are increasingly available today.

Therapeutic massage is used mainly for stress reduction and relaxation. It also serves as a complementary therapy for a broad range of conditions. Relaxation and massage stimulation distract the patient from pain. In some cases, massage is used to stretch fibrous scar tissue that's causing pain.

Pain-related disorders that may benefit from massage include:
• muscle spasms
• fibromyalgia
• headache
• arthritic joints
• back and shoulder pain.

Oh yeah... I kneaded this.

How it works

The main physiologic effect of massage is improved blood circulation. Kneading and stretching of muscles increases blood return to the heart. It also aids removal of lactic acid and other toxins from the muscle tissues for excretion from the body.

Straight to the brain

Improved circulation enhances tissue perfusion and oxygenation. When more blood circulates through the brain, thinking becomes clearer and the person feels more alive. Improved perfusion and oxygenation of other organ systems leads to better digestion and elimination and speeds wound healing.

Massage may relieve pain by stimulating specific parts of the body or by shutting the "gate" to transmission of pain messages to the brain. Some researchers suspect massage also triggers endorphin release.

Special considerations
• To avoid causing pain or discomfort, closely observe the patient's body language and note his verbal responses.
• Don't perform massage within 6″ (15 cm) of a bruise, cyst, skin break, or broken bone.
• Know that massage is contraindicated in patients with diabetes, varicose veins, phlebitis or other vascular problems, pitting edema, or swollen limbs.
• Avoid massaging the abdomen of a patient with hypertension or gastric or duodenal ulcers.

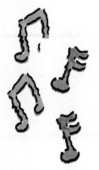

Music therapy
A form of sound therapy, music therapy takes advantage of the universal appeal of rhythmic sound to communicate, relax, encourage healing, and create a feeling of well-being. Music therapy can take the form of listening to music, creating music, singing, moving to music, and music and imagery exercises.

Music therapy can be effective in reducing chronic pain and as an adjunctive therapy for patients with burns, cancer, cerebral palsy, stroke and other brain injuries, Parkinson's disease, and substance abuse problems. Studies show that music decreases pain associated with dental and medical procedures.

I'll be signing autographs after I finish my gig on the unit today.

Musical preference?
A comfortable environment and enjoyable music are the two necessary ingredients for music therapy. The music should be appropriate for the patient and the session goal. As you might expect, fast music stimulates and slow music calms. Music selection can also be based on the patient's ethnic, cultural, or religious background. Whatever the choice, the music should be meaningful to the patient.

How it works
Various theories attempt to explain how music affects the body. One proposes that the resonance emitted by sound waves restores the body's natural rhythm and encourages healing. Another theory proposes that the brain reacts to sound waves by sending out instructions to control the heart rate, respiratory rate, and other body functions. These effects may lower blood pressure and decrease muscle tension. Also, sound impulses may trigger release of endorphins, which help relieve pain and lift mood. This combination of factors may create a state of total relaxation, possibly allowing the body to heal itself.

Special considerations
• After a music therapy session, encourage the patient to discuss the feelings he had while listening to the music.
• If a musical selection brings back an unpleasant memory or experience, comfort the patient and help him change his focus to more pleasant thoughts.

Therapeutic Touch

Developed in the 1970s, Therapeutic Touch is a widely used complementary therapy developed by and for health care providers in an attempt to bring a more humane and holistic approach to their practice. It's best known for its use in relieving pain and anxiety.

I have the touch

Therapeutic Touch is founded on the premise that the body, mind, emotions, and intuition form a complex, dynamic human energy field. During periods of health, the energy field is governed by pattern and order. During periods of stress and disease, it's unbalanced and disordered. Pain is thought to create a disorder in the person's energy field. Therapeutic Touch is said to reduce pain by restoring balance to the energy field.

A typical session lasts 10 to 30 minutes. The patient lies fully clothed on a massage table or hospital bed. The session starts with the health care provider "centering" herself and ends after she completes "interventions" aimed at balancing the energy field and removing obstructions. (See *Basic steps of Therapeutic Touch*, page 404.)

Proof is in the pudding

Although the existence of a human energy field remains unproven, practitioners claim they can feel something best described as energy when performing the technique. Many patients who receive Therapeutic Touch report that the treatment helps them feel deeply relaxed and reduces their pain.

How it works
By using their hands to manipulate the energy field above patients' skin, practitioners say they can restore equilibrium, which reactivates the mind-body-spirit connection and empowers patients to fully participate in their own healing.

Special considerations
• Therapeutic Touch rarely causes complications. However, practitioners must take care to moderate the length and strength of the treatment for elderly patients and young children because of their more fragile physiology.

Basic steps of Therapeutic Touch

A Therapeutic Touch practitioner applies her hands to the energy field around a patient's body. This method involves several steps.

Centering

In the first step, called *centering,* the practitioner achieves a calm, meditative state that helps her sense the patient's signs and symptoms and perceive subtle changes in the patient's energy field.

Assessment

Next, the practitioner begins her assessment. She slowly moves her hands over the patient's body, 2" to 6" (5 to 15 cm) away from the skin's surface, to detect alterations in the energy field, such as cold, heat, vibration, or blockages.

Unruffling

Depending on assessment findings, the practitioner then performs interventions aimed at balancing the energy field and removing any obstructions. Typically, these interventions involve "unruffling," which attempts to restore order to the patient's energy field.

To perform unruffling, the practitioner uses hand movements from the midline while continuing to move her hands in a rhythmic, symmetrical, head-to-toe fashion. Where an energy deficit occurs, energy is thought to transfer from the practitioner's hands to the patient.

Other interventions include eliminating "congestion" or acting as a conduit to direct the "life energy" from the environment into the patient.

Closure

The last step, closure, ends the treatment. Using intuitive judgment, the practitioner determines when to end the session. Cues come largely from continuous reassessment of the patient's energy field during the treatment to determine balance and obtain feedback.

Yoga

One of the oldest known health practices, yoga integrates physical, mental, and spiritual energies to promote health and wellness. Its basic components are proper breathing, movement, meditation, and posture. Yoga is used to relieve pain and anxiety in such disorders as heart disease, diabetes, migraine headaches, hypertension, cancer, arthritis, and back and neck pain.

What's your style?

Various yoga styles exist. Hatha yoga, the type most commonly taught in the West, encompasses a unique combination of physical postures and exercise (known as *asanas*), breathing techniques (called *pranayamas*), relaxation, diet, and proper thinking. Hatha yoga focuses on removing toxins from the body, cleansing the mind, energizing and realigning the body, releasing muscle tension, and increasing strength and flexibility.

How it works

While practicing specific postures, the person closely observes his breathing, exhaling at certain times and inhaling at others. Yoga breathing techniques are believed to help maintain the postures as well as to promote relaxation and enhance the flow of vital energy, known as *prana.* (See *Understanding yoga.*)

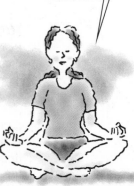

Yoga is one of the oldest known health practices.

Understanding yoga

Yoga practitioners believe that *prana,* or the life force, circulates throughout the body in a system of 72,000 subtle nerves. Improper diet, stress, or toxins can interrupt the flow of *prana,* affecting a person's physical or mental health. Chronic blockages can lead to illness. By promoting an even flow of *prana* and removing blockages, yoga breathing exercises are thought to maintain and restore health.

A boost to body systems

Other yoga practices are believed to stimulate the endocrine and nervous systems:

• Assuming certain body positions and contracting specific muscles during particular postures supposedly boosts circulation to the glands.

• Breathing exercises manipulate the respiratory system and presumably benefit the nervous system.

Relaxation response

Many scientific studies show that practicing yoga regularly can produce the same physiologic changes as meditation. Called the *relaxation response,* these changes include:

• decreased heart and respiratory rates
• improved heart and respiratory function
• lower blood pressure
• reduced oxygen consumption
• brain wave changes found only during deep meditation.

Special considerations

• Advise your patient to consult the doctor before starting a yoga program. Some yoga postures can be stressful to people with certain pain disorders.

• Be aware that yoga may cause muscle injury if done improperly or if the patient tries to force his body into a certain position.

• Inform the patient that yoga requires regular practice to be effective and that few people can perform all the movements in the beginning.

• Remind the patient that yoga is a complementary therapy — not a cure for pain or disease. Instruct him to continue conventional treatments.

Cognitive and behavioral therapies

Cognitive approaches to pain management focus on influencing the patient's interpretation of the pain experience. Behavioral approaches help the patient develop skills for managing pain and changing his reaction to it. These techniques improve the patient's sense of control over pain and allow him to participate actively in pain management.

Cognitive and behavioral approaches to managing pain include biofeedback, hypnosis, and meditation.

Biofeedback

Biofeedback uses electronic monitors to teach patients how to exert conscious control over various autonomic functions. By watching the fluctuations of various body functions (such as breathing, heart rate, and blood pressure) on a monitor, patients eventually learn how to change a particular body function by adjusting thoughts, breathing pattern, posture, or muscle tension.

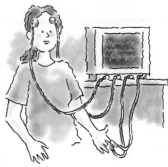

I wonder if this biofeedback machine can read my mind, too?

Modify at will

As they learn to modify vital functions at will, patients may develop the ability to control pain and certain other conditions without using drugs or other conventional medical treatments.

Everybody loves biofeedback

Biofeedback is used to treat various chronic pain states, such as headache, back pain, TMJ, stress-related disorders, and GI disorders. Approved by both conventional and alternative practitioners, it's popular with patients because it gives them a sense of control over their health problem.

Common types of biofeedback used to treat pain disorders include electromyography (EMG), which measures muscle tension and thermal biofeedback, which measures skin temperature.

EMG for you and me

In EMG, the patient is connected to a device with electrodes that pick up signals from muscles. The device changes the signals into a form the patient can understand, such as flashing lights or beeping, when the muscles tense up. A biofeedback practitioner interprets the signals and guides the patient in mental and physical exercises that help him achieve the desired result. Eventually, the patient trains himself to control physiologic functions by adjusting muscle tension. Decreasing muscle tension can reduce pain. With experience, patients become increasingly more self-aware and can learn how to relax muscle groups even without the device attached.

Temperature tip-off

Used most commonly to treat migraine, thermal biofeedback measures skin temperature (usually of a finger) as an indication of changes in peripheral blood flow. (See *Biofeedback: Migraine buster.*)

How it works

Scientists aren't sure how biofeedback produces its positive effects. Several studies have shown that biofeedback can be beneficial when no physical changes occur, or even when the patient learns to increase muscle tension.

Positive feedback

One possible explanation is that for some people, biofeedback reduces maladaptive physiologic activity, whereas for others it instills the belief that they can exert some control over their bodies and symptoms. This belief might lead to other coping behaviors that reduce emotional distress and help relieve pain.

Special considerations

• If your patient is seeking biofeedback therapy, help him find a qualified practitioner. Practitioners should be licensed, board-certified, or both.
• Instruct the patient to keep taking prescribed medications while receiving biofeedback training.
• Minimize distractions during the biofeedback session because they can prevent the patient from focusing and gaining optimal results.
• Know that biofeedback is contraindicated in patients with hypotension, psychiatric disorders, impaired memory, or dementia.

Hypnosis

Hypnosis harnesses the power of suggestion and altered levels of consciousness to produce positive behavior changes and treat various health conditions. Under hypnosis, a patient typically relaxes and experiences changes in respiration, which may lead to a positive shift in behavior and a greater sense of well-being.

You're getting sleepy...

Defined as a state of attentive, focused concentration, hypnosis leaves a person relatively unaware of surroundings and highly susceptible to suggestion. However, he must be willing to follow the suggestions offered. He can't be hypnotized to follow suggestions that go against his wishes.

...and your pain is vanishing

Hypnosis aids pain management by helping the patient gain control over the fear and anxiety that may accompany pain. It has been used to treat chronic pain, headaches, rheumatoid arthritis, and menstrual pain.

How it works

The hypnotic state may increase the patient's control over autonomic nervous system functions ordinarily considered beyond conscious control. The physiologic effects of hypnosis are similar to those seen in other states of deep relaxation and include:
• decreased sympathetic nervous system activity

Biofeedback: Migraine buster

In biofeedback, the patient learns to change a specific body function, such as heart rate or skin temperature, by changing his thoughts, breathing pattern, posture, or muscle tension.

Halting a migraine
To treat a patient with a migraine, for example, a special probe monitors skin temperature, which reflects the amount of blood flowing beneath the skin. Temperature changes, reflecting vasoconstriction and vasodilation, indicate the stress response.

As skin temperature fluctuates, lights on the monitor indicate the patient's response: black if he's tense, blue if he's relaxed. (Environmental conditions must be constant when monitoring skin temperature.)

Open to interpretation
The therapist helps the patient interpret the signals and teaches him relaxation and imagery techniques designed to maintain a blue light. The patient repeats this process until he achieves the desired response—migraine relief.

- reduced oxygen consumption
- lower blood pressure
- slower heart rate
- increases in certain types of brain wave activity.

Special considerations
- Because hypnosis deals with the subconscious mind, it may elicit disturbing emotions or memories. If the patient becomes upset or aggressive or exhibits strong negative feelings, the hypnotherapist should redirect him to a safe memory and end the session.
- Be aware that some patients experience light-headedness or psychological reactions to hypnosis.
- Know that patients with organic psychiatric conditions, psychosis, or antisocial personality disorders shouldn't be treated with hypnosis.

Meditation

Meditation—focusing one's attention on a single sound or image or the rhythm of one's own breathing—has been found to have positive effects on health. It may be especially helpful in chronic pain. By directing attention away from pain and other negative stimuli, it reduces stress, which commonly accompanies or worsens pain. Stress reduction has a wide range of physiologic and mental health benefits, ranging from decreased oxygen consumption and slower heart and respiratory rates to improved mood, spiritual calm, and heightened awareness.

More bennies

In addition to helping patients cope better with pain and anxiety, meditation may enhance immune function in patients with cancer, AIDS, and autoimmune disorders.

Mind the gap

However, meditation should be considered strictly an adjunct to pain management—not a substitute for medical treatment—because it doesn't always decrease pain intensity.

Most meditation techniques fall into one of two categories:
- *concentrative*, in which the person focuses on an image, a sound, or his own breathing to achieve a state of calm and heightened awareness (see *The focusing breath*)
- *mindful*, in which the person remains aware of all sensations, feelings, images, thoughts, sounds, and smells that pass through his mind but doesn't actually think about them in order to achieve a calmer, clearer, nonreactive mental state.

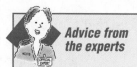

Advice from the experts

The focusing breath

When teaching your patient the proper technique for relaxation and breathing to promote pain relief, cover these points:
- Sit in a comfortable position with eyes closed.
- Focus on a sound or an image (such as an image of a peaceful scene or of white light entering the body).
- Breathe in through the nose to a count of 4.
- Hold your breath for a count of 2.
- Breathe out through your mouth for a count of 6.
- Repeat this cycle for 30 seconds to 5 minutes.

How it works

Meditation is thought to relieve stress and reduce pain through an effect called the *relaxation response,* a natural protective mechanism against overstress. Learning to activate the relaxation response through meditation may offset some of the negative physiologic effects of stress.

Transcends tension

Transcendental meditation, for instance, has been shown to reduce oxygen consumption, slow the heart and respiratory rates, lower blood lactose levels, increase alpha waves (brain waves indicating a deeply relaxed state), and ease hypertension.

Special considerations

• Know that teaching meditation and other relaxation exercises to patients, family members, and other caregivers is considered an independent health care activity.
• Before providing teaching, assess what the patient knows and how he feels about meditation.
• Inform the patient that learning to meditate takes some practice.

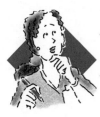

Quick quiz

1. Which of the following factors may influence a person's pain?
   A. Cultural background
   B. Weather
   C. Family's response to pain
   D. Nurse's response

Answer: A. Although pain may seem like a simple sensation, it's actually a complex experience influenced by a person's cultural background, the anticipation of pain, previous experience with pain, the context in which pain occurs, and emotional and cognitive responses.

2. The first stage of nociception is:
   A. modulation.
   B. perception.
   C. transmission.
   D. transduction.

Answer: D. Transduction—the first stage of nociception— refers to the conversion of mechanical, chemical, or thermal information into electrical activity in the nervous system.

3. The type of pain that comes on suddenly and may trigger sweating, fast heart and respiratory rates, and elevated blood pressure is:

    A.   chronic pain.
    B.   cancer pain.
    C.   acute pain.
    D.   moderate pain.

Answer: C. Acute pain comes on suddenly — for instance, after trauma, surgery, or an acute disease — and lasts from a few days to a few weeks.

4. When assessing pain in a 5-year-old child, which scale would be most appropriate to use?

    A.   Visual analog scale
    B.   Verbal descriptor scale
    C.   Numeric pain intensity rating scale
    D.   Faces pain intensity rating scale

Answer: D. You can evaluate pain in a nonverbal manner for pediatric patients ages 3 and older or for adult patients with language difficulties. The faces pain rating scale consists of six faces with expressions ranging from happy and smiling to sad and teary.

5. The questionnaire that consists of multiple true and false questions that may be helpful in assessing pain is the:

    A.   self-monitoring record.
    B.   Minnesota Multiphasic Personality Inventory.
    C.   brief pain inventory.
    D.   McGill pain questionnaire.

Answer: B. Used particularly for patients with chronic pain, the Minnesota Multiphasic Personality Inventory consists of 566 true-or-false questions that help assess personality characteristics in patients. Its main value lies in predicting responses to pain interventions.

Scoring

☆☆☆ If you answered all five questions correctly, fantastic! You're managing pain without any complications!

☆☆ If you answered four questions correctly, keep up the good work! You're well on your way to blocking those nosy nociceptors.

☆ If you answered fewer than four questions correctly, don't fret! A quick review of this chapter will be painless.

Wound care

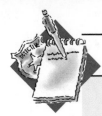

Just the facts

In this chapter, you'll learn:

♦ types of wound healing and the phases of wound healing

♦ factors that affect wound healing and potential complications

♦ proper wound assessment techniques

♦ types of wounds

♦ basic wound care procedures.

A look at wounds

Any break in the skin is considered a wound. Wounds can result from a planned event, such as surgery, or from an unexpected event, such as an accident, trauma, or exposure to pressure, heat, sun, or chemicals. Tissue damage in wounds varies widely, from a superficial break in the epithelium to deep trauma that involves the muscle and bone. A "clean" wound is a wound produced by surgery. A wound is described as "dirty" if it might contain bacteria or debris. Trauma typically produces dirty wounds. The rate of recovery is influenced by the extent and type of damage incurred as well as other intrinsic factors, such as patient circulation, nutrition, and hydration. Regardless of the cause of a wound, the healing process is much the same in all cases.

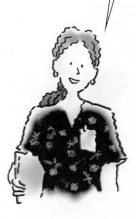

Healing occurs pretty much the same way no matter what caused the wound.

Types of wound healing

Wounds are classified by the way the wound closes. A wound can close by primary intention, secondary intention, or tertiary intention.

Primary intention

Primary intention, or *primary healing*, involves reepithelialization, in which the skin's outer layer grows closed. Cells grow in from the margins of the wound and out from epithelial cells lining the hair follicles and sweat glands.

Just a scratch

Wounds that heal through primary intention are, most commonly, superficial wounds that involve only the epidermis and don't involve the loss of tissue — a first-degree burn, for example. However, a wound that has well-approximated edges (edges that can be pulled together to meet neatly), such as a surgical incision, also heals through primary intention. Because there's no loss of tissue and little risk of infection, the healing process is predictable. These wounds usually heal in 4 to 14 days and result in minimal scarring.

Secondary intention

A wound that involves some degree of tissue loss heals by secondary intention. The edges of these wounds can't be easily approximated, and the wound itself is described as partial thickness or full thickness, depending on its depth:
• *Partial-thickness* wounds extend through the epidermis and into, but not through, the dermis.
• *Full-thickness* wounds extend through the epidermis and dermis and involve subcutaneous tissue, muscle and, possibly, bone.

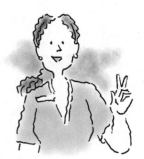

Secondary intention healing results in scarring and is more likely to be accompanied by complications than primary healing.

Getting under the skin

During healing, wounds that heal by secondary intention fill with granulation tissue, a scar forms, and reepithelialization occurs, primarily from the wound edges. Pressure ulcers, burns, dehisced surgical wounds, and traumatic injuries are examples of this type of wound. These wounds also take longer to heal, result in scarring, and have a higher rate of complications than do wounds that heal by primary intention.

Tertiary intention

When a wound is intentionally kept open to allow edema or infection to resolve or to permit removal of exudate, the wound heals by tertiary intention, or *delayed primary intention*. These wounds result in more scarring than wounds that heal by primary intention but less than wounds that heal by secondary intention.

Phases of wound healing

The healing process is the same for all wounds, whether the cause is mechanical, chemical, or thermal.

Don't let it phase you

Health care professionals discuss the process of wound healing in four specific phases:

Hemostasis occurs immediately after the injury. The body releases chemical mediators and intercellular messengers to stop bleeding and begin the cleaning process.

Inflammation, characterized by redness, swelling, heat, and pain, typically lasts 4 to 6 days, during which time bleeding is controlled and bacteria are destroyed.

Proliferation typically lasts 4 to 24 days. Granulation tissue, consisting of macrophages, fibroblasts, immature collagen, blood vessels, and ground substance is formed and the wound appears red, beefy, and shiny with a granular appearance. As this type of tissue forms, fibroblasts stimulate collagen production, which gives tissue its strength and structure.

Maturation, the final stage of wound healing, happens when the collagen fibers reorganize, remodel, and mature and gain tensile strength. This phase can last from 21 days to 2 years.

> Fibroblasts play an important role in the proliferation stage. We build collagen, which is important for proper wound healing.

All together now

Although this categorization is useful, it's important to remember that healing rarely occurs in this strict order. Typically, the phases of wound healing overlap.

Factors that affect healing

The healing process is affected by many factors. The most important influences include:
- nutrition
- oxygenation
- infection
- age
- chronic health conditions
- medications
- smoking.

Nutrition

Proper nutrition is arguably the most important factor affecting wound healing. Unfortunately, malnutrition is a common finding among patients with wounds. Poor nutrition prolongs hospitalization and increases the risk of medical complications, and the severity of complications is directly related to the severity of the malnutrition. In older patients, malnutrition is known to increase the risk of pressure ulcers and delay wound healing. It may also contribute to poor tensile strength in healing wounds, with an associated increase in the risk of wound dehiscence. (See *Tips for detecting nutritional problems.*)

Protein is key...

Protein is critical for wounds to heal properly. In fact, a person needs to double the recommended dietary allowance of protein (from 0.8 g/kg/day to 1.6 g/kg/day) before tissue even begins to heal. If a significant amount of body weight has been lost in connection with the injury, as much as 50% of the lost weight must be regained before healing will begin. A patient who lacks reserves of

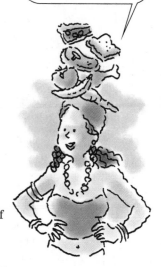

Because nutrition plays a critical role in wound healing, you need to make sure that your patient eats a balanced diet.

Tips for detecting nutritional problems

Nutritional problems may stem from physical conditions, drugs, diet, or lifestyle factors. The list below can help you identify risk factors that make your patient particularly susceptible to nutritional problems.

Physical condition
• Chronic illnesses, such as diabetes and neurologic, cardiac, or thyroid problems
• Family history of diabetes or heart disease
• Draining wounds or fistulas
• Weight issues—weight loss of 5% of normal body weight; weight less than 90% of ideal body weight; weight gain or loss of 10 lb or more in last 6 months; obesity; or weight gain of 20% above normal body weight
• History of GI disturbances
• Anorexia or bulimia
• Depression or anxiety
• Severe trauma

• Recent chemotherapy or radiation therapy
• Physical limitations, such as paresis or paralysis
• Recent major surgery
• Pregnancy, especially teen or multiple-birth pregnancy

Drugs and diet
• Fad diets
• Steroid, diuretic, or antacid use
• Mouth, tooth, or denture problems
• Excessive alcohol intake
• Strict vegetarian diet
• Liquid diet or nothing by mouth for more than 3 days

Lifestyle factors
• Lack of support from family or friends
• Financial problems

protein heals slowly, if at all, and a patient who's borderline malnourished can easily become malnourished under this demand.

The body needs protein to form collagen during the proliferation phase. Without adequate protein, collagen formation is reduced or delayed and the healing process slows.

...but other nutrients are also necessary

Fatty acids (lipids) are used in cell structures and play a role in the inflammatory process. Also, vitamins C, B-complex, A, and E and the minerals iron, copper, zinc, and calcium are important in the healing process. A zinc deficiency adversely affects the proliferation phase and, thus, the strength of the wound.

Oxygenation

Healing depends on a regular supply of oxygen. For example, oxygen is critical for leukocytes to destroy bacteria and for fibroblasts to stimulate collagen synthesis. If the supply is hindered by poor blood flow to the area of the wound or if the patient's ability to take in adequate oxygen is impaired, the result is the same — impaired healing.

Possible causes of inadequate blood flow to the area of the wound include pressure, arterial occlusion, or prolonged vasoconstriction, possibly associated with such medical conditions as peripheral vascular disease and atherosclerosis. Possible causes of a lower than necessary systemic blood oxygenation include:
- inadequate oxygen intake
- hypothermia or hyperthermia
- anemia
- alkalemia
- other medical conditions such as chronic obstructive pulmonary disease.

Infection

Infection can be systemic or localized in the wound. A systemic infection, such as pneumonia or tuberculosis, increases the patient's metabolism and thus consumes the fluids, nutrients, and oxygen the body needs for healing.

A localized infection in the wound itself is more common. Remember, any break in the skin allows bacteria to enter. The infection may occur as part of the injury or may develop later in the healing process.

Age

Skin changes that occur with aging cause healing time to be prolonged in elderly patients. Although delayed healing is partially

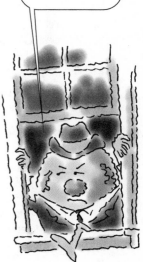

Pay no attention to me! I'm just looking for a way to get under your skin.

Ages and stages

Effects of aging on wound healing

In older adults, these factors impede wound healing:
• slower turnover rate in epidermal cells
• poorer oxygenation at the wound due to increasingly fragile capillaries and a reduction in skin vascularization
• altered nutrition and fluid intake resulting from physical changes that can accompany aging, such as reduced saliva production, a declining sense of smell and taste, or decreased stomach motility
• altered nutrition and fluid intake attributable to troubling personal or social issues, such as loose-fitting dentures, financial concerns, eating alone after the death of a spouse, or problems preparing or obtaining food
• impaired function of the respiratory or immune systems
• reduced dermal and subcutaneous mass leading to an increased risk of chronic pressure ulcers
• healed wounds that lack tensile strength and are prone to reinjury.

due to physiologic changes, it's usually complicated by other problems associated with aging, such as poor nutrition and hydration, the presence of a chronic condition, or the use of multiple medications. (See *Effects of aging on wound healing*.)

Chronic health conditions

Respiratory problems, atherosclerosis, diabetes, and malignancies can increase the risk of wounds and interfere with wound healing. These conditions can interfere with systemic and peripheral oxygenation and nutrition, which affect healing.

Getting complicated

Impaired circulation, a common problem for patients with diabetes and other disorders, can cause tissue hypoxia (lack of oxygen). Neuropathy associated with diabetes reduces a person's ability to sense pressure. As a result, a diabetic patient may experience trauma, especially to the feet, without realizing it. Insulin dependency can impair leukocyte function, which adversely affects cell proliferation.

Hemiplegia and quadriplegia involve the breakdown of muscle tissue and reduction in the padding around the large bones of the lower body. Because a patient with one of these conditions lacks sensation, he's at risk for developing chronic pressure ulcers.

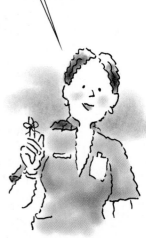

Don't forget that such health problems as respiratory disorders, atherosclerosis, diabetes, and malignancies not only increase the risk of wounds but also hinder healing.

Night and day shifts

Normally, a healthy person shifts position every 15 minutes or so, even during sleep. This shifting prevents tissue damage due to ischemia. Anything that impairs the ability to sense pressure, including the use of pain medications, spinal cord lesions, or cognitive impairment, puts the patient at risk (the patient can't feel the growing discomfort of pressure and respond to it).

Other conditions that can delay healing include dehydration, end-stage renal disease, thyroid disease, heart failure, peripheral vascular disease, and vasculitis and other collagen vascular disorders.

Medications

Any medication that reduces a patient's movement, circulation, or metabolic function, such as sedatives and tranquilizers, has the potential to inhibit the patient's ability to sense and respond to pressure. Also, because movement promotes adequate oxygenation, lack of motion means that peripheral blood delivers less oxygen to the extremities than it should. Lack of motion is especially problematic for older adults. Remember, oxygen is important; without it, the healing process slows and the potential for complications rises.

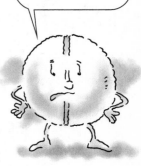

Medications, particularly sedatives, can also complicate wound healing. Sorry about that!

Some medications, such as steroids and chemotherapeutic agents, reduce the body's ability to mount an appropriate inflammatory response. This interference interrupts the inflammatory phase of healing and can dramatically lengthen healing time, especially in patients with compromised immune systems, such as those with acquired immunodeficiency syndrome.

Smoking

Carbon monoxide, a component of cigarette smoke, binds to the hemoglobin in blood in the place of oxygen. This binding significantly reduces the amount of oxygen circulating in the bloodstream, which can impede wound healing. To some extent, this reaction also occurs in people regularly exposed to second-hand smoke.

Complications of wound healing

The most common complications associated with wound healing are hemorrhage, dehiscence and evisceration, infection, and fistula formation.

Hemorrhage

Internal hemorrhage (bleeding) can result in the formation of a hematoma—a blood clot that solidifies to form a hard lump under the skin. Hematomas are commonly found around bruises.

External hemorrhage is visible bleeding from the wound. External bleeding during healing isn't unusual because the newly developed blood vessels are fragile and rupture easily. Thus, a wound needs to be protected by a dressing. However, each time the new blood vessels suffer damage, healing is delayed while repairs are made.

Dehiscence and evisceration

Dehiscence is a separation of skin and tissue layers. It's most likely to occur 3 to 11 days after the injury was sustained and may follow surgery. Evisceration is similar but involves protrusion of underlying visceral organs as well. Dehiscence and evisceration may constitute a surgical emergency, especially if they involve an abdominal wound. If a wound opens without evisceration, it may need to heal by secondary intention. Poor nutrition and advanced age are two factors that increase a patient's risk of dehiscence and evisceration. (See *Recognizing dehiscence and evisceration*.)

Infection

Infection is a relatively common complication of wound healing that should be addressed promptly. Infection can lead to a cellulitis or bacterial infection that spreads to surrounding tissue. Signs that infection may be at work include:
• redness and warmth of the margins and tissue around the wound
• fever
• edema
• pain (or a sudden increase in pain)
• pus
• increase in exudate or a change in its color
• odor
• discoloration of granulation tissue
• further wound breakdown or lack of progress toward healing.

Fistula

A fistula is an abnormal passage between two organs or between an organ and the skin. In a wound, it may appear as undermining or a sinus tract in the skin around the wound. If a sinus tract (or tunneling) is present, it's important to determine its extent and direction.

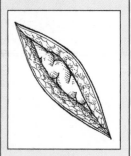
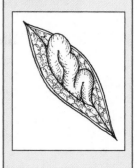

Wound assessment

Each time you assess a wound, remember that you're assessing a patient with a wound — not simply the wound itself. Remembering the patient will help keep you focused on the big picture as you perform your initial assessment and will set the stage for effective monitoring and successful healing.

Key considerations

Several factors influence the body's ability to heal itself, regardless of the type of injury suffered. You should include these elements in your wound assessment:

- immune status
- blood glucose levels
- hydration
- nutrition
- blood albumin levels
- oxygen and vascular supply
- pain.

Immune status

The immune system plays a central role in wound healing. If the immune system is impaired due to such diseases as human immunodeficiency virus (HIV) infection or as a result of chemotherapy or radiation, the wound should be closely monitored for impaired healing.

Blood glucose levels

Blood glucose levels should range from 70 to 120 mg/dl for satisfactory healing, regardless of the cause of the wound. Levels above 120 mg/dl can impair the function of white blood cells (WBCs), which help prevent infection and are important in wound healing.

Hydration

Be sure to closely monitor and optimize the patient's hydration status — successful healing depends on it. Skin and subcutaneous tissues need to be well hydrated from the inside. Dehydration impairs the healing process by slowing the body's metabolism. Dehydration also reduces skin turgor, leaving skin vulnerable to new wounds.

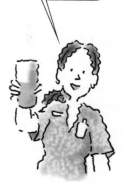

Encourage the patient to keep hydrated. Successful healing depends on it!

Nutrition

Nutritional status helps you determine the patient's vulnerability to skin breakdown as well as the body's overall ability to heal. A comprehensive assessment of your patient's nutritional status also helps you plan effective care.

Blood albumin levels

Blood albumin levels are an essential factor in wound assessment for two important reasons:

Skin is primarily constructed of protein, and albumin is a protein. If albumin levels are low, the body lacks an important building block for skin repair.

Albumin is the blood component that provides colloid osmotic pressure (the force that prevents fluid from leaking out of blood vessels into nearby tissues). If albumin levels fall below 3.5 g/dl, the patient can develop edema (fluid leakage into tissues), which compromises wound healing. The patient also risks developing hypotension (low blood pressure) as fluid leaks out of the bloodstream into tissues. If blood pressure falls to the point where adequate blood flow is no longer maintained through the capillaries near the wound, healing slows or stops.

Oxygen and vascular supply

Healing requires oxygen—it's that simple. Therefore, anything that impedes full oxygenation also impedes healing. Your assessment should consider any factor that has the potential to reduce the amount of oxygen available for healing. Possible problems include:
• impaired gas exchange, causing decreased oxygen levels in the blood
• hemoglobin levels that are too low to transport adequate oxygen
• low blood pressure that fails to drive oxygenated blood through capillaries
• insufficient arterial and capillary supply in the area of the wound.

Any of these problems, or a combination of these problems, can deprive the wound of the oxygen needed for successful healing.

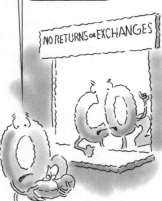

Impaired gas exchange can impede wound healing.

Smoke bomb

Smoking is a modifiable factor that impedes oxygenation of the wound. If your patient is a smoker, explain to him that smoking adversely affects wound healing.

Pain

In order to promote patient comfort, you should control your patient's pain to the best of your ability. However, pain control has a practical purpose as well. In response to pain, the body releases epinephrine, a powerful vasoconstrictor. Vasoconstriction reduces blood flow to the wound. When you relieve pain, vasoconstriction subsides, blood vessels dilate, and blood flow to the wound improves.

Wound classification

The words you choose to describe your observations of a specific wound have to communicate the same thing to other members of the health care team, insurance companies, regulators, the patient's family and, ultimately, the patient himself. Communicating to so many different people is a tall order when you consider that even wound care experts debate the descriptive phrases they use. The best way to classify wounds is to use the basic system described here, which focuses on three categories with fundamental characteristics:
• wound age
• wound depth
• wound color.

Wound age

When determining the age of a wound, you must first determine if the wound is acute or chronic. However, this determination can present a problem if you adhere solely to a time line. For instance, just how long is it before an acute wound becomes a chronic wound?

A different way of thinking

Rather than base your determination solely on time, consider a wound an acute wound if it's new or making progress as expected and a chronic wound if it isn't healing in a timely fashion. The main idea is that, in a chronic wound, healing has slowed or stopped and the wound is no longer getting smaller and shallower. Even if the wound bed appears healthy, red, and moist, if healing fails to progress, consider it a chronic wound.

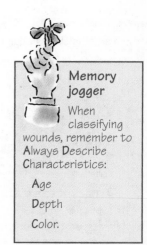

Memory jogger

When classifying wounds, remember to Always Describe Characteristics:

Age

Depth

Color.

More bad than good

Chronic wounds don't heal as easily as acute wounds. The drainage in chronic wounds contains a greater amount of destructive enzymes, and fibroblasts—the cells that function as the architects in wound healing—seem to lose their "oomph." They're less effective at producing collagen, divide less often, and send fewer signals to other cells telling them to divide and fill the wound. In other words, the wound changes from one that's vigorous and ready to heal, to one that's downright lazy!

Wound depth

Wound depth is another fundamental characteristic used to classify wounds. In your assessment, record wound depth as partial-thickness or full-thickness. (See *Classifying wound depth*.)

Partial-thickness

Partial-thickness wounds normally heal very quickly because they involve only the epidermal layer of the

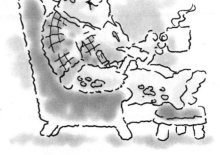

Break time! When a wound becomes chronic, fibroblasts slow down.

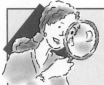

A closer look

Classifying wound depth

Wounds are classified as partial-thickness or full-thickness according to the depth of the wound. Partial-thickness wounds involve only the epidermis or extend into the dermis but not through it. Full-thickness wounds extend through the dermis into tissues beneath and may expose adipose tissue, muscle, or bone. The diagrams below illustrate the relative depth of both classifications.

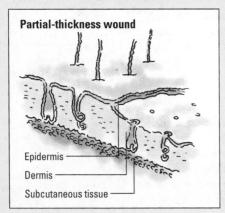

Partial-thickness wound

Epidermis
Dermis
Subcutaneous tissue

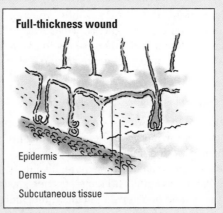

Full-thickness wound

Epidermis
Dermis
Subcutaneous tissue

skin or extend through the epidermis into (but not through) the dermis. The dermis remains at least partially intact to generate the new epidermis needed to close the wound. Partial-thickness wounds are also less susceptible to infection because part of the body's first level of defense (the skin) is still intact. These wounds tend to be painful, however, and need protection from the air to reduce pain.

Full-thickness

Full-thickness wounds penetrate completely through the skin into underlying tissues. The wound may expose adipose tissue (fat), muscle, tendon, or bone. In the abdomen, you may see adipose tissue or omentum (the covering of the bowel). If the omentum is penetrated, the bowel may protrude through the wound (evisceration). Granulation tissue may be visible if the wound has started to heal.

Full-thickness wounds heal by granulation and contraction, which require more body resources and more time than the healing of partial-thickness wounds. When assessing a full-thickness wound, report the depth as well as the length and width of the wound. .

The added pressure of pressure ulcers

In the case of pressure ulcers, wound depth allows you to stage the ulcer according to the classification system developed by the National Pressure Ulcer Advisory Panel (NPUAP).

> Pressure ulcer depth is staged according to the National Pressure Ulcer Advisory Panel classification system.

Wound color

Wounds are also classified by the color of the wound bed. Wound color helps the wound care team determine whether debridement is appropriate. (See *Tailoring wound care to wound color*, page 424.)

Be picky about wound bed color! Only red will do, and the best shade is blood red — not pale pink or grayish red. There are literally thousands of words to describe colors; however, you can simplify your assessment by sticking to the Red-Yellow-Black Classification System. This system is a useful tool for developing effective wound care management plans.

Red means you're ahead

If the wound bed is red (the color of healthy granulation tissue), the wound is healthy and normal healing is under way. When a wound begins to heal, a layer of pale pink granulation tissue covers the wound bed. As this layer thickens, it becomes beefy red.

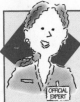

Advice from the experts

Tailoring wound care to wound color

With any wound, you can promote healing by keeping the wound moist, clean, and free from debris. For open wounds, using wound color can guide the specific management approach to aid healing.

Wound color	Management technique
Red	• Cover the wound, keep it moist and clean, and protect it from trauma. • Use a transparent dressing (such as Tegaderm or OpSite) over a gauze dressing moistened with normal saline solution or use a hydrogel, foam, or hydrocolloid dressing to insulate and protect the wound.
Yellow	• Clean the wound and remove the yellow layer. • Cover the wound with a moisture-retentive dressing, such as a hydrogel or foam dressing or a moist gauze dressing with or without a debriding enzyme. • Consider hydrotherapy with whirlpool or pulsatile lavage.
Black	• Debride the wound as ordered. Use an enzyme product (such as Accuzyme or Panafil), conservative sharp debridement, or hydrotherapy with whirlpool or pulsatile lavage. • For wounds with inadequate blood supply and noninfected heel ulcers, don't debride. Keep them clean and dry.

Not so mellow yellow

If the wound bed is yellow, beware! A yellow color in the wound bed may be a film of fibrin on the tissue. Fibrin is a sticky substance that normally acts as a glue in tissue rebuilding. However, if the wound is unhealthy or too dry, fibrin builds up into a layer that can't be rinsed off and may require debridement. Tissue that has recently died due to ischemia or infection may also be yellow and must be debrided.

Black = debridement

If the wound bed is black, be alarmed. A black wound bed signals necrosis (tissue death). Eschar (dead, avascular tissue) covers the wound, slowing the healing process and providing microorganisms with a site in which to proliferate. When eschar covers a wound, accurate assessment of wound depth is difficult and should be deferred until eschar is removed.

Typically, debridement is indicated for black wounds; however, ulcers caused by ischemia (damage due to inadequate blood supply) and uninfected heel pressure ulcers are exceptions. Ischemic wounds won't heal until blood supply is improved, and they're less likely to become infected if kept dry. The wound can be debrided and kept moist after blood supply is reestablished. (The body can then fend off infection and heal the wound.) As long as they're un-infected, heel pressure ulcers tend to heal from beneath the ulcer and don't require debridement.

Multicolored wounds

If you note two or even all three colors in a wound, classify the wound according to the least healthy color present. For example, if your patient's wound appears both red and yellow, classify it as a yellow wound.

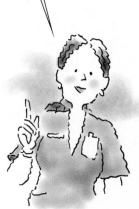

Remember to classify wounds according to the least healthy color present.

Assessing drainage

To begin collecting information about wound drainage, inspect the dressing as it's removed and record answers to such questions as:
• Is the drainage well contained, or is it oozing from the edges? If it's oozing, consider using a more absorbent dressing.
• In the case of an occlusive dressing, were the dressing edges well sealed? If the patient has fecal incontinence, it's even more important to note the seal status.
• Is the dressing saturated or dry?
• How much drainage is there? Is the amount scant, moderate, or large?
• What are the color and consistency of the drainage? (See *Drainage descriptors*.)

Drainage descriptors

The chart below provides terminology that you can use to describe the color and consistency of wound drainage.

Description	Color and consistency
Serous	• Clear or light yellow • Thin and watery
Sanguineous	• Red (with fresh blood) • Thin
Serosanguineous	• Pink to light red • Thin • Watery
Purulent	• Creamy yellow, green, white, or tan • Thick and opaque

Skipping the swab?

Also consider the texture of the drainage. If the drainage has a thick, creamy texture, the wound contains an excessive amount of bacteria. However, this texture doesn't necessarily mean a clinically significant infection is present. Document the characteristics of the drainage. Drainage might be creamy because it contains WBCs that have killed bacteria. The drainage is also contaminated with surface bacteria that naturally live in moist environments on the human body. Because of this bacterial colonization, guidelines developed by the Agency for Health Care Policy and Research (now the Agency for Healthcare Research and Quality) recommend against using swab cultures to identify wound infections. Nonetheless, some doctors still order swab cultures because they're easy to collect and inexpensive.

Ideally, obtain a swab of the clear fluid expressed from the wound tissue after it has been thoroughly cleaned. This culture is more likely to produce a sample of the bacteria in question. Punch biopsy of tissue or needle aspiration of fluid may also be used. These methods require more skill but are more likely to reveal accurate results.

Assessing the wound bed

As you assess the wound bed, record information about:
• wound dimensions, including size and depth
• tunneling and undermining
• bed texture and moisture
• wound odor
• margins and surrounding skin.

Dimensions

Because accurately recording wound dimensions is important, many health care facilities use photography as a tool in wound assessment. If photography is available in your facility, it should be included in your assessment of wound characteristics. Some photographic techniques produce a picture with a grid overlay that's useful for measuring. Remember, however, that there are qualities of the wound that a camera simply can't record. (See *What's missing?*)

Get out your ruler

The most common method of measuring wound dimensions is to use a tape measure. Make sure it's a disposable device to prevent contamination and cross-contamination. Record the length of the wound as the longest overall distance across the wound (regard-

What's missing?

If wound photography is a routine part of your wound documentation system, remember that a picture may be worth a thousand words but your assessment skills and personal observations are still essential. Many wound characteristics can't be recorded accurately—or at all—on film. These include:

- location
- depth
- tunnel measurement
- odor
- feel of surrounding tissue
- pain.

All of this information is needed if the health care team is to make sound treatment decisions.

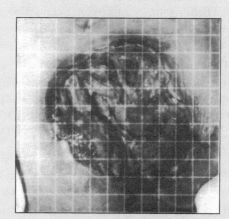

less of orientation), and record the width as the longest measurement perpendicular (at a right angle) to your length measurement. Be sure to record observed areas of discoloration of the intact skin around the wound opening separately—not as part of the wound bed. Record all measurements in centimeters.

Trace the wound

Another way to measure the wound is to use wound tracing (wound margins are traced on a sheet of clear plastic). You use the tracing to calculate an approximate wound area. This method provides only a rough estimate but is simple and fairly quick.

How deep

To measure the depth of the wound, you'll need a cotton-tipped swab. Gently insert the swab into the deepest portion of the wound and then carefully mark the stick where it meets the edge of the skin. Remove the swab and measure the distance from your mark to the end to determine depth.

Tunneling and undermining

It's also important to measure tunnels, or *sinus tracts* (extensions of the wound bed into adjacent tissue), and undermining (areas of the wound bed that extend under the skin). Measure these features just as you would the depth. Carefully insert a cotton-tipped swab to the bottom of the tunnel or to the end of the undermined area; then mark the stick and measure the distance from your mark to the end of the swab. If a tunnel is large, palpate it with a gloved finger rather than a swab because you can sense the end of the tunnel better with your finger. Palpating also avoids damaging the tissue.

Texture

The texture of the wound bed provides just as much information about the wound and healing as its color does. If you note very smooth red tissue in a partial-thickness wound, it's most likely the dermis. In a full-thickness wound, it's probably muscle tissue — not granulation tissue. In a full-thickness wound, healthy granulation tissue — which has a soft, bumpy appearance that's like the surface of a bowl of tapioca, only red — is a sign of proper healing.

Moisture

The wound bed should be moist but not overly moist. Moisture allows the cells and chemicals needed for healing to move about the wound surface.

Desert storm

In dry wound beds, cells involved in healing, which normally exist in a fluid environment, are a bit like fish in a desert — they can't move. WBCs can't fight infection, enzymes such as collagenase can't break down dead material, and macrophages can't carry away debris. The wound edges curl up to preserve moisture remaining in the edge and epithelial cells (new skin cells) fail to grow over and cover the wound. Healing grinds to a halt and necrotic tissue builds up.

Flood watch

Too much moisture poses a different problem. It floods the wound and spills out onto the skin, where the constant moisture causes the death of skin cells.

Odor

If kept clean, a noninfected wound usually produces little, if any, odor. (One exception is the odor normally present under a hydrocolloid dressing that develops as a by-product of the degradation process.) A newly detected odor might be a sign of infection. Record a new odor in your findings and report it to the doctor. When documenting wound odor, it's important to include when the odor was noted and whether it went away with wound cleaning.

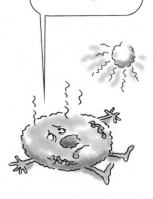

> Gasp! Dryness is a drag. If the wound bed is too dry, I can't move. This makes it hard for me to advance healing…

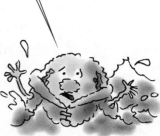

> …Make sure I'm not swimming either, though. Too much moisture can be the death of me.

Margins and surrounding skin

When assessing wound margins, you'll want to see skin that's smooth—not rolled—and tightly adherent to the wound bed. Rolled skin may indicate that the wound bed is too dry. Loose skin at the edges may indicate additional shearing injury (separation of skin layers), possibly due to a rough transfer or repositioning. In this case, improve transfer and repositioning techniques to prevent recurrence.

Rainbow connections

The color of the skin around the wound can alert you to impending problems that can impede healing:
• White skin indicates maceration, or too much moisture, and signals the need for a protective barrier around the wound and a more absorbent dressing.
• Red skin can indicate inflammation, injury (for example, tape burn, excessive pressure, or chemical exposure), or infection. Remember that inflammation is healthy only during the inflammatory phase of healing—not after!
• Purple skin can indicate bruising, one sign of trauma.

Let your fingers do the talking

Your fingers are invaluable tools you may be taking for granted. During your assessment of the area around the wound, your fingers will tell you much. For example, gently probe the tissue around the wound bed to determine if it's soft or hard (indurated). Indurated tissue, even in the absence of erythema (redness), is one indication of infection. Similarly, if your patient has dark skin, it may be impossible to see color cues. Again, your fingers can help. Probe the area around the wound bed and compare the feel to surrounding healthy skin. A tender area of skin that appears shiny and feels hard may indicate inflammation in such a patient.

Assessing pain

Assessing patient pain is an important part of wound assessment. You'll want to note not only pain associated with the injury itself, but also pain associated with healing and with therapies employed to promote healing. To fully understand your patient's pain, talk with him and ask about his pain. Then, independently, watch to see how he responds to pain and the therapies provided. As always, remember to record your findings. (See *How to assess pain*, page 430.)

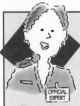

Advice from the experts

How to assess pain

To properly assess patient pain, consider the patient's descriptions and your own observations of his reaction to pain and treatments.

Talk to your patient
Begin your pain assessment by asking your patient the following questions:
• Where is the pain located? How long does it last? How often does it occur?
• What does the pain feel like? (Let the patient describe it; don't prompt.)
• What relieves the pain? What makes it worse?
• How do you usually get relief?
• How would you rate your pain on a scale of 0 to 10, with 0 representing no pain and 10 representing the worst pain?
    Talking with the patient about his pain in this manner helps him define his pain—for himself and you—and helps

you evaluate the effectiveness of therapies used to relieve pain.

Monitor and observe your patient
As you work with the patient, observe his responses to pain and to interventions intended to relieve pain.
    Behavioral responses to watch for include:
• altered body position
• crying
• grimacing
• immobility
• moaning
• muscle twitching
• sighing
• restlessness
• withdrawing from painful stimuli.

Sympathetic responses, normally associated with mild to moderate pain, include:
• diaphoresis (sweating)
• dilated pupils
• dyspnea (shortness of breath)
• elevated blood pressure
• pallor
• tachycardia (rapid heart beat)
• tension in skeletal muscles.
    Parasympathetic responses, which are more common in cases of severe, deep pain, include:
• bradycardia (slower than normal heartbeat)
• dizziness
• loss of consciousness
• lower than normal blood pressure
• nausea and vomiting
• pallor
• weakness.

Listen and learn

If your patient is conscious and can communicate, have him rate his pain before and during each dressing change. If your notes reveal that his pain is higher before the dressing change, it may indicate an impending infection, even before other signs appear.

If your patient says the dressing change itself is painful, you might consider administering pain medication before the procedure or changing the dressing technique itself. For example, if treatment calls for a wet-to-dry debridement technique, you can anticipate that the patient will experience pain, and it makes sense to provide some measure of preprocedure pain medication. However, remember to document this pain and report it to the doctor. Less painful methods of removing dead tissue exist but, if the patient's pain isn't documented and communicated, wet-to-dry debridement orders may stand and the patient may suffer unnecessary discomfort.

Useful tips for removal

In general, when removing adherent dressings, it's less painful if you soak the dressing or, over intact skin, use an adhesive remover. Also, keep the skin taut. Press down on the skin to release the dressing, rather than just pulling the dressing off. If the patient still says that dressing removal is painful, the team may wish to choose a less adherent dressing type.

Documenting assessment findings

In the course of a wound assessment, you amass quite a bit of useful information about the patient, his environment, the characteristics of his wound, and his current status in the healing process. In fact, your assessment creates a picture of the wound that accurately depicts your patient and his current status.

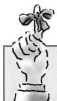

Memory jogger

Use the mnemonic device **WOUND PICTURE** to help you recall and organize all of the key facts that should be included in your documentation:

Wound or ulcer location

Odor? (in room or just when wound is uncovered?)

Ulcer category, stage (for pressure ulcer) or classification (for diabetic ulcer), and depth (partial-thickness or full-thickness)

Necrotic tissue?

Dimension of wound (shape, length, width, depth); drainage color, consistency, and amount (scant, moderate, large)

Pain? (if so, what relieves it, patient's description, patient's rating on scale of 0 to 10)

Induration? (surrounding tissue hard or soft)

Color of wound bed (red, yellow, black, or combination)

Tunneling? (length and direction — toward patient's right, left, head, or feet)

Undermining? (length and direction, using clock references to describe)

Redness or other discoloration in surrounding skin?

Edge of skin (loose or tightly adhered? flat or rolled under?)

Wound monitoring

The next step is to monitor the patient throughout the healing process, periodically reassessing his status and documenting progress to full healing. Not only is this monitoring an excellent way to determine progress and the usefulness of interventions, but it's also a requirement for some regulatory agencies such as the Centers for Medicare and Medicaid Services (CMS).

Your initial assessment sets the benchmark for subsequent monitoring and reassessment activities. One assessment is a static report. A series of assessments, however, becomes a moving picture illustrating the dynamic aspect of the healing process. In this way, all members of the health care team can see progress toward healing (or failure to thrive), developing complications, and the relative success of interventions. The view will depend on the accuracy, quality, and consistency of your documentation.

The prospect of monitoring, reassessing, and documenting over time may seem exciting or daunting, depending on your current energy level — but take heart. Several good research-based documentation tools are available — or your facility may have its own — to help you manage the task. Let's take a look.

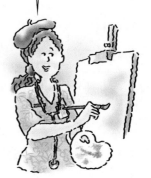

The picture of the wound that you paint during your initial assessment plays an important role in wound monitoring. It serves as a benchmark for wound healing.

Documentation tools

Most wound documentation tools in use in the United States focus on pressure ulcers. Pressure ulcers were selected as the basis of documentation because of the tremendous impact they've had on countless patients' lives and the health care system itself. Pressure ulcers are painful, typically chronic, life-disrupting, and expensive to treat in dollars and in amount of time spent by providers. They're also preventable.

Pressure Ulcer Scale for Healing

The Pressure Ulcer Scale for Healing (PUSH) tool was developed and revised by NPUAP and is only applicable to pressure ulcers. (See *PUSH tool.*)

When working with this tool, you develop three scores: one for the surface area (length × width), one for the drainage amount, and one for the tissue type in the wound during each review. The sum of these scores yields a total score for the wound on a given day. This score is then plotted on a pressure ulcer healing record and healing graph. By recording and reviewing scores over time, you can determine the pace of progress toward healing. NPUAP is working with CMS to incorporate the PUSH tool into the Mini-

PUSH tool

The beauty of the Pressure Ulcer Scale for Healing (PUSH) tool is its simplicity. It's quick and easy to score.

Patient name _David Quinn_   User location _Sunview Nursing Home_

Patient I.D. # _0162386_   Date _1/3/06_

Directions

Observe and measure the pressure ulcer. Categorize the ulcer with respect to surface area, exudate, and type of wound tissue. Record a subscore for each of the ulcer characteristics. Add the subscores to obtain the total score. A comparison of total scores measured over time provides an indication of the improvement or deterioration in pressure ulcer healing.

Length × width

0	1	2	3	4	5	6	7	8	9	10
0 cm^2	<0.3 cm^2	0.3 to 0.6 cm^2	0.7 to 1.0 cm^2	1.1 to 2.0 cm^2	2.1 to 3.0 cm^2	3.1 to 4.0 cm^2	4.1 to 8.0 cm^2	8.1 to 12.0 cm^2	12.1 to 24.0 cm^2	> 24.0 cm^2

Subscore: 3

Exudate amount

0	1	2	3
None	Light	Moderate	Heavy

Subscore: 1

Tissue type

0	1	2	3	4
Closed	Epithelial tissue	Granulation tissue	Slough	Necrotic tissue

Subscore: 1

Total score: 5

Length × width

Measure the greatest length (head-to-toe) and the greatest width (side-to-side) using a centimeter ruler. Multiply these two measurements (length × width) to obtain an estimate of surface area in square centimeters (cm^2). Don't guess! Always use a centimeter ruler and always use the same method each time the ulcer is measured.

Exudate amount

Estimate the amount of exudate (drainage) present after removal of the dressing and before applying any topical agent to the ulcer. Estimate the exudate as none, light, moderate, or heavy.

Tissue type

Tissue type refers to the types of tissue present in the wound (ulcer) bed. Score as a 4 if necrotic tissue is present. Score as a 3 if slough is present and necrotic tissue is absent. Score as a 2 if the wound is clean and contains granulation tissue. Score a superficial wound that's reepithelializing as a 1. When the wound is closed, score it as a 0.

4—Necrotic tissue (eschar): Black, brown, or tan tissue that adheres firm-ly to the wound bed or ulcer edges and may be firmer or softer than surrounding tissue

3—Slough: Yellow or white tissue that adheres to the ulcer bed in strings or thick clumps or is mucinous

2—Granulation tissue: Pink or beefy red tissue with a shiny, moist, granular appearance

1—Epithelial tissue: For superficial ulcers, new pink or shiny tissue (skin) that grows in from the edges or as islands on the ulcer surface

0—Closed or resurfaced: Completely covered wound with epithelium (new skin)

Adapted with permission from PUSH tool version 3.0, © 1998 National Pressure Ulcer Advisory Panel, Reston, Va.

mum Data Set, a required documentation form in long-term care facilities.

Pressure Sore Status Tool

The Pressure Sore Status Tool (PSST) allows you to track scores for 11 factors over time. These factors are each scored based on a number scale, and the scores are added. The total score reflects overall wound status. The PSST is a precise record of wound changes and is fairly time consuming to fill out. Consequently, it's used more in research than in clinical practice.

Wound Healing Scale

The Wound Healing Scale is a simple classification system that combines a designation for wound stage, or *thickness*, with a tissue descriptor. For example, a stage 3 pressure ulcer containing necrotic tissue is recorded as *3N*. Using this tool, you can track the general direction of healing by noting, for example, that this week the wound is an *FG* (full-thickness with granulation tissue), whereas last week it was an *FN* (full-thickness with necrotic tissue). The tool includes modifiers that allow you to use it for all types of wounds, although it was developed initially for use with pressure ulcers.

Sussman Wound Healing Tool

The Sussman Wound Healing Tool was developed to help physical therapists track pressure ulcer healing. This tool lists 10 wound attributes and classifies each as "good" or "not good" in terms of wound healing. For example, granulation tissue is classified "good" and undermining is classified "not good." During each assessment, record your findings for each of the 10 attributes that apply to your patient. Over time, this record provides a picture of healing or failure to thrive.

> In wound care, you may be able to foresee problems by recognizing signs of complications or failure to heal.

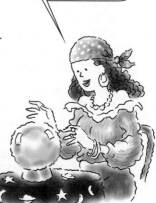

Recognizing complications

It's important to monitor and track, or *reassess*, wound status to identify signs and symptoms of complications or failure to heal as early in the process as possible. Early intervention improves the likelihood of resolving complications successfully and getting the healing process back on track.

Oh say, can you see?

You'll conduct your reassessments using the same criteria used in the initial assessment, with one added advantage—

perspective. Careful monitoring can help you catch failure to heal early so you can intervene appropriately. (See *Recognizing failure to heal.*)

Recognizing failure to heal

This chart presents the most common signs of failure to heal and associated probable causes and appropriate interventions.

Sign	Cause	Interventions
Wound bed		
Too dry	• Exposure of tissue and cells normally in a moist environment to air • Inadequate hydration	• Add moisture regularly. • Use a dressing that maintains moisture, such as a hydrocolloid or hydrogel dressing.
No change in size or depth for 2 weeks	• Pressure or trauma to the area • Poor nutrition, poor circulation, inadequate hydration, or medications • Poor control of disease processes such as diabetes • Inadequate pain control • Infection	• Reassess the patient for local or systemic problems that impair wound healing, and intervene as necessary.
Increase in size or depth	• Ischemia due to excess pressure or poor circulation • Infection	• Poor circulation may not be resolvable, but consider adding warmth to the area and administering a vasodilator or antiplatelet medication.
Necrosis	• Ischemia	• Perform debridement if the remaining living tissue has adequate circulation.
Increase in drainage or change of drainage color from clear to purulent	• Autolytic or enzymatic debridement • Infection	• No intervention is necessary if caused by autolytic or enzymatic debridement. Increase in drainage or change of drainage color is expected because of the breakdown of dead tissue. • If debridement isn't the cause, assess the wound for infection.
Tunneling	• Pressure over bony prominences • Presence of foreign body • Deep infection	• Protect the area from pressure. • Irrigate and inspect the tunnel as carefully as possible for a hidden suture or leftover bit of dressing material. • If the tunnel doesn't shorten in length each week, thoroughly clean and obtain a tissue biopsy for infection and — with a chronic wound — possible malignancy.

(continued)

Recognizing failure to heal *(continued)*

Sign	Cause	Interventions
Wound edges		
Red, hot skin; tenderness; and induration	• Inflammation due to excess pressure or infection	• If pressure relief doesn't resolve the inflammation within 24 hours, topical antimicrobial therapy may be indicated.
White skin (maceration)	• Excess moisture	• Protect the skin with petrolatum ointment or barrier wipe. • If practical, obtain an order for a more absorptive dressing.
Rolled skin edges	• Too-dry wound bed	• Obtain an order for moisture-retentive dressings. • If rolling isn't resolved in 1 week, debridement of the edges may be necessary.
Undermining or ecchymosis of surrounding skin (loose or bruised skin edges)	• Excess shearing force to the area	• Initiate measures to protect the area, especially during patient transfers.

The sooner, the better

Success or failure of the healing process has a tremendous impact on quality of life for the patient and his family. Early intervention can mean that a patient with a diabetic foot ulcer can avoid amputation or a paraplegic patient with an ischial ulcer can once again sit up and lead an active life.

Chronic ulcers pose a particularly difficult problem, not only for individual practitioners but also for the health care industry as a whole. Treating chronic ulcers is expensive because they're difficult or impossible to heal. Consequently, the people footing the largest portion of the bill—the government and insurance companies—are placing increased emphasis on early intervention and prevention.

Types of wounds

You may encounter many types of wounds in practice. The main types of wounds are acute wounds, vascular ulcers, pressure ulcers, and diabetic foot ulcers.

(Text continues on page 437.)

Recognizing skin ulcers

Vascular ulcers

Vascular ulcers typically result from some form of peripheral vascular disease, which can affect the venous, lymphatic, and arterial systems.

Venous ulcers

Venous ulcers result from venous hypertension. These ulcers, the most frequently occurring lower leg ulcers, are typically found around the ankle, as shown in the photo below.

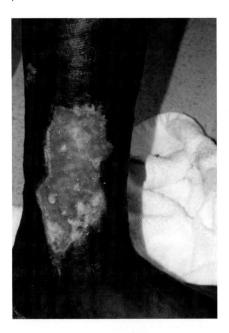

Lymphatic ulcers

Lymphatic ulcers result from lymphedema, in which the capillaries are compressed by thickened tissue, which occludes blood flow to the skin. Lymphatic ulcers are extremely difficult to treat because of this reduced blood flow. The photo below shows a patient with lymphedema of the leg and a large lymphatic ulcer.

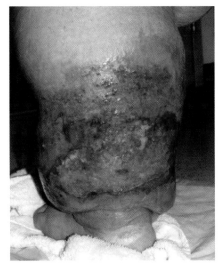

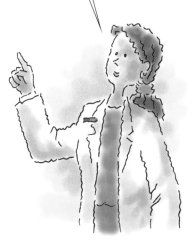

Note that vascular ulcers differ in appearance and severity, depending on the part of the vascular system that's affected.

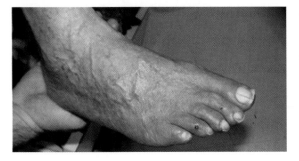

Arterial ulcers

Arterial ulcers result from insufficient blood flow to tissue due to arterial insufficiency. They're commonly found at the distal ends of arterial branches, especially at the tips of the toes, the corners of nail beds, or over bony prominences, as shown in the photo at left.

Pressure ulcers

You can use pressure ulcer characteristics gained from your assessment to stage a pressure ulcer, as described here. Staging reflects the anatomic depth of exposed tissue. Keep in mind that if the wound contains necrotic tissue, you won't be able to determine the stage until you can see the wound base.

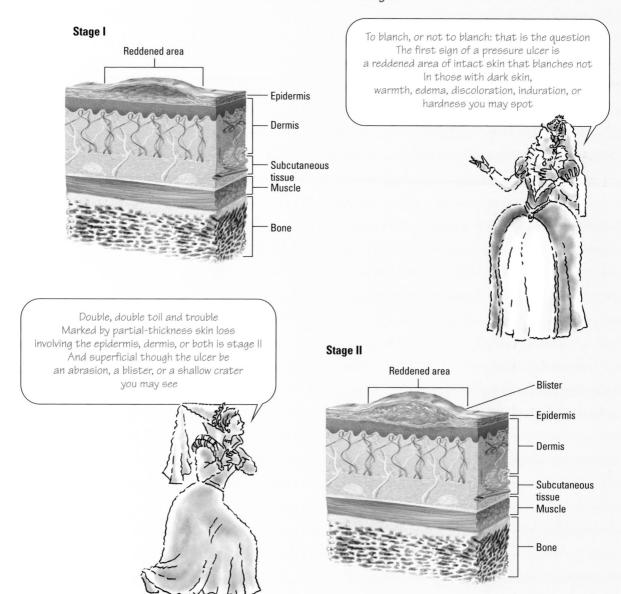

Welcome hither, and learn thee of pressure ulcer stages. As Shakespeare knew, all the world's a stage...

Stage I

Reddened area

— Epidermis

— Dermis

— Subcutaneous tissue
— Muscle

— Bone

To blanch, or not to blanch: that is the question
The first sign of a pressure ulcer is
a reddened area of intact skin that blanches not
In those with dark skin,
warmth, edema, discoloration, induration, or
hardness you may spot

Double, double toil and trouble
Marked by partial-thickness skin loss
involving the epidermis, dermis, or both is stage II
And superficial though the ulcer be
an abrasion, a blister, or a shallow crater
you may see

Stage II

Reddened area

— Blister

— Epidermis

— Dermis

— Subcutaneous tissue
— Muscle

— Bone

Stage III

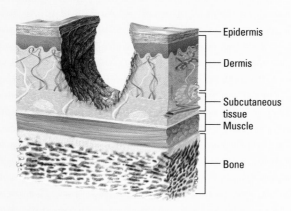

- Epidermis
- Dermis
- Subcutaneous tissue
- Muscle
- Bone

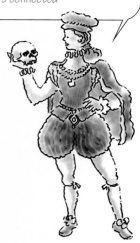

Now is the winter of our discontent
In stage III, the ulcer is a full-thickness wound
that appears like a deep crater when inspected
Underlying fasciae it may extend to
and thou might find undermining of the tissue
that's connected

That it should come to this!
As through the skin the ulcer extends,
damage to muscle, bone, and supporting structures
accompany necrosis of tissues
Alas, undermining and sinus tracts
may also be issues

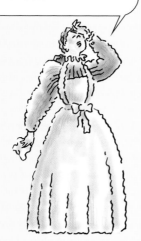

Stage IV

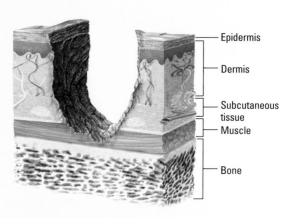

- Epidermis
- Dermis
- Subcutaneous tissue
- Muscle
- Bone

Parting is such sweet sorrow, that I shall say, "Go forth and provide
good wound care for all morrows!"

Diabetic foot ulcers

Because of the neurologic and vascular complications associated with diabetes, patients with this disorder are prone to foot ulcers. As with other pressure ulcers, diabetic foot ulcers typically develop over bony prominences when pressure is unrelieved.

This photo shows a patient with diabetes who has a pressure wound to the right lateral malleoli. Note the characteristic tissue changes associated with arterial insufficiency: thin, shiny skin; pale coloring; and muscular atrophy in the lower extremity.

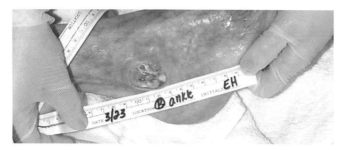

This photo shows a patient with type 2 diabetes who has developed a pressure ulcer from impaired protective sensation and poor mobility.

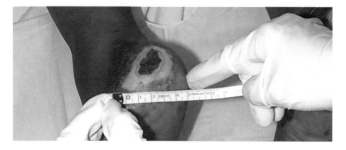

This photo shows a patient who has a diabetic foot ulcer on the plantar surface of the fifth metatarsal head. The circular shape of the wound is consistent with a wound created by pressure over a bony prominence.

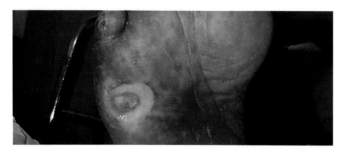

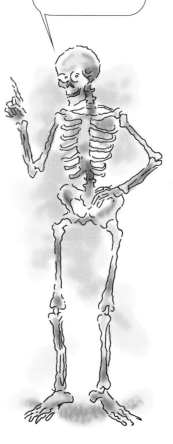

> Pressure over bony prominences can cause all sorts of problems. For patients who have diabetes, the feet are at greatest risk.

Acute wounds

As you know, three aspects are used to classify wounds and determine wound severity: age, depth, and color. Wound age is typically described as acute or chronic. Seems simple enough until you ask, "At what point does an acute wound become a chronic wound?" Time alone is not the distinguishing factor. Progress toward complete healing is also a component. Therefore, an acute wound is better characterized by these criteria:
- it's a new or relatively new wound
- it occurred suddenly (as opposed to developing over time)
- healing is progressing in a timely and predictable manner.

Intent or accident?

Acute wounds can occur by intention or trauma. A surgical incision is an example of an acute wound that's caused intentionally. Traumatic wounds can range from simple to severe. Burns are a category of traumatic wound that have a unique set of causes. Regardless of the cause, caring for a patient with an acute wound focuses on restoring normal anatomic structure, physiologic function, and appearance to the wound area.

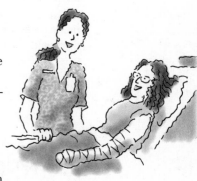

Surgical wounds typically respond well to postoperative care.

Surgical wound

An acute surgical wound is a healthy, uncomplicated break in the skin's continuity resulting from surgery. In an otherwise healthy individual, this type of wound responds well to postoperative care and heals without incident. Surgical wounds may be closed with sutures, staples, or adhesive skin closures.

Traumatic wound

A traumatic wound is a sudden, unplanned injury to the skin that can range from minor (such as a skinned knee) to severe (such as a gunshot wound). This category of wounds includes abrasions, lacerations, skin tears, bites, and penetrating trauma wounds.

Abrasions

Abrasions occur when a mechanical force, such as friction or shearing, scrapes away a partial thickness of the skin. Unless an unusually large amount of skin is involved or an infection develops, an abrasion is one of the least complicated traumatic wounds.

Lacerations

Lacerations are tears in the skin caused by a sharp object, such as metal, glass, or wood. They can also be caused by trauma that produces high shearing force. These wounds have jagged, irregular edges and their severity depends on the cause, size, depth, and location.

All about friction

Skin tears are a specific type of laceration that most commonly affects older adults. In a skin tear, friction alone — or shearing force plus friction — separate layers of skin. A partial-thickness wound occurs if the epidermis separates from the dermis. A full-thickness wound occurs if the epidermis and dermis separate from underlying tissue. This type of injury may be preventable through careful handling by members of the health care team. (See *Preventing skin tears.*)

Bites

When assessing a bite wound, it's important to quickly discover the bite's source — cat, dog, bat, snake, spider, human. This helps the health care team determine which bacteria or toxins may be present and the likely type of tissue trauma.

Preventing skin tears

As aging occurs, the skin becomes more prone to skin tear injuries. With a little effort and education, you can substantially reduce a patient's risk. Here are nine ways to prevent skin tears:
• Use proper lifting, positioning, transferring, and turning techniques to reduce or eliminate friction or shear.
• Pad support surfaces where risk is greatest, such as bed rails and limb supports on a wheelchair.
• Use pillows or cushions to support the patient's arms and legs.
• Tell the patient to add protection by wearing long-sleeved shirts and long pants, as weather permits.
• Use nonadhering dressings or those with minimal adherent, such as paper tape, and use a skin barrier wipe before applying dressings.
• Remove tape cautiously using the push-pull technique.
• Use wraps, such as a stockinette or soft gauze, to protect areas of skin where the risk of tearing is high.
• Tell the patient to avoid sudden or brusque movements that can pull the skin and possibly cause a skin tear.
• Apply skin lotion twice per day to areas at risk.

Hannibal the cannibal?

For example, a human bite can cause a puncture wound and introduce one of the innumerable organisms present in the human mouth into the wound. *Staphylococcus aureus* and streptococci are two such organisms that can be transmitted to the wound or into the victim's bloodstream. Other serious diseases that can be transmitted in this way include HIV infection, hepatitis B, hepatitis C, syphilis, and tuberculosis. Some evidence suggests that a human bite can also cause necrotizing fasciitis.

Animal house

A bite from a dog, cat, or rodent can introduce deadly infectious diseases, such as rabies, into the wound.

Penetrating trauma wounds

Penetrating trauma wounds are puncture wounds. This type of wound may be the result of an accident or a personal attack, as in the case of a stabbing or gunshot wound.

Be aware that bites from such animals as dogs, cats, and rabbits can cause rabies in addition to possible tissue damage.

Not so nice knife

Stab wounds are low-velocity wounds that generally present as classic puncture wounds or lacerations. In some cases, however, they may involve organ damage beneath the site of the wound. X-rays, computed tomography scanning, and magnetic resonance imaging are used to evaluate possible organ damage. If the weapon used is contaminated, the patient is at risk for, and should be treated for, local infection, sepsis, and tetanus.

Bullet wound blues

A gunshot wound is a high-velocity wound. Factors that affect the severity of tissue damage include the caliber of the weapon, the velocity of the projectile, and the patient's position at the time of injury.

In most cases, a small-caliber weapon firing a relatively low-velocity projectile creates a small, clean punctate lesion with little or no bleeding. If the projectile is no longer in the patient's body, treat this lesion as you would any other open wound.

A large-caliber, relatively high-velocity projectile typically causes massive tissue destruction, a large gaping wound, profuse bleeding and wound contamination. In this case, the patient usually requires immediate surgical intervention. After surgery, treat the wound as a surgical wound. (See *Caring for a traumatic wound*, page 440.)

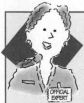

Advice from the experts

Caring for a traumatic wound

When treating a patient with a traumatic wound, always begin by assessing the ABCs: airway, breathing, and circulation. Move on to the wound itself only after ABCs are stable. Here are the basic steps to follow in caring for each type of traumatic wound.

Abrasion
• Flush the area of the abrasion with normal saline solution or wound cleaning solution.
• Use a sterile 4″ × 4″ gauze pad moistened with normal saline solution to remove dirt or gravel, and gently rub toward the entry point to work contaminants back out the way they entered.
• If the wound is extremely dirty, you may need to scrub it with a surgical brush. Be as gentle as possible and keep in mind that this is a painful process for your patient.
• Allow a small wound to dry and form a scab. Cover larger wounds with a nonadherent pad or petroleum gauze and a light dressing. Apply antibacterial ointment if ordered.

Laceration
• Moisten a sterile 4″ × 4″ gauze pad with normal saline solution or wound cleaning solution. Gently clean the wound, beginning at the center and working out to approximately 2″ (5 cm) beyond the edge of the wound. Whenever the pad becomes soiled, discard it and use a new one. Continue until the wound appears clean.
• If necessary, irrigate the wound using a 50-ml catheter-tip syringe and normal saline solution.

• Assist the doctor in suturing the wound if necessary. Apply sterile strips of porous tape if suturing isn't needed.
• Apply antibacterial ointment as ordered to prevent infection.
• Apply a dry sterile dressing over the wound to absorb drainage and help prevent bacterial contamination.

Bite
• Immediately irrigate the wound with copious amounts of normal saline solution. Don't immerse and soak the wound because this may allow bacteria to float back into the tissue.
• Clean the wound with sterile 4″ × 4″ gauze pads and an antiseptic solution such as povidone-iodine.
• Assist with debridement if ordered.
• Apply a loose dressing. If the bite is on an extremity, elevate it to reduce swelling.
• Ask the patient about the animal that bit him to determine whether there's a risk of rabies. Administer rabies and tetanus shots as needed.

Penetrating wound
• If the wound is minor, allow it to bleed for a few minutes before cleaning it. A larger puncture wound may require irrigation.
• Cover the wound with a dry dressing.
• If the wound contains an embedded foreign object, such as a shard of glass or metal, stabilize the object until the doctor can remove it. When the object is removed and bleeding is under control, clean the wound as you would a laceration.

Burns

Burns are acute wounds caused by exposure to thermal extremes, caustic chemicals, electricity, or radiation. The degree of tissue damage depends on the strength of the source and the duration of contact or exposure. (See *Visualizing burn depth*.)

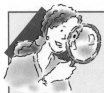

A closer look

Visualizing burn depth

The most widely used system of classifying burn depth and severity categorizes burns by degree. However, it's important to remember that most burns involve tissue damage of different degrees and thicknesses. This illustration may help you visualize burn damage at the various degrees.

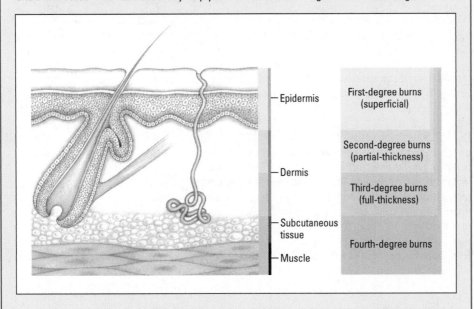

— Epidermis

— Dermis

— Subcutaneous tissue

— Muscle

First-degree burns (superficial)

Second-degree burns (partial-thickness)

Third-degree burns (full-thickness)

Fourth-degree burns

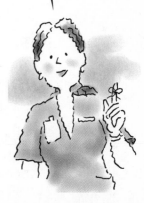

Remember, when determining burn severity, you must take into account not only the size of the wound but also the depth.

Thermal burns

Thermal burns, the most common type of burn, can result from virtually any misuse or mishandling of fire or a combustible product. Thermal burns can also result from kitchen accidents, house or office fires, automobile accidents, or physical abuse. Although less common, exposure to extreme cold can also cause a thermal burn.

Chemical burns

Chemical burns most commonly result from contact (skin contact or inhalation) with a caustic agent, such as an acid, an alkali, or a vesicant.

Biological dressings

Biological dressings function much like skin grafts, preventing infection and fluid loss and easing patient discomfort. However, biological dressings are only temporary measures; the body eventually rejects them. If the underlying wound hasn't healed, the dressing must be replaced with a graft of the patient's own skin. Here's a comparison of the four types of biological dressings and their uses.

Type and source	Use and duration	Special considerations
Amnion Made from amnion and chorionic membranes	Used to protect burns and to temporarily cover granulation tissue awaiting a graft. Must be changed every 48 hours.	• Apply only to clean wounds. • Leave open to the air or cover with a dressing.
Biosynthetic Woven from man-made fibers	Used to cover donor sites; protect clean, superficial burns and excised wounds awaiting grafts; and cover meshed grafts. Must be reapplied every 3 to 4 days.	• Don't remove to treat the wound. (Biosynthetic dressings are permeable to antimicrobials.)
Heterograft (xenograft) Harvested from animals (usually pigs)	Used to protect granulation tissue after escharotomy, protect excisions, serve as a test graft before skin grafting, and temporarily cover burns when the patient doesn't have sufficient skin for immediate grafting. Also used to cover meshed grafts, protect exposed tendons, and cover burns that are eschar-free and only slightly contaminated. This type is usually rejected in 7 to 10 days.	• Dress or leave open. • Watch for signs of rejection.
Homograft (allograft) Harvested from cadavers	Used for same purposes as a heterograft and is usually rejected in 7 to 10 days.	• Observe wound for exudate. • Watch for local and systemic signs of rejection.

Electrical burns

Electrical burns result from contact with flowing electrical current. Household current, high-voltage transmission lines, and lightning are sources of electrical burns.

Radiation burns

The most common radiation burn is sunburn, which follows excessive exposure to the sun. Almost all other burns due to radiation exposure occur as a result of radiation treatment or in specific industries that use or process radioactive materials.

Minor or severe?

Regardless of the type of burn, a minor burn may heal by itself without complications or extraordinary means. However, if the burn is severe, it may require skin grafting with biological dressings and prolonged hospitalization and rehabilitation may be necessary. (See *Biological dressings*.)

Vascular ulcers

The vascular system is composed of arteries, veins, capillaries, and lymphatics. Pressure from the beating heart carries blood away from the heart through the arteries into progressively smaller vessels until they connect with the capillaries. On the other side of the capillaries, small veins receive blood and pass it into progressively larger veins on its return trip to the heart. The lymphatic system is a separate system of vessels that collect waste products and deliver them to the venous system.

A group of disorders that affect the blood vessels outside the heart, or the lymphatic vessels, are known collectively as peripheral vascular disease (PVD). Vascular ulcers are chronic wounds that stem from PVD in the venous, arterial, and lymphatic systems. Venous and arterial ulcers are most common in the distal lower extremities, whereas lymphatic ulcers occur in the arms or the legs.

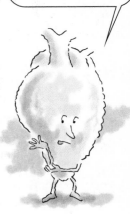

The cardiovascular system is complicated! Nearly 60,000 miles of arteries, arterioles, capillaries, venules, and veins keep blood circulating to and from every functioning cell in the body.

Venous ulcers

Venous ulcers, which result from venous hypertension, occur on the lower leg. They're most common in older adults, affecting 3.5% of the population over age 65. Venous ulcers account for 70% to 90% of all leg ulcers. (See *Signs of venous insufficiency*.)

Signs of venous insufficiency

In a patient with venous insufficiency, check for ulcerations around the ankle. Pulses are present but may be difficult to find if edema is present. The foot may become cyanotic when dependent.

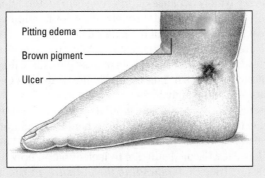

Pitting edema

Brown pigment

Ulcer

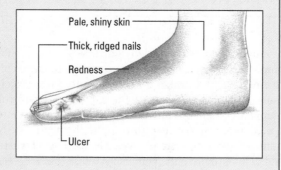

Signs of arterial insufficiency

Arterial ulcers most commonly occur in the area around the toes. In a patient with arterial insufficiency, the foot usually turns deep red when dependent and the nails may be thick and ridged. In addition, pulses may be faint or absent; the skin is cool, pale, and shiny; and the patient may report pain in his legs and feet.

Pale, shiny skin
Thick, ridged nails
Redness
Ulcer

Arterial ulcers

Arterial ulcers, which are also called *ischemic ulcers*, are the result of tissue ischemia due to arterial insufficiency. They can occur at the distal (farthest) end of any arterial branch, and they account for 5% to 20% of all leg ulcers. (See *Signs of arterial insufficiency*.)

Lymphatic ulcers

Lymphatic ulcers, which result from injury in the presence of lymphedema, occur most commonly on the arms and legs. Lymphedema leaves the skin vulnerable to infection and creates skin folds that trap moisture. These conditions cause ulcerations that become difficult to treat. (See *Dressings for vascular ulcers*.)

Pressure ulcers

Pressure ulcers are a serious health problem. Although incidence figures vary widely because of differences in methodology, setting, and subjects, data gathered through 10 years of nationwide studies reveal that 10% to 15% of the general population suffers from chronic pressure ulcers. Although this finding is significant in itself, prevalence in some groups — such as patients with spinal cord injuries, patients in intensive care units, and nursing home residents — is shockingly higher.

Pressure ulcers are chronic wounds resulting from tissue death due to prolonged, irreversible ischemia brought on by compression of soft tissue. Pressure ulcers are the clinical manifestation of localized tissue death due to lack of blood flow in areas under pressure. (See *Understanding the pressure gradient*, page 446.)

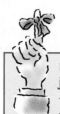

Memory jogger

To remember the five factors commonly used to determine a patient's risk of developing pressure ulcers, think of the 5 I's:

Immobility

Inactivity

Incontinence

Improper nutrition (malnutrition)

Impaired mental status or sensation.

Dressings for vascular ulcers

Choosing the best type of dressing for your patient's vascular ulcer depends not only on the ulcer type but also on its condition. The chart below lists indications and contraindications for each dressing according to ulcer type.

To use the chart, find the type of ulcer you're trying to dress and then look down the column for indications and contraindications for each dressing type. For example, the chart indicates that an alginate dressing can be used to manage copious drainage in a venous ulcer but isn't indicated for arterial ulcers.

Dressing	Indications and contraindications		
	Venous ulcers	*Arterial ulcers*	*Lymphatic ulcers*
Alginates	• Use to manage copious drainage.	• Not indicated	• Not indicated
Foam	• Use to protect the ulcer. • Use for absorption underneath a compression dressing.	• Use to protect the ulcer. • Use with dry gangrene. • Use for a moist, revascularized ulcer.	• Use to protect the ulcer. • Use to absorb drainage.
Gauze	• Use for absorption.	• Use for protection and to allow dry gangrene to maintain its dryness.	• Use for absorption or padding. (Don't allow to dry out on the ulcer.)
Hydrocolloids	• Use to promote granulation. • Use to manage pain. • Don't use when copious drainage is present.	• Use for autolytic debridement. • Use for primary dressing after revascularization. • Don't use on ischemic tissue.	• Use to protect the skin. • Use to promote epithelialization. • Don't use when copious drainage is present. • Don't use when cellulitis is present.
Hydrogel	• Don't use when copious drainage is present.	• Use to maintain a moist wound bed. • Use to debride.	• Use to manage pain. • Use to debride.
Transparent films	• Not indicated	• Use only after the ulcer is almost completely healed.	• Use to protect fragile skin. • Don't use when cellulitis is present.

Pressure ulcers are most common in areas where pressure compresses soft tissue over a bony prominence in the body — the tissue is pinched between the outer pressure and the hard underlying surface. Other factors that contribute to the problem include shearing, friction, and moisture.

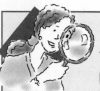

A closer look

Understanding the pressure gradient

In this illustration, the V-shaped pressure gradient results from the upward force exerted by the supporting surface and the downward force of the bony prominence. Pressure is greatest on tissues at the apex of the gradient, and lessens to the right and left of this point.

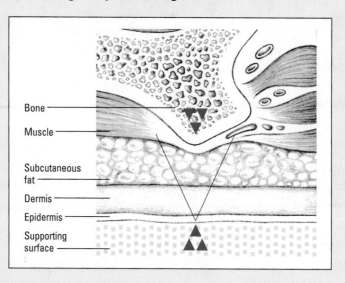

Bone

Muscle

Subcutaneous fat

Dermis

Epidermis

Supporting surface

Diabetic foot ulcers

Diabetes mellitus is a metabolic disorder characterized by hyperglycemia resulting from lack of insulin, lack of insulin effect, or both. High plasma glucose levels caused by diabetes can damage blood vessels and nerves. Therefore, patients with diabetes are prone to developing foot ulcers due to nerve damage and poor circulation to the lower extremities. Good diabetes control may help prevent these potentially chronic problems or make them less serious. (See *Keeping it toe-gether: Proper foot care.*)

Basic wound care procedures

Wound care orders are typically written by doctors, podiatrists, nurse practitioners, and physician assistants. However, policies and procedures related to skin and wound care activities are commonly written by and carried out by registered nurses. The doctor in charge reviews and approves these policies and procedures. Many facilities now have specific policies and procedures for different types of wounds.

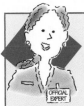

Advice from the experts

Keeping it toe-gether: Proper foot care

With proper skin care and frequent position changes, patients and their caregivers can keep the patient's skin healthy—a crucial element in pressure ulcer prevention. Here are some important do's and don'ts to pass along to patients.

Foot care
• Check feet daily for injury or pressure areas. (A long-handled mirror can help.)
• Wash feet with a mild soap and dry thoroughly between toes.
• Check bath water to make sure it isn't too hot. Test water with your elbow, if able. Otherwise, use a thermometer or ask a family member to help.
• Apply a moisturizing cream (such as Vaseline, which is cheap and effective) to prevent dry, cracking skin on the feet and to balance skin pH. Don't apply moisturizer between the toes.
• Cut toenails off squarely. See a podiatrist if they're dystrophic (deformed and thickened).
• Don't go barefooted—the risk of injury is too great.

Socks
• Use silver ion-lined socks for fungus control.
• Wear white or light-colored socks so that bleeding from trauma can be detected quickly.
• Wear natural fiber socks. They breathe better than synthetics.
• Wear socks that wick perspiration away from feet to prevent maceration.
• Use diabetic padded socks for shear and friction control.

Shoes
• Wear well-fitting shoes, not shoes that are too tight or loose.
• Wear shoes that breathe to reduce maceration and fungal infections.
• Wear new shoes for short periods (under 1 hour) each day initially. Gradually increase the time as your feet adjust.
• If deformities are present or you have a history of ulceration, wear professionally fitted shoes.
• If possible, wash shoes to destroy microorganisms.
• Check shoes before putting them on to make sure nothing fell in that could cause harm.

Basic wound care

Basic wound care centers on cleaning and dressing the wound. Because open wounds are colonized (or contaminated) with bacteria, observe clean technique using clean, nonsterile gloves during wound care unless sterile dressing changes are specified. Always follow standard precautions.

No need to keep it under wraps. Everyone should know that basic wound care involves cleaning and dressing the wound.

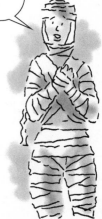

The goal of wound cleaning is to remove debris and contaminants from the wound without damaging healthy tissue. The wound should be cleaned initially; repeat cleaning as needed or before a new dressing is applied.

The basic purpose of a dressing, to provide an optimal environment in which the body can heal itself, should be considered before one is selected. Functions of a wound dressing include:
• protecting the wound from contamination and trauma
• providing compression if bleeding or swelling is anticipated

- applying medications
- absorbing drainage or debrided necrotic tissue
- filling or packing the wound
- protecting the skin surrounding the wound.

The cardinal rule is to keep moist tissue moist and dry tissue dry. Ideally, a dressing should keep the wound moist, absorb drainage or debris, conform to the wound, and be adhesive to surrounding skin yet also be easily removable. It should also be user-friendly, require minimal changes, decrease the need for a secondary dressing layer, and be cost-effective and comfortable for the patient.

What you need

Hypoallergenic tape or elastic netting ✳ overbed table ✳ piston-type irrigating system ✳ two pairs of gloves ✳ cleaning solution (such as normal saline solution) as ordered ✳ sterile gauze pads ✳ selected topical dressing ✳ linen-saver pads ✳ impervious plastic trash bag ✳ disposable wound-measuring device

Getting ready

Assemble the equipment at the patient's bedside. Use clean or sterile technique, depending on facility policy and wound care orders. Cut tape into strips for securing dressings. Loosen lids on cleaning solutions and medications for easy removal. Attach an impervious plastic trash bag to the overbed table to hold used dressings and refuse.

How you do it

Before a dressing change, wash your hands and review the principles of standard precautions.

Cleaning the wound

- Provide privacy and explain the procedure to the patient to allay his fears and promote cooperation.
- Position the patient in a way that maximizes his comfort while allowing easy access to the wound site.
- Cover bed linens with a linen-saver pad to prevent soiling.

No splashing

- Open the cleaning solution container and carefully pour cleaning solution into a bowl to avoid splashing. The bowl may be clean or sterile, depending on facility policy. (See *Choosing a cleaning agent.*)
- Open the packages of supplies.
- Put on gloves.

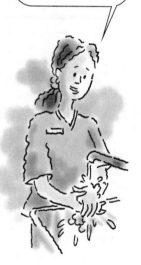

Before any dressing change, be sure to wash your hands. Follow standard precautions during the procedure.

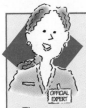

Advice from the experts

Choosing a cleaning agent

The most commonly used wound cleaning agent is sterile normal saline solution, which provides a moist environment, promotes granulation tissue formation, and causes minimal fluid shifts in healthy adults.

Antiseptic solutions may damage tissue and delay healing but are sometimes used for cleaning infected or newly contaminated wounds. Here are some examples of antiseptic solutions:

• *Hydrogen peroxide* (commonly used half-strength) irrigates the wound and aids in mechanical debridement. Its foaming action also warms the wound, promoting vasodilation and reducing inflammation.

• *Acetic acid* treats *Pseudomonas* infection.

• *Sodium hypochlorite* (Dakin's fluid) is an antiseptic that also slightly dissolves necrotic tissue. This unstable solution must be freshly prepared every 24 hours.

• *Povidone-iodine* is a broad-spectrum, fast-acting antimicrobial agent. Watch for patient sensitivity to this solution. Also, protect the surrounding skin from contact because this solution can dry and stain the skin.

• Gently roll or lift an edge of the soiled dressing to obtain a starting point. Support adjacent skin while gently releasing the soiled dressing from the skin. When possible, remove the dressing in the direction of hair growth.

• Discard the soiled dressing and your contaminated gloves in the impervious plastic trash bag to avoid contaminating the clean or sterile field.

• Put on a clean pair of gloves (sterile or nonsterile, depending on facility policy or the wound care order).

• Inspect the wound. Note the color, amount, and odor of drainage and necrotic debris.

• Fold a sterile gauze pad into quarters and grasp it with your fingers. Make sure the folded edge faces outward.

• Dip the folded gauze into the cleaning solution. Alternatively, use a wound cleaning solution in a spray gun bottle.

Circles on the skin

• When cleaning, be sure to move from the least-contaminated area to the most-contaminated area. For a linear shaped wound, such as an incision, gently wipe from top to bottom in one motion, starting directly over the wound and moving outward. For an open wound, such as a pressure ulcer, gently wipe in concentric circles, again starting directly over the wound and moving outward.

• Discard the gauze pad in the plastic trash bag.

• Using a clean gauze pad for each wiping motion, repeat the procedure until you've cleaned the entire wound.
• Dry the wound with gauze pads, using the same procedure as for cleaning. Discard the used gauze pads in the plastic trash bag.

Examining the wound

• Measure the perimeter of the wound with a disposable wound-measuring device (for example, a square, transparent card with concentric circles arranged in bull's-eye fashion and bordered with a straight-edge ruler). Measure the longest length and the widest width.
• Measure the depth of a full-thickness wound. Insert a sterile cotton-tipped applicator gently into the deepest part of the wound bed, and place a mark on the applicator where it meets the skin level. Measure the marked applicator to determine wound depth.
• Gently probe the wound bed and edges with your finger or a sterile cotton-tipped applicator to assess for wound tunneling or undermining. Tunneling usually signals wound extension along fascial planes. Gauge tunnel depth by determining how far you can insert your finger or the cotton-tipped applicator.
• Next, reassess the condition of the skin and wound. Note the character of the clean wound bed and the surrounding skin.
• If you observe adherent necrotic material, notify a wound care specialist or a doctor to ensure appropriate debridement.
• Prepare to apply the appropriate topical dressing. Instructions for applying topical moist saline gauze, hydrocolloid, transparent, alginate, foam, and hydrogel dressings follow.
• For other dressings or topical agents, follow your facility's protocol or the manufacturer's instructions.

Applying a moist saline gauze dressing

• Moisten the gauze dressing with normal saline solution. Wring out excess fluid.
• Gently place the dressing into the wound surface. To separate surfaces within the wound, gently guide the gauze between opposing wound surfaces. To avoid damage to tissues, don't pack the gauze tightly.
• To protect the surrounding skin from moisture, apply a sealant or barrier.
• Change the dressing often enough to keep the wound moist.

Applying a hydrocolloid dressing

• Choose a clean, dry, presized dressing, or cut one to overlap the wound by about 1″ (2.5 cm). Remove the dressing from its package, pull the release paper from the adherent side of the dressing, and apply the dressing to the wound. Hold the dressing in place with your hand. (The warmth will mold the dressing to the skin.)

Smooth operator

- As you apply the dressing, carefully smooth out wrinkles and avoid stretching the dressing.
- If the dressing's edges need to be secured with tape, apply a skin sealant to the intact skin around the wound. After the area dries, tape the dressing to the skin. The sealant protects the skin from tape burns and skin stripping and promotes tape adherence. Avoid using tension or pressure when applying the tape.
- Remove your gloves and discard them in the impervious plastic trash bag. Dispose of refuse according to facility policy, and wash your hands.
- Change a hydrocolloid dressing every 2 to 7 days as necessary. Change it immediately if the patient complains of pain, the dressing no longer adheres, or leakage occurs.

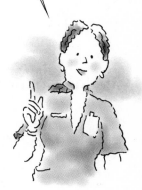

Carefully smooth out wrinkles as you apply the dressing to minimize irritation.

Applying a transparent dressing
- Clean and dry the wound as described above.
- Select a dressing to overlap the wound by 1″ to 2″ (2.5 to 5 cm).
- Gently lay the dressing over the wound; avoid wrinkling the dressing. To prevent shearing force, don't stretch the dressing over the wound. Press firmly on the edges of the dressing to promote adherence. Although this type of dressing is self-adhesive, you may have to tape the edges to prevent them from curling.
- Change the dressing every 3 to 5 days, depending on the amount of drainage. If the seal is no longer secure, or if accumulated tissue fluid extends beyond the edges of the wound and onto the surrounding skin, change the dressing.

Applying an alginate dressing
- Apply the alginate dressing to the wound surface. Cover the area with a secondary dressing (such as gauze pads or transparent film), as ordered. Secure the dressing with tape or elastic netting.
- If the wound is draining heavily, change the dressing once or twice daily for the first 3 to 5 days. As drainage decreases, change the dressing less frequently—every 2 to 4 days or as ordered. When the drainage stops or the wound bed looks dry, stop using alginate dressing.

Applying a foam dressing
- Gently lay the foam dressing over the wound.
- Use tape, elastic netting, or gauze to hold the dressing in place.
- Change the dressing when the foam no longer absorbs the exudate.

Applying a hydrogel dressing

• Apply a moderate amount of gel to the wound bed.
• Cover the area with a secondary dressing (gauze, transparent film, or foam).
• Change the dressing daily or as needed to keep the wound bed moist.
• If the hydrogel dressing you select comes in sheet form, cut the dressing to overlap the wound by 1″ (2.5 cm). Then apply it as you would a hydrocolloid dressing.
• Hydrogel dressings also come in a prepackaged, saturated gauze for wounds with cavities that require "dead space" to be filled. Follow the manufacturer's directions.

Practice pointers

• Be aware that infection may cause foul-smelling drainage, persistent pain, severe erythema, induration, and elevated skin and body temperatures. Advancing infection or cellulitis can lead to septicemia.
• Severe erythema may signal worsening cellulitis, which means the offending organisms have invaded the tissue and are no longer localized.

Irrigating wounds

Irrigation cleans tissues and flushes cell debris and drainage from an open wound. It also helps prevent premature surface healing over an abscess pocket or infected tract. After irrigation, pack open wounds to absorb additional drainage. Always follow the standard precaution guidelines of the Centers for Disease Control and Prevention (CDC).

What you need

Waterproof trash bag ✳ linen-saver pad ✳ emesis basin ✳ clean gloves ✳ sterile gloves, if indicated per facility policy ✳ goggles ✳ gown, if indicated ✳ prescribed irrigant such as sterile normal saline solution ✳ sterile water or normal saline solution ✳ soft rubber or plastic catheter ✳ sterile container ✳ materials as needed for wound care ✳ sterile irrigation and dressing set ✳ commercial wound cleaner ✳ 35-ml piston syringe with 19G needle or catheter ✳ skin protectant wipe (skin sealant) or other protective skin barrier

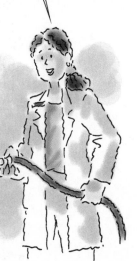

Irrigation cleans tissues and flushes away cell debris from an open wound.

Getting ready

Assemble equipment in the patient's room. Check the expiration date on each sterile package and inspect for tears. Don't use any solution that has been open longer than 24 hours. As needed, dilute the prescribed irrigant to the correct proportions with sterile water or normal saline solution. Allow the solution to reach room temperature, or warm it to 90° to 95° F (32.2° to 35° C). Open the waterproof trash bag and place it near the patient's bed. Form a cuff by turning down the top of the trash bag.

How you do it

• Check the doctor's order, assess the patient's condition, and identify allergies. Explain the procedure to the patient, provide privacy, and position the patient correctly for the procedure. Place the linen-saver pad under the patient, and place the emesis basin below the wound so that the irrigating solution flows from the wound into the basin.
• Wash your hands and put on a gown and gloves.
• Remove the soiled dressing; then discard the dressing and gloves in the trash bag.
• Establish a clean or sterile field with all the equipment and supplies you'll need for wound irrigation and dressing. Pour the prescribed amount of irrigating solution into a clean or sterile container. Put on a new pair of clean gloves and a gown and goggles, if indicated.

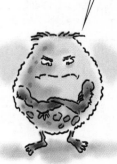

If you aren't careful during irrigation, my pathogenic friends and I will run rampant.

From clean to dirty

• Fill the syringe with the irrigating solution and connect the catheter to the syringe. Gently instill a slow, steady stream of solution into the wound until the syringe empties. Make sure the solution flows from the clean to the dirty area of the wound to prevent contamination of clean tissue by exudate. Also make sure the solution reaches all areas of the wound.
• Refill the syringe, reconnect it to the catheter, and repeat the irrigation. Continue to irrigate the wound until you've administered the prescribed amount of solution or until the solution returns clear. Note the amount of solution administered. Then remove and discard the catheter and syringe in the waterproof trash bag. (See *Wound irrigation tips*, page 454.)

Positioned for success

• Keep the patient positioned to allow further wound drainage into the basin.
• Clean the area around the wound with normal saline solution and pat dry with gauze; wipe intact surrounding skin with a skin protectant wipe, and allow it to dry.

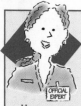

Advice from the experts

Wound irrigation tips

How can you avoid mess or spillage when irrigating a wound in a hard-to-reach location? Here are some tips you can follow.

Limb wounds
An arm or leg wound may be soaked in a large vessel of warm irrigating fluid, such as water, normal saline solution, or an appropriate antiseptic. An agitator can help dislodge bacteria and loosen debris.

If possible, rinse the wound several times, and carefully dispose of the contaminated liquid. Reserve the equipment you used for that particular patient. Dry and store it after soaking it in disinfectant.

Trunk or thigh wounds
Because they're difficult to irrigate, trunk or thigh wounds require some ingenuity. One device uses Stomahesive and a plastic irrigating chamber applied over the wound. (Run warm solution through an infusion set and collect it in a drainage bag.)

A syringe irrigation is another alternative. Where possible, direct the flow at right angles to the wound, and allow the fluid to drain by gravity. Doing so requires careful positioning of the patient in bed or on a chair. The patient may need analgesia during the treatment.

If irrigation isn't possible, you'll have to swab-clean the wound, which is time-consuming. Swab away exudate before using antiseptic or saline solution to clean the wound, taking care not to push loose debris into the wound. Facility policy permitting, use sharp scissors to snip off loose dead tissue—never pull it off.

• Pack the wound lightly and loosely if ordered, and apply a dressing.
• Remove and discard your gloves and gown.
• Make sure the patient is comfortable.
• Dispose of drainage, solutions, trash bag, and soiled equipment and supplies according to facility policy and CDC guidelines.

Practice pointers

• Try to coordinate wound irrigation with the doctor's visit so that he can inspect the wound.
• Irrigate with a bulb syringe if the wound is small or not particularly deep, or if a piston syringe is unavailable. However, use a bulb syringe cautiously because this type of syringe doesn't deliver enough pressure to adequately clean the wound.

Debriding wounds

Debridement of nonviable tissue is the most important factor in wound management. Wound healing can't take place until necrotic tissue is removed. Necrotic tissue may appear as moist yellow or gray tissue that's separating from viable tissue. If this moist, necrotic tissue becomes dry, it appears as thick, hard, leathery black eschar. Areas of necrotic tissue may mask underlying fluid collections or abscesses. Although debridement can be painful (especially with burns), it's necessary to prevent infection and promote healing of burns and other wounds.

Types of debridement

Debridement of necrotic tissue may be accomplished by sharp, autolytic, chemical, or mechanical techniques.

Sharp debridement

Sharp debridement, which is categorized as *conservative* or *surgical*, involves removing necrotic tissue from the wound bed with the use of a cutting tool, such as a scalpel, scissors, or a laser. Conservative sharp debridement involves the removal of necrotic tissue only and is usually done by a doctor, a physician assistant, an advanced practice nurse, or another certified wound specialist. It involves careful prying and cutting of loosened eschar with forceps and scissors to separate it from viable tissue beneath. One of the most painful types of debridement, conservative sharp debridement may require topical or systemic analgesic administration.

Eschar-go

Surgical sharp debridement involves the removal of necrotic and healthy tissue, converting a chronic wound to a clean, acute wound. Surgical sharp debridement is typically beyond the practice of nonphysician providers. Caution should be used when performing conservative or surgical sharp debridement on patients who have low platelet counts or who are taking anticoagulants.

Because you're more likely to be involved in the process of mechanical debridement and conservative sharp debridement, these procedures are covered here in detail.

Autolytic debridement

Autolytic debridement involves the use of moisture-retentive dressings to cover the wound bed. Necrotic tissue is then dissolved through self-digestion of enzymes in the wound fluid. Although autolytic debridement takes longer than other debridement methods, it isn't painful, it's easy to do, and it's appropriate for patients who can't tolerate any other method. If the wound is infected, autolytic debridement isn't the treatment of choice.

Chemical debridement

Chemical debridement with enzymatic agents is a selective method of debridement. Enzymes are applied topically to areas of necrotic tissue only, breaking down necrotic tissue elements. En-

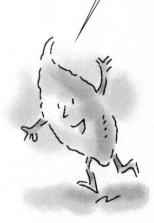

In autolytic debridement, moisture-retentive dressings are placed over the wound and necrotic tissue dissolves in the wound fluid.

zymes digest only necrotic tissue — they don't harm healthy tissue. These agents require specific conditions that vary from product to product. Effectiveness is achieved by carefully following each manufacturer's guidelines. Stop using the enzymes when the wound is clean and has red granulation tissue.

Mechanical debridement

Mechanical debridement includes wet-to-dry dressings, irrigation, and hydrotherapy. Wet-to-dry dressings, typically used for wounds with extensive necrotic tissue and minimal drainage, require an appropriate technique and the dressing materials used are critical to the outcome. The nurse or doctor places a wet dressing in contact with the lesion and covers it with an outer layer of bandaging. As the dressing dries, it sticks to the wound. When the dried dressing is removed, the necrotic tissue comes off with it.

Irrigation of a wound with a pressurized antiseptic solution cleans tissue and removes wound debris and excess drainage.

Hydrotherapy — commonly referred to as *tubbing*, *tanking*, or *whirlpool* — involves placing the patient or just the affected body part in a tank of warm water, with intermittent agitation of the water. It's usually performed on large wounds with a significant amount of nonviable tissue covering the wound surface.

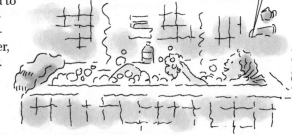

In hydrotherapy, the patient is immersed in a tank of warm water. Where's my rubber ducky?

What you need

Ordered pain medication ✳ two pairs of sterile gloves ✳ two gowns or aprons ✳ mask ✳ cap ✳ sterile scissors ✳ sterile forceps ✳ sterile 4″ × 4″ gauze pads ✳ sterile solutions and medications as ordered ✳ hemostatic agent as ordered

Hemorrhage emergency

Also have the following equipment immediately available to control bleeding: needle holder ✳ gut suture with needle.

How you do it

• Explain the procedure to the patient to allay his fears and promote cooperation. Teach him distraction and relaxation techniques, if possible, to minimize his discomfort.
• Provide privacy. Per orders, administer an analgesic 20 minutes before debridement begins, or give an I.V. analgesic immediately before the procedure.

Wet-to-dry dressings

• Put on clean nonsterile gloves.

• Slowly and gently remove the old dressing, using saline solution to moisten portions of the dressing that don't easily pull away. Discard the old dressing and gloves in a waterproof trash bag.
• Put on clean gloves.
• Using sterile technique, moisten an open-weave cotton gauze dressing with saline solution and loosely pack it into the wound. Make sure the entire wound surface is lightly covered with moistened gauze.
• Apply an outer dressing and secure it with tape or an adhesive bandage.
• Remove the dressing after it completely dries and becomes adherent to the necrotic tissue (typically in 4 to 6 hours).

Irrigation
• Use sterile technique to instill a slow, steady stream of solution into the wound with an irrigating syringe or catheter. (For more information, see the irrigation procedure earlier in this chapter.)

Hydrotherapy
• Prepare the tub and obtain the patient's vital signs.
• Assist the patient into the tub.
• After the affected body part has been placed in the swirling water for the prescribed amount of time (10 to 20 minutes), put on clean gloves, remove the old dressings, and discard all items in a waterproof trash bag.
• Spray rinse and pat dry the patient before reapplying sterile dressings.

Conservative sharp debridement
• Keep the patient warm. Expose only the area to be debrided to prevent chilling and fluid and electrolyte loss.
• Wash your hands and put on clean gloves.
• Remove the wound dressings and clean the wound.
• Remove your dirty gloves and change into sterile gloves.
• Lift loosened edges of eschar with sterile forceps. Holding the necrotic tissue taut with the forceps, visualize where to cut. Cut the dead tissue from the wound with the scissors.
• Irrigate the wound.

Slim to none

• Because debridement removes only dead tissue, bleeding should be minimal. If bleeding occurs, apply gentle pressure on the wound with sterile 4″ × 4″ gauze pads. Then apply the hemostatic agent. If bleeding persists, notify the doctor and maintain pressure on the wound. Excessive bleeding or spurting vessels may warrant ligation.

• Perform additional procedures, such as application of topical medications and dressing replacements, as ordered.

Practice pointers

• Acknowledge the patient's discomfort and provide pain control and emotional support.
• Work quickly — with an assistant if possible — to complete this painful procedure as quickly as possible. Try to limit procedure time to 20 minutes. Serial debridement may be necessary to rid the wound of necrotic tissue.

Wound care products

When selecting wound care products for your patient, let the findings of a thorough assessment guide your product selection. (See *Product selection: Let the big picture be your guide.*)

New products arrive almost daily, and others are updated or improved regularly. Because the quality of the care that you provide depends on your level of knowledge, it's imperative that you stay up-to-date by periodically reviewing the products available.

> The abundance of commercially prepared dressings and adjunct products — and the fact that many have similar names and functions — can make choosing the right product a daunting task.

Wound dressings

If we held a wound dressing endurance contest, gauze would win hands-down. Gauze has been a core wound dressing for more years than any other material. However, as medical research has afforded a better understanding of wounds and the healing process, medical manufacturers have developed new materials and sophisticated dressing options that better promote healing.

Moisture level, tissue adherence, infection control, and wound dimensions are just some of the factors that affect wound dressing selection. The level of moisture in the wound bed is critical to the success or failure of healing. Consequently, one fundamental way to classify dressings is by their effect on wound moisture. In other words, do they add, absorb, or not affect wound moisture? (See *Dressing for the occasion*, page 460.)

Gauze but not forgotten

Although gauze remains a good choice for secondary dressings, it no longer represents the most effective choice for a primary dressing. Let's take a close look at the dressings you'll use when providing wound care.

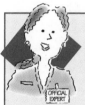

Advice from the experts

Product selection: Let the big picture be your guide

When selecting wound care products, let the big picture guide your choices. Ask yourself these important questions.

• Which companies have contracts to supply wound care products to your facility? (Learn about these products first.)

• What's the simplest method of closing the wound? Which is most cost-effective?

• Can the patient afford the supplies he needs? (Simple and affordable aren't necessarily synonymous.) If not, is financial assistance available?

• Who provides wound care at home? If the patient can't perform this important task, can family members or friends? Is home health care an option? If so, is the patient eligible?

• What caused the wound, and how can the cause best be alleviated? (Answering this question is especially important when treating chronic wounds; less so when treating acute wounds.)

• How often does the dressing need to be changed? (It takes several hours—figure at least 8 hours—for a wound to achieve homeostasis after a dressing change. Therefore, less often is better.)

• How much drainage is present?

• Does the wound need more moisture?

• Should the wound be debrided? If so, which method is best for the patient?

• After cleaning and drying, does the wound (not the dressing) have an unpleasant odor? Do you suspect infection? If so, is a culture warranted?

• Is there tunneling, undermining, or a cavity that needs to be filled?

• Are the wound edges open or closed? (Wound edges must be open for complete healing to occur.)

• How large is the wound? Would it be more cost-effective to use an advanced wound care product to facilitate granulation tissue or closure?

Alginate dressings

Made from seaweed, these nonwoven, absorptive dressings are available as soft, white, sterile pads or ropes. Alginate dressings absorb excessive exudate and may be used on infected wounds. As the dressing absorbs exudate, it turns into a gel that keeps the wound bed moist and promotes healing. Alginates are also nonadhesive and nonocclusive, and they promote autolysis. Examples of alginate products include AlgiSite M, KALTOSTAT Wound Dressing, Maxorb CMC/Alginate Dressing, and Sorbsan Topical Wound Dressing.

Worth their weight in fluid

Alginate dressings are used on wounds with moderate to heavy drainage as they hold 7 to 10 times their own weight in fluid. They may be cut to fit wound dimensions and may be layered for more absorption. They also come in ropes that are useful for deep wound packing.

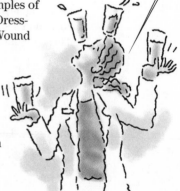

Try absorbing this! Alginate dressings are good for wounds with moderate to heavy drainage because they can hold 7 to 10 times their own weight in fluid.

Dressing for the occasion

Some dressings absorb moisture from a wound bed, whereas others add moisture to it. Use the chart below to quickly determine the category of dressing that's appropriate for your patient.

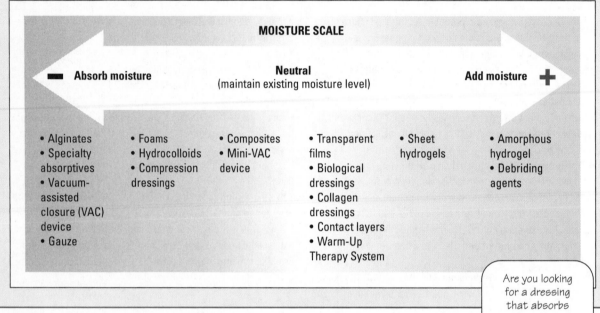

MOISTURE SCALE

— **Absorb moisture**   **Neutral**
(maintain existing moisture level)   **Add moisture** +

• Alginates • Specialty absorptives • Vacuum-assisted closure (VAC) device • Gauze	• Foams • Hydrocolloids • Compression dressings	• Composites • Mini-VAC device	• Transparent films • Biological dressings • Collagen dressings • Contact layers • Warm-Up Therapy System	• Sheet hydrogels	• Amorphous hydrogel • Debriding agents

> Are you looking for a dressing that absorbs moisture? Check out the piece above!

Biological dressings

Biological dressings are temporary dressings that function similarly to skin grafts. They may be made from amnionic or chorionic membranes, woven from manmade fibers, harvested from animals (usually pigs), or harvested from cadavers. These dressings are good only for temporary use because the body eventually rejects them. If rejection occurs before the underlying wound heals, the dressing must be replaced with a skin graft. Examples of biological dressings include Hyalofill Biopolymeric Wound Dressing, Inerpan, and Oasis.

What's the use?

Biological dressings should be used as temporary dressings for skin grafting donor sites and burns. The biggest advantage of biological dressings is that they can shorten healing times. They also prevent infection and fluid loss and ease patient discomfort.

Collagen dressings

Collagen dressings, which are made with bovine or avian collagen, accelerate wound healing by encouraging the organization of new collagen fibers and granulation tissue. Examples include FIBRA-COL PLUS Collagen Wound Dressing with Alginate and Kollagen-Medifil Pads.

For the clean, chronic kind

Collagen dressings should be used on chronic, nonhealing, granulated wound beds. They're available in gel, granule, and sheet forms. Some also contain alginate. These dressings are effective on chronic, clean wounds.

Composite dressings

Composite dressings are hybrids that combine two or more types of dressings into one. For example, a three-layer composite dressing can include a bacterial barrier; an absorbent foam, a hydrocolloid, or a hydrogel layer; and an adherent or a nonadherent outer layer. Examples of composite dressings include Alldress, Comp-Dress Island Dressing, COVADERM Plus, MPM Multi-Layered Dressing, and TELFA PLUS Island Dressing.

Composite sketch

Composite dressings can be used as the primary or secondary dressings on wounds with light to moderate drainage. They can also be used to protect peripheral and central I.V. lines. Composite dressings are all-in-one dressings that come in various combinations, depending on the patient's wound care needs. They are available in multiple sizes and shapes.

Contact layer dressings

Contact layer dressings are single layers of woven or perforated material suitable for direct contact with the wound's surface. The nonadherent contact layer prevents other dressings from sticking to the surface of the wound. Examples include Conformant 2 Wound Veil, Mepitel, Profore Wound Contact Layer, and Telfa Clear.

We have contact!

A contact layer dressing is used to allow the flow of drainage to a secondary dressing while preventing that dressing from adhering to the wound. On the plus side, contact layer dressings decrease the pain experienced during dressing changes. They can also be cut to fit or overlap the wound edges.

Foam dressings

Foam dressings are spongelike polymer dressings that provide a moist wound environment. These dressings are somewhat absorptive and may include an adhesive border. Examples of foam dressing include Allevyn Cavity Wound Dressing, CarraSmart Foam Dressing, Hydrasorb Foam Wound Dressing, Mepilex, PolyTube Tube-Site Dressing, and Tielle Plus Hydropolymer Dressing.

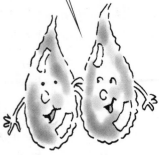

Foam dressings provide a moist wound environment.

Nonstick coating

Use a foam dressing as a primary or secondary dressing on wounds with minimal to moderate drainage (including around tubes) when a nonadherent surface is important. Those with an adhesive border don't require a secondary dressing. However, foam dressings may be used in combination with other products Hydropolymer foam dressings can manage heavier drainage as they wick moisture from the wound and allow evaporation.

Hydrocolloid dressings

Hydrocolloid dressings are adhesive, moldable wafers made of a carbohydrate-based material. Most have a waterproof backing. They're impermeable to oxygen, water, and water vapor, and most hydrocolloid dressings provide some degree of absorption. These dressings turn to gel as they absorb moisture, help maintain a moist wound bed, and promote autolytic debridement. Examples of hydrocolloid dressings include BandAid Advanced Healing Bandages (available over-the-counter), DuoDERM CGF, Restore Cx Wound Care Dressing, and 3M Tegasorb Hydrocolloid Dressing.

Calling all hydrocolloids

Hydrocolloid dressings should be used for wounds with minimal to moderate drainage, including wounds with necrosis or slough. Hydrocolloid sheet dressings may also be used as secondary dressings. They're beneficial because they don't stick to a moist wound base and maintain moisture by becoming gel as they absorb drainage. They may require changing only two to three times each week and can be easily removed from the wound base. They're available in contoured forms, in several varieties (sheets, powder, or gel), and in thin and traditional thickness.

Hydrogel dressings

Hydrogel dressings are water- or glycerin-based polymer dressings. They're nonadherent, provide limited absorption (some are 96% water themselves), and come as tubes of gel or in flexible sheets. Hydrogel dressings add moisture and promote autolytic debridement. Examples include Aquasorb Hydrogel Wound Dressing, Carrasyn Gel Wound Dressing with Acemannan Hydrogel, CURASOL Gel Wound Dressing, Hypergel, Phyto Derma Wound Gel, SAF-Gel Hydrating Dermal Wound Dressing, and TOE-AID Toe and Nail Dressing.

Say gel-lo to hydrogel dressings

Hydrogel dressings should be used on dry wounds or wounds with minimal drainage. One advantage of hydrogel dressings is that they come in sheet or amorphous gel form. In addition, when applied, they may provide cooling that soothes and eases pain.

Specialty absorptive dressings

Specialty absorptive dressings have multiple layers of a highly absorbent material, such as cotton or rayon, and may have adhesive borders. Various forms are available, including gels, pads, gauze, or pillows. Examples include AQUACEL, BreakAway Wound Dressing, Sofsorb Wound Dressing, and TENDERSORB WET-PRUF Abdominal Pads.

For a heavy order

A specialty absorptive dressing should be used on infected or non-infected wounds with heavy drainage. The advantages of specialty absorptive dressings are that they're highly absorptive, require less frequent changes (in most cases), and are available in a variety of forms.

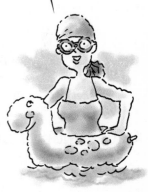

As their name suggests, specialty absorptive dressings are made for wounds with heavy drainage.

Transparent film dressings

Transparent film dressings are clear, adherent, nonabsorptive, polyurethane dressings. They're semipermeable to oxygen and water vapor, but not to water itself. Transparency allows visual inspection of the wound while the dressing is in place. Transparent film dressings maintain a moist wound environment and promote autolysis. Examples of transparent film dressings include BIO-CLUSIVE Transparent Dressing, BlisterFilm, ClearSite Transparent Membrane, OpSite FLEXIGRID, 3M NexCare Waterproof Bandages (available over-the-counter), and 3M Tegaderm Transparent Dressing.

A clear view

Transparent film dressings should be used on partial-thickness wounds with minimal exudate and on wounds with eschar to promote autolysis. Transparent film dressings may require less frequent changes and allow you to see the wound without removing the dressing. In addition, they're adherent but won't stick to the wound and aren't bulky. Transparent film dressings don't absorb drainage, so they should be used only on partial-thickness wounds with minimal exudate.

Wound fillers

As the name suggests, wound fillers are specialized dressings used to fill deeper wounds. They're made of various materials and come in many forms, such as pastes, granules, powders, beads, and gels. Wound fillers can add moisture to the wound bed or absorb drainage, depending on the product. Examples include Acry-Derm STRANDS Absorbent Wound Filler, Bard Absorption Dressing, Catrix Wound Dressing, and Multidex Maltodextrin Wound Dressing Gel or Powder.

Packing material

Wound filler can be used as a primary dressing on an infected or a noninfected wound with minimal to moderate drainage that requires packing. These dressings come in various forms and absorptive abilities. Wound fillers can't be used on third-degree burns, dry wounds, or wounds with tunnels and sinuses.

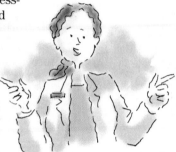

Wound fillers can go both ways. Some add moisture to the wound bed while others absorb drainage.

Adjunct wound care products

An entire universe of topical skin and wound care aids is available to complement the function of dressings. Because a comprehensive listing would require several companion volumes, we'll limit our discussion to several categories of products and devices that directly impact a wound's ability to heal.

Provant Wound Closure System

The Provant Wound Closure System is a noninvasive treatment that stimulates healing. A treatment signal is directed $2\frac{3}{4}''$ to $3\frac{1}{8}''$ (7 to 8 cm) into the tissues around the wound to induce the proliferation of fibroblasts and epithelial cells as well as the secretion of multiple growth factors. The result is faster healing. Treatment doesn't require removal of existing dressings. Clinical studies indicate that the Provant system is effective in promoting healing, even in cases of chronic, severe pressure ulcers.

A system in place

The Provant system is beneficial to wounds in the inflammatory phase of healing. It requires no special training (patients may be able to perform therapy at home) and requires only two 30-minute treatments per day (duration is pre-set in the device so it turns off automatically at the end of a session). In addition, it may be used over existing dressings.

Vacuum-assisted closure device

The vacuum-assisted closure (VAC) device uses negative air pressure to promote wound closure. This system consists of a special open-cell polyurethane ether foam dressing cut to the size of the wound, a vacuum tube, and a vacuum pump. One end of the vacuum tube is embedded in the foam dressing and the other connects to the vacuum pump. The dressing is sealed securely in place with adhesive tape that extends 1½″ to 2″ (3 to 5 cm) over adjacent skin all around the dressing. When turned on, the pump gently reduces air pressure beneath the dressing, drawing off exudate and reducing edema in surrounding tissues. This process reduces bacterial colonization, promotes granulation tissue development, increases the rate of cell mitosis, and spurs the migration of epithelial cells within the wound. Special training is required to operate this device. (See *Understanding VAC therapy*.)

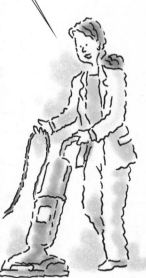

Suck this up! The VAC device aids healing by removing infectious drainage, promoting granulation tissue formation, and drawing wounds closed.

Understanding VAC therapy

Vacuum-assisted closure (VAC) therapy, also called *negative pressure wound therapy,* is an option to consider when a wound fails to heal in a timely manner. VAC therapy encourages healing by applying localized subatmospheric pressure at the site of the wound, as shown below. This pressure reduces edema and bacterial colonization and stimulates the formation of granulation tissue.

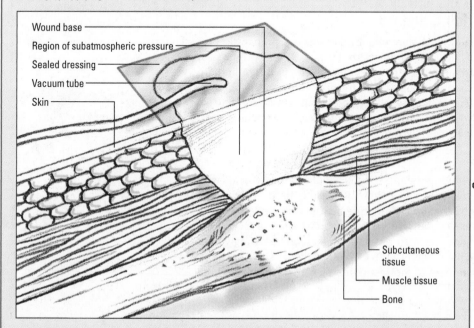

Wound base
Region of subatmospheric pressure
Sealed dressing
Vacuum tube
Skin

Subcutaneous tissue
Muscle tissue
Bone

Keeping cavities clean

VAC therapy is useful in managing slow-healing acute, subacute, or chronic exudative wounds with cavities. It's ideal for pressure ulcers or surgical wounds with depths greater than 1 cm.

Warm-Up Therapy System

The Warm-Up Therapy System for wounds, or *noncontact normothermic wound therapy*, is a temporary therapy that increases the temperature of the wound bed, thereby promoting increased blood flow in the area of the wound. The dressing in this system contains a special electronic warming card. Once in place, the card heats to 100.4° F (38° C), bathing the wound in radiant heat. The closely sealed wound covering promotes a moist environment in the wound bed. This system is designed to remain in place for 72 hours.

Warming up to the Warm-Up System

The Warm-Up Therapy System may be used for acute or chronic, full- or partial-thickness wounds, regardless of etiology, that have failed to thrive with traditional therapies, including wounds with compromised blood flow, such as arterial or diabetic foot ulcers. The wound covering can absorb a small to moderate amount of drainage.

Debriding agents

Debriding agents are chemical or enzyme preparations used to debride necrotic or devitalized tissues. These products are applied directly to the offending tissues in the wound. In wounds containing eschar, the eschar is crosshatched so the agent can penetrate the tissue. Examples of debriding agents include ACCUZYME, Collagenase Santyl Ointment, and PANAFIL.

Here comes debride

These products should be used in debriding wounds with moderate to large amounts of necrotic tissue, especially in cases where surgical debridement isn't an option. Some products contain chlorophyll, which helps control odor. (Drainage may turn green, however, and be wrongly interpreted as infection.) Effective debridement requires only a small amount of the agent; more isn't necessarily better.

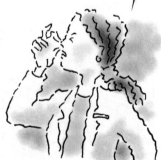

The chlorophyll found in some debriding agents helps to control wound odor.

Other treatment options

Some old and new therapeutic methods widely embraced by today's wound care practitioners are:
- biotherapy (growth factors, living skin equivalents)
- hydrotherapy (pulsatile lavage, whirlpool)
- therapeutic light (UV treatment, laser therapy)
- ultrasound
- electrical stimulation
- hyperbaric oxygen.

Biotherapy

Two biotherapy methods used in wound treatment include growth factors and living skin equivalents.

Growth factors

Because of the important role that growth factors play in the healing process (stimulating cell proliferation), they're one important form of biotherapy currently used.

The master factor

In the past decade, growth factors have been studied to determine exactly how they function in healing and how they may be used in the treatment of chronic wounds. Particular focus has been placed on platelet-derived growth factor (PDGF), which some experts call the *master factor*. Although the specific growth factor or other mechanism that initiates wound healing isn't known, PDGF is known to play a central role by attracting fibroblasts and inducing them to divide. The presence of fibroblasts is central to wound healing because they're responsible for collagen formation and are one of the components of granulation tissue.

A few more factors

Other key growth factors that play roles in wound healing include:
- *transforming growth factor beta (TGF-β)*, which controls movement of cells to sites of inflammation and stimulates extracellular matrix formation
- *basic fibroblast growth factor (bFGF)*, which stimulates angiogenesis (the development of blood vessels)
- *vascular endothelial growth factor (VEGF)*, which stimulates angiogenesis
- *insulin-like growth factor (IGF)*, which increases collagen synthesis

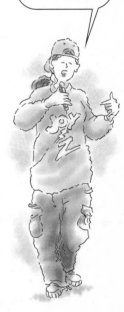

Yo, yo, yo. I say that PDGF is the master factor, dawg!

• *epidermal growth factor (EGF)*, which stimulates epidermal regeneration.

Growth factors on trial

Of these growth factors, PDGF, TGF-β, bFGF, and EGF have been through or are undergoing testing in clinical trials. At this time, the only synthetic growth factor approved for use in wound care is becaplermin (Regranex Gel 0.01%), which has a biological activity similar to that of endogenous PDGF. Regranex increases wound closure by 43%. It's recommended for use on lower-extremity diabetic neuropathic ulcers that have adequate blood flow and involve tissues at and below the subcutaneous level.

A put-on

Regranex can be applied to wounds using a sterile applicator, such as a swab, tongue blade, or saline-moistened gauze. A dime-size thickness of Regranex is all that's needed. The wound can then be dressed with a saline-moistened gauze.

Living skin equivalents

Living skin equivalents are living constructs derived from biological substances such as bovine collagen and human neonatal foreskin. Two living skin equivalents approved by the Food and Drug Administration in the United States are Dermagraft and graftskin (Apligraf). Dermagraft is used in treating patients with partial-thickness burns and diabetic foot ulcers. Apligraf is approved for use in venous and diabetic foot ulcers. All living skin equivalents should be used on wounds that are free from infection and necrosis, and have adequate blood flow to support healing.

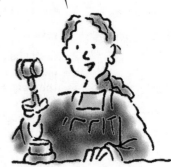

On trial today are the growth factors PDGF, TGF-β, bFGF, and EGF. Only becaplermin — a substance similar to PDGF — has been approved for use in wound care.

One singular solution

Dermagraft is a dermal substitute and, as such, is a single layer composed of human neonatal fibroblasts seeded on a polyglactin mesh (dissolvable suture material). The fibroblasts secrete and fill in this mesh with extracellular matrix. Dermagraft is contraindicated for use on clinically infected wounds and wounds with sinus tracks and in individuals with known allergies to bovine products.

A two-layered solution

Apligraf is a bilayered skin substitute consisting of an epidermal layer and a dermal layer. The dermal layer is composed of type 1 collagen and human neonatal fibroblasts; the epidermal layer is formed from human keratinocytes (the epidermal cells that synthesize keratin).

When applied to venous ulcers, Apligraf is used along with standard compression therapy. For a patient with diabetic foot ulcers, appropriate off-loading devices are also used.

Contraindications for Apligraf include use on wounds that are infected and use in individuals with known allergies to bovine collagen or other components in the medium in which Apligraf is shipped.

Hydrotherapy

Hydrotherapy, one of the oldest therapeutic modalities, is used in wound care by members of many disciplines.

Getting wet

As with most treatments, the type of therapy used depends on the patient's wound type. There are various forms of hydrotherapy, including:

- pulsatile lavage with concurrent suction
- whirlpool therapy
- jet irrigation
- irrigation with a bulb syringe or a syringe with an attached angiocatheter.

Pulsatile lavage

Today, most hydrotherapy treatments are delivered by pulsatile lavage. Pulsatile lavage cleans and debrides wounds by combining pulse irrigation with suction. Advantages of pulsatile lavage include improved comfort for the patient and mobility of the apparatus. (This treatment can be performed in a hospital, clinic, or home setting.) It's effective in reaching deep, tunneling wounds and there's a minimal chance of cross-contamination.

Puttin' on the spritz

Sterile normal saline solution at room temperature is typically used for pulsatile lavage. It's applied by spray gun using a plastic, disposable fan tip. A tunneling tip is used for deep wounds with tunnels or extensive undermining.

The solution is delivered under pressure to the wound bed and concurrently aspirated by negative pressure through a separate plastic tube in the spray gun. The therapist can control the delivery or impact pressure of the sterile saline and the suction pressure for aspiration of the contaminated fluid.

Versatility is a virtue

Pulsatile lavage can be used with almost any wound type—acute or chronic, large or small, infected or noninfected, and clean or necrotic.

Whirlpool therapy

In whirlpool therapy, part of the body is immersed in a tank of water that has been heated to a prescribed temperature and circulated by an agitator. This therapy softens tissue, removes debris and drainage, and improves blood flow to the area, enhancing the delivery of oxygen and nutrients. Treatment times range from 10 to 20 minutes.

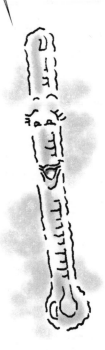

Don't just heat it all the way up! Water temperature in whirlpool therapy varies, depending on the patient's wound type.

Large, light, and no local

Whirlpools are useful for large surface area treatments, especially when these areas are covered with tough necrotic tissue. Whirlpool treatments are useful with painful ulcers when the patient can't tolerate the pressure of a pulsatile lavage head or when allergies to local anesthetics prevent the use of pulsatile lavage.

Tepid, neutral, warm

The water temperature depends on the patient's wound type:
• For arterial wounds, a neutral temperature is recommended, along with shorter treatment times (2 to 5 minutes) to avoid increasing tissue metabolism in an ischemic limb.
• Tepid whirlpool temperature and short treatment times (2 to 5 minutes) are recommended for venous ulcers because the edema associated with venous ulcers may increase with warm or hot whirlpool for extended treatments due to heat exposure and the dependent position of the lower extremities.
• Pressure ulcers and other types of wounds can tolerate neutral to warm temperatures. Warm temperatures may inactivate the harmful enzymes in chronic wound beds.

When to whirl

Whirlpool treatment indications include large surface area wounds, wounds with tough black eschar, wounds with particulate (such as "road rash") and painful wounds.

Everybody else, out of the pool!

Contraindications to whirlpool include:
• bowel or bladder incontinence
• cardiovascular, pulmonary, or renal failure
• deep vein thrombosis or acute phlebitis
• edema
• unresponsiveness or dementia

- wounds with dry gangrene
- wound infections.

Therapeutic light

Therapeutic light modalities include UV treatment and laser therapy.

UV treatment

Although not a form of light, UV energy or radiation is commonly categorized as *therapeutic light*. UV energy lies between X-rays and visible light on the electromagnetic spectrum.

Battle of the bands

UV radiation is typically divided into three bands: UVA, UVB, and UVC. Chronic pressure ulcers treated with UVA and UVB energy have exhibited increased wound healing in clinical studies. In addition, UVA and UVB energy has been found to enhance WBC accumulation and lysosomal activity, possibly offering an explanation for UV-mediated debridement. UV radiation also stimulates the production of interleukin-1 alpha, a cytokine that plays a role in epithelialization.

UVC is killer

The utility of UVC has been demonstrated in various wound types. It's primarily used for treatment in patients with infected wounds. An added benefit of UVC is that it kills a broad spectrum of microorganisms with low exposure times and isn't likely to generate resistant microorganisms. Recent research has shown that UVC can kill antibiotic-resistant strains of bacteria such as methicillin-resistant *Staphylococcus aureus*. UVC is easily administered with minimal intervention time and is inexpensive, too.

Laser therapy

The word *laser* is actually an acronym for *light amplification by stimulated emission of radiation*.

Hot- and cold-running radiation

Lasers can be divided into two groups: cold and hot. Cold lasers include the helium-neon laser, also called a *red laser*, and the gallium-arsenide laser. Hot lasers consist of the carbon dioxide laser and other lasers used for surgical dissection. In wound healing, cold lasers promote wound closure and nerve regeneration. The treatment consists of placing the laser probe directly over selected treatment points for a specific time, according to the dose required, or using a gridlike pattern and continuously moving the probe over this grid for a specific treatment time.

Let the laser go

Indications for laser therapy include slow healing wounds, nerve regeneration, and pain relief.

Ultrasound

Ultrasound (mechanical pressure waves) is used in treating open and closed wounds due to its nonthermal and thermal effects.

Bubbles with no heat

Nonthermal effects of ultrasound include acoustic cavitation and microstreaming. In acoustic cavitation, gas bubbles expand and contract rhythmically in the tissues being treated. These bubbles are thought to stimulate biological phenomena such as the activation of ionic channels in cellular membranes. Microstreaming occurs as a result of this cavitation. In cavitation, fluids close to the bubbles stream by, thus stimulating the cells in close proximity. In this way, ultrasound increases calcium conductance in fibroblasts, which is important because collagen secretion is a calcium-dependent process.

Warm up and get the blood flowing

Ultrasound's thermal effects include increased blood flow to tissues, which results in increased tissue healing. Ultrasound also increases WBC migration and promotes a more orderly arrangement of collagen in open and closed wounds. Ultrasound appears to have optimal effects when used early on, during the inflammatory phase of wound healing. It speeds the wound's progress through the healing phases.

Sounds like a job for ultrasound

Ultrasound is indicated to increase wound healing, enhance blood flow, decrease pain and decrease inflammation.

Electrical stimulation

Electrical stimulation is used to enhance healing of recalcitrant wounds, especially chronic pressure ulcers. The types of electrical stimulation used in wound healing include high-voltage and low-voltage pulsed current. Electrical stimulation is delivered through a device that has conductive electrodes, which are applied to the skin.

Electrical stimulation may use high- or low-voltage pulsed current. Yowza!

Zap it!

Electrical stimulation can be used to orient cells and promote cellular migration. This treatment also enhances blood flow, increases protein synthesis and wound bed formation, destroys microorganisms, and provides pain relief.

Stimulate to oxygenate (among other things)

Electrical stimulation is indicated to promote wound healing and increase blood flow, angiogenesis, and tissue oxygenation. It also reduces pain and wound microbial content.

Hyperbaric oxygen

Hyperbaric oxygen (HBO) is the delivery of 100% oxygen through a sealed chamber.

In whole or part

Two forms of HBO are used for wound healing. One form involves a large multipatient or single patient chamber, such as that used for decompression therapy for divers, and the other involves a smaller chamber used just for the limbs. (The effectiveness of topical HBO through small-limb chambers hasn't yet been proven through research.)

Extra O_2

HBO delivered by a large chamber increases the amount of dissolved oxygen in the blood that's available for wound healing. This increased availability of readily usable oxygen in the blood provides extra oxygen for use by cells such as neutrophils that employ oxygen-dependent processes. (The processes by which neutrophils destroy microorganisms are oxygen-based, as is cellular metabolism in general). The increased availability of oxygen for tissues apparently relieves relative hypoxia in wounded tissues.

Evidence supporting systemic or whole body HBO treatment for patients with chronic wounds is evolving. Patients with venous ulcers that don't improve with traditional therapies may benefit when compression therapy is paired with systemic HBO treatment. Another possible use for HBO is treating patients with diabetic foot ulcers. HBO increases nitric oxide production in the wound. Nitric oxide is a unique free radical that's important in vasodilation and neurotransmission, which play major roles in diabetic wound healing. Indications for HBO include diabetic foot ulcers and venous ulcers.

> We have oxygen on our side! Extra oxygen in the blood aids us in battling microorganisms in wounded tissues.

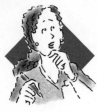

Quick quiz

1. Wounds that fill with granulation tissue and form a scar heal by:
- A. primary intention.
- B. secondary intention.
- C. tertiary intention.
- D. escharotomy.

Answer: B. During healing, wounds that heal by secondary intention fill with granulation tissue, form a scar, and undergo reepithelialization, primarily from the wound edges.

2. The phase of wound healing marked by shrinking and strengthening of the scar is:
- A. hemostasis.
- B. inflammation.
- C. proliferation.
- D. maturation.

Answer: D. The final phase of wound healing is maturation, which is marked by the shrinking and strengthening of the scar. This phase of healing is gradual and transitional and can continue for months or even years after the wound has closed.

3. The complication associated with wound healing that occurs when skin and tissue layers separate is:
- A. hemorrhage.
- B. dehiscence.
- C. evisceration.
- D. fistula formation.

Answer: B. Dehiscence, a separation of skin and tissue layers, is most likely to occur 3 to 11 days after the injury was sustained and may follow surgery.

Scoring

⭐⭐⭐ If you answered all three questions correctly, congrats! You obviously have the skinny on wound care.

⭐⭐ If you answered two questions correctly, take a bow! You've transparently absorbed all of the information on wound care.

⭐ If you answered fewer than two questions correctly, don't despair. You've just skinned the surface of wound care. Go back and review the chapter.

8

Disorders

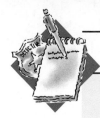

Just the facts

In this chapter, you'll learn:

♦ pathophysiology behind common disorders

♦ signs and symptoms associated with each disorder

♦ diagnostic tests used to diagnose each disorder

♦ treatments for each disorder.

A look at disorders

Although the terms *disease* and *illness* aren't synonymous, they're commonly used interchangeably. *Disease* occurs when homeostasis isn't maintained. *Illness* occurs when a person is no longer in a state of "normal health." This chapter discusses common disorders that you're likely to encounter in your clinical practice.

Acidosis, metabolic

A physiologic state of excess acid accumulation and deficient base bicarbonate, metabolic acidosis is produced by an underlying pathologic disorder. Symptoms result from the body's attempts to correct the acidotic condition through compensatory mechanisms in the lungs, kidneys, and cells.

Oh no, acidosis!

Metabolic acidosis is more prevalent among children, who are vulnerable to acid-base imbalance because their metabolic rates are faster and their ratios of water to total body weight are lower. Severe or untreated metabolic acidosis can be fatal.

> The cells, kidneys, and lungs attempt to compensate for an acidotic condition.

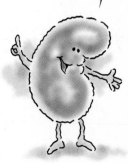

What causes it

Metabolic acidosis usually results from excessive burning of fats in the absence of usable carbohydrates, causing the production of more keto acids than the metabolic process can handle. Conditions that cause metabolic acidosis through excessive fat burning include:

- diabetic ketoacidosis (DKA)
- chronic alcoholism
- malnutrition
- a low-carbohydrate, high-fat diet.
    Other causes of metabolic acidosis include:
- anaerobic carbohydrate metabolism
- renal insufficiency
- diarrhea and intestinal malabsorption.
    Less commonly, metabolic acidosis results from salicylate intoxication (overuse of aspirin), exogenous poisoning, or Addison's disease with increased sodium and chloride excretion and potassium ion retention (due to a deficiency of glucocorticoids and mineralocorticoids).

What to look for

With mild acidosis, symptoms of the underlying disease may obscure any direct clinical evidence. Metabolic acidosis typically begins with headache and lethargy, progressing to drowsiness, central nervous system (CNS) depression, Kussmaul's respirations (as the lungs attempt to compensate by "blowing off" carbon dioxide), stupor and, if the condition is severe and goes untreated, coma and death.

Gut reactions

Associated GI distress usually produces anorexia, nausea, vomiting, and diarrhea and may lead to dehydration. Underlying diabetes mellitus may cause fruity breath from catabolism of fats and excretion of accumulated acetone through the lungs.

What tests tell you

Arterial pH below 7.35 confirms metabolic acidosis. With severe acidotic states, pH may fall to 7.10 and partial pressure of arterial carbon dioxide ($Paco_2$) may be normal or less than 34 mm Hg as compensatory mechanisms take hold. Bicarbonate level may be less than 22 mEq/L. Supportive findings include:

- urine pH—less than 4.5 in the absence of renal disease
- serum potassium levels—greater than 5.5 mEq/L from chemical buffering

• glucose level — greater than 150 mg/dl in those with diabetes mellitus
• serum ketone body level — elevated in those with diabetes mellitus
• plasma lactic acid level — elevated in those with lactic acidosis
• anion gap — greater than 14 mEq/L, indicating metabolic acidosis.
  These values result from increased acid production or renal insufficiency. (See *Crossing the great anion gap*.)

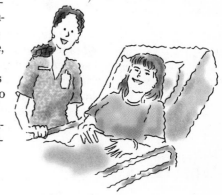

Patients with metabolic acidosis should be positioned to prevent aspiration.

How it's treated

Treatment for metabolic acidosis consists of administering sodium bicarbonate I.V. for severe cases, evaluating and correcting electrolyte imbalances and, ultimately, correcting the underlying cause. For example, in a patient with DKA, a low-dose continuous I.V. infusion of insulin is recommended. If the patient has diabetic acidosis, watch for secondary changes due to hypovolemia, such as decreasing blood pressure.

Because metabolic acidosis commonly causes vomiting, position the patient to prevent aspiration. In addition, follow these steps:
• Keep sodium bicarbonate handy for emergency administration. Frequently monitor vital signs, laboratory results, and level of consciousness (LOC) because changes can occur rapidly. Record intake and output accurately to monitor renal function.

Crossing the great anion gap

This illustration represents the normal anion gap. It's calculated by adding the chloride level and the bicarbonate level and then subtracting that total from the sodium level. The value normally ranges from 8 to 14 mEq/L and represents the level of unmeasured anions in extracellular fluid.

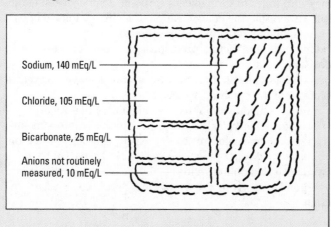

Sodium, 140 mEq/L

Chloride, 105 mEq/L

Bicarbonate, 25 mEq/L

Anions not routinely measured, 10 mEq/L

• Watch for signs of excessive serum potassium — weakness, flaccid paralysis, and arrhythmias, possibly leading to cardiac arrest. After treatment, check for overcorrection to hypokalemia.
• Prepare for the possibility of seizures by taking seizure precautions.
• To prevent metabolic acidosis, carefully observe patients who are receiving I.V. therapy or who have intestinal tubes in place as well as those suffering from shock, hyperthyroidism, hepatic disease, circulatory failure, or dehydration.

Acidosis, respiratory

Respiratory acidosis is an acid-base disturbance. It occurs as a result of reduced alveolar ventilation, which produces hypercapnia ($Paco_2$ greater than 45 mm Hg). Hypercapnia is a key finding in respiratory acidosis. It can be acute (from a sudden failure in ventilation) or chronic (as in long-term pulmonary disease). The prognosis depends on the severity of the underlying disturbance and the patient's general condition.

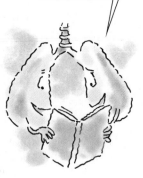

Oh no! Hypercapnia is a key finding in respiratory acidosis.

What causes it

Respiratory acidosis can result from airway obstruction, parenchymal lung disease, chronic obstructive pulmonary disease (COPD), asthma, severe acute respiratory distress syndrome (ARDS), chronic bronchitis, large pneumothorax, extensive pneumonia, or pulmonary edema.

Hypoventilation compromises excretion of carbon dioxide produced through metabolism. The retained carbon dioxide then combines with water to form excess carbonic acid, decreasing the blood pH. As a result, the concentration of hydrogen ions in body fluids, which directly reflects acidity, increases.

In addition, several factors predispose the patient to respiratory acidosis, including:
• *drugs* — opioids, anesthetics, hypnotics, and sedatives decrease the sensitivity of the respiratory center
• *CNS trauma* — medullary injury may impair ventilatory drive
• *chronic metabolic alkalosis* — respiratory compensatory mechanisms attempt to normalize pH by decreasing alveolar ventilation
• *neuromuscular disease* (such as myasthenia gravis, Guillain-Barré syndrome, and poliomyelitis) — failure of respiratory muscles to respond properly to respiratory drive reduces alveolar ventilation.

What to look for

Acute respiratory acidosis produces CNS disturbances that reflect changes in the pH of cerebrospinal fluid (CSF) rather than increased carbon dioxide levels in cerebral circulation. Effects range from restlessness, confusion, and apprehension to somnolence with a fine or flapping tremor (asterixis) or coma. The patient may complain of headaches and exhibit dyspnea and tachypnea with papilledema and depressed reflexes. Unless the patient is receiving oxygen, hypoxemia accompanies respiratory acidosis.

Headed for a heartache

This disorder may also cause cardiovascular abnormalities, such as tachycardia, hypertension, atrial and ventricular arrhythmias and, in severe acidosis, hypotension with vasodilation (bounding pulses and warm periphery).

What tests tell you

The following arterial blood gas (ABG) levels confirm respiratory acidosis:
- $Paco_2$ exceeds the normal level of 45 mm Hg
- pH is usually below the normal range of 7.35 to 7.45
- bicarbonate level is normal in the acute stage but elevated in the chronic stage.

Chest X-ray, computed tomography (CT) scanning, or pulmonary function tests (PFTs) may help diagnose lung disease.

How it's treated

Effective treatment of respiratory acidosis is designed to correct the underlying source of alveolar hypoventilation. Significantly reduced alveolar ventilation may require mechanical ventilation until the underlying condition can be treated. Here are some other treatments for respiratory acidosis:
- In a patient with COPD, treatment includes a bronchodilator, oxygen, a corticosteroid and, commonly, an antibiotic; drug therapy for such conditions as myasthenia gravis; removal of foreign bodies from the airway; an antibiotic for pneumonia; dialysis or charcoal to remove toxic drugs; and correction of metabolic alkalosis. Elevated $Paco_2$ may persist in a patient with COPD despite optimal treatment.
- Closely monitor the patient's blood pH level. If it drops below 7.15, profound CNS and cardiovascular deterioration may result, requiring administration of I.V. sodium bicarbonate. However, this should be reserved for only the most critical cases because it can cause a paradoxical worsening of CNS effects.

• Stay alert for critical changes in the patient's respiratory, CNS, and cardiovascular function. Also, watch closely for variations in ABG values and electrolyte status. Maintain adequate hydration. If acidosis requires mechanical ventilation, maintain a patent airway and provide adequate humidification.

• Perform tracheal suctioning regularly and vigorous chest physiotherapy, if needed. Continuously monitor ventilator settings and the patient's respiratory status.

If the patient has COPD and chronic carbon dioxide retention, closely monitor him for signs of respiratory acidosis. Also, administer oxygen at low flow rates, and closely monitor the patient if he's receiving an opioid or a sedative. Instruct the patient who has received a general anesthetic to turn, cough, and perform deep-breathing exercises frequently to prevent the onset of respiratory acidosis.

Alkalosis, metabolic

A clinical state marked by decreased amounts of acid or increased amounts of base bicarbonate, metabolic alkalosis causes metabolic, respiratory, and renal responses, producing characteristic symptoms—most notably, hypoventilation. This condition always occurs secondary to an underlying cause. With early diagnosis and prompt treatment, the prognosis is good. However, untreated metabolic alkalosis may lead to coma and death.

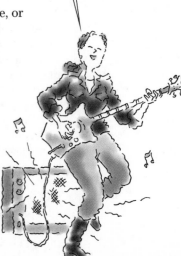

Did someone say something about retaining base? I'm sorry; I couldn't hear.

What causes it

Metabolic alkalosis results from loss of acid, retention of base, or renal mechanisms associated with decreased serum levels of potassium and chloride.

Losing acid...

Each of the following leads to a loss of acid:
• vomiting
• nasogastric (NG) tube drainage or lavage without adequate electrolyte replacement
• fistulas
• steroid use
• diuretics, such as furosemide, thiazides, and ethacrynic acid
• hyperadrenocorticism.

...retaining base

Retention of base occurs with:

- excessive intake of bicarbonate of soda or other antacids
- excessive intake of absorbable alkali (as in milk-alkali syndrome)
- administration of excessive amounts of I.V. fluids with high concentrations of bicarbonate or lactate
- respiratory insufficiency.

On the lower level

The following conditions are associated with decreased serum levels of potassium and chloride related to excessive urinary loss:
- Cushing's disease
- primary hyperaldosteronism
- Bartter syndrome (hyperplasia of the cells within the kidneys).

What to look for

Signs and symptoms of metabolic alkalosis result from the body's attempt to correct the acid-base imbalance, primarily through hypoventilation. Other signs and symptoms include irritability, picking at bedclothes (carphology), twitching, confusion, nausea, vomiting, and diarrhea (which aggravates alkalosis).

More metabolic mishaps

Cardiovascular abnormalities, such as atrial tachycardia, and respiratory disturbances, such as cyanosis and apnea, also occur. In the alkalotic patient, diminished peripheral blood flow during repeated blood pressure checks may provoke carpopedal spasm in the hand — a possible sign of impending tetany (Trousseau's sign). Uncorrected metabolic alkalosis may progress to seizures and coma.

What tests tell you

A blood pH greater than 7.45 and a bicarbonate level above 29 mEq/L confirm the diagnosis. A partial pressure of carbon dioxide greater than 45 mm Hg indicates attempts at respiratory compensation. Serum electrolyte levels show a potassium level of 3.5 mEq/L and a chloride level of 98 mEq/L. Other characteristic findings include:
- urine pH of about 7 (usually)
- urinalysis revealing alkalinity after the renal compensatory mechanism begins to excrete bicarbonate
- an electrocardiogram (ECG) that may show a low T wave merging with a P wave and atrial tachycardia.

How it's treated

The goal of treatment is to correct the underlying cause of metabolic alkalosis:

• Therapy for severe alkalosis may include cautious administration of ammonium chloride I.V. to release hydrogen chloride and restore the concentration of extracellular fluid and chloride levels.

• Potassium chloride and normal saline solution (except in the presence of heart failure) are usually sufficient to replace losses from gastric drainage. Electrolyte replacement with potassium chloride and discontinuation of diuretics correct metabolic alkalosis resulting from potent diuretic therapy.

• When administering 0.9% ammonium chloride, limit the infusion rate to 75 minutes; faster administration may cause hemolysis of red blood cells (RBCs). Avoid overdosage because it may cause overcorrection to metabolic acidosis. Don't give ammonium chloride to a patient with signs of hepatic or renal disease.

• Dilute potassium when giving I.V. potassium salts. Monitor the infusion rate to prevent damage to blood vessels and watch for signs of phlebitis.

• Monitor vital signs frequently and record intake and output to evaluate respiratory, fluid, and electrolyte status. Remember, respiratory rate usually decreases in an effort to compensate for alkalosis. Hypotension and tachycardia may indicate electrolyte imbalance, especially hypokalemia.

Alkalosis, respiratory

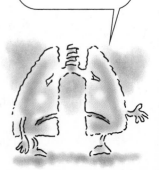

When I can't eliminate carbon dioxide as fast as cells can produce it, respiratory alkalosis results.

Caused by alveolar hyperventilation, respiratory alkalosis is a condition marked by a decrease in Pa_{CO_2} to less than 35 mm Hg. Uncomplicated respiratory alkalosis leads to a decrease in hydrogen ion concentration, which causes elevated blood pH. Hypocapnia occurs when the elimination of carbon dioxide by the lungs exceeds the production of carbon dioxide at the cellular level.

What causes it

Respiratory alkalosis can result from pulmonary or nonpulmonary causes:

• Pulmonary causes include pneumonia, interstitial lung disease, pulmonary vascular disease, and acute asthma.

• Nonpulmonary causes include anxiety, fever, aspirin toxicity, metabolic acidosis, CNS disease (inflammation or tumor), sepsis, hepatic failure, and pregnancy.

What to look for

The cardinal sign of respiratory alkalosis is deep, rapid breathing, possibly exceeding 40 breaths/minute and much like the Kussmaul's respirations that characterize diabetic acidosis. Such hyperventilation usually leads to:
• light-headedness or dizziness
• agitation
• circumoral and peripheral paresthesia
• carpopedal spasms
• twitching
• muscle weakness.

Severe respiratory alkalosis may cause cardiac arrhythmias that fail to respond to conventional treatment and seizures.

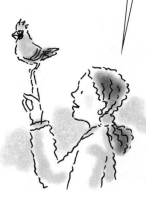

The cardinal sign of respiratory alkalosis is deep, rapid breathing.

What tests tell you

ABG analysis confirms respiratory alkalosis and rules out respiratory compensation for metabolic acidosis. Findings include:
• $Paco_2$ below 35 mm Hg
• pH that's elevated in proportion to the fall in $Paco_2$ in the acute stage but that drops toward normal in the chronic stage
• bicarbonate level that's normal in the acute stage but below normal in the chronic stage.

How it's treated

The goal of treatment is to eradicate the underlying condition— for example, to remove ingested toxins or treat fever, sepsis, or CNS disease. With severe respiratory alkalosis, the patient may be instructed to breathe into a paper bag, which helps relieve acute anxiety and increases carbon dioxide level. Here are other treatment measures for respiratory alkalosis:
• Prevent hyperventilation in patients receiving mechanical ventilation by monitoring ABG values and adjusting dead space or minute ventilation volume.
• Watch for and report changes in neurologic, neuromuscular, or cardiovascular function. Monitor ABG and serum electrolyte levels closely, watching for variations.

Alzheimer's disease

Alzheimer's disease is a progressive degenerative disorder of the cerebral cortex. It accounts for more than one-half of all cases of dementia. Cortical degeneration is most marked in the frontal lobes, but atrophy occurs in all areas of the cortex. Because this is a primary progressive dementia, the prognosis is poor.

Sometimes it's all in the family

Researchers recognize two forms of Alzheimer's disease. In familial Alzheimer's, genes directly cause the disease. These cases are rare and have been identified in a relatively small number of families, with many people in multiple generations affected.

Sometimes sporadic

In sporadic Alzheimer's, the most common form of the disease, genes don't cause the disease but may influence the risk of developing the disease. The incidence of sporadic Alzheimer's disease is less predictable than the familial type and occurs in fewer family members.

What causes it

The cause of Alzheimer's disease is unknown, but four factors are thought to contribute:
• neurochemical factors, such as deficiencies in the neurotransmitters acetylcholine, somatostatin, substance P, and norepinephrine
• viral factors such as slow-growing CNS viruses
• trauma
• genetic factors.

An issue of brain tissue

The brain tissue of patients with Alzheimer's disease has three distinguishing features:
• neurofibrillary tangles formed out of proteins in the neurons
• beta-amyloid plaques
• granulovascular degeneration of neurons.
   The disease causes degeneration of neuropils (dense complexes of interwoven cytoplasmic processes of nerve cells and neuroglial cells), especially in the frontal, parietal, and occipital lobes. It also causes enlargement of the ventricles (cavities within the brain filled with CSF).

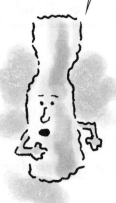

In familial Alzheimer's disease, genes are the direct cause of the disease.

Early cerebral changes include formation of microscopic plaques, consisting of a core surrounded by fibrous tissue. Later on, atrophy of the cerebral cortex becomes strikingly evident.

The part plaques play

If a patient has many beta-amyloid plaques, his dementia will be more severe. The amyloid in the plaques may exert neurotoxic effects. Evidence suggests that plaques play an important part in bringing about the death of neurons.

Absence of acetylcholine

Problems with neurotransmitters and the enzymes associated with their metabolism may play a role in the disease. The severity of dementia is directly related to a reduced amount of the neurotransmitter acetylcholine. On autopsy, the brains of patients with Alzheimer's disease may contain as little as 10% of the normal amount of acetylcholine.

What to look for

Alzheimer's disease has an insidious onset. At first, changes are barely perceptible, but they gradually lead to serious problems. Patient history is almost always obtained from a family member or caregiver.

Early changes may include forgetfulness, subtle memory loss without a loss of social skills or behavior patterns, difficulty learning and retaining new information, an inability to concentrate, and deterioration in personal hygiene and appearance. As the disease progresses, signs and symptoms indicate a degenerative disorder of the frontal lobe. They may include:
• difficulty with abstract thinking and activities that require judgment
• progressive difficulty in communicating
• severe deterioration of memory, language, and motor function progressing to coordination loss and an inability to speak or write
• repetitive actions
• restlessness
• irritability, depression, mood swings, paranoia, hostility, and combativeness
• nocturnal awakenings
• disorientation.

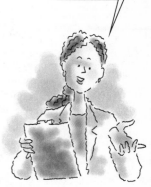

Early changes in Alzheimer's disease may be subtle.

The proof is in the...

Neurologic examination confirms many of the problems revealed during the history. In addition, it commonly reveals an impaired sense of smell (usually an early symptom), an inability to recognize and understand the form and nature of objects by touching them, gait disorders, and tremors. The patient will also have a positive snout reflex; in response to a tap or stroke of the lips or the area just under the nose, the patient grimaces or puckers his lips.

In the final stages, urinary or fecal incontinence, twitching, and seizures commonly occur.

What tests tell you

Alzheimer's disease can't be confirmed until death, when an autopsy reveals pathologic findings. These tests help rule out other disorders:
• Positron emission tomography (PET) scan measures the metabolic activity of the cerebral cortex and may help confirm early diagnosis.
• CT scan may show more brain atrophy than occurs in normal aging.
• Magnetic resonance imaging (MRI) evaluates the condition of the brain and rules out intracranial lesions as the source of dementia.
• EEG evaluates the brain's electrical activity and may show brain wave slowing late in the disease. It also identifies tumors, abscesses, and other intracranial lesions that might cause symptoms.
• CSF analysis helps determine whether signs and symptoms stem from a chronic neurologic infection.
• Cerebral blood flow studies may detect abnormalities in blood flow to the brain.

How it's treated

No cure for Alzheimer's disease exists. Although current drugs can't alter the progressive loss of brain cells, the drugs listed here may help minimize or stabilize symptoms:
• Cholinesterase inhibitors, such as donepezil, rivastigmine, and galantamine, prevent the breakdown of acetylcholine, a chemical messenger in the brain that's important for memory and other thinking skills.
• Memantine, an uncompetitive low to moderate affinity N-methyl-D-aspartate receptor antagonist, is sometimes prescribed. It appears to work by regulating the activity of glutamate, one of the brain's chemicals that's involved in information processing, storing, and retrieval.
• Vitamin E supplements are commonly prescribed because they may help defend the brain against damage.

There is no cure for Alzheimer's disease.

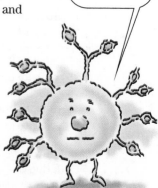

Arterial occlusive disease

With arterial occlusive disease, the obstruction or narrowing of the lumen of the aorta and its major branches causes an interruption of blood flow, usually to the legs and feet. Arterial occlusive disease may affect the carotid, vertebral, innominate, subclavian, mesenteric, or celiac artery. Occlusions, which may be acute or chronic, commonly cause severe ischemia, skin ulceration, and gangrene. Arterial occlusive disease is more common in males than in females.

> Arterial occlusive disease is more common in males.

What causes it

Arterial occlusive disease is a common complication of atherosclerosis. The occlusive mechanism may be endogenous (due to embolus formation or thrombosis) or exogenous (due to trauma or fracture). Predisposing factors include:
• smoking
• aging
• hypertension
• hyperlipidemia
• diabetes
• family history of vascular disorders
• myocardial infarction (MI)
• stroke.

What to look for

Evidence of this disease varies widely, according to the occlusion site. (See *Types of arterial occlusive disease*, page 488.)

What tests tell you

With arterial occlusive disease, the diagnosis is usually based on patient history and physical examination. Diagnostic tests include:
• Arteriography demonstrates the type (thrombus or embolus), location, and degree of obstruction and collateral circulation.
• Doppler ultrasonography and plethysmography are noninvasive tests that, in acute disease, show decreased blood flow distal to the occlusion.
• Ophthalmodynamometry helps determine the degree of obstruction in the internal carotid artery by comparing ophthalmic artery pressure with brachial artery pressure on the affected side. A more than 20% difference between pressures suggests insufficiency.
• EEG and CT scanning may be necessary to rule out brain lesions.

Types of arterial occlusive disease

The signs and symptoms of arterial occlusive disease depend on the location of the occlusion. Use the chart below to help determine the site of your patient's occlusion.

Site of occlusion	Signs and symptoms
Carotid arterial system • Internal carotids • External carotids	Neurologic dysfunction: transient ischemic attacks (TIAs) due to reduced cerebral circulation producing unilateral sensory or motor dysfunction (transient monocular blindness, hemiparesis), possible aphasia or dysarthria, confusion, decreased mentation, and headache, all of which usually last 5 to 10 minutes but may persist up to 24 hours and may herald a stroke; absent or decreased pulsation with an auscultatory bruit over the affected vessels
Vertebrobasilar system • Vertebral arteries • Basilar arteries	Neurologic dysfunction: TIAs of the brain stem and cerebellum, producing binocular vision disturbances, vertigo, dysarthria, and "drop attacks" (falling down without loss of consciousness); less common than a carotid TIA
Innominate • Brachiocephalic artery	Neurologic dysfunction: signs and symptoms of vertebrobasilar occlusion; indications of ischemia (claudication) of right arm; possible bruit over right side of neck
Subclavian artery	Subclavian steal syndrome, characterized by blood backflow from the brain through the vertebral artery on the same side as the occlusion, into the subclavian artery distal to the occlusion; clinical effects of vertebrobasilar occlusion and exercise-induced arm claudication; possible gangrene, usually limited to the digits
Mesenteric artery • Superior (most commonly affected) • Celiac axis • Inferior	Bowel ischemia, infarct necrosis, and gangrene; sudden, acute abdominal pain; nausea and vomiting; diarrhea; leukocytosis; and shock due to massive intraluminal fluid and plasma loss
Aortic bifurcation (saddle block occlusion, a medical emergency associated with cardiac embolization)	Sensory and motor deficits (such as muscle weakness, numbness, paresthesia, and paralysis) and signs of ischemia (such as sudden pain and cold, pale legs with decreased or absent peripheral pulses) in both legs
Iliac artery (Leriche's syndrome)	Intermittent claudication of lower back, buttocks, and thighs, relieved by rest; absent or reduced femoral or distal pulses; possible bruit over femoral arteries; and impotence in males
Femoral and popliteal artery (associated with aneurysm formation)	Intermittent claudication of the calves on exertion; ischemic pain in feet; pretrophic pain (heralds necrosis and ulceration); leg pallor and coolness; blanching of feet on elevation; gangrene; and no palpable pulses in ankles and feet

How it's treated

Effective treatment depends on the cause, location, and size of the obstruction. The goal of medical management is to impede progression of peripheral arterial occlusive disease.

Take a walk on the mild side

For mild chronic disease, supportive measures include elimination of smoking, control of hypertension, and initiation of a walking program. For carotid artery occlusion, antiplatelet therapy may begin with aspirin. For intermittent claudication of chronic occlusive disease, pentoxifylline may improve blood flow through the capillaries, particularly in patients who are poor candidates for surgery. Exercise also plays a vital role in treating claudication.

Fast intervention required

Acute arterial occlusive disease usually requires surgery to restore circulation to the affected area. Treatment may include one or a combination of the following procedures:
• Embolectomy with a balloon-tipped catheter to remove thrombotic material from the artery. It's used mainly for mesenteric, femoral, or popliteal artery occlusion.
• Thromboendarterectomy is performed when the occluded artery is opened and the obstructing thrombus and the medial layer of the arterial wall are removed. It's usually performed after angiography and is commonly used with autogenous vein or Dacron bypass surgery (femoral-popliteal or aortofemoral).
• Patch grafting involves removal of the thrombosed arterial segment and replacement with an autogenous vein or Dacron graft.
• Bypass graft is performed when blood flow is diverted through an anastomosed autogenous or Dacron graft past the thrombosed segment.
• Thrombolytic therapy is done for a clot around or in the plaque through lysis with streptokinase or alteplase.
• Arthrectomy is excision of the plaque by a drilling or slicing mechanism.
• Balloon angioplasty is when the obstruction is compressed using using balloon inflation.
• Laser angioplasty is vaporization of the obstruction through excision and use of hot-tip lasers.
• Stents are a mesh of wires that stretch and mold to the arterial wall; they're inserted to prevent reocclusion.

Other treatments include heparin to prevent embolus formation (for embolic occlusion) and bowel resection after restoration of blood flow (for mesenteric artery occlusion). Amputation becomes necessary with failure of arterial reconstructive surgery or with the development of gangrene, persistent infection, or intractable pain.

Asthma

Asthma is a chronic reactive airway disorder that can manifest as an acute attack. It causes episodic airway obstruction resulting from bronchospasms, increased mucus secretion, and mucosal edema. Cases of asthma continue to rise. It currently affects an estimated 17 million Americans; children account for 4.8 million asthma sufferers in the United States. Twice as many boys than girls are affected.

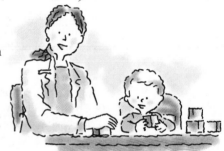

Approximately 30% of asthma sufferers in the United States are children.

It's a family affair

About one-third of patients develop asthma between ages 10 and 30. In this group, incidence is the same in both sexes. About one-third of all patients share the disease with at least one immediate family member.

In asthma, bronchial linings overreact to various stimuli, causing episodic smooth-muscle spasms that severely constrict the airways. Mucosal edema and thickened secretions further block the airways. (See *Understanding asthma.*)

What causes it

Asthma can be described as *extrinsic* or *intrinsic:*
• Extrinsic asthma is sensitive to specific external allergens, which include pollen, animal dander, house dust or mold, kapok or feather pillows, food additives containing sulfites, cockroach allergen, and any other sensitizing substance. It begins in childhood and is commonly accompanied by other hereditary allergies, such as eczema and allergic rhinitis.
• Intrinsic, or *nonatopic*, asthma is a reaction to internal, nonallergenic factors — no external substance can be implicated in intrinsic asthma. Most episodes occur after a severe respiratory tract infection, especially in adults.

Many patients with asthma, especially children, have both intrinsic and extrinsic asthma.

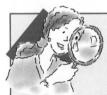

A closer look

Understanding asthma

Asthma is an inflammatory disease characterized by hyperresponsiveness of the airway and bronchospasm. These illustrations show the progression of an asthma attack.

When the patient inhales a substance he's hypersensitive to, abnormal antibodies stimulate the mast cells in the lung interstitium to release histamine and slow-reacting substance of anaphylaxis.

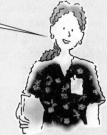

1. Histamine (H) attaches to receptor sites in the larger bronchi, where it causes swelling in smooth muscles.

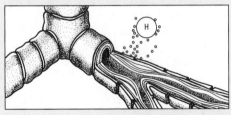

2. Slow-reacting substance of anaphylaxis (SRS-A) attaches to receptor sites in the smaller bronchi and causes swelling of smooth muscle there. SRS-A also causes fatty acids called *prostaglandins* to travel through the bloodstream to the lungs, where they enhance histamine's effects.

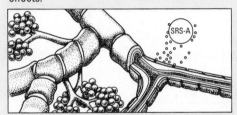

3. Histamine stimulates the mucous membranes to secrete excessive mucus, further narrowing the bronchial lumen, as shown below.

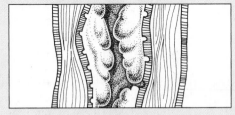

4. On inhalation, the narrowed bronchial lumen can still expand slightly, allowing air to reach the alveoli. On exhalation, increased intrathoracic pressure closes the bronchial lumen completely.

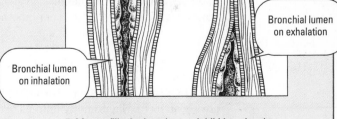

Bronchial lumen on inhalation

Bronchial lumen on exhalation

5. Mucus fills the lung bases, inhibiting alveolar ventilation, as shown below. Blood, shunted to alveoli in other lung parts, still can't compensate for diminished ventilation.

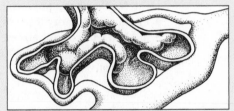

What to look for

Signs and symptoms vary depending on the severity of a patient's asthma.

From mild...

Patients with mild asthma have adequate air exchange and are asymptomatic between attacks. Mild asthma is classified as either mild intermittent asthma or mild persistent asthma. With mild intermittent asthma, the patient experiences symptoms of cough, wheezing, chest tightness, or difficulty breathing less than twice per week. Flare-ups are brief but may vary in intensity. Nighttime symptoms occur less than twice per month.

In mild persistent asthma, symptoms of cough, wheezing, chest tightness, or difficulty breathing occur three to six times per week. Flare-ups may affect the patient's activity level. Nighttime symptoms occur three or four times per month.

> Looking for signs and symptoms of asthma? They vary depending on the severity of the disease.

...to not so bad...

Patients with moderate persistent asthma have normal or below-normal air exchange as well as signs and symptoms that include cough, wheezing, chest tightness, or difficulty breathing daily. Flare-ups may affect the patient's level of activity. Nighttime symptoms occur five or more times per month.

...to worse...

Patients with severe persistent asthma have below-normal air exchange and experience continual symptoms of cough, wheezing, chest tightness, and difficulty breathing. Their activity level is greatly affected. Nighttime symptoms occur frequently.

...to the very worst

Patients with any type of asthma may develop status asthmaticus, a severe acute attack that doesn't respond to conventional treatment. Signs and symptoms include:
- marked respiratory distress
- marked wheezing or absent breath sounds
- pulsus paradoxus greater than 10 mm Hg
- chest wall contractions.

What tests tell you

These tests are used to diagnose asthma:

• PFTs reveal signs of obstructive airway disease, low-normal or decreased vital capacity, and increased total lung and residual capacities. Pulmonary function may be normal between attacks. Partial pressure of arterial oxygen (PaO_2) and $PaCO_2$ are usually decreased, except in severe asthma, when $PaCO_2$ may be normal or increased, indicating severe bronchial obstruction.

• Serum immunoglobulin (Ig) E levels may increase from an allergic reaction.

• Complete blood count (CBC) with differential reveals an increased eosinophil count.

• Chest X-rays can diagnose or monitor asthma's progress and may show hyperinflation with areas of atelectasis.

• ABG analysis detects hypoxemia and guides treatment.

• Skin testing may identify specific allergens. Test results are read in 1 to 2 days to detect an early reaction and again after 4 to 5 days to reveal a late reaction.

• Bronchial challenge testing evaluates the clinical significance of allergens identified by skin testing.

• Pulse oximetry may show a reduced arterial oxygen saturation (SaO_2) level.

How it's treated

The best treatment for asthma is prevention by identifying and avoiding precipitating factors, such as environmental allergens or irritants. Usually, such stimuli can't be removed entirely, so desensitization to specific antigens may be helpful, especially in children. Other common treatments are medication and oxygen.

Medication

Three types of drugs are usually given:

Bronchodilators (theophylline, aminophylline, epinephrine, albuterol, metaproterenol, and terbutaline) decrease bronchoconstriction, reduce bronchial airway edema, and increase pulmonary ventilation. Albuterol and terbutaline cause fewer adverse reactions than epinephrine.

Corticosteroids (hydrocortisone and methylprednisolone) have the same effects as bronchodilators as well as anti-inflammatory and immunosuppressive effects.

Mast cell stabilizers (cromolyn and nedocromil) are effective in patients with atopic asthma who have seasonal disease. When given prophylactically, they block the acute obstructive effects of antigen exposure by inhibiting the degranulation of mast cells, thereby preventing the release of the chemical mediators responsible for anaphylaxis.

Oxygen

Low-flow humidified oxygen may be needed to treat dyspnea, cyanosis, and hypoxemia. The amount delivered is designed to maintain Pao_2 between 65 and 85 mm Hg, as determined by ABG analysis. Mechanical ventilation is necessary if the patient doesn't respond to initial ventilatory support and medication or if he develops respiratory failure.

Alternative therapy

Relaxation exercises, such as yoga, may help increase circulation and help a patient recover from an asthma attack.

Breast cancer

Breast cancer is the most common cancer among females in the United States and the second leading cause of cancer deaths in women ages 35 to 54. Breast cancer also occurs in men, although it's rare.

Thanks to earlier diagnosis and expanded treatment options, the 5-year survival rate for patients with localized breast cancer is now 92%. For noninvasive cancer in situ (confined to the origin site without invading neighboring tissue), the survival rate is near 100%. If the cancer has spread regionally, the survival rate is 71%. With distant metastasis, it falls to 18%.

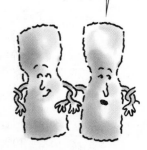

Specific genes are linked to 5% of all cases of breast cancer.

What causes it

The exact causes of breast cancer remain elusive. Scientists have discovered specific genes linked to approximately 5% of all cases of breast cancer (called *BRCA1* and *BRCA2*), which confirms that the disease can be inherited from a person's mother or father. Those who inherit either of these genes have an 80% chance of developing breast cancer.

Other significant risk factors have been identified. These include:
• family history of breast cancer

- radiation exposure
- being a premenopausal woman older than age 45
- obesity
- age
- recent use of hormonal contraceptives
- early onset of menses or late menopause
- nulligravida (never pregnant)
- first pregnancy after age 30
- high-fat diet
- colon, endometrial, or ovarian cancer
- postmenopausal progestin and estrogen therapy
- alcohol use (one or more alcoholic beverages per day)
- benign breast disease.

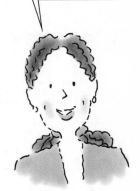

Dimples may be a good feature for a smile, but they shouldn't appear on the breasts.

What to look for

Breast cancer is more commonly found in the left breast than the right. It's also more common in the upper outer quadrant. Typically, the patient discovers a thickening of the breast tissue or a painless lump or mass in her breast. Other signs and symptoms include:
- changes in breast symmetry or size
- changes in breast skin, such as dimpling (called *peau d'orange*), edema, or ulcers
- changes in nipples — for instance, itching, burning, erosion, or retraction
- skin temperature changes (warm, hot, or pink area).

What tests tell you

These tests are used to diagnose breast cancer:
- Regular breast self-examination, followed by a clinical breast examination, is one method for detecting breast lumps early.
- Mammography — the primary test for breast cancer — can be used to detect tumors that are too small to palpate.
- Fine-needle aspiration and excisional biopsy provide cells for histologic examination to confirm diagnosis.
- Hormone receptor assay can be used to pinpoint whether the tumor is estrogen- or progesterone-dependent so that appropriate therapy can be chosen.
- Ultrasonography can be used to distinguish between a fluid-filled cyst and a solid mass.
- Ductoscopy reveals small intraductal lesions that aren't palpable or visible on mammography.
- Ductal lavage identifies cancerous cells in the milk ducts of the breast.

How it's treated

Treatment for breast cancer may include a combination of surgery, radiation, chemotherapy, and hormonal therapy, depending on the disease stage and type, the woman's age and menopausal status, and the disfiguring effects of the surgery. Each treatment is explained here.

Lumpectomy

In lumpectomy, a surgeon removes the tumor through a small incision. This surgery may be done on an outpatient basis and may be the only surgery needed, especially if the tumor is small and there's no evidence of axillary node involvement. Radiation therapy is commonly combined with this surgery. Lumpectomy and radiation are as effective as mastectomy in early-stage breast cancer.

Two-stage procedure

A two-stage procedure in which the surgeon removes the lump and confirms that it's malignant and then discusses treatment options with the patient is desirable because it allows the patient to participate in her treatment plan. Sometimes if the tumor is diagnosed as malignant, such planning can be done before surgery. In lumpectomy and dissection of the axillary lymph nodes, the tumor and the axillary lymph nodes are removed, leaving the breast intact.

Mastectomy procedures

Mastectomy procedures vary by the size and location of the tumor.

Simple

Simple mastectomy involves removal of the breast tissue but not the lymph nodes or pectoral muscles.

Modified radical

Modified radical mastectomy involves removal of the breast and the axillary nodes.

Radical

A radical mastectomy, the performance of which has declined, involves removal of the breast, the pectoralis major and minor, and the axillary lymph nodes.

Road to recovery

After a mastectomy, reconstructive surgery can create a breast mound if the patient desires it and doesn't have evidence of advanced disease.

Chemotherapy

Cytotoxic drugs may be used either as adjuvant therapy or primary therapy. Decisions to start chemotherapy are based on several factors, such as the stage of the cancer and hormone receptor assay results. Chemotherapy commonly involves the use of a combination of drugs. A typical regimen includes cyclophosphamide, methotrexate, doxorubicin, and fluorouracil.

Hormone therapy

Hormone therapy lowers the levels of estrogen and other hormones suspected of nourishing breast cancer cells. Anti-estrogen therapy, with tamoxifen or raloxifene, is used in women at increased risk for developing breast cancer. Other commonly used drugs include the antiandrogen aminoglutethimide, the androgen fluoxymesterone, the estrogen diethylstilbestrol, and the progestin megestrol.

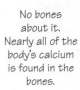

Chemotherapy typically involves the use of several drugs.

Calcium imbalance

Calcium plays an indispensable role in cell permeability, formation of bones and teeth, blood coagulation, transmission of nerve impulses, and normal muscle contraction. Nearly all (99%) of the body's calcium is found in the bones. The remaining 1% exists in ionized form in serum, and it's the maintenance of the 1% of ionized calcium in the serum that's critical to healthy neurologic function.

The parathyroid glands regulate ionized calcium and determine its resorption into bone, absorption from the GI mucosa, and excretion in urine and stool.

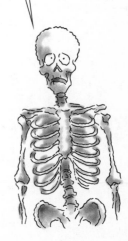

No bones about it. Nearly all of the body's calcium is found in the bones.

What causes it

Causes of calcium imbalance vary by the type of imbalance.

The low side...

Hypocalcemia can be caused by any of these factors:
• Inadequate intake of calcium and vitamin D results in inhibited intestinal absorption of calcium.

- Hypoparathyroidism as a result of injury, disease, or surgery decreases or eliminates parathyroid hormone (PTH) secretion, which is necessary for calcium absorption and normal serum calcium levels.
- Malabsorption or loss of calcium from the GI tract can result from increased intestinal motility from severe diarrhea or laxative abuse. Malabsorption of calcium from the GI tract can also result from inadequate levels of vitamin D or PTH or a reduction in gastric acidity, which decreases the solubility of calcium salts.
- Severe infections or burns can lead to diseased and burned tissue trapping calcium from the extracellular fluid.
- Overcorrection of acidosis can lead to alkalosis, which causes decreased ionized calcium and induces symptoms of hypocalcemia.
- Pancreatic insufficiency may cause calcium malabsorption and subsequent calcium loss in stool. In pancreatitis, participation of calcium ions in saponification contributes to calcium loss.
- Renal failure results in excessive calcium excretion secondary to increased phosphate retention. Renal failure also results in a loss of the active metabolite of vitamin D, which impairs calcium absorption.
- Hypomagnesemia causes decreased PTH secretion and blocks the peripheral action of that hormone.

...the high side

Hypercalcemia may be caused by any of these factors:
- Hyperparathyroidism increases serum calcium levels by promoting calcium absorption from the intestine, resorption from bone, and reabsorption from the kidneys.
- Hypervitaminosis D can promote increased absorption of calcium from the intestine.
- Tumors raise serum calcium levels by destroying bone or releasing PTH or a PTH-like substance, osteoclast-activating factor, prostaglandins and, perhaps, a vitamin D–like sterol.
- Multiple fractures and prolonged immobilization release bone calcium and raise the serum calcium level.
- Multiple myeloma promotes calcium loss from bone.

What to look for

Indications of calcium imbalance depend on the type of imbalance. (See *Signs and symptoms of calcium imbalance.*)

Hypo...Oh, no

Characteristic signs and symptoms of hypocalcemia include perioral paresthesia, twitching, carpopedal spasm, tetany, seizures and,

Signs and symptoms of calcium imbalance

The chart below lists possible signs and symptoms of hypocalcemia and hypercalcemia by body system dysfunction.

Dysfunction	Hypocalcemia	Hypercalcemia
Cardiovascular	Arrhythmias, hypotension	Signs of heart block, cardiac arrest in systole, hypertension
Central nervous system	Anxiety, irritability, twitching around mouth, laryngospasm, seizures, Chvostek's sign, Trousseau's sign	Drowsiness, lethargy, headaches, depression or apathy, irritability, confusion, coma
GI	Increased GI motility, diarrhea	Anorexia, nausea, vomiting, constipation, dehydration, polydipsia
Musculoskeletal	Paresthesia (tingling and numbness of the fingers), tetany or painful tonic muscle spasms, facial spasms, abdominal cramps, muscle cramps, spasmodic contractions	Weakness, muscle flaccidity, bone pain, pathologic fractures
Other	Blood clotting abnormalities (rare)	Polyuria, flank pain, renal calculi and, eventually, azotemia

possibly, cardiac arrhythmias. Although Chvostek's and Trousseau's signs are reliable indicators of hypocalcemia, they aren't specific.

Hyper...

Signs and symptoms of hypercalcemia include muscle weakness, decreased muscle tone, lethargy, anorexia, constipation, nausea, vomiting, dehydration, polydipsia, and polyuria. When calcium levels are greater than 13 mg/dl (3.2 mmol/L), renal insufficiency may develop, especially if blood phosphate levels are normal or elevated due to impaired renal function. Severe hypercalcemia (serum levels that exceed 18 mg/dl [4.5 mmol/L]) may produce cardiac arrhythmias and, eventually, coma.

What tests tell you

A serum calcium level below 8.2 mg/dl confirms hypocalcemia; a level above 10 mg/dl confirms hypercalcemia. (However, because about half of serum calcium is bound to albumin, changes in serum protein must be considered when interpreting serum calcium level.)

In patients with hypocalcemia, an ECG reveals a lengthened QT interval, a prolonged ST segment, and arrhythmias; in those with hypercalcemia, an ECG reveals a shortened QT interval and heart block.

How it's treated

An acute imbalance requires immediate correction, followed by maintenance therapy and correction of the underlying cause:
• A mild calcium deficit may require nothing more than an adjustment in diet to allow adequate calcium intake, vitamin D, and protein, possibly with oral calcium supplements.
• Acute hypocalcemia is an emergency that needs immediate correction by I.V. administration of calcium gluconate or calcium chloride.
• Chronic hypocalcemia requires vitamin D supplements to facilitate GI absorption of calcium.
• Treatment of hypercalcemia primarily eliminates excess serum calcium through hydration with normal saline solution, which promotes calcium excretion in urine. Loop diuretics, such as ethacrynic acid and furosemide, also promote calcium excretion. (Because thiazide diuretics inhibit calcium excretion, they're contraindicated in hypercalcemic patients.)
• Plicamycin can lower the serum calcium level and is especially effective against hypercalcemia secondary to certain tumors. Calcitonin may also be helpful in certain instances.
• Sodium phosphate solution administered by mouth or by retention enema promotes calcium deposits in bone and inhibits its absorption from the GI tract.
• If the patient is receiving massive transfusions of citrated blood or has chronic diarrhea, severe infection, or insufficient dietary intake of calcium or protein (common in elderly patients), monitor him for hypocalcemia.

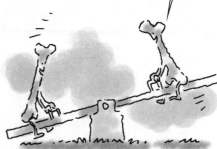

An acute calcium imbalance requires immediate correction.

Chronic obstructive pulmonary disease

COPD, also called *chronic obstructive lung disease*, results from emphysema, chronic bronchitis, asthma, or any combination of these disorders. Usually more than one of these underlying conditions coexist; most commonly, bronchitis and emphysema occur together.

(Text continues on page 501.)

Neurologic disorders

Alzheimer's disease

In Alzheimer's disease, amyloid plaques develop in the cerebral cortex and cause the death of neurons. Later, atrophy of the cerebral cortex becomes evident.

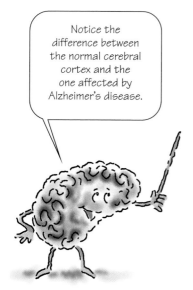

Notice the difference between the normal cerebral cortex and the one affected by Alzheimer's disease.

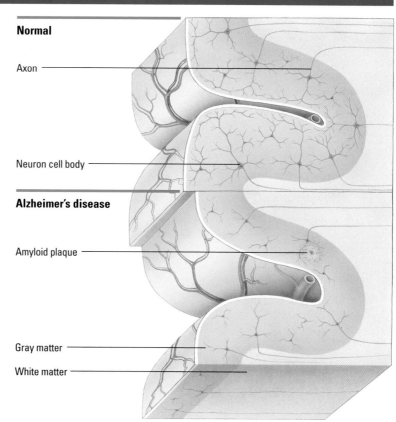

Normal

Axon

Neuron cell body

Alzheimer's disease

Amyloid plaque

Gray matter

White matter

Normally, neurons communicate via a chemical message that passes between two cells across a synapse. A neuron receives messages from its dendrites and passes the information to the cell body, where the message is received. The message can then be sent to the end of the axon, where sacs containing neurotransmitters are released. The sacs empty the neurotransmitter into the synapse between the two cells. The other cell picks up the chemical message and the process continues. This process is disrupted in patients with Alzheimer's disease.

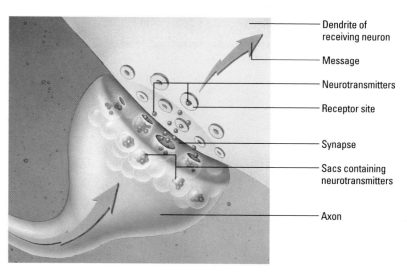

Dendrite of receiving neuron

Message

Neurotransmitters

Receptor site

Synapse

Sacs containing neurotransmitters

Axon

Stroke

Stroke occurs when cerebral circulation is suddenly impaired in one or more blood vessels that supply the brain. When circulation is impaired, oxygen supply to the brain is diminished or interrupted, causing damage or death in the brain tissues. The cause can be ischemic or hemorrhagic.

Ischemic stroke

With ischemic stroke, a thrombus and plaque form in a vessel (shown at right), interrupting cerebral circulation. Thrombi develop in different areas of the heart according to the underlying condition. Sometimes, a piece called an *embolus* dislodges and travels into the cerebral circulation.

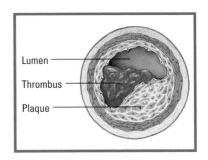

Lumen
Thrombus
Plaque

Common sites of cardiac thrombosis

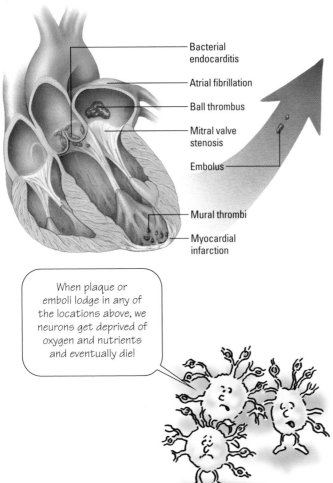

Bacterial endocarditis
Atrial fibrillation
Ball thrombus
Mitral valve stenosis
Embolus
Mural thrombi
Myocardial infarction

When plaque or emboli lodge in any of the locations above, we neurons get deprived of oxygen and nutrients and eventually die!

Common sites of plaque formation, embolism, and infarction

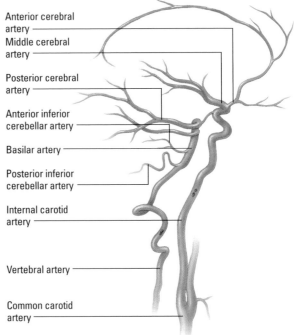

Anterior cerebral artery
Middle cerebral artery
Posterior cerebral artery
Anterior inferior cerebellar artery
Basilar artery
Posterior inferior cerebellar artery
Internal carotid artery
Vertebral artery
Common carotid artery

Hemorrhagic stroke

In hemorrhagic stroke, bleeding occurs within and around the brain. Bleeding may be caused by a ruptured aneurysm, arteriovenous malformation (AVM), hypertension, or head trauma. An abnormality of the brain's blood vessels, an AVM may dilate and rupture, causing bleeding that results in stroke. Intracerebral hemorrhage, bleeding within the brain tissue itself, can also cause stroke. It may result from hypertension. Lacunar infarcts are miniature infarcts that occur in the brain, also as a result of hypertension.

Aneurysms usually occur where the artery branches. I better keep an eye on my branches!

Common sites of cerebral hemorrhage

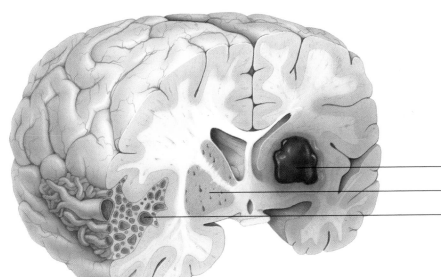

- Intracerebral hemorrhage
- Lacunar infarcts
- AVM

Confused about hemorrhage? When an aneurysm ruptures, blood fills the spaces between the brain and the skull, causing a subarachnoid hemorrhage, as shown at right.

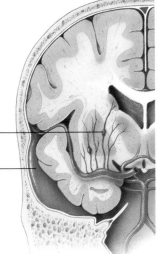

- Aneurysm
- Subarachnoid hemorrhage

Parkinson's disease

Parkinson's disease affects the extrapyramidal system, which influences body movement. The extrapyramidal system consists of the corpus striatum, globus pallidus, and substantia nigra. In Parkinson's disease, a dopamine deficiency occurs in the basal ganglia, the dopamine-releasing pathway that connects the substantia nigra to the corpus striatum.

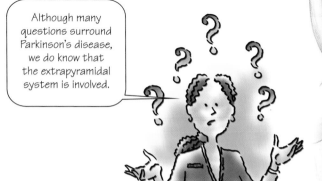

Although many questions surround Parkinson's disease, we do know that the extrapyramidal system is involved.

Motor cortex

Thalamus

Corpus striatum

Globus pallidus

Subthalamic nucleus

Substantia nigra

Cerebellum

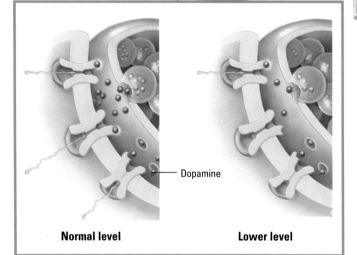

Dopamine

Normal level

Lower level

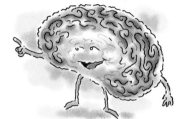

Look at the difference between my normal dopamine levels and the lower levels found with Parkinson's disease.

The most common chronic lung disease, COPD doesn't always produce symptoms and causes only minimal disability in many patients. However, COPD tends to worsen with time.

What causes it

Predisposing factors include:
- cigarette smoking
- recurrent or chronic respiratory tract infections
- air pollution
- occupations involving exposure to dusts or noxious gases
- allergies
- familial and hereditary factors (deficiency of alpha$_1$-antitrypsin).

What to look for

The typical patient with COPD is asymptomatic until middle age, when the following signs and symptoms may occur:
- reduced ability to exercise or do strenuous work
- productive cough
- dyspnea with minimal exertion.

What tests tell you

X-rays rule out associated problems and may show emphysema, hyperinflation, and pulmonary hypertension as COPD advances. PFTs reflect the degree of impairment.

How it's treated

The main goal of treatment is to relieve symptoms and prevent complications:
- Bronchodilators can help alleviate bronchospasm and enhance mucociliary clearance of secretions. Effective coughing, postural drainage, and chest physiotherapy can help mobilize secretions.
- Administration of low concentrations of oxygen helps relieve symptoms; ABG analysis helps determine oxygen need and helps avoid carbon dioxide narcosis.
- Antibiotics help treat respiratory tract infections.
- Pneumococcal vaccination and annual influenza vaccinations are important preventive measures.

Some patients benefit from inhaled corticosteroids as maintenance therapy. Oral corticosteroids are occasionally needed for acute exacerbations.

Colorectal cancer

Colorectal cancer accounts for 10% to 15% of all new cancer cases in the United States. It occurs equally in both sexes and is the third most common cause of cancer death. It's most common among people older than age 50.

Early warning

Because colorectal cancer progresses slowly and remains localized for a long time, early detection is key to recovery. Unless the tumor metastasizes, the 5-year survival rate is 80% for rectal cancer and 85% for colon cancer.

What causes it

The primary risk factor for colorectal cancer is age. Colorectal polyps are also closely tied to colorectal cancer—the larger the polyp, the greater the risk. Several disorders and preexisting conditions are also linked to colorectal cancer, including:

- familial adenomatous polyposis, such as Gardner's and Peutz-Jeghers syndromes
- ulcerative colitis
- Crohn's disease
- Turcot's syndrome
- hereditary nonpolyposis colorectal carcinoma
- other pelvic cancers treated with abdominal radiation
- genetic abnormality.

Slow passage

A high-fat, low-fiber diet is thought to contribute to colorectal cancer by slowing fecal movement through the bowel. This slowed movement results in prolonged exposure of the bowel mucosa to digested materials and may encourage mucosal cells to mutate.

What to look for

In its early stages, colorectal cancer usually causes no symptoms. Rectal bleeding, blood in the stool, a change in bowel habits, and cramping pain in the lower abdomen may signal advanced disease.

What tests tell you

Several tests are used to diagnose colorectal cancer:
• Digital rectal examination (DRE) is used to detect 15% of colorectal cancers.
• Fecal occult blood test is used to detect blood in stool.
• Proctoscopy or sigmoidoscopy is used to visualize the lower GI tract and aids in the detection of two-thirds of all colorectal cancers.
• Colonoscopy is used to visualize and photograph the colon up to the ileocecal valve and provides access for polypectomies and biopsies.
• Barium enema is used to locate lesions that aren't visible or palpable.
• CT scanning helps to detect cancer spread.
• Carcinoembryonic antigen, a tumor marker, which becomes elevated in about 70% of patients with colorectal cancer, is used to monitor the patient before and after treatment to detect metastasis or recurrence.
• Liver function studies determine whether liver metastasis has occurred.

How it's treated

The most effective treatment for colorectal cancer is surgical removal of the malignant tumor, adjacent tissues, and cancerous lymph nodes. The surgical site depends on the location of the tumor. Different locations in the colon may be resected for tumor removal. A permanent colostomy is rarely needed in a patient with colorectal cancer.

Chemotherapy or chemotherapy in combination with radiation therapy is given before or after surgery to most patients whose cancer has deeply perforated the bowel wall or has spread to the lymph nodes. Commonly used drugs include oxaliplatin in combination with fluorouracil followed by leucovorin for patients with metastatic carcinoma.

Coronary artery disease

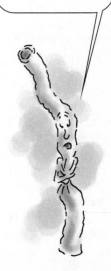

In CAD, poor coronary blood flow decreases the delivery of oxygen and nutrients to myocardial tissue.

Coronary artery disease (CAD) causes the loss of oxygen and nutrients to myocardial tissue because of poor coronary blood flow. This disease is nearly epidemic in the Western world. About 250,000 people a year die in the United States of CAD without being hospitalized—about one-half of all deaths caused by CAD.

What causes it

Atherosclerosis is the most common cause of CAD. In this condition, fatty, fibrous plaques, possibly including calcium deposits, progressively narrow the coronary artery lumens, which reduces the volume of blood that can flow through them. This reduction in flow can lead to myocardial ischemia (a temporary deficiency of blood flow to the heart) and eventually necrosis (heart tissue death).

What you can and can't control

Many risk factors are associated with atherosclerosis and CAD. Some are modifiable and some are nonmodifiable.

Nonmodifiable risk factors include being older than age 40, being male, being white, and having a family history of CAD. (See *Genes implicated in CAD.*)

Modifiable risk factors include:
• systolic blood pressure greater than 119 mm Hg or diastolic blood pressure greater than 79 mm Hg
• increased low-density and decreased high-density lipoprotein levels

---

Genes implicated in CAD

Overwhelming evidence confirms a genetic link to coronary artery disease (CAD). Researchers have identified more than 250 genes that may play a role in CAD. It commonly results from combined effects of multiple genes. These effects make the genetics of CAD very complicated because many genes can influence a person's risk.

Here are some of the best understood genes linked to CAD:
• Low-density lipoprotein (LDL) receptor is a protein that removes LDL from the bloodstream. A mutation in this gene is responsible for familial hypercholesterolemia.
• Apolipoprotein E is commonly called *apo E.* Mutations in this gene also affect blood levels of LDL.
• Apolipoprotein B-100—commonly called *apo B-100*—is a component of LDL. Mutations

of this gene cause LDL to stay in the blood longer than normal, leading to a very high LDL level.
• Apolipoprotein A is a glycoprotein that combines with LDL to form a particle called *Lp(a).* Lp(a) appears as part of plaque on blood vessels.
• Methylenetetrahydrofolate (MTHFR) reductase is one of the enzymes that clears homocysteine from the blood. Mutations in MTHFR genes may cause a higher homocysteine level.
• Cystathionine B-synthase—also known as *CBS*—is another enzyme involved in homocysteine metabolism. CBS mutations cause a condition known as *homocystinuria* in which homocysteine levels are so high that homocysteine can be detected in urine.

- elevated homocysteine levels
- smoking (risk dramatically drops within 1 year of quitting)
- stress
- obesity, which increases the risk of diabetes mellitus, hypertension, and high cholesterol
- inactivity
- diabetes mellitus, especially in women.

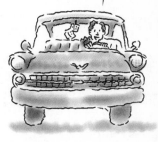

Angina is the classic sign of CAD.

What to look for

Angina is the classic sign of CAD. The patient may describe a burning, squeezing, or crushing tightness in the substernal or precordial area that radiates to the left arm, neck, jaw, or shoulder blade. Pain is commonly accompanied by nausea, vomiting, fainting, sweating, and cool extremities.

Angina commonly occurs after physical exertion but may also follow emotional excitement, exposure to cold, or the consumption of a large meal. Sometimes, it develops during sleep and awakens the patient.

When to label it stable or unstable

If the pain is predictable and relieved by rest or nitrates, it's called *stable angina*. If it increases in frequency and duration and is more easily induced, it's called *unstable angina*. Left untreated, either type of angina may progress to MI.

What tests tell you

These diagnostic tests confirm CAD:
- ECG during an episode of angina shows ischemia, as demonstrated by T-wave inversion, ST-segment depression and, possibly, arrhythmias such as premature ventricular contractions.
- Treadmill or bicycle exercise stress test may provoke chest pain and ECG signs of myocardial ischemia. The ECG rhythm may show T-wave inversion or ST-segment depression in ischemic areas.
- Coronary angiography reveals the location and extent of coronary artery stenosis or obstruction, collateral circulation, and the arteries' condition beyond the narrowing.
- Myocardial perfusion imaging with thallium-201 during treadmill exercise test detects ischemic areas of the myocardium, visualized as "cold spots."

How it's treated

The goals of treatment involve controlling risk factors and reducing myocardial demand or increasing oxygen supply and alleviating pain.

Controlling risk

Patients should limit calories and their intake of salt, fats, and cholesterol as well as stop smoking. Regular exercise is important, although it may need to be done more slowly to prevent pain. If stress is a known pain trigger, patients should learn stress reduction techniques.

Other preventive actions include controlling hypertension with diuretics, beta-adrenergic blockers, or angiotensin-converting enzyme (ACE) inhibitors; controlling elevated serum cholesterol or triglyceride levels with antilipemics; and minimizing platelet aggregation and blood clot formation with aspirin.

Noninvasive measures

Drug therapy also consists of nitrates, such as nitroglycerin, isosorbide dinitrate, or beta-adrenergic blockers that dilate vessels.

Invasive measures

Three invasive treatments are commonly used:
• coronary artery bypass graft (CABG) surgery which bypasses the site of occlusion using a graft
• percutaneous transluminal coronary angioplasty (PTCA) to compress fatty deposits, relieve occlusion and, possibly, allow placement of a stent
• laser angioplasty to dissolve the occlusion using a laser beam.

Deep vein thrombosis

Deep vein thrombosis (DVT) affects small veins, such as the soleal venous sinuses, or large veins, such as the vena cava and the femoral, iliac, and subclavian veins. It's an acute condition characterized by inflammation and thrombus formation. This disorder is commonly progressive, leading to pulmonary embolism, a potentially lethal complication.

What causes it

DVT may be idiopathic but may also result from endothelial damage, accelerated blood clotting, and reduced blood flow. Predisposing factors include:
• prolonged bed rest
• trauma
• surgery
• childbirth
• hormonal contraceptive use.

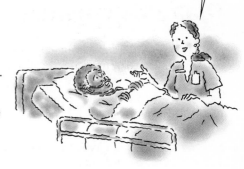

Prolonged bed rest increases the risk of DVT.

What to look for

In thrombosis, clinical features vary with the site and length of the affected vein. Although DVT may occur asymptomatically, it may also produce:
• severe pain
• fever
• chills
• malaise
• possibly swelling and cyanosis of the affected arm or leg.

What tests tell you

Some patients may display signs of inflammation and, possibly, a positive Homans' sign (pain on dorsiflexion of the foot) during physical examination; others are asymptomatic. Essential laboratory tests include:
• Doppler ultrasonography is used to identify reduced blood flow to a specific area and any obstruction to venous flow, particularly in iliofemoral deep vein thrombophlebitis.
• Plethysmography shows decreased circulation distal to the affected area; it's more sensitive than ultrasound in detecting DVT.
• Phlebography can show filling defects and diverted blood flow and usually confirms the diagnosis.

How it's treated

The goals of treatment for DVT are to control thrombus development, prevent complications, relieve pain, and prevent recurrence. Symptomatic measures include bed rest with elevation of the affected arm or leg, analgesics, and warm, moist soaks to the affected area.

Treatment may also include anticoagulants (initially, heparin; later, warfarin) to prolong clotting time. Prophylactic doses of anticoagulants may reduce the risk of DVT and pulmonary embolism after surgery. For lysis of acute, extensive DVT, treatment should include streptokinase.

Diabetes mellitus

Diabetes mellitus is a disease in which the body doesn't produce or properly use insulin, leading to hyperglycemia. The disease occurs in two primary forms:

✌ type 1 (formerly referred to as *insulin-dependent diabetes mellitus*)

✌ type 2 (formerly referred to as *non-insulin-dependent diabetes mellitus*), the more prevalent form.

Several secondary forms also exist, caused by such conditions as pancreatic disease, pregnancy (gestational diabetes mellitus), hormonal or genetic problems, and certain drugs or chemicals.

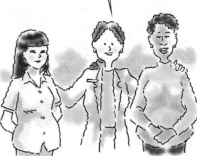

Diabetes mellitus in pregnant women is known as gestational diabetes mellitus.

What causes it

Insulin transports glucose into the cell for use as energy and storage as glycogen. It also stimulates protein synthesis and free fatty acid storage. Insulin deficiency or resistance compromises the body tissues' access to essential nutrients for fuel and storage. The effects of diabetes mellitus result from insulin deficiency.

Type 1 diabetes can result from autoimmune beta-cell destruction, resulting in insulin deficiency or ketosis. Risk factors for type 2 diabetes include:
• obesity (body mass index $\geq 27 \text{ kg/m}^2$)
• high-density lipoprotein level ≤ 35 mg/dl or triglyceride level ≥ 250 mg/dl
• hypertension (blood pressure $\geq 140/90$ mm Hg)
• family history of diabetes
• age ≥ 45.

Acute danger

Two acute metabolic complications of diabetes are DKA and hyperosmolar hyperglycemic nonketotic syndrome (HHNS). These life-threatening conditions require immediate medical intervention. (See *Comparing HHNS and DKA.*)

Comparing HHNS and DKA

Hyperosmolar hyperglycemic nonketotic syndrome (HHNS) and diabetic ketoacidosis (DKA) both are acute complications of diabetes. Although they share some similarities, they're two distinct conditions. Use the flowchart below to determine which condition your patient has.

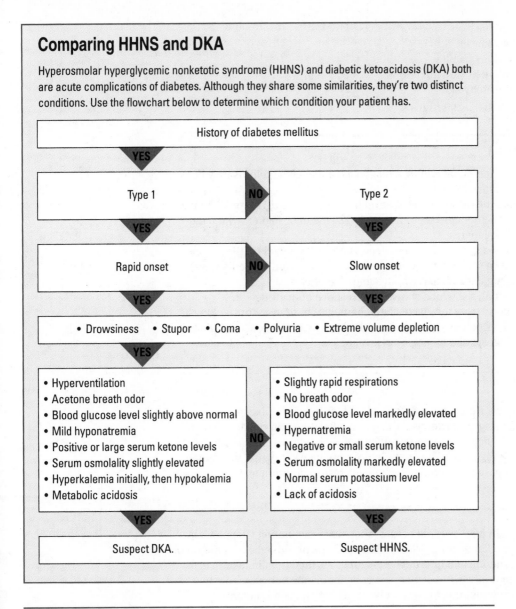

History of diabetes mellitus

YES

| Type 1 | **NO** | Type 2 |

YES — **YES**

| Rapid onset | **NO** | Slow onset |

YES — **YES**

• Drowsiness   • Stupor   • Coma   • Polyuria   • Extreme volume depletion

YES

• Hyperventilation
• Acetone breath odor
• Blood glucose level slightly above normal
• Mild hyponatremia
• Positive or large serum ketone levels
• Serum osmolality slightly elevated
• Hyperkalemia initially, then hypokalemia
• Metabolic acidosis

NO

• Slightly rapid respirations
• No breath odor
• Blood glucose level markedly elevated
• Hypernatremia
• Negative or small serum ketone levels
• Serum osmolality markedly elevated
• Normal serum potassium level
• Lack of acidosis

YES — **YES**

| Suspect DKA. | Suspect HHNS. |

What to look for

Patients with type 1 or type 2 diabetes may report symptoms related to hyperglycemia, such as:
• excessive urination (polyuria)
• excessive thirst (polydipsia)
• excessive eating (polyphagia)
• weight loss

- fatigue
- weakness
- vision changes
- frequent skin infections
- dry, itchy skin
- vaginal discomfort.

What tests tell you

In nonpregnant adults, a diagnosis of diabetes mellitus may be confirmed by:
- fasting plasma glucose level between 100 and 125 mg/dl, which signals prediabetes, or a level of 126 mg/dl or higher, which indicates diabetes
- blood glucose level between 140 and 199 mg/dl on the second hour of the glucose tolerance test, which signifies prediabetes, or 200 mg/dl or higher, which signifies diabetes
- urinalysis, which shows the presence of acetone
- blood tests for glycosylated hemoglobin to monitor the long-term effectiveness of diabetes therapy, with the goal of achieving a glycosylated hemoglobin level of 7%.

How it's treated

In type 1 diabetes, treatment includes insulin replacement, meal planning, and exercise. Current forms of insulin replacement include single-dose, mixed-dose, split-mixed-dose, and multiple-dose regimens. The multiple-dose regimens may use an insulin pump. In some patients, pancreas transplantation may be an option.

Insulin action

Insulin may be rapid-acting (Humalog), fast-acting (Regular), intermediate-acting (NPH and Lente), or a premixed combination of fast-acting and intermediate-acting. Purified human insulin is used commonly today. Patients may inject insulin subcutaneously throughout the day or receive it through an insulin pump.

Personalized meal plan

Treatment for both types of diabetes also requires a meal plan to meet nutritional needs, control blood glucose levels, and help the patient reach and maintain his ideal body weight. A dietitian estimates the total amount of energy a patient needs per day based on his ideal body weight. Then she plans meals with the appropriate carbohydrate, fat, and protein content. For the diet to work, the patient must follow it consistently and eat at regular times.

Other treatments

Exercise is also useful in managing type 2 diabetes because it increases insulin sensitivity, improves glucose tolerance, and promotes weight loss. In addition, patients with type 2 diabetes may need oral antidiabetic drugs to stimulate endogenous insulin production and increase insulin sensitivity at the cellular level.

Gastroenteritis

Also called *intestinal flu*, *traveler's diarrhea*, *viral enteritis*, and *food poisoning*, gastroenteritis is a self-limiting disorder characterized by diarrhea, nausea, vomiting, and abdominal cramping. It can be life-threatening in elderly and debilitated people.

What causes it

Gastroenteritis has many possible causes, including:
• bacteria (responsible for acute food poisoning), such as *Staphylococcus aureus*, *Salmonella*, *Shigella*, *Clostridium botulinum*, *Escherichia coli*, and *Clostridium perfringens*
• amoebae—especially *Entamoeba histolytica*
• parasites, such as *Ascaris*, *Enterobius*, and *Trichinella spiralis*
• viruses (which may be responsible for traveler's diarrhea), including adenovirus, echovirus, or coxsackievirus
• ingestion of toxins, such as plants and toadstools (mushrooms)
• reactions to such drugs as antibiotics
• enzyme deficiencies
• food allergens.
    The bowel reacts to any of these enterotoxins with hypermotility, producing severe diarrhea and secondary depletion of intracellular fluid.

What to look for

Signs and symptoms of gastroenteritis vary, depending on the organism and the level of GI tract involved. Signs and symptoms include diarrhea, abdominal discomfort (ranging from cramping to pain), nausea, and vomiting. Other possible symptoms include fever, malaise, and borborygmi. (See *Low tolerance*.)

Low tolerance

In children, the elderly, and debilitated people, gastroenteritis produces the same symptoms. However, the inability of these patients to tolerate electrolyte and fluid losses leads to a higher mortality.

What tests tell you

Patient history can aid in the diagnosis of gastroenteritis. A stool culture should be obtained. Blood cultures are indicated in febrile patients.

How it's treated

Treatment of gastroenteritis is supportive and consists of nutritional support and increased fluid intake. An episode of acute gastroenteritis is self-limiting. When an episode is severe and produces symptoms for more than 3 or 4 days, hospitalization may be necessary. Treatment may include fluid and electrolyte replacement, antibiotic therapy, and antiemetics.

Gastroesophageal reflux disease

Popularly known as *heartburn*, gastroesophageal reflux disease (GERD) involves backflow of gastric or duodenal contents or both into the esophagus and past the lower esophageal sphincter (LES), without associated belching or vomiting. The reflux of gastric contents causes acute epigastric pain, usually after a meal. The pain may radiate to the chest or arms.

Most estimates show that approximately 2% of the adult population suffers from GERD. The incidence of GERD increases markedly after age 40. It commonly occurs in pregnant or obese people.

What causes it

Various factors can lead to GERD, including:
• weakened esophageal sphincter
• increased abdominal pressure, such as with obesity or pregnancy
• hiatal hernia
• medications, such as morphine, diazepam, and calcium channel blockers
• food or alcohol ingestion or cigarette smoking that lowers LES pressure
• NG intubation for more than 4 days.

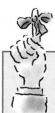

Memory jogger

Remember these facts about **GERD**:

Generally known as heartburn.

Epigastric pain and spasm usually follow a meal.

Radiating pain to arms and chest is common.

Diet therapy, antacids and smoking cessation can help alleviate symptoms.

Less LES pressure means more reflux

Normally, the LES maintains enough pressure around the lower end of the esophagus to close it and prevent reflux. Typically, the sphincter relaxes after each swallow to allow food into the stomach. In GERD, the sphincter doesn't remain closed (usually because of deficient LES pressure or pressure within the stomach that exceeds LES pressure), and the pressure in the stomach pushes the stomach contents into the esophagus. The high acidity of the stomach contents causes pain and irritation when the contents enter the esophagus.

What to look for

Patients with GERD typically complain of a burning pain in the epigastric area. The pain may radiate to the arms and chest. Pain usually occurs after meals or when the patient lies down. The patient may also complain of a feeling of fluid accumulating in the throat. The fluid doesn't have a sour or bitter taste because of the hypersecretion of saliva.

What tests tell you

Diagnostic tests are aimed at determining the underlying cause of GERD:
• Esophageal acidity test evaluates the competence of the LES and provides an objective measure of reflux.
• Acid perfusion test confirms esophagitis and distinguishes it from cardiac disorders.
• Esophagoscopy allows visual examination of the lining of the esophagus to reveal the extent of disease and confirm pathologic changes in mucosa.
• Barium swallow identifies hiatal hernia as the cause.
• Upper GI series detects hiatal hernia or motility problems.
• Esophageal manometry evaluates the resting pressure of the LES and determines sphincter competence.

How it's treated

Treatment of GERD may include:
• diet therapy with frequent, small meals and avoidance of eating before going to bed
• positioning—sitting up during and after meals and sleeping with the head of the bed elevated
• increased fluid intake
• antacids

- histamine-2 (H_2) receptor antagonists
- proton pump inhibitors
- cholinergic agents
- smoking cessation (because nicotine lowers LES pressure)
- surgery if hiatal hernia is the cause or if the patient has refractory symptoms.

Heart failure

When the myocardium can't pump effectively enough to meet the body's metabolic needs, heart failure occurs. Pump failure usually occurs in a damaged left ventricle, but it may also happen in the right ventricle. Usually, left-sided heart failure develops first.

Heart failure is classified as:
- high-output or low-output
- acute or chronic
- left-sided or right-sided
- forward or backward. (See *Classifying heart failure.*)

Classifying heart failure

Heart failure may be classified different ways according to its pathophysiology.

Right-sided or left-sided

Right-sided heart failure is a result of ineffective right ventricular contractile function. It may be caused by an acute right ventricular infarction or pulmonary embolus. However, the most common cause is profound backward flow due to left-sided heart failure.

Left-sided heart failure is the result of ineffective left ventricular contractile function. It may lead to pulmonary congestion or pulmonary edema and decreased cardiac output. Left ventricular myocardial infarction, hypertension, and aortic and mitral valve stenosis or insufficiency are common causes.

As the decreased pumping ability of the left ventricle persists, fluid accumulates, backing up into the left atrium and then into the lungs. If this accumulation worsens, pulmonary edema and right-sided heart failure may also result.

Systolic or diastolic

In systolic heart failure, the left ventricle can't pump enough blood out to the systemic circulation during systole and the ejection fraction falls. Consequently, blood backs up into the pulmonary circulation, pressure rises in the pulmonary venous system, and cardiac output falls.

In diastolic heart failure, the left ventricle can't relax and fill properly during diastole and the stroke volume falls. Therefore, larger ventricular volumes are needed to maintain cardiac output.

Acute or chronic

Acute refers to the timing of the onset of symptoms and whether compensatory mechanisms kick in. Typically, fluid status is normal or low, and sodium and water retention don't occur.

In *chronic* heart failure, signs and symptoms have been present for some time, compensatory mechanisms have taken effect, and fluid volume overload persists. Drugs, diet changes, and activity restrictions usually control symptoms.

What causes it

Heart failure may result from a primary abnormality of the heart muscle caused by an MI that impairs ventricular function and prevents the heart from pumping enough blood.

Heart failure may also be caused by:
• atrial fibrillation
• aortic insufficiency
• aortic stenosis
• mitral stenosis secondary to rheumatic heart disease or constrictive pericarditis
• systemic hypertension.

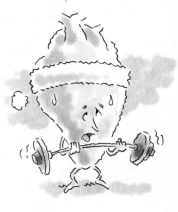

I fail when the myocardium can't pump effectively enough to meet the body's metabolic needs.

Factors favorable to failure

Certain conditions can predispose a patient to heart failure, especially if he has underlying heart disease. These conditions include:
• arrhythmias
• pregnancy
• thyrotoxicosis
• pulmonary embolism
• infections
• anemia
• increased physical activity
• increased salt or water intake
• emotional stress
• failure to comply with the prescribed treatment regimen for the underlying heart disease.

Getting complicated

Eventually, sodium and water may enter the lungs, causing pulmonary edema, a life-threatening condition. Decreased perfusion to the brain, kidneys, and other major organs can cause them to fail. MI can occur because the oxygen demands of the overworked heart can't be met.

What to look for

The early signs and symptoms of heart failure include:
• fatigue
• exertional, paroxysmal, and nocturnal dyspnea
• jugular vein engorgement
• hepatomegaly.

Later signs and symptoms include:
• tachypnea
• palpitations

- dependent edema
- unexplained, steady weight gain
- nausea
- chest tightness
- slowed mental response
- anorexia
- hypotension
- diaphoresis
- narrow pulse pressure
- pallor
- oliguria
- gallop rhythm
- inspiratory crackles on auscultation
- dullness over the lung bases
- hemoptysis
- cyanosis
- marked hepatomegaly
- pitting ankle enema
- sacral edema in bedridden patients.

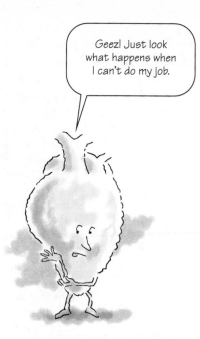

Geez! Just look what happens when I can't do my job.

What tests tell you

These tests help diagnose heart failure:
- ECG reveals ischemia, tachycardia, and extrasystole.
- Echocardiogram identifies the underlying cause as well as the type and severity of heart failure.
- Laboratory studies, such as B-type natriuretic peptide, confirm the presence of heart failure.
- Chest X-ray shows increased pulmonary vascular markings, interstitial edema, or pleural effusion and cardiomegaly.
- Pulmonary artery pressure (PAP) monitoring shows elevated PAP, pulmonary artery wedge pressure, and left ventricular end-diastolic pressure in left-sided heart failure; elevated right atrial pressure or elevated central venous pressure in right-sided heart failure.

How it's treated

The goal of treatment for heart failure is to improve pump function, thereby reversing the compensatory mechanisms that produce or intensify the clinical effects. Heart failure can usually be controlled quickly with treatment, including:
- bed rest
- supplemental oxygen
- drug therapy that includes diuretics, such as furosemide, bumetanide, and ethacrynic acid; inotropic drugs, such as digoxin

or nesiritide; sympathomimetics, such as dobutamine, inamrinone, or milrinone; vasodilators, such as nitroglycerin; and ACE inhibitors
• antiembolism stockings to prevent venostasis and thromboembolism formation.

Acute pulmonary edema

As a result of decreased contractility and elevated fluid volume and pressure, fluid may be driven from the pulmonary capillary beds into the alveoli, causing pulmonary edema. Treatment for acute pulmonary edema includes:
• drug therapy that includes morphine; vasodilators, such as nitroglycerin and nitroprusside; dobutamine; dopamine; inamrinone; nesiritide; milrinone; or diuretics to reduce fluid volume)
• administration of supplemental oxygen
• placement of the patient in high Fowler's position.

Continued care

After recovery, the patient must continue medical care and usually must continue taking digoxin, diuretics, and potassium supplements. The patient with valve dysfunction who has recurrent, acute heart failure may need surgical valve replacement.

What's left?

Left ventricular remodeling surgery may also be performed. This surgical procedure involves cutting a wedge about the size of a small slice of pie out of the left ventricle of an enlarged heart and then repairing the left ventricle. The result is a smaller ventricle that can pump blood more efficiently. The only option for some patients is heart transplantation. A left ventricular assist device may be necessary until a heart is available for transplantation.

Hepatitis, viral

Viral hepatitis is a common infection of the liver. Marked by liver cell destruction, tissue death (necrosis), and self-destruction of cells (autolysis), it leads to anorexia, jaundice, and hepatomegaly. In most patients, damaged liver cells eventually regenerate with little or no permanent damage. However, old age and serious underlying disorders make complications more likely.

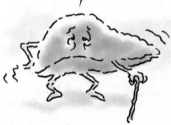

Old age and serious underlying disorders can prevent the regeneration of damaged liver cells.

What causes it

Five types of viral hepatitis are commonly recognized, each caused by a different virus:

• Type A is transmitted almost exclusively by the fecal-oral route, and outbreaks are common in areas of overcrowding and poor sanitation. Day care centers and other institutional settings are common sources of outbreaks. The incidence is also increasing among homosexuals and in people with human immunodeficiency virus (HIV) infection.

• Type B, also increasing among HIV-positive people, accounts for 5% to 10% of posttransfusion hepatitis cases in the United States. Vaccinations are available and are now required for health care workers and school children in many states.

• Type C accounts for about 20% of all viral hepatitis as well as most cases that follow transfusion.

• Type D, in the United States, is confined to people frequently exposed to blood and blood products, such as I.V. drug users and patients with hemophilia.

• Type E was formerly grouped with type C under the name *non-A, non-B hepatitis*. In the United States, this type mainly occurs in people who have visited an endemic area, such as India, Africa, Asia, or Central America.

The forms of viral hepatitis result from infection with the causative viruses A, B, C, D, and E. (See *Viral hepatitis from A to E.*)

Type G is a newly identified virus, transmitted by the blood-borne route, similar to hepatitis C. Detection of hepatitis G antigen supports diagnosis; the patient may be otherwise asymptomatic.

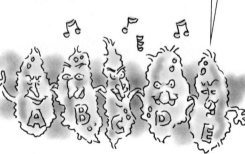

Now you know your ABCs and also how we cause disease.

What to look for

Signs and symptoms of viral hepatitis progress in three stages:

 prodromal

 clinical

 recovery.

Prodromal stage

During the prodromal stage, the infection is highly transmissible. In this stage, signs and symptoms include:

• fatigue

Viral hepatitis from A to E

This chart compares the features of each type of viral hepatitis.

Feature	Hepatitis A	Hepatitis B	Hepatitis C	Hepatitis D	Hepatitis E
Incubation	15 to 45 days	30 to 180 days	15 to 160 days	14 to 64 days	14 to 60 days
Onset	Acute	Insidious	Insidious	Acute	Acute
Age-group most affected	Children, young adults	Any age	More common in adults	Any age	Ages 20 to 40
Transmission	Fecal-oral, sexual (especially oral-anal contact), nonpercutaneous (sexual, maternal-neonatal), percutaneous (rare)	Blood-borne; parenteral route, sexual, maternal-neonatal; virus is shed in all body fluids	Blood-borne; parenteral route	Parenteral route; most people infected with hepatitis D are also infected with hepatitis B	Primarily fecal-oral
Severity	Mild	Usually severe	Moderate	Can be severe and lead to fulminant hepatitis	Highly virulent with common progression to fulminant hepatitis and hepatic failure, especially in pregnant patients
Prognosis	Generally good	Worsens with age and debility	Moderate	Fair; worsens in chronic cases; can lead to chronic hepatitis D and chronic liver disease	Good unless pregnant
Progression to chronicity	None	Occasional	10% to 50% of cases	Occasional	None

- anorexia
- mild weight loss
- generalized malaise
- depression
- headache
- weakness
- joint pain (arthralgia)
- muscle pain (myalgia)
- intolerance of light (photophobia)
- nausea and vomiting

- changes in the senses of taste and smell
- temperature of 100° to 102° F (37.8° to 38.9° C)
- right upper quadrant tenderness
- dark-colored urine and clay-colored stools (1 to 5 days before the onset of the clinical jaundice stage).

Clinical stage

The clinical stage begins 1 to 2 weeks after the prodromal stage. It's the phase of actual illness. If the patient progresses to this stage, he may have these signs and symptoms:
- itching
- abdominal pain or tenderness
- indigestion
- appetite loss (in early clinical stage)
- jaundice.

Color my world

Jaundice lasts for 1 to 2 weeks and indicates that the damaged liver can't remove bilirubin from the blood. However, jaundice doesn't indicate disease severity and, occasionally, hepatitis occurs without jaundice.

Recovery stage

Recovery begins with the resolution of jaundice and lasts 2 to 6 weeks in uncomplicated cases. The prognosis is poor if edema and hepatic encephalopathy develop.

What tests tell you

These tests are used to diagnose viral hepatitis:
- Hepatitis profile establishes the type of hepatitis.
- Liver function studies show disease stage.
- Prothrombin time (PT) is prolonged.
- White blood cell (WBC) count is elevated.
- Liver biopsy may be performed if chronic hepatitis is suspected.

How it's treated

Hepatitis C has been treated somewhat successfully with interferon alfa. No specific drug therapy has been developed for other types of viral hepatitis. Instead, the patient is advised to rest in the early stages of the illness and combat anorexia by eating small, high-calorie, high-protein meals.

Protein intake should be reduced if signs of precoma — lethargy, confusion, or mental changes — develop. Large meals are usually better tolerated in the morning because many patients have nausea late in the day.

Acute cases

In acute viral hepatitis, hospitalization is usually required only if severe symptoms or complications occur. Parenteral nutrition may be needed if the patient can't eat because of persistent vomiting.

Human immunodeficiency virus disease

HIV is the infectious agent responsible for the immune system disorder HIV disease. The disease, characterized by progressive immune system impairment, destroys T cells and, therefore, the cell-mediated response. This immunodeficiency makes the patient more susceptible to infections and unusual cancers. The course of HIV disease can vary, but it usually results in death from opportunistic infections. Most experts believe that virtually everyone infected with HIV will eventually develop acquired immunodeficiency syndrome (AIDS).

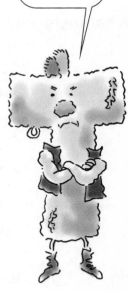

I'd better watch out. It sounds like HIV disease has it in for me.

What causes it

HIV is a ribonucleic acid–based retrovirus that requires a human host to replicate. The average time between HIV infection and the development of AIDS is 8 to 10 years. HIV destroys CD4+ cells— also known as *helper T cells*—that regulate the normal immune response. The CD4+ antigen serves as a receptor for HIV and allows it to invade the cell. Afterward, the virus replicates within the CD4+ cell, causing cell death.

Modes of transmission

HIV is transmitted three ways:

👆 through contact with infected blood or blood products during transfusion or tissue transplantation or by sharing a contaminated needle

✌ through contact with infected body fluids, such as semen and vaginal fluids, during unprotected sex

🤟 across the placental barrier from an infected mother to a fetus or from an infected mother to an infant either through cervical or blood contact at delivery or through breast milk.

What to look for

After initial exposure, the infected person may have no signs or symptoms, or he may have a flulike illness (primary infection) and then remain asymptomatic for years. As the syndrome progresses, he may have neurologic symptoms from HIV encephalopathy or symptoms of an opportunistic infection, such as *Pneumocystis carinii* pneumonia, cytomegalovirus, or cancer. Eventually, repeated opportunistic infections overwhelm the patient's weakened immune defenses, invading every body system.

Little ones

In children, the incubation period averages only 17 months. Signs and symptoms resemble those for adults, except that children are more likely to have a history of bacterial infections, such as otitis media and lymphoid interstitial pneumonia, as well as sepsis, types of pneumonia not caused by *P. carinii*, and chronic salivary gland enlargement.

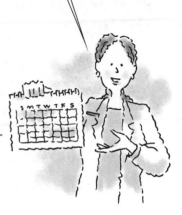

An infected person can test negative for HIV antibodies for up to 35 months after exposure.

What tests tell you

Standard HIV testing typically consists of the enzyme immunoassay, Western blot, or immunofluorescence assay. If the results are positive, they're confirmed at the next health care visit, typically in 1 to 2 weeks.

Other blood tests support the diagnosis and are used to evaluate the severity of immunosuppression. They include CD4+ and CD8+ cell (killer T cell) subset counts, erythrocyte sedimentation rate (ESR), CBC, serum beta microglobulin, p24 antigen, neopterin levels, and anergy testing.

Many opportunistic infections in patients with AIDS are reactivations of previous infections. Therefore, patients may also be tested for syphilis, hepatitis B, tuberculosis, toxoplasmosis, and histoplasmosis.

How it's treated

There's no cure for HIV disease; however, several types of drugs are used to treat the disease and prolong life, including antiretrovirals, anti-infectives, and antineoplastics.

Antiretrovirals

Antiretroviral drugs are used to control reproduction of the virus and slow the progression of HIV-related disease. Highly active antiretroviral therapy (HAART) is the recommended treatment for

HIV infection. HAART combines three or more antiretroviral medications in a daily regimen. The Food and Drug Administration has approved four classes of antiretroviral drugs:

Nonnucleoside reverse transcriptase inhibitors bind to and disable reverse transcriptase, a protein that HIV needs to make more copies of itself. Such drugs as delavirdine, efavirenz, and nevirapine are included in this class.

Nucleoside reverse transcriptase inhibitors are faulty versions of building blocks that HIV requires to make more copies of itself. When HIV uses one of these drugs instead of a normal building block, reproduction of the virus is halted. Abacavir, didanosine, emtricitabine, lamivudine, stavudine, tenofovir, zalcitabine, and zidovudine are included in this class.

Protease inhibitors disable protease, a protein that HIV needs to make more copies of itself. These drugs include amprenavir, atazanivir, fosamprenavir, indinavir, lopinavir, nelfinavir, ritonavir, and saquinavir.

Fusion inhibitors block HIV entry into cells. Enfuvirtide is the only currently approved fusion inhibitor.

Anti-infectives and antineoplastics

In addition to antiretroviral drugs, anti-infective drugs are prescribed to treat opportunistic infections. Antineoplastic drugs are used to treat associated cancers.

Hypertension

Hypertension is an intermittent or sustained elevation of diastolic or systolic blood pressure. Generally, a sustained systolic blood pressure of 140 mm Hg or higher or a diastolic blood pressure of 90 mm Hg or higher indicates hypertension. If a patient's blood pressure is between 120/80 mm Hg and 139/89 mm Hg, the patient is considered to have prehypertension.

Listen up — this is essential

The two major types of hypertension are essential (also called *primary* or *idiopathic*) and secondary. The etiology of essential hypertension, the most common type, is complex. It involves several interacting homeostatic mechanisms. Hypertension is classified as secondary if it's related to a systemic disease that raises peripheral vascular resistance or cardiac output. Malignant hypertension is a severe, fulminant form of the disorder that may arise from either type.

What causes it

Hypertension may be caused by increases in cardiac output, total peripheral resistance, or both. Family history, race, stress, obesity, a diet high in fat or sodium, use of tobacco or hormonal contraceptives, a sedentary lifestyle, and aging may all play a role.

Secondary hypertension

Secondary hypertension may be caused by:
- renovascular disease
- renal parenchymal disease
- pheochromocytoma
- primary hyperaldosteronism
- Cushing's syndrome
- diabetes mellitus
- dysfunction of the thyroid, pituitary, or parathyroid glands
- coarctation of the aorta
- pregnancy
- neurologic disorders.

What to look for

Hypertension usually doesn't produce signs or symptoms until vascular changes in the heart, brain, or kidneys occur. Severely elevated blood pressure damages the intima of small vessels, resulting in fibrin accumulation in the vessels, local edema and, possibly, intravascular clotting.

Location, location, location

Symptoms depend on the location of the damaged vessels, for example:
- brain—stroke, transient ischemic attacks (TIAs)
- retina—blindness
- heart—MI
- kidneys—proteinuria, edema and, eventually, renal failure.

A heavy heart workload

Hypertension increases the heart's workload. This increase causes left ventricular hypertrophy and, later, left-sided heart failure, pulmonary edema, and right-sided heart failure.

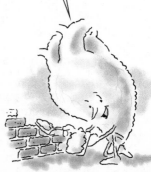

I already have enough work to do. Lay off, hypertension!

What tests tell you

According to the new classification for hypertension, people with serial systolic blood pressures between 120 to 139 mm Hg or diastolic blood pressures between 80 to 89 mm Hg are diagnosed with prehypertension. Those with blood pressures of 140/90 mm Hg or higher are diagnosed with hypertension.

Hypertension detectives

The following tests may reveal predisposing factors and help identify the cause of hypertension:
• Urinalysis may show protein, RBCs, or WBCs, suggesting renal disease, or glucose, suggesting diabetes mellitus.
• Serum potassium levels less than 3.5 mEq/L may indicate adrenal dysfunction (primary hyperaldosteronism).
• A blood urea nitrogen (BUN) level that's elevated to more than 20 mg/dl and a serum creatinine level that's elevated to more than 1.5 mg/dl suggest renal disease.

These tests may help detect cardiovascular damage and other complications:
• ECG may show left ventricular hypertrophy or ischemia.
• Chest X-ray may demonstrate cardiomegaly.

How it's treated

Although essential hypertension has no cure, drugs and modifications in diet and lifestyle can control it. Generally, lifestyle modification is the first treatment used, especially in those with prehypertension. If these modifications don't work, the doctor may prescribe drugs, such as diuretics, ACE inhibitors, angiotensin receptor blockers, beta-adrenergic blockers, calcium channel blockers, or a combination.

Influenza

Influenza is an acute, highly contagious infection of the respiratory tract that results from three types of *Myxovirus influenzae*. It occurs sporadically in epidemics (usually during the colder months). Epidemics tend to peak within 2 to 3 weeks after initial cases and subside within 1 month. Although influenza affects all age-groups, its incidence is highest in school children. Its severity is greatest in the very young, the elderly, and those with chronic disease. In these groups, influenza may even lead to death.

What causes it

Transmission occurs through inhalation of a respiratory droplet from an infected person or by indirect contact such as using a contaminated drinking glass. Influenza may be caused by one of the three following groups of viruses:
• Type A, the most prevalent, strikes every year with new serotypes causing epidemics every 3 years.
• Type B also strikes annually, but only causes epidemics every 4 to 6 years.
• Type C is endemic and causes only sporadic cases.

> One good respiratory droplet is all I need to make my way in.

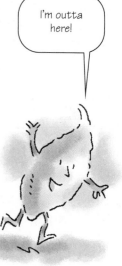

What to look for

After an incubation period of 24 to 48 hours, signs and symptoms appear, including:
• sudden onset of chills
• temperature of 101° to 104° F (38.3° to 40° C)
• headache
• malaise
• myalgia (particularly in the back and limbs)
• nonproductive cough
• occasionally, laryngitis, hoarseness, conjunctivitis, rhinitis, and rhinorrhea.

These signs and symptoms usually subside in 3 to 5 days, but cough and weakness may persist. Fever is usually higher in children than in adults. Also, cervical adenopathy and croup are likely to be associated with influenza in children. In some patients (especially the elderly), lack of energy and easy fatigability may persist for weeks.

Fever that persists longer than 5 days signals the onset of complications. The most common complication is pneumonia.

> I'm outta here!

What tests tell you

At the beginning of an influenza epidemic, early cases are usually mistaken for other respiratory disorders. Because signs and symptoms aren't diagnostic, isolation of *M. influenzae* through the inoculation of chicken embryos (with nasal secretions from infected patients) is essential at the first sign of an epidemic. Nose and throat cultures and increased serum antibody titers help confirm the diagnosis.

After these measures confirm an influenza epidemic, diagnosis requires only observation of clinical signs and symptoms. Uncomplicated cases show a decreased WBC count with an increased lymphocyte count.

How it's treated

Uncomplicated influenza is treated with bed rest, adequate fluid intake, aspirin (or acetaminophen in children) to relieve fever and muscle pain, and guaifenesin or another expectorant to relieve nonproductive coughing.

Amantadine and rimantadine (antiviral drugs) have proven effective in reducing the duration of signs and symptoms in influenza A infection. The neuraminidase inhibitors zanamivir and oseltamivir are available for influenza A and B. If influenza is complicated by pneumonia, supportive care (fluid and electrolyte supplements, oxygen, and assisted ventilation) and treatment of bacterial superinfection with appropriate antibiotics are necessary. No specific therapy exists for cardiac, CNS, or other complications.

Irritable bowel syndrome

Irritable bowel syndrome (IBS) is characterized by chronic symptoms of abdominal pain, alternating constipation and diarrhea, and abdominal distention. This disorder is common, although about 20% of patients never seek medical attention. It's twice as common in women as in men.

What causes it

IBS is generally associated with psychological stress; however, it may result from physical factors, such as diverticular disease, ingestion of irritants (coffee, raw vegetables, or fruits), laxative abuse, food poisoning, and colon cancer.

What to look for

The most commonly reported symptom is intermittent, crampy, lower abdominal pain, usually relieved by defecation or passage of flatus. It usually occurs during the day and intensifies with stress or 1 to 2 hours after meals. The patient may experience constipation alternating with diarrhea, with one being the dominant problem. Mucus is usually passed through the rectum. Abdominal distention and bloating are common.

What tests tell you

There are no tests that are specific for diagnosing IBS. Other disorders, such as diverticulitis, colon cancer, and lactose intolerance, should be ruled out by these tests:
• Stool samples for ova, parasites, bacteria, and blood rule out infection.
• Lactose intolerance test rules out lactose intolerance.
• Barium enema may reveal colon spasm and tubular appearance of descending colon without evidence of cancers and diverticulosis.
• Sigmoidoscopy or colonoscopy may reveal spastic contractions without evidence of colon cancer or inflammatory bowel disease.
• Rectal biopsy rules out malignancy.

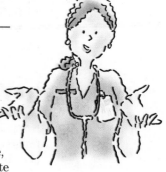

There are no tests that are specific for diagnosing IBS.

How it's treated

Treatment for IBS aims to relieve symptoms.

Medical therapy

Therapy aims to relieve symptoms and includes counseling to help the patient understand the relation between stress and his illness. Dietary restrictions haven't proven to be effective, but the patient is encouraged to be aware of foods that exacerbate symptoms. Rest and heat applied to the abdomen are usually helpful.

In the case of laxative overuse, bowel training is sometimes recommended.

Drug therapy

Antispasmodics, such as propantheline and diphenoxylate with atropine, are commonly prescribed.

Lyme disease

Lyme disease occurs chiefly in the United States and is named for the Connecticut town in which it was first recognized in 1975. It affects multiple body systems and usually appears in summer or early fall with a skin lesion called *erythema chronicum migrans*. Weeks or months later, cardiac, neurologic, or joint abnormalities may develop, sometimes followed by arthritis. The incidence has increased in most states over the past 10 years.

What causes it

Lyme disease is caused by the spirochete *Borrelia burgdorferi*, which is carried by deer ticks. Here's how the disease develops:
• The tick injects spirochete-laden saliva into the bloodstream or deposits fecal matter on the skin.
• After incubating for 3 to 32 days, the spirochetes migrate outward, causing a rash.
• Spirochetes disseminate to other skin sites or organs through the bloodstream or lymphatic system. They may survive for years in the joints, or they may die after triggering an inflammatory response in the host.

What to look for

Lyme disease occurs in three stages. Signs and symptoms may take years to fully develop.

Stage 1

In stage one, a red lesion forms at the site of the tick bite — usually the axilla, thigh, or groin — and may expand to more than 20″ (50.8 cm) in diameter. The lesion has a white center and a bright red outer rim, and it may itch, sting, or burn. It usually disappears within 1 month.

After a few days, more lesions may erupt in addition to a migratory, ringlike rash and conjunctivitis. In 3 to 4 weeks, the lesions fade to small red blotches, which persist for several more weeks.

The rash is commonly accompanied by fatigue, headache, chills, fever, sore throat, stiff neck, nausea, and muscle and joint pain. In children, body temperature may rise to 104° F (40° C) accompanied by chills. At this stage, 10% of patients report symptoms, such as palpitations and mild dyspnea. Severe headache and stiff neck, which suggest meningeal irritation, may also occur.

Stage 2

Weeks to months later, patients who aren't treated may enter the second stage of the disease. Meningitis, cranial nerve palsies, and peripheral neuropathy may occur. Fewer than 10% of patients have cardiac signs and symptoms. With neurologic involvement, neck stiffness usually occurs only with extreme flexion.

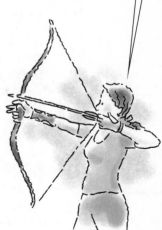

The bull's-eye-shaped rash is the beginning of the Lyme disease syndrome.

Stage 3

In the final stage, arthritis occurs 6 weeks to several years after the tick bite. Usually, only one or a few joints are affected, especially large ones such as the knees. Recurrent attacks may lead to chronic arthritis with severe cartilage and bone erosion. One-half of patients who aren't treated progress to this stage.

What tests tell you

These tests are used to diagnose Lyme disease:
• Blood tests, including antibody titers, enzyme immunoassay, and Western blot assay, may be used to identify *B. burgdorferi*. Mild anemia and elevated ESR, WBC count, serum IgM level, and aspartate aminotransferase level support the diagnosis.
• CSF analysis may be used to detect antibodies to *B. burgdorferi* if the disease has affected the CNS.

How it's treated

A 3- to 4-week course of oral amoxicillin or doxycycline is the treatment of choice for adults infected with Lyme disease. Cefuroxime or erythromycin can be used for patients who are allergic to penicillin or who can't take tetracyclines. In later stages of the disease, particularly when neurologic symptoms are present, treatment with I.V. ceftriaxone or penicillin for 4 weeks or more may be necessary. Analgesics and antipyretics reduce inflammation and fever.

Multiple sclerosis

Multiple sclerosis (MS) results from progressive demyelination of the white matter of the brain and spinal cord, leading to widespread neurologic dysfunction. The structures usually involved are the optic and oculomotor nerves and the spinal nerve tracts. The disorder doesn't affect the peripheral nervous system.

The ups and downs of MS

Characterized by exacerbations and remissions, MS is a major cause of chronic disability in people ages 18 to 40. The incidence is highest in women, people who live in northern urban areas, people in higher socioeconomic groups, and people with a family history of the disease.

What causes it

The exact cause of MS is unknown. It may be caused by a slow-acting viral infection, an autoimmune response of the nervous system, or an allergic response. Other possible causes include trauma, anoxia, toxins, nutritional deficiencies, vascular lesions, and anorexia nervosa, all of which may help destroy axons and the myelin sheath.

In addition, emotional stress, overwork, fatigue, pregnancy, or an acute respiratory tract infection may precede the onset of this illness. Genetic factors may also play a part.

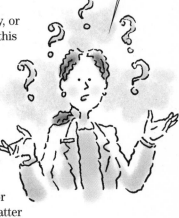

The exact cause of MS is unknown.

What to look for

Symptoms may be unpredictable and difficult for the patient to describe. They may be transient or may last for hours or weeks. Usually, the patient history reveals two initial symptoms: vision problems (caused by optic neuritis) and sensory impairment such as paresthesia. After the initial episode, findings may vary. They may include blurred vision or diplopia, emotional lability (from involvement of the white matter of the frontal lobes), and dysphagia.

Other signs and symptoms include:
• poorly articulated speech
• muscle weakness and spasticity
• hyperreflexia
• urinary problems
• intention tremor
• gait ataxia
• paralysis, ranging from monoplegia to quadriplegia
• vision problems, such as scotoma (an area of lost vision in the visual field), optic neuritis, and ophthalmoplegia (paralysis of the eye muscles).

What tests tell you

Diagnosing MS may take years because of remissions. These tests help diagnose the disease:
• EEG shows abnormalities in one-third of patients.
• CSF analysis reveals elevated IgG levels but normal total protein levels. This elevation is significant only when serum gamma globulin levels are normal, and it reflects hyperactivity of the immune system due to chronic demyelination. The WBC count may be slightly increased.
• Evoked potential studies demonstrate slowed conduction of nerve impulses in 80% of patients.

- CT scan may disclose lesions within the brain's white matter.
- MRI is the most sensitive method of detecting lesions and is also used to evaluate disease progression. More than 90% of patients show lesions when this test is performed.

How it's treated

Treatment for MS aims to shorten exacerbations and, if possible, relieve neurologic deficits so the patient can resume a near-normal lifestyle.

Drug options

Because MS may have allergic and inflammatory causes, cortico-tropin, prednisone, or dexamethasone is used to relieve symptoms and hasten remissions. However, these drugs don't prevent future exacerbations.

Currently, the preferred treatment during an acute attack is a short course of methylprednisolone, with or without a short pred-nisone taper. Interferon beta-1a or interferon beta-1b may also be given to decrease the frequency of relapses.

The Others

Other useful drugs include chlordiazepoxide to mitigate mood swings, baclofen or dantrolene to relieve spasticity, and bethane-chol or oxybutynin to relieve urine retention and minimize urinary frequency and urgency.

Supportive measures

During acute exacerbations, supportive measures include bed rest, massage, prevention of fatigue and pressure ulcers, bowel and bladder training, treatment of bladder infections with antibi-otics, physical therapy, and counseling.

Myocardial infarction

MI, an acute coronary syndrome, results from reduced blood flow through one of the coronary arteries. In non-ST-segment elevation MI, an imbalance exists between myocardial oxygen supply and de-mand, typically caused by narrowing of a coronary artery. In ST-seg-ment elevation MI, blood flow is impeded by an occlusive thrombus.

Leading the way

In North America and Western Europe, MI is one of the leading causes of death. Death usually results from cardiac damage or complications. Mortality is about 25% in men and 38% in women within 1 year of experiencing an MI. However, more than 50% of sudden deaths occur within 1 hour after the onset of symptoms—before the patient reaches the hospital.

What causes it

MI results from occlusion of one or more of the coronary arteries. Occlusion can stem from atherosclerosis, thrombosis, platelet aggregation, or coronary artery stenosis or spasm. Predisposing factors include:
- aging
- diabetes mellitus
- elevated serum triglyceride, low-density lipoprotein, cholesterol, and homocysteine levels and decreased serum high-density lipoprotein levels
- excessive intake of saturated fats, carbohydrates, or salt
- hypertension
- obesity
- family history of CAD
- sedentary lifestyle
- smoking
- stress
- use of amphetamines or cocaine.

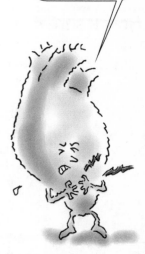

The cardinal symptom of MI is persistent, crushing substernal pain.

What to look for

The cardinal symptom of MI is persistent, crushing substernal pain that may radiate to the left arm, jaw, neck, or shoulder blades. The pain is commonly described as heavy, squeezing, or crushing and may persist for 12 hours or more. However, in some patients—particularly elderly or diabetic patients—pain may not occur at all. In others, it may be mild and confused with indigestion.

An infarction on the horizon?

In patients with CAD, angina of increasing frequency, severity, or duration (especially if not provoked by exertion, a heavy meal, or cold and wind) may signal an impending MI.

Other clinical effects include a feeling of impending doom, fatigue, nausea and vomiting, shortness of breath, cool extremities, diaphoresis, anxiety, and restlessness. Fever is unusual at the onset of an MI, but a low-grade temperature may develop during the next few days. Blood pressure varies. Hypotension or hypertension may occur.

What tests tell you

These tests help diagnose MI:
• Serial 12-lead ECG may be normal or inconclusive during the first few hours after an MI. Abnormalities include serial ST-segment depression or ST-segment elevation and Q waves.
• Serum creatine kinase (CK) levels are elevated, especially the CK-MB isoenzyme, the cardiac muscle fraction of CK.
• Echocardiography shows ventricular wall dyskinesia with a ST-segment elevation MI and is used to evaluate the ejection fraction.
• Radionuclide scans using I.V. technetium 99m can show acutely damaged muscle by picking up accumulations of radionuclide, which appear as a "hot spot" on the film. Myocardial perfusion imaging with thallium-201 reveals a "cold spot" in most patients during the first few hours after a Q-wave MI.
• Cardiac troponin levels are elevated 4 to 6 hours after an MI.

How it's treated

Arrhythmias, the most common problem during the first 48 hours after MI, require antiarrhythmics, a pacemaker (possibly), and cardioversion (rarely).

Drug therapy

Drugs are the mainstay of therapy for MI. Typical drugs include:
• thrombolytic agents (such as tissue plasminogen activator [tPA] and streptokinase) to revascularize myocardial tissue
• procainamide or another antiarrhythmic, such as amiodarone, for ventricular arrhythmias
• I.V. atropine for heart block or bradycardia
• sublingual, topical, transdermal, or I.V. nitroglycerin and calcium channel blockers (such as diltiazem), given by mouth or I.V. to relieve angina
• I.V. morphine (drug of choice) or hydromorphone for pain and sedation
• drugs that increase myocardial contractility (such as dobutamine, inamrinone, and milrinone)
• beta-adrenergic blockers (such as propranolol, metoprolol, and timolol) after acute MI to help prevent reinfarction by decreasing myocardial workload and oxygen demand
• antiplatelet therapy with such agents as clopidogrel, aspirin, or the glycoprotein IIb/IIIa inhibitors abciximab, eptifibatide, or tirofiban.

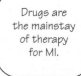

Drugs are the mainstay of therapy for MI.

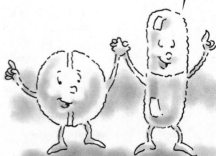

Revascularization therapy

Revascularization therapy may be performed on patients under age 70 who don't have a history of stroke, bleeding, GI ulcers, marked hypertension, recent surgery, or chest pain lasting longer than 6 hours. It must begin within 6 hours after the onset of symptoms, using I.V. intracoronary or systemic streptokinase or tPA. The best response occurs when treatment begins within 1 hour after symptoms first appear.

Other therapies

Other therapies include:
• temporary pacemaker for heart block or bradycardia
• oxygen administered by face mask or nasal cannula at a modest flow rate for 24 to 48 hours, or at a lower concentration if the patient has COPD
• bed rest with a bedside commode to decrease cardiac workload
• intra-aortic balloon pump for cardiogenic shock
• cardiac catheterization, PTCA, stent placement, and CABG surgery.

Obesity

Obesity is defined as an excess of body fat with a body mass index (BMI) greater than or equal to 30. In the United States, obesity has risen at an epidemic rate during the past 20 years. Research indicates that the situation is worsening rather than improving. Obesity leads to many health problems including heart disease and diabetes.

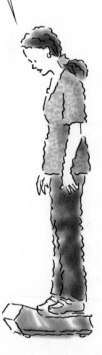

Obesity is rising at an epidemic rate in the United States.

What causes it

It may result from excessive calorie intake and inadequate expenditure of energy. Explanatory theories include hypothalamic dysfunction of hunger and satiety centers, genetic predisposition, abnormal absorption of nutrients, impaired action of GI growth hormones and hormonal regulators (such as insulin), and hypothyroidism.

What to look for

In addition to the BMI, other indices may support the diagnosis of obesity, such as anthropometric parameters and a standard detailed examination of the person. The degree and distribution of obesity may be estimated by standard skin thicknesses, such as subscapular, triceps, biceps, and suprailiac. Various anthropometric measurements of the waist and hip circumferences are most important. A chronic multisystemic disorder may be found in some individuals. In the skin examination, include a search for rashes, contact dermatoses, or other indications of problems related to obesity.

What tests tell you

In addition to anthropometric measurements and skin thickness estimates, supportive laboratory studies include:
• full lipid panel, which may be normal or elevated
• hepatic panel, which may be normal or abnormal if liver problems exist
• thyroid function tests to detect cases of primary hypothyroidism
• 24-hour urinary free cortisol when Cushing's syndrome or another state that causes cortisol levels to rise is suspected
• fasting glucose and insulin because obesity is associated with insulin resistance.

How it's treated

An obese patient must increase his activity level while reducing daily calorie intake through a balanced, low-calorie diet that reduces fat and sugar intake. Fat substitutes may be used, such as Olestra (Olean) and Sitostanol (Benecol). Olestra, however, has been shown to cause abdominal cramping and loose stools in some individuals, and it inhibits the body's absorption of certain fat-soluble vitamins and nutrients, making its use controversial. Treatment options may include hypnosis, behavior modification techniques, and psychotherapy.

Amphetamines, amphetamine congeners, and sibutramine may be used temporarily to enhance compliance by suppressing appetite and creating a feeling of well-being.

The mor-bid, the more treatment

Morbid obesity (BMI greater than 40) may be treated surgically with bariatric surgery. If a patient undergoes surgery for obesity, micronutrient deficiencies can occur, especially calcium, vitamin B_{12}, folate, and iron. In malabsorptive operations, a portion of the stomach is removed that plays a role in the absorption process, which results in such complications as uncontrolled diarrhea, potassium or magnesium deficiency, gallstone development, and metabolic encephalopathy.

Osteoarthritis

Osteoarthritis, the most common form of arthritis, is widespread, occurring equally in both sexes. Incidence occurs after age 40; its earliest symptoms generally begin in middle age and may progress with advancing age.

The degree of disability depends on the site and severity of involvement; it can range from minor limitation of the fingers to severe disability in a person with hip or knee involvement. The rate of progression varies, and joints may remain stable for years in an early stage of deterioration.

What causes it

Primary osteoarthritis, a normal part of aging, results from many things, including metabolic factors, genetics, chemical factors, and mechanical factors.

The wear and tear

Secondary osteoarthritis usually follows an identifiable predisposing event — most commonly trauma, congenital deformity, or obesity — and leads to degenerative changes.

Osteoarthritis is chronic, causing deterioration of the joint cartilage and formation of reactive new bone at the margins and subchondral (below the cartilage) areas of the joints. This degeneration results from a breakdown of chondrocytes (cartilage cells), most commonly in the hips and knees.

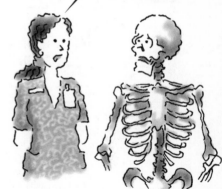

I'm afraid I've got some bad news. The normal aging process commonly leads to osteoarthritis.

What to look for

The most common symptom of osteoarthritis is a deep, aching joint pain, particularly after exercise or weight bearing, that's usually relieved by rest. Other signs and symptoms of osteoarthritis include:

- stiffness in the morning and after exercise (relieved by rest)
- aching during changes in weather
- "grating" of the joint during motion
- altered gait contractures
- limited movement.

These signs and symptoms increase with poor posture, obesity, and occupational stress.

A close look at the effects of osteoarthritis

Involvement of the interphalangeal (finger bone) joints produces irreversible changes in the distal joints (Heberden's nodes) and the proximal joints (Bouchard's nodes), as shown below.

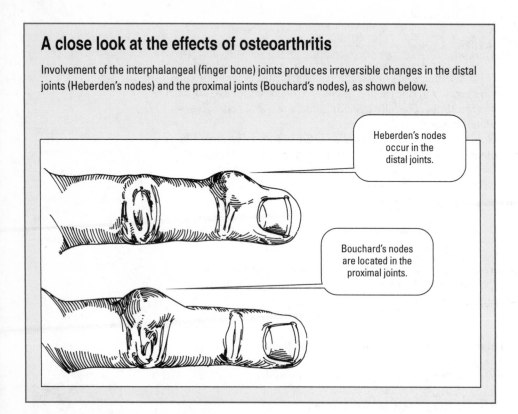

Heberden's nodes occur in the distal joints.

Bouchard's nodes are located in the proximal joints.

The nodes know

Osteoarthritis involving the joints of the fingers produces irreversible changes in the distal joints (Heberden's nodes) and proximal joints (Bouchard's nodes). These nodes may be painless at first but eventually become red, swollen, and tender, causing numbness and loss of dexterity. (See *A close look at the effects of osteoarthritis*.)

What tests tell you

A thorough physical examination confirms typical symptoms, and the absence of systemic symptoms rules out an inflammatory joint disorder. X-rays of the affected joint help confirm the diagnosis of osteoarthritis but may be normal in the early stages.

X-rays may require many views and typically show:
• narrowing of the joint space or margins
• cystlike bony deposits in the joint space and margins
• sclerosis of the subchondral space
• joint deformity due to degeneration or articular damage

• bony growths at weight-bearing areas
• fusion of joints.
  No laboratory test is specific for osteoarthritis.

How it's treated

The goal of osteoarthritis treatment is to:
• relieve pain
• maintain or improve mobility
• minimize disability.

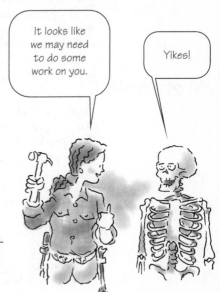

Drug therapy

Drug therapy for osteoarthritis includes:
• acetaminophen
• aspirin (or other nonopioid analgesics)
• celecoxib
• meloxicam
• ibuprofen.
  In some cases, intra-articular injections of cortico-steroids given every 4 to 6 months may delay the development of nodes in the hands.

Surgical interventions

Surgical treatment of osteoarthritis is reserved for patients who have severe disability or uncontrollable pain and may include:
• arthroplasty — replacement of the deteriorated part of the joint with a prosthetic appliance
• arthrodesis — surgical fusion of the bones; used primarily in the spine (laminectomy)
• osteoplasty — scraping and lavage of deteriorated bone from the joint
• osteotomy — change in alignment of the bone to relieve stress by excision of a bone wedge or cutting of the bone.

Noninvasive interventions

Noninvasive interventions may also be used:
• Weight loss helps decrease stress on joints.
• Strengthening exercises for muscles around the knee and hip help stabilize these joints and improve alignment of the articular surfaces, preventing further cartilage deterioration. Exercise may also help with weight management.
• Effective treatment also reduces stress by supporting or stabilizing the joint with crutches, braces, a cane, a walker, a cervical collar, or traction.

Osteoporosis

Osteoporosis is a metabolic bone disorder in which the rate of bone resorption accelerates and the rate of bone formation decelerates. The result is decreased bone mass. Bones affected by this disease lose calcium and phosphate and become porous, brittle, and abnormally prone to fracture.

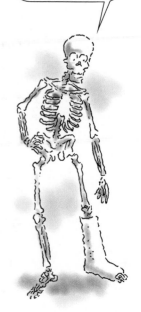

Bones affected by osteoporosis are porous and brittle, making them prone to fracture.

What causes it

Osteoporosis is four times more common in women than in men. White and Asian women are more likely to develop the disease than Black or Hispanic women. It may be a primary disorder or occur secondary to an underlying disease.

At the primaries

The cause of primary osteoporosis is unknown. However, contributing factors include:
• mild but prolonged lack of calcium due to poor dietary intake or poor absorption by the intestine secondary to age
• hormonal imbalance due to endocrine dysfunction
• faulty metabolism of protein due to estrogen deficiency
• sedentary lifestyle.

On secondary thought

Secondary osteoporosis may result from:
• prolonged therapy with steroids or heparin
• bone immobilization or disuse (such as paralysis)
• alcoholism
• malnutrition
• rheumatoid arthritis
• liver disease
• calcium malabsorption
• scurvy
• lactose intolerance
• hyperthyroidism
• osteogenesis imperfecta (an inherited condition that causes brittle bones)
• trauma leading to atrophy in the hands and feet, with recurring attacks (Sudeck's disease)
• smoking.

What to look for

Bone fractures are the major complication of osteoporosis. Fractures occur mostly in the vertebrae, femur, and distal radius. Signs of redness, warmth, and new sites of pain may indicate new fractures.

Patient profile

The patient with osteoporosis is typically postmenopausal or has one of the conditions that cause secondary osteoporosis. She may report that she heard a snapping sound and felt a sudden pain in her lower back when she bent down to lift something. Alternatively, she may say that the pain developed slowly over several years. If the patient has vertebral collapse, she may describe a backache and pain radiating around the trunk. Movement or jarring aggravates the pain.

Don't get bent out of shape

The patient may have a humped back (dowager's hump); the curvature worsens as repeated vertebral fractures increase spinal curvature. The abdomen eventually protrudes to compensate for the changed center of gravity. The patient commonly reports a gradual loss of height, decreased exercise tolerance, and trouble breathing. Palpation may reveal muscle spasm. The patient may also have decreased spinal movement, with flexion more limited than extension.

What tests tell you

A diagnosis excludes other causes of bone disease, especially those that affect the spine, such as cancer and tumors. These tests help confirm a diagnosis of osteoporosis:
• X-ray studies show characteristic degeneration in the lower vertebrae.
• Serum calcium, phosphorus, and alkaline phosphatase levels remain within normal limits; PTH level may be elevated.
• Bone biopsy allows direct examination of changes in bone cells.
• CT scanning allows accurate assessment of spinal bone loss.
• Radionuclide bone scans display injured or diseased areas as darker portions.
• Dual photon or dual energy X-ray absorptiometry can detect bone loss in a safe, noninvasive test.
• Bone density measurements confirm the diagnosis.

How it's treated

Treatment measures may include supportive devices such as a back brace and, possibly, surgery to correct fractures. Estrogen may be prescribed within 3 years after menopause to decrease the rate of bone resorption. A balanced diet should be rich in nutrients, such as vitamin D, calcium, and protein, that support skeletal metabolism. Low-impact weight-bearing exercises can help stimulate osteoblast formation. Heat may be applied to relieve pain.

Drug therapy

These drugs may be prescribed for osteoporosis:
• Analgesics may be given to relieve pain.
• Alendronate, risedronate, or raloxifene may be prescribed to treat and prevent osteoporosis.
• Calcium and vitamin D supplements may help to support normal bone metabolism.
• Calcitonin may be used to reduce bone resorption and slow the decline in bone mass.
• Etidronate is the first agent proved to increase bone density and restore lost bone by inhibiting osteoblast activity.
• Teriparatide, an injectable form of human PTH, may be prescribed for postmenopausal women and men with osteoporosis who are at high risk for developing fractures; the drug stimulates bone formation in the spine and hips.

Otitis media

Inflammation of the middle ear, otitis media may be suppurative or secretory, acute or chronic. Acute otitis media is common in children; its incidence rises during the winter months, paralleling the seasonal rise in nonbacterial respiratory tract infections.

What causes it

Each type of otitis media has its own cause.

Suppurative otitis media

In the suppurative form, respiratory tract infection, allergic reaction, nasotracheal intubation, or positional changes allow nasopharyngeal flora to reflux through the Eustachian tube and colonize the middle ear. Suppurative otitis media usually results from bacterial infection with pneumococci, *Haemophilus influenzae* (the most common cause in children younger than age 6), *Morax-ella catarrhalis*, beta-hemolytic streptococci, staphylococci (most common cause in children age 6 or older), or gram-negative bacteria.

Predisposing factors include genetic factors, such as susceptibility to infection; the normally wider, shorter, more horizontal eustachian tubes and increased lymphoid tissue in children; and anatomic anomalies. Chronic suppurative otitis media results from inadequate treatment of acute otitis episodes, infection by resistant strains of bacteria or, rarely, tuberculosis.

Secretory otitis media

With secretory otitis media, obstruction of the eustachian tube causes a buildup of negative pressure in the middle ear that promotes transudation of sterile serous fluid from blood vessels in the membrane of the middle ear. Such effusion may be secondary to eustachian tube dysfunction from viral infection or allergy. It may also follow barotrauma (pressure injury caused by an inability to equalize pressures between the environment and the middle ear), as can occur during rapid aircraft descent in a person with an upper respiratory tract infection or during rapid underwater ascent in scuba diving (barotitis media).

Chronic otitis media

Chronic secretory otitis media follows persistent eustachian tube dysfunction from mechanical obstruction (such as adenoidal tissue overgrowth and tumors), edema (such as allergic rhinitis and chronic sinus infection), or inadequate treatment of acute suppurative otitis media.

What to look for

Signs and symptoms vary with the specific type of the disorder.

Suppurative otitis media

Signs and symptoms of acute suppurative otitis media include severe, deep, throbbing pain (from pressure behind the tympanic membrane); signs of upper respiratory tract infection (such as sneezing and coughing); mild to very high fever; hearing loss (usually mild and conductive); dizziness; nausea; and vomiting.

Other possible effects include bulging of the tympanic membrane with concomitant erythema and purulent drainage in the ear canal from tympanic membrane rupture. However, many patients are asymptomatic.

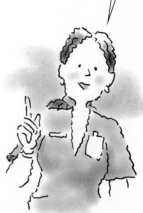

Signs and symptoms of otitis media vary depending on the type.

Secretory otitis media

With acute secretory otitis media, a severe conductive hearing loss varies, depending on the thickness and amount of fluid in the middle ear cavity, and possibly, a sensation of fullness in the ear and popping, crackling, or clicking sounds on swallowing or with jaw movement. Accumulation of fluid may also cause the patient to hear an echo when he speaks and to experience a vague feeling of top-heaviness.

Chronic otitis media

The cumulative effects of chronic otitis media include thickening and scarring of the tympanic membrane, decreased or absent tympanic membrane mobility, cholestearoma (a cystlike mass in the middle ear) and, in patients with chronic suppurative otitis media, a painless, purulent discharge. The extent of associated conductive hearing loss varies with the size and type of tympanic membrane perforation and ossicular destruction.

If the tympanic membrane has ruptured, the patient may state that the pain has suddenly stopped.

What tests tell you

Diagnostic tests vary with the specific type of otitis media.

Suppurative otitis media

With acute suppurative otitis media, otoscopy reveals obscured or distorted bony landmarks of the tympanic membrane. Pneumatoscopy can show decreased tympanic membrane mobility, but this procedure is painful with an obviously bulging, erythematous tympanic membrane. The pain pattern is diagnostically significant. With acute suppurative otitis media, for example, pulling the auricle doesn't exacerbate the pain.

Secretory otitis media

With acute secretory otitis media, otoscopic examination reveals tympanic membrane retraction, which causes the bony landmarks to appear more prominent. Examination also detects clear or amber fluid behind the tympanic membrane. If hemorrhage into the middle ear has occurred, as in barotrauma, the tympanic membrane appears blue-black.

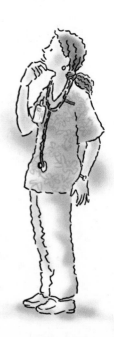

Chronic otitis media

In patients with chronic otitis media, the history discloses recurrent or unresolved otitis media. Otoscopy shows thickening (and sometimes scarring) and decreased mobility of the tympanic membrane, whereas pneumatoscopy shows decreased or absent tympanic membrane movement. Mastoid X-rays or CT scans may show spreading infection beyond the middle ear. History of recent travel or scuba diving suggests barotitis media.

How it's treated

The type of otitis media dictates treatment guidelines.

Suppurative otitis media

With acute suppurative otitis media, antibiotic therapy may be prescribed if the disease is bacterial in origin. Nasal spray, nose drops, oral decongestants, or antihistamines may be used to promote fluid drainage through the eustachian tube. Eardrops may be prescribed to relieve pain, as may analgesics such as acetaminophen. Oral corticosteroids may be used to reduce inflammation.

Severe, painful bulging of the tympanic membrane usually necessitates myringotomy. Broad-spectrum antibiotics can help prevent acute suppurative otitis media in high-risk patients. In patients with recurring otitis, antibiotics must be used with discretion to prevent resistant strains of bacteria from developing.

Secretory otitis media

For patients with acute secretory otitis media, inflation of the eustachian tube by performing Valsalva's maneuver several times per day may be the only treatment required. Otherwise, nasopharyngeal decongestant therapy may be helpful. It should continue for at least 2 weeks and, sometimes, indefinitely with periodic evaluations.

If decongestant therapy fails, myringotomy and aspiration of middle ear fluid are necessary. This procedure is followed by insertion of a polyethylene tube into the tympanic membrane for immediate and prolonged equalization of pressure. The tube falls out spontaneously after 9 to 12 months. Concomitant treatment of the underlying cause, such as elimination of allergens, or adenoidectomy for hypertrophied adenoids, may also be helpful in correcting this disorder.

Chronic otitis media

Treatment of chronic otitis media includes broad-spectrum antibiotics for exacerbations of acute otitis media, elimination of eustachian tube obstruction, treatment of otitis externa, myringoplasty and tympanoplasty to reconstruct middle ear structures when thickening and scarring are present, and mastoidectomy. Cholesteatoma requires excision.

Parkinson's disease

Parkinson's disease produces progressive muscle rigidity, loss of muscle movement (akinesia), and involuntary tremors. The patient's condition may deteriorate for more than 10 years. Eventually, aspiration pneumonia or some other infection causes death.

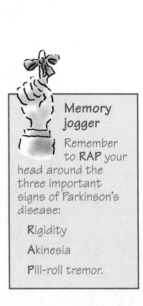

A deficiency of dopamine isn't good news.

What causes it

Although the cause of Parkinson's disease is unknown, study of the extrapyramidal brain nuclei (corpus striatum, globus pallidus, and substantia nigra) has established that a dopamine deficiency prevents affected brain cells from performing their normal inhibitory function within the CNS.

What to look for

Important signs of Parkinson's disease include muscle rigidity, akinesia, and a unilateral "pill-roll" tremor:
• Muscle rigidity results in resistance to passive muscle stretching, which may be uniform (lead-pipe rigidity) or jerky (cogwheel rigidity).
• Akinesia causes gait and movement disturbances. The patient walks with his body bent forward, takes a long time initiating movement when performing a purposeful action, pivots with difficulty, and easily loses his balance. Akinesia may also cause other signs that include masklike facial expression and blepharospasm, in which the eyelids stay closed.
• "Pill-roll" tremor is insidious. It begins in the fingers, increases during stress or anxiety, and decreases with purposeful movement and sleep.

Also be on the lookout for...

Other signs and symptoms of Parkinson's disease include:
• high-pitched, monotone voice

Memory jogger

Remember to **RAP** your head around the three important signs of Parkinson's disease:

Rigidity

Akinesia

Pill-roll tremor.

- drooling
- dysarthria (impaired speech due to a disturbance in muscle control)
- dysphagia (difficulty swallowing)
- fatigue
- muscle cramps in the legs, neck, and trunk
- oily skin
- increased perspiration
- insomnia
- mood changes.

What tests tell you

Diagnosis of Parkinson's disease is based on the patient's age, history, and signs and symptoms, so laboratory tests are generally of little value. However, urinalysis may reveal decreased dopamine levels, and CT scan or MRI may rule out other disorders such as intracranial tumors.

How it's treated

Treatment for Parkinson's disease aims to relieve symptoms and keep the patient functional as long as possible. It consists of drugs, physical therapy, and stereotactic neurosurgery in extreme cases.

Looking to levodopa and other drugs

Drug therapy usually includes levodopa, a dopamine replacement that's most effective in the first few years after it's initiated. It's given in increasing doses until signs and symptoms are relieved or until adverse reactions develop. Because adverse effects can be serious, levodopa is commonly given along with carbidopa to halt peripheral dopamine synthesis. Bromocriptine may be given as an additive to reduce the levodopa dose.

When levodopa is ineffective or too toxic, anticholinergics, such as trihexyphenidyl or benztropine, and antihistamines, such as diphenhydramine, are given. Anticholinergics may be used to control tremors and rigidity. They may also be used in combination with levodopa. Antihistamines may help decrease tremors because of their central anticholinergic and sedative effects.

Amantadine, an antiviral agent, is used early in treatment to reduce rigidity, tremors, and akinesia. Patients with mild disease are given deprenyl to slow the disease progression and ease symptoms. Tricyclic antidepressants may be given to decrease depression.

Stalevo, the new drug that combines carbidopa, levodopa, and entacapone, is used when carbidopa and levodopa are no longer effective throughout the dosing interval. The added component entacapone prolongs the time that levodopa is active in the brain.

Deep brain stimulation

In the past, pallidotomy and thalamotomy were the only available surgical options. However, deep brain stimulation is now the preferred surgical option. With deep brain stimulation, electrodes are implanted into the targeted brain area. These electrodes are connected to wires attached to an impulse generator that's implanted under the collarbone. The electrodes control symptoms on the opposite side of the body by sending electrical impulses to the brain.

Come on...do the range of motion

Physical therapy helps maintain the patient's normal muscle tone and function. It includes active and passive range-of-motion (ROM) exercises, routine daily activities, walking, and baths and massage to help relax muscles.

Peptic ulcer

A peptic ulcer is a circumscribed lesion in the mucosal membrane of the upper GI tract. Peptic ulcers can develop in the lower esophagus, stomach, duodenum, or jejunum.

The two major forms of peptic ulcer are duodenal and gastric. Both forms are chronic conditions. Duodenal ulcers affect the upper part of the small intestine. This type of ulcer accounts for about 80% of peptic ulcers and follows a chronic course of remissions and exacerbations.

What causes it

There are three major causes of peptic ulcers:
• bacterial infection with *Helicobacter pylori* is the cause of 90% of peptic ulcers
• use of nonsteroidal anti-inflammatory drugs (NSAIDs)
• hypersecretory states such as Zollinger-Ellison syndrome.
    Predisposing factors include:
• blood type A (common in people with gastric ulcers) and blood type O (common in those with duodenal ulcers)
• genetic factors
• exposure to irritants
• trauma
• stress and anxiety
• normal aging.

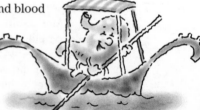

Try to relax. Stress and anxiety can lead to peptic ulcers.

What to look for

The patient with a gastric ulcer may report a recent loss of weight or appetite; pain, heartburn, or indigestion; a feeling of abdominal fullness or distention; and pain triggered or aggravated by eating. The patient with a duodenal ulcer may describe the pain as sharp, gnawing, burning, boring, aching, or hard to define. He may liken it to hunger, abdominal pressure, or fullness. Typically, pain occurs 90 minutes to 3 hours after eating. However, eating usually reduces the pain, so the patient may report a recent weight gain. The patient may also have pale skin from anemia caused by blood loss.

What tests tell you

These tests are used to diagnose peptic ulcer:
• Upper GI endoscopy or esophagogastroduodenoscopy confirms an ulcer and permits cytologic studies and biopsy to rule out *H. pylori* or cancer. Endoscopy is the major diagnostic test for peptic ulcers.
• Barium swallow and upper GI or small-bowel series may pinpoint the ulcer in a patient whose symptoms aren't severe.
• Upper GI tract X-ray reveals mucosal abnormalities.
• Stool analysis may detect occult blood.
• WBC count is elevated; other blood tests may also disclose clinical signs of infection.
• Gastric secretory studies show excess hydrochloric acid (hyperchlorhydria).
• Carbon-13 urea breath test reflects activity of *H. pylori*.

How it's treated

Drug therapy for *H. pylori* infection consists of 1 to 2 weeks of antibiotic therapy using amoxicillin, tetracycline, metronidazole, or clarithromycin. Antibiotics should be used in combination with ranitidine, famotidine, bismuth citrate, bismuth subsalicylate, or a proton pump inhibitor.

More drastic measures

Gastroscopy allows visualization of the bleeding site and coagulation by laser or cautery to control bleeding. Surgery is indicated if the patient doesn't respond to other treatment or has a perforation, suspected cancer, or other complications.

Pneumonia

Pneumonia is an acute infection of the lung parenchyma that commonly impairs gas exchange. The prognosis is good for patients with normal lungs and adequate immune systems. However, bacterial pneumonia is the leading cause of death in debilitated patients.

Pneumonia is classified three ways:

☝ by *origin*—Pneumonia may be viral, bacterial, fungal, or protozoal in origin.

✌ by *location*—Bronchopneumonia involves distal airways and alveoli; lobular pneumonia, part of a lobe; and lobar pneumonia, an entire lobe.

🖐 by *type*—Primary pneumonia results from inhalation or aspiration of a pathogen, such as bacteria or a virus, and includes pneumococcal and viral pneumonia. Secondary pneumonia may follow lung damage from a noxious chemical or other insult or may result from hematogenous spread of bacteria. Aspiration pneumonia results from inhalation of foreign matter, such as vomitus or food particles, into the bronchi.

What causes it

In general, the lower respiratory tract can be exposed to pathogens by inhalation, aspiration, vascular dissemination, or direct contact with contaminated equipment such as suction catheters. After pathogens get inside, they begin to colonize and infection develops.

Stasis report

In bacterial pneumonia, which can occur in any part of the lungs, an infection initially triggers alveolar inflammation and edema. This condition produces an area of low ventilation with normal perfusion. Capillaries become engorged with blood, causing stasis. As the alveolocapillary membrane breaks down, alveoli fill with blood and exudate, resulting in atelectasis (lung collapse). (See *A close look at atelectatic alveoli.*)

In severe bacterial infections, the lungs look heavy and liver-like—reminiscent of ARDS.

We bacteria can sneak into the lower respiratory tract through inhalation, aspiration, or vascular dissemination.

A close look at atelectatic alveoli

Normally, air-filled alveoli exchange oxygen and carbon dioxide with capillary blood. However, in atelectasis, airless, shrunken alveoli can't accomplish gas exchange.

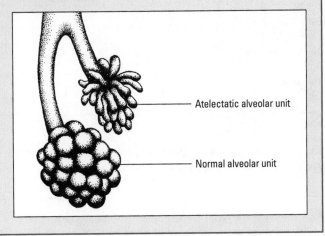

Atelectatic alveolar unit

Normal alveolar unit

Virus attack!

In viral pneumonia, the virus first attacks bronchiolar epithelial cells. This attack causes interstitial inflammation and desquamation. The virus also invades bronchial mucous glands and goblet cells. It then spreads to the alveoli, which fill with blood and fluid. In advanced infection, a hyaline membrane may form. Like bacterial infections, viral pneumonia clinically resembles ARDS.

Subtracting surfactant

In aspiration pneumonia, inhalation of gastric juices or hydrocarbons triggers inflammatory changes and also inactivates surfactant over a large area. Decreased surfactant leads to alveolar collapse. Acidic gastric juices may damage the airways and alveoli. Particles containing aspirated gastric juices may obstruct the airways and reduce airflow, leading to secondary bacterial pneumonia.

Risky business

Certain predisposing factors increase the risk of pneumonia. For bacterial and viral pneumonia, these factors include:
• abdominal and thoracic surgery
• alcoholism
• aspiration
• atelectasis
• cancer (particularly lung cancer)
• chronic illness and debilitation
• colds or other viral respiratory infections
• chronic respiratory disease, such as COPD, bronchiectasis, or cystic fibrosis

- exposure to noxious gases
- immunosuppressive therapy
- influenza
- malnutrition
- premature birth
- sickle cell disease
- smoking
- tracheostomy.

What to look for

The clinical manifestations of different types of pneumonia vary. (See *Distinguishing among types of pneumonia*.)

What tests tell you

These tests are used to diagnose pneumonia:
- Chest X-rays confirm the diagnosis by disclosing infiltrates.
- Sputum specimen, Gram stain, and culture and sensitivity tests help differentiate the type of infection and the drugs that are effective in treatment.
- WBC count indicates leukocytosis in bacterial pneumonia and a normal or low count in viral or mycoplasmal pneumonia.
- Blood cultures reflect bacteremia and are used to determine the causative organism.
- ABG levels vary, depending on the severity of pneumonia and the underlying lung state.
- Bronchoscopy or transtracheal aspiration allows the collection of material for culture.
- Pulse oximetry may show a reduced SaO_2 level.

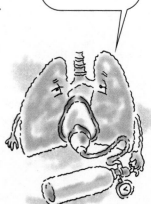

Patients with pneumonia may require ventilatory support.

How it's treated

The patient with pneumonia needs antimicrobial therapy based on the causative agent. Reevaluation should be done early in treatment. Supportive measures include:
- humidified oxygen therapy for hypoxia
- bronchodilator therapy
- antitussives
- mechanical ventilation for respiratory failure
- positive end-expiratory pressure ventilation to maintain adequate oxygenation for patients with severe pneumonia on mechanical ventilation
- high-calorie diet and adequate fluid intake
- bed rest
- analgesics to relieve pleuritic chest pain.

Distinguishing among types of pneumonia

The characteristics and prognosis of the different types of pneumonia vary. The chart below lists each type along with its characteristics.

Type	Characteristics	Type	Characteristics
Viral		**Viral** (continued)	
Influenza	• Prognosis poor even with treatment • 50% mortality from cardiopulmonary collapse • Cough (initially nonproductive; later, purulent sputum), marked cyanosis, dyspnea, high fever, chills, substernal pain and discomfort, moist crackles, frontal headache, myalgia	Chickenpox (varicella pneumonia)	• Uncommon in children but present in 30% of adults with varicella • Characteristic rash, cough, dyspnea, cyanosis, tachypnea, pleuritic chest pain, and hemoptysis and rhonchi 1 to 6 days after onset of rash
Adenovirus	• Insidious onset • Generally affects young adults • Good prognosis; usually clears with no residual effects • Sore throat, fever, cough, chills, malaise, small amounts of mucoid sputum, retrosternal chest pain, anorexia, rhinitis, adenopathy, scattered crackles, and rhonchi	Cytomegalovirus	• Difficult to distinguish from other non-bacterial pneumonias • In adults with healthy lung tissue, resembles mononucleosis and is generally benign; in neonates, occurs as devastating multisystemic infection; in immunocompromised hosts, varies from clinically inapparent to fatal infection • Fever, cough, shaking chills, dyspnea, cyanosis, weakness, and diffuse crackles
Respiratory syncytial virus	• Most prevalent in infants and children • Complete recovery in 1 to 3 weeks; may cause death in premature infants younger than age 6 months • Listlessness, irritability, tachypnea with retraction of intercostal muscles, slight sputum production, fever, severe malaise, possible cough or croup, and fine, moist crackles	**Bacterial**	
		Streptococcus	• Sudden onset of a single, shaking chill, and sustained temperature of 102° to 104° F (38.9° to 40° C); commonly preceded by upper respiratory tract infection
Measles (rubeola)	• Typically more severe in adults than in children • Fever, dyspnea, cough, small amounts of sputum, rash, cervical adenopathy, and profusely runny nose	*Klebsiella*	• More likely in patients with chronic alcoholism, pulmonary disease, and diabetes • Fever and recurrent chills; cough producing rusty, bloody, viscous sputum (currant jelly); cyanosis of lips and nail beds from hypoxemia; and shallow, grunting respirations

(continued)

Distinguishing among types of pneumonia (continued)

Type	Characteristics	Type	Characteristics
Bacterial (continued)		**Aspiration**	
Staphylococcus	• Commonly occurs in patients with viral illness, such as influenza or measles, and in those with cystic fibrosis • Temperature of 102° to 104° F (38.9° to 40° C), recurrent shaking chills, bloody sputum, dyspnea, tachypnea, and hypoxemia		• Results from vomiting and aspiration of gastric or oropharyngeal contents into trachea and lungs • Noncardiogenic pulmonary edema possible with damage to respiratory epithelium from contact with gastric acid • Subacute pneumonia possible with cavity formation • Lung abscess possible if foreign body present • Crackles, dyspnea, cyanosis, hypotension, and tachycardia

Potassium imbalance

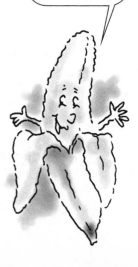

Because many foods contain potassium, hypokalemia rarely results from a dietary deficiency.

Potassium, a cation that's the dominant cellular electrolyte, facilitates contraction of skeletal and smooth muscles—including myocardial contraction—and figures prominently in nerve impulse conduction, acid-base balance, enzyme action, and cell-membrane function. Because the normal serum potassium level has such a narrow range (3.5 to 5 mEq/L), a slight deviation in either direction can produce profound clinical consequences.

Paradoxically, both hypokalemia (potassium deficiency) and hyperkalemia (potassium excess) can lead to muscle weakness and flaccid paralysis because they create an ionic imbalance in neuromuscular tissue excitability. Both conditions also diminish excitability and conduction rate of the heart muscle, which may lead to cardiac arrest.

What causes it

Because many foods contain potassium, hypokalemia rarely results from a dietary deficiency. Instead, potassium loss results from:
• excessive GI or urinary losses, such as vomiting, gastric suction, diarrhea, dehydration, anorexia, or prolonged laxative use

• trauma (injury, burns, or surgery) in which damaged cells release potassium, which enters serum or extracellular fluid to be excreted in urine
• chronic renal disease with tubular potassium wasting
• certain drugs, especially potassium-wasting diuretics, steroids, and certain sodium-containing antibiotics (carbenicillin)
• acid-base imbalances, which cause potassium shifting into cells without true depletion in alkalosis
• prolonged potassium-free I.V. therapy
• hyperglycemia, causing osmotic diuresis and glycosuria
• Cushing's syndrome, primary hyperaldosteronism, excessive ingestion of licorice, and severe serum magnesium deficiency.

Generally, hyperkalemia results from the kidneys' inability to excrete excessive amounts of potassium infused I.V. or administered orally; decreased urine output, renal dysfunction, or renal failure; or the use of potassium-sparing diuretics, such as triamterene, by patients with renal disease. It may also result from injuries or conditions that release cellular potassium or favor its retention, such as burns, crushing injuries, failing renal function, adrenal gland insufficiency, dehydration, or diabetic acidosis.

What to look for

Signs and symptoms of hypokalemia and hyperkalemia will vary depending on the cause. (See *Signs and symptoms of potassium imbalance*, page 556.)

What tests tell you

• Serum potassium level less than 3.5 mEq/L indicate hypokalemia.
• Serum potassium level greater than 5 mEq/L indicate hyperkalemia.

Additional tests may be necessary to determine the underlying cause of the imbalance.

How it's treated

Treatment depends on the imbalance.

Hypokalemia

Replacement therapy with potassium chloride (I.V. or by mouth) is the primary treatment for hypokalemia. When diuresis is necessary, spironolactone, a potassium-sparing diuretic, may be administered concurrently with a potassium-wasting diuretic to minimize potassium loss. Hypokalemia can be prevented by giving a

Signs and symptoms of potassium imbalance

The chart below lists possible signs and symptoms of hypokalemia and hyperkalemia by body system dysfunction.

Dysfunction	Hypokalemia	Hyperkalemia
Acid-base balance	Metabolic alkalosis	Metabolic acidosis
Cardiovascular	Dizziness, hypotension, arrhythmias, electrocardiogram (ECG) changes (flattened T waves, elevated U waves, depressed ST segment), cardiac arrest (with serum potassium levels < 2.5 mEq/L)	Tachycardia and later bradycardia, ECG changes (tented and elevated T waves, widened QRS complex, prolonged PR interval, flattened or absent P waves, depressed ST segment), cardiac arrest (with levels > 7 mEq/L)
Central nervous system	Malaise, irritability, confusion, mental depression, speech changes, decreased reflexes, respiratory paralysis	Hyperreflexia progressing to weakness, numbness, tingling, and flaccid paralysis
GI	Nausea and vomiting, anorexia, diarrhea, abdominal distention, paralytic ileus, or decreased peristalsis	Nausea, diarrhea, abdominal cramps
Genitourinary	Polyuria	Oliguria, anuria
Musculoskeletal	Muscle weakness and fatigue, leg cramps	Muscle weakness, flaccid paralysis

maintenance dose of potassium I.V. to patients who may not take anything by mouth and to others predisposed to potassium loss.

Hyperkalemia

For the management of hyperkalemia, rapid infusion of 10% calcium gluconate decreases myocardial irritability and temporarily prevents cardiac arrest but doesn't correct serum potassium excess; it's also contraindicated in patients receiving a cardiac glycoside.

Potassium power

As an emergency measure, sodium bicarbonate I.V. increases pH and causes potassium to shift back into the cells. Insulin and 10% to 50% glucose I.V. also move potassium back into the cells. Infusions should be followed by dextrose 5% in water because an infusion of 10% to 15% glucose stimulates the secretion of endogenous insulin.

Sodium shifter

Sodium polystyrene sulfonate (Kayexalate) with 70% sorbitol produces an exchange of sodium ions for potassium ions in the intes-

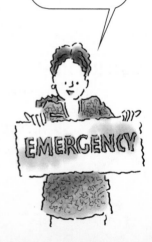

Give sodium bicarbonate stat for emergency treatment of hyperkalemia.

tine. Hemodialysis or peritoneal dialysis also help remove excess potassium.

Prostate cancer

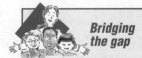

Incidence of prostate cancer

Black men have the highest prostate cancer incidence in the world. The disease is common in North America and northwestern Europe and is rare in Asia and South America.

Prostate cancer is the most common cancer affecting men and the second cause of cancer death. About 85% of these cancers originate in the posterior prostate gland; the rest grow near the urethra. Adenocarcinoma is the most common form. Prostate cancer grows slowly. When primary lesions spread beyond the prostate gland, they invade the prostatic capsule and then spread along the ejaculatory ducts in the space between the seminal vesicles or perivesicular fascia. When prostate cancer is treated in its localized form, the 5-year survival rate is 70%; after metastasis, it's lower than 35%. Fatal prostate cancer usually results from widespread bone metastasis.

What causes it

Risk factors for prostate cancer include:
• age (more than 70% of all prostate cancer cases are diagnosed in men older than age 65)
• diet high in saturated fats
• ethnicity (see *Incidence of prostate cancer*).

What to look for

Prostate cancer seldom produces signs and symptoms until it's advanced. Signs of advanced disease include a slow urinary stream, urinary hesitancy, incomplete bladder emptying, and dysuria. These symptoms are due to obstruction caused by tumor progression.

What tests tell you

These tests and results are common in prostate cancer:
• DRE is performed to determine prostate location, size, and the presence of nodules.
• Biopsy of the prostate may distinguish between a benign or malignant mass.
• Blood tests may show elevated levels of prostate-specific antigen (PSA). Although an elevated PSA level occurs with metastasis, it also occurs with other prostate diseases.
• Transrectal prostatic ultrasonography may be used for patients with abnormal DRE and PSA findings.

• Bone scan and excretory urography determine the extent of the disease.
• MRI and CT scanning help define the tumor's extent.

How it's treated

Therapy varies depending on the stage of the cancer and may include radiation, prostatectomy, and hormone therapy. Because most prostate cancers are androgen- or hormone-dependent, the main treatments are antiandrogens to suppress adrenal function or medical castration with estrogen or gonadotropin-releasing hormone analogs.

Docetaxel, a chemotherapy agent, is approved for men with advanced prostate cancer that doesn't respond to hormone therapy. The drug is administered along with the steroid prednisone. Docetaxel is the first drug shown to improve the survival rate in men with the advanced stage of the disease.

Radical prostatectomy usually works for localized lesions without metastasis. Transurethral resection of the prostate may be used to relieve an obstruction.

Nonsurgical treatments

Radiation therapy may cure locally invasive lesions in early disease and may relieve bone pain from metastatic skeletal involvement. It's also used prophylactically to prevent tumor growth for patients with tumors in regional lymph nodes. Radioactive "seeds" may also be implanted into the prostate. This treatment increases radiation to the area while minimizing exposure to surrounding tissues.

Chemotherapy with combinations of cyclophosphamide, doxorubicin, fluorouracil, methotrexate, estramustine, vinblastine, and cisplatin reduce pain from metastasis but hasn't helped patients live longer.

Pulmonary embolism

Pulmonary embolism is an obstruction of the pulmonary arterial bed by a dislodged thrombus, heart valve growths, or a foreign substance. Although pulmonary infarction that results from embolism may be so mild as to produce no symptoms, massive embolism (more than a 50% obstruction of pulmonary arterial circulation) and the accompanying infarction can be rapidly fatal.

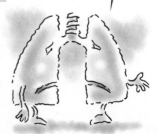

Massive pulmonary embolism can be rapidly fatal.

What causes it

Pulmonary embolism generally results from dislodged thrombi originating in the leg veins or pelvis. More than one-half of such thrombi arise in the deep veins of the legs.

Predisposing factors include long-term immobility, chronic pulmonary disease, heart failure, atrial fibrillation, thrombophlebitis, polycythemia vera, thrombocytosis, autoimmune hemolytic anemia, sickle cell disease, and varicose veins. Other factors include recent surgery, advanced age, pregnancy, lower-extremity fractures or surgery, burns, obesity, vascular injury, cancer, I.V. drug abuse, and hormonal contraceptives.

What to look for

Total occlusion of the main pulmonary artery is rapidly fatal; smaller or fragmented emboli produce symptoms that vary with the size, number, and location of the emboli. Usually, the first symptom of pulmonary embolism is dyspnea, which may be accompanied by anginal or pleuritic chest pain.

Now featuring...

Other clinical features include tachycardia, productive cough (sputum may be blood-tinged), low-grade fever, and pleural effusion. Less common signs include massive hemoptysis, splinting of the chest, leg edema and cyanosis, syncope, and distended jugular veins (with a large embolus). In addition, pulmonary embolism may cause pleural friction rub, signs of circulatory collapse (weak, rapid pulse and hypotension), and hypoxia (restlessness and anxiety).

What tests tell you

The patient history should reveal predisposing conditions for pulmonary embolism as well as risk factors, including long car or plane trips, cancer, pregnancy, hypercoagulability, and previous DVT or pulmonary emboli. These tests support the diagnosis of pulmonary embolism:
• Chest X-rays help to rule out other pulmonary diseases.
• Lung scan shows perfusion defects in areas beyond occluded vessels; however, it doesn't rule out microemboli.
• Pulmonary angiography is the most definitive test, but it poses some risk to the patient. Its use depends on the uncertainty of the diagnosis and the need to avoid unnecessary anticoagulant therapy in a high-risk patient.

• ECG is inconclusive but helps distinguish pulmonary embolism from MI.
• Auscultation occasionally reveals a right ventricular S_3 gallop and increased intensity of a pulmonic component of S_2. Also, crackles and a pleural rub may be heard at the embolism site.
• ABG values showing decreased Pao_2 and $Paco_2$ are characteristic, but don't always occur.

How it's treated

Treatment of pulmonary embolism is designed to maintain adequate cardiovascular and pulmonary function during resolution of the obstruction as well as prevent embolus recurrence.

Treatment consists of oxygen therapy, as needed, and anticoagulation with heparin to inhibit new thrombus formation. Nonpharmacologic therapies include pneumatic compression devices.

Fibrin busters

Patients with massive pulmonary embolism and shock may need fibrinolytic therapy with streptokinase or alteplase to enhance fibrinolysis of the pulmonary emboli and remaining thrombi.

Filtering umbrella

Surgery is performed on patients who can't take anticoagulants (because of recent surgery or blood dyscrasias) or who have recurrent emboli during anticoagulant therapy. Surgery typically consists of inserting of a device (umbrella filter) to filter blood returning to the heart and lungs.

Renal failure, acute

Acute renal failure is the sudden interruption of renal function. It can be caused by obstruction, poor circulation, or kidney disease. It's potentially reversible; however, if left untreated, permanent damage can lead to chronic renal failure.

What causes it

Acute renal failure may be classified as prerenal, intrarenal, or postrenal. Each type has separate causes:
• Prerenal failure results from conditions that diminish blood flow to the kidneys (hypoperfusion). Examples include hypovolemia, hypotension, vasoconstriction, or inadequate cardiac output. One condition, prerenal azotemia (excess nitrogenous waste prod-

ucts in the blood), accounts for 40% to 80% of all cases of acute renal failure. Azotemia occurs as a response to renal hypoperfusion. Usually, it can be rapidly reversed by restoring renal blood flow and glomerular filtration.

• Intrarenal failure, also called *intrinsic* or *parenchymal renal failure*, results from damage to the filtering structures of the kidneys, usually from acute tubular necrosis, a disorder that causes cell death, or from nephrotoxic substances such as certain antibiotics.

• Postrenal failure results from bilateral obstruction of urine outflow, as in prostatic hyperplasia or bladder outlet obstruction.

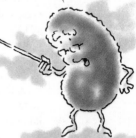

Postrenal failure is caused by any condition that blocks urine flow from both kidneys.

Going through the phases

With treatment, each type of acute renal failure passes through three distinct phases:

 oliguric (decreased urine output, less than 400 ml/24 hours)

 diuretic (increased urine output, 4 to 5 L/day)

recovery (glomerular filtration rate [GFR] normalizes).

What to look for

The signs and symptoms of prerenal failure depend on the cause. If the underlying problem is a change in blood pressure and volume, the patient may have:

• decreased cardiac output and cool, clammy skin in a patient with heart failure
• dry mucous membranes
• flat jugular veins
• hypotension
• lethargy progressing to coma
• oliguria
• tachycardia.

As renal failure progresses, the patient may show signs and symptoms of uremia, including:

• confusion
• fluid in the lungs
• GI complaints
• infection.

General hospital

About 5% of all hospitalized patients develop acute renal failure. The condition is usually reversible with treatment but, if it isn't treated, it may progress to end-stage renal disease, excess urea in the blood (prerenal azotemia or uremia), and death.

What tests tell you

These tests are used to diagnose acute renal failure:
- Blood studies reveal elevated BUN, serum creatinine, and potassium levels and decreased hematocrit and blood pH, bicarbonate, and hemoglobin levels.
- Urine specimens show casts, cellular debris, decreased specific gravity and, in glomerular diseases, proteinuria and urine osmolality close to serum osmolality. Urine sodium level is less than 20 mEq/L if oliguria results from decreased perfusion and more than 40 mEq/L if it results from an intrarenal problem.
- Creatinine clearance test measures the GFR and is used to estimate the number of remaining functioning nephrons.
- ECG shows tall, peaked T waves, a widening QRS complex, and disappearing P waves if an increased serum potassium (hyperkalemia) level is present.
- Other studies that help determine the cause of renal failure include kidney ultrasonography, plain films of the abdomen, kidney-ureter-bladder (KUB) radiography, excretory urography, renal scan, retrograde pyelography, CT scan, and nephrotomography.

How it's treated

Supportive measures for acute renal failure include:
- high-calorie diet that's low in protein, sodium, and potassium
- fluid and electrolyte balance
- monitoring for signs and symptoms of uremia
- fluid restriction
- diuretic therapy during the oliguric phase
- prevention of infection
- renal-dose dopamine to improve renal perfusion.

Meticulous electrolyte monitoring is needed to detect excess potassium in the blood (hyperkalemia). If symptoms occur, hypertonic glucose, insulin, and sodium bicarbonate are given I.V., and sodium polystyrene sulfonate is given by mouth or enema. If these measures fail to control uremia, the patient may need hemodialysis, continuous renal replacement therapy, or peritoneal dialysis.

Renal failure, chronic

Chronic renal failure, usually a progressive, irreversible deterioration, is the end result of gradual tissue destruction and loss of kidney function. Occasionally, however, chronic renal failure results from a rapidly progressing disease of sudden onset that destroys the nephrons and causes irreversible kidney damage. (See *Stages of chronic renal failure.*)

What causes it

Chronic renal failure may result from:
• chronic glomerular disease, such as glomerulonephritis, which affects the capillaries in the glomeruli
• chronic infections, such as chronic pyelonephritis and tuberculosis
• congenital anomalies such as polycystic kidney disease
• vascular diseases, such as hypertension and nephrosclerosis, which cause hardening of the kidneys
• obstructions such as renal calculi
• collagen diseases such as lupus erythematosus
• nephrotoxic agents such as long-term aminoglycoside therapy
• endocrine diseases such as diabetic neuropathy.

What to look for

Few symptoms develop until more than 75% of glomerular filtration is lost. Then the remaining normal tissue deteriorates progressively. Symptoms worsen as kidney function decreases. Profound changes affect all body systems. Major findings include hypervolemia (abnormal increase in plasma volume), peripheral edema, hyperphosphatemia, hyperkalemia, hypocalcemia, azotemia, metabolic acidosis, anemia, and peripheral neuropathy.

Body count

Other signs and symptoms, by body system, include:
• renal — dry mouth, fatigue, nausea, hypotension, loss of skin turgor, listlessness that may progress to somnolence and confusion, decreased or dilute urine, irregular pulses, and edema
• cardiovascular — hypertension, irregular pulse, life-threatening arrhythmias, and heart failure
• respiratory — infection, crackles, and pleuritic pain
• GI — gum sores and bleeding, hiccups, metallic taste, anorexia, nausea, vomiting, ammonia smell to the breath, and abdominal pain on palpation
• skin — pallid, yellowish-bronze color; dry, scaly skin; thin, brittle nails; dry, brittle hair that may change color and fall out easily; severe itching; and white, flaky urea deposits (uremic frost) in critically ill patients
• neurologic — altered LOC, muscle cramps and twitching, and pain, burning, and itching in the legs and feet (restless leg syndrome)

Stages of chronic renal failure

Chronic renal failure typically progresses through four stages:

Reduced renal reserve — Glomerular filtration rate (GFR) is 35% to 50% of the normal rate.

Renal insufficiency — GFR is 20% to 35% of the normal rate.

Renal failure — GFR is 20% to 25% of the normal rate.

End-stage renal disease — GFR is less than 20% of the normal rate.

• endocrine — growth retardation in children, infertility, decreased libido, amenorrhea, and impotence
• hematologic — GI bleeding and hemorrhage from body orifices and easy bruising
• musculoskeletal — fractures, bone and muscle pain, abnormal gait, and impaired bone growth and bowed legs in children.

What tests tell you

These tests are used to diagnose chronic renal failure:
• Blood studies show decreased arterial pH and bicarbonate levels, low hematocrit, low hemoglobin level, and elevated BUN, serum creatinine, sodium, and potassium levels.
• ABG analysis reveals metabolic acidosis.
• Urine specific gravity becomes fixed at 1.010; urinalysis may show proteinuria, glycosuria, RBCs, leukocytes, casts, or crystals, depending on the cause.
• X-ray studies, including KUB radiography, excretory urography, nephrotomography, renal scan, and renal arteriography, show reduced kidney size.
• Renal biopsy is used to identify underlying disease.
• EEG shows changes that indicate brain disease (metabolic encephalopathy).

How it's treated

Treatment for chronic renal failure may consist of one or more of these treatments, depending on the stage of failure. Conservative treatment includes:
• low-protein diet to reduce end products of protein metabolism that the kidneys can't excrete
• high-protein diet for patients on continuous peritoneal dialysis
• high-calorie diet to prevent ketoacidosis (the accumulation of ketones, such as acetone, in the blood) and tissue atrophy
• sodium and potassium restrictions
• phosphorus restriction
• fluid restrictions to maintain fluid balance.

Drug therapy

Drugs used to treat chronic renal failure include:
• loop diuretics such as furosemide (if some renal function remains) to maintain fluid balance
• antihypertensives to control blood pressure and edema
• antiemetics to relieve nausea and vomiting

• H_2-receptor antagonists, such as famotidine, to decrease gastric irritation
• stool softeners to prevent constipation
• iron and folate supplements or RBC infusion for anemia
• synthetic erythropoietin to stimulate the bone marrow to produce RBCs
• antipruritics, such as trimeprazine or diphenhydramine, to relieve itching
• aluminum hydroxide gel to lower serum phosphate levels
• supplementary vitamins, particularly vitamins B and D, and essential amino acids.

Dialysis

When the kidneys fail, kidney transplantation or dialysis may be the patient's only chance for survival. Dialysis options include hemodialysis, which filters blood through a dialysis machine, or peritoneal dialysis, in which a catheter is placed in the peritoneal cavity for instillation of dialysate.

Rheumatoid arthritis

A chronic, systemic, inflammatory disease, rheumatoid arthritis usually attacks peripheral joints and surrounding muscles, tendons, ligaments, and blood vessels. Spontaneous remissions and unpredictable exacerbations mark the course of this potentially crippling disease. Rheumatoid arthritis usually requires lifelong treatment and sometimes surgery. In most patients, the disease is intermittent, allowing for periods of normal activity. However, 10% of patients suffer total disability from severe joint deformity, associated symptoms, or both.

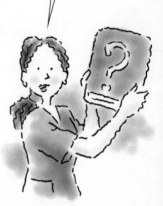

Genetics? Infections? Hormones? The cause of rheumatoid arthritis is unknown.

What causes it

The cause of rheumatoid arthritis isn't known, but infections, genetics, and endocrine factors may play a part.

What to look for

At first, the patient may complain of nonspecific symptoms, including fatigue, malaise, anorexia, persistent low-grade fever, weight loss, and vague articular symptoms. As inflammation progresses, specific symptoms develop, frequently in the fingers. They usually occur bilaterally and symmetrically and may extend to the wrists, elbows, knees, and ankles.

What tests tell you

Although no test can be used to definitively diagnose rheumatoid arthritis, these tests are useful:

• X-rays may show bone demineralization and soft-tissue swelling and help determine the extent of cartilage and bone destruction, erosion, subluxations, and deformities.

• Rheumatoid factor test is positive in 75% to 80% of patients, as indicated by a titer of 1:160 or higher. Although the presence of rheumatoid factor doesn't confirm the disease, it helps in determining the prognosis. A patient with a high titer usually has more severe and progressive disease with extra-articular signs and symptoms.

• Synovial fluid analysis shows increased volume and turbidity but decreased viscosity and complement levels. The WBC count commonly exceeds 10,000/mm^3.

• Serum protein electrophoresis may show elevated serum globulin levels.

• ESR is elevated in 85% to 90% of patients. Because an elevated rate commonly parallels disease activity, this test helps monitor the patient's response to therapy.

How it's treated

Treatment measures are used to reduce pain and inflammation and preserve the patient's functional capacity and quality of life.

Drug therapy

NSAIDs, which include the traditional NSAIDs (such as ibuprofen), COX-2 inhibitors (such as celecoxib), and salicylates (aspirin), are the mainstay of therapy because they decrease inflammation and relieve joint pain. Other drugs that can be used are hydroxychloroquine, gold salts, penicillamine, and corticosteroids such as prednisone. Immunosuppressants — cyclophosphamide, methotrexate, and azathioprine — are used in the early stages of the disease.

Protein-A immunoadsorption therapy

Patients with moderate to severe rheumatoid arthritis who haven't responded well to drug therapy may opt for protein-A immunoadsorption therapy. During this therapy, blood is drawn from a vein in the patient's arm and pumped into an apheresis machine, which separates plasma from the blood cells. Plasma then passes through a PROSORBA column (a plastic cylinder about the size of a coffee mug that contains a sandlike substance coated with protein A). Protein A in the cylinder binds with the antibodies produced in rheumatoid arthritis. After the plasma passes through the PROSORBA column, it's returned to the body through a vein in the patient's other arm. This procedure typically lasts 2 hours. The recommended regimen is one treatment weekly for 12 weeks.

Physical and other therapies

Joint function can be preserved through ROM exercises and a carefully individualized physical and occupational therapy program. Surgery is available for joints that are damaged or painful.

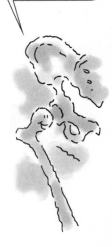

Joint function can be preserved in patients with rheumatoid arthritis through ROM exercises.

Seizure disorder

Also known as *epilepsy*, seizure disorder is a brain condition characterized by recurrent seizures. Seizures are paroxysmal events associated with abnormal electrical discharges of neurons in the brain. The discharge may trigger a convulsive movement, an interruption of sensation, an alteration in LOC, or a combination of these symptoms. In most cases, seizure disorder doesn't affect intelligence.

From young to old

This condition affects people of all ages, races, and ethnic backgrounds. The condition appears most commonly in early childhood and advanced age. About 80% of patients have good seizure control with strict adherence to prescribed treatment.

What causes it

In seizure disorder, a group of neurons may lose afferent stimulation (ability to transmit impulses from the periphery toward the CNS) and function as an epileptogenic focus. These neurons are hypersensitive and easily activated. In response to changes in the cellular environment, the neurons become hyperactive and fire abnormally.

Don't know why

About one-half of seizure disorder cases are idiopathic. No specific cause can be found, and the patient has no other neurologic abnormality. In other cases, however, possible causes of seizure disorder include:
• genetic abnormalities, such as tuberous sclerosis (tumors and sclerotic patches in the brain) and phenylketonuria (inability to convert phenylalanine into tyrosine)
• perinatal injuries

• metabolic abnormalities, such as hyponatremia, hypocalcemia, hypoglycemia, and pyridoxine deficiency
• brain tumors or other space-occupying lesions of the cortex
• infections, such as meningitis, encephalitis, or brain abscess
• traumatic injury, especially if the dura mater has been penetrated
• ingestion of toxins, such as mercury, lead, or carbon monoxide
• stroke
• hereditary abnormalities (some seizure disorders appear to run in families)
• fever.

What to look for

Signs and symptoms of seizure disorder vary depending on the type and cause of the seizure. (See *Understanding types of seizures.*)

Physical findings may be normal if the patient doesn't have a seizure during assessment and the cause is idiopathic. If the seizure is caused by an underlying problem, the patient's history and physical examination should uncover related signs and symptoms.

In many cases, the patient's history shows that seizures are unpredictable and unrelated to activities. Occasionally, a patient may report precipitating factors. For example, the seizures may always take place at a certain time, such as during sleep, or after a particular circumstance, such as lack of sleep or emotional stress. He may also report nonspecific symptoms, such as headache, mood changes, lethargy, and myoclonic jerking up to several hours before a seizure.

Aural report

Some patients report an aura a few seconds or minutes before a generalized seizure. An aura signals the beginning of abnormal electrical discharges within a focal area of the brain. Typical auras include:
• pungent smell
• nausea or indigestion
• rising or sinking feeling in the stomach
• dreamy feeling
• unusual taste
• visual disturbance such as a flashing light.

What tests tell you

These tests are used to diagnose seizure disorder:
• EEG showing paroxysmal abnormalities may confirm the diagnosis by providing evidence of continuing seizure tendency. A neg-

Understanding types of seizures

Use these guidelines to understand different seizure types. Remember that patients may be affected by more than one type of seizure.

Partial seizures

Arising from a localized area in the brain, partial seizure activity may spread to the entire brain, causing a generalized seizure. Several types and subtypes of partial seizures exist:
• simple partial, which includes jacksonian and sensory
• complex partial
• secondarily generalized partial seizure (partial onset leading to generalized tonic-clonic seizure).

Jacksonian seizure

A jacksonian seizure begins as a localized motor seizure, characterized by a spread of abnormal activity to adjacent areas of the brain. The patient experiences a stiffening or jerking in one extremity, accompanied by a tingling sensation in the same area. Although the patient in a jacksonian seizure seldom loses consciousness, the seizure may progress to a generalized tonic-clonic seizure.

Sensory seizure

Symptoms of a sensory seizure include hallucinations, flashing lights, tingling sensations, vertigo, déjà vu, and smelling a foul odor.

Complex partial seizure

Signs and symptoms of a complex partial seizure are variable but usually involve purposeless behavior, including a glassy stare, picking at clothes, aimless wandering, lip-smacking or chewing motions, and unintelligible speech. An aura may occur first, and seizures may last from a few seconds to 20 minutes. Afterward, mental confusion may last several minutes, and an observer may mistakenly suspect alcohol or drug intoxication or psychosis. The patient has no memory of his actions during the seizure.

Secondarily generalized seizure

A secondarily generalized seizure can be simple or complex and can progress to a generalized seizure. An aura may occur first, with loss of consciousness occurring immediately or 1 to 2 minutes later.

Generalized seizures

Generalized seizures cause a generalized electrical abnormality within the brain. Types include:
• absence or petit mal
• myoclonic
• generalized tonic-clonic
• akinetic.

Absence seizure

Absence seizure occurs most commonly in children. This type of seizure usually begins with a brief change in the level of consciousness, signaled by blinking or rolling of the eyes, a blank stare, and slight mouth movements. The patient retains his posture and continues pre-seizure activity without difficulty. Seizures last from 1 to 10 seconds, and impairment is so brief that the patient may be unaware of it. However, if not properly treated, these seizures can recur up to 100 times per day and progress to a generalized tonic-clonic seizure.

Myoclonic seizure

Also called *bilateral massive epileptic myoclonus,* myoclonic seizure is marked by brief, involuntary muscular jerks of the body or extremities, which may occur in a rhythmic manner, and a brief loss of consciousness.

Generalized tonic-clonic seizure

Typically, a generalized tonic-clonic seizure begins with a loud cry, caused by air rushing from the lungs through the vocal cords. The patient falls to the ground, losing consciousness. The body stiffens (tonic phase) and then alternates between episodes of muscle spasm and relaxation (clonic phase). Tongue biting, incontinence, labored breathing, apnea, and cyanosis may also occur.

The seizure stops in 2 to 5 minutes, when abnormal electrical conduction of the neurons is completed. Afterward, the patient regains consciousness but is somewhat confused. He may have difficulty talking and may have drowsiness, fatigue, headache, muscle soreness, and arm or leg weakness. He may fall into a deep sleep afterward.

Akinetic seizure

Characterized by a general loss of postural tone and a temporary loss of consciousness, akinetic seizure occurs in young children. Sometimes it's called a "drop attack" because the child falls.

ative EEG doesn't rule out seizure disorder because paroxysmal abnormalities occur intermittently. EEG also helps determine the prognosis and can help classify the disorder.
• CT scan and MRI provide density readings of the brain and may indicate abnormalities in internal structures.

Other tests include serum glucose and calcium studies, skull X-rays, lumbar puncture, brain scan, and cerebral angiography.

How it's treated

Treatment for seizures seeks to reduce the frequency of them and prevent recurrence.

Drug therapy

Drug therapy is specific to the type of seizure. The most commonly prescribed drugs for generalized tonic-clonic and complex partial seizures are phenytoin, carbamazepine, phenobarbital, and primidone, administered individually. Valproic acid, clonazepam, and ethosizimide are commonly prescribed for absence seizures. Lamotrigine is also given as adjunct therapy for partial seizures.

Surgery

If drug therapy fails, treatment may include surgical removal of a demonstrated focal lesion to try to stop seizures. Surgery is also performed when seizure disorder results from an underlying problem, such as an intracranial tumor, a brain abscess or cyst, and vascular abnormalities.

Sodium imbalance

Sodium is the major cation (90%) in extracellular fluid. Potassium is the major cation in intracellular fluid. During repolarization, the sodium-potassium pump continually shifts sodium into the cells and potassium out of the cells; during depolarization, it does the reverse. Sodium cation functions include maintaining tonicity and concentration of extracellular fluid, acid-base balance (reabsorption of sodium ions and excretion of hydrogen ions), nerve conduction and neuromuscular function, glandular secretion, and water balance.

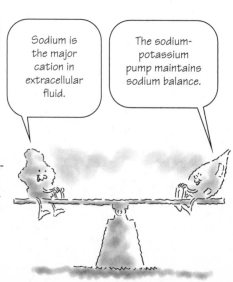

Sodium is the major cation in extracellular fluid.

The sodium-potassium pump maintains sodium balance.

What causes it

Sodium imbalance can result from several causes. A low-sodium diet or excessive use of diuretics may induce hyponatremia (decreased serum sodium concentration). Dehydration may induce hypernatremia (increased serum sodium concentration).

Hyponatremia

One of the main causes of hyponatremia is excessive GI loss of water and electrolytes. This loss can result from vomiting, suctioning, or diarrhea; excessive perspiration or fever; potent diuretics; or the use of tap-water enemas. Excessive drinking of water, infusion of I.V. dextrose in water without other solutes, malnutrition or starvation, and a low-sodium diet can also cause hyponatremia, usually in combination with one of the other causes.

Trauma, surgery (wound drainage), and burns, which cause sodium to shift into damaged cells, can lead to decreased serum sodium levels, as can adrenal gland insufficiency (Addison's disease), hypoaldosteronism, and cirrhosis of the liver with ascites.

Syndrome of inappropriate antidiuretic hormone (SIADH), resulting from a brain tumor, a stroke, pulmonary disease, or a neoplasm with ectopic antidiuretic hormone (ADH) production can also lead to hyponatremia. Certain drugs, such as chlorpropamide and clofibrate, may produce an SIADH-like syndrome.

Hypernatremia

Decreased water intake can cause hypernatremia. When severe vomiting and diarrhea cause water loss that exceeds sodium loss, serum sodium levels rise but overall extracellular fluid volume decreases.

Other causes include excess adrenocortical hormones, as in Cushing's syndrome, and ADH deficiency (diabetes insipidus). Salt intoxication—an uncommon cause—may result from excessive ingestion of table salt.

What to look for

Sodium imbalance has profound physiologic effects and can induce severe CNS, cardiovascular, and GI abnormalities. (See *Signs and symptoms of sodium imbalance*, page 572.)

For example, hyponatremia may result in renal dysfunction or, if serum sodium loss is abrupt or severe, seizures. Hypernatremia may produce pulmonary edema, circulatory disorders, and a decreased LOC.

Signs and symptoms of sodium imbalance

The chart below lists possible signs and symptoms of hyponatremia and hypernatremia by body system dysfunction.

Dysfunction	Hyponatremia	Hypernatremia
Cardiovascular	Hypotension, tachycardia; with severe deficit, vasomotor collapse, thready pulse	Hypertension, tachycardia, pitting edema, excessive weight gain
Central nervous system	Anxiety, headaches, muscle twitching and weakness, seizures	Fever, agitation, restlessness, seizures
Cutaneous	Cold, clammy skin; decreased skin turgor	Flushed skin; dry, sticky mucous membranes
GI	Nausea, vomiting, abdominal cramps	Rough, dry tongue; intense thirst
Genitourinary	Oliguria or anuria	Oliguria
Respiratory	Cyanosis with severe deficiency	Dyspnea, respiratory arrest, and death (from dramatic rise in osmotic pressure)

What tests tell you

Hyponatremia is defined as a serum sodium level less than 135 mEq/L; hypernatremia, as a serum sodium level greater than 145 mEq/L. However, additional laboratory studies are necessary to determine etiology and differentiate between a true deficit and an apparent deficit resulting from a sodium shift or from hypervolemia or hypovolemia.

True grit

In true hyponatremia, supportive values include urine sodium greater than 100 mEq/24 hours, with low serum osmolality; in true hypernatremia, urine sodium is less than 40 mEq/24 hours, with high serum osmolality.

How it's treated

The type of treatment varies with the severity of the imbalance.

Hyponatremia

Treatment for mild hyponatremia usually consists of restricted electrolyte-free water intake when it results from hemodilution, SIADH, or such conditions as heart failure, cirrhosis of the liver, and renal failure. If fluid restriction alone fails to normalize serum sodium levels, demeclocycline or lithium, which blocks ADH action in the renal tubules, can be used to promote water excretion.

Rare or well-done?

In extremely rare instances of severe, symptomatic hyponatremia when the serum sodium level falls below 110 mEq/L, treatment may include an infusion of 3% or 5% saline solution. Treatment with saline infusion requires careful monitoring of venous pressure to prevent potentially fatal circulatory overload. The aim of treatment of secondary hyponatremia is to correct the underlying disorder.

Hypernatremia

Primary treatment of hypernatremia is administration of salt-free solutions (such as dextrose in water), which returns serum sodium level to normal, followed by infusion of half-normal saline solution to prevent hyponatremia. Other measures include a sodium-restricted diet and discontinuation of drugs that promote sodium retention.

Stroke

Previously known as *cerebrovascular accident*, stroke is a sudden impairment of cerebral circulation in one or more of the blood vessels supplying the brain. It interrupts or diminishes oxygen supply, causing serious damage or necrosis in brain tissues. The sooner circulation returns to normal after stroke, the better chances are for complete recovery. About one-half of those who survive remain permanently disabled and suffer another stroke within weeks, months, or years.

Transient, progressive, or completed

Stroke is classified according to how it progresses:
• TIA, the least severe type, is caused by a temporary interruption of blood flow, usually in the carotid and vertebrobasilar arteries. (See *Understanding TIA*, page 574.)
• Progressive stroke, also called *stroke-in-evolution* or *thrombus-in-evolution*, begins with a slight neurologic deficit and worsens in a day or two.
• Completed stroke, the most severe type, causes maximum neurologic deficits at the onset.

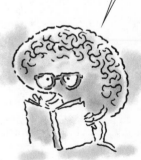

Oh, no! Says here that in stroke, circulation is impaired in the vessels that supply me with blood.

Understanding TIA

A transient ischemic attack (TIA) is a recurrent episode of neurologic deficit, lasting from seconds to hours, that clears within 12 to 24 hours. TIA is usually considered a warning sign of an impending thrombotic stroke. In fact, TIAs have been reported in 50% to 80% of patients who have had a cerebral infarction from thrombosis. The age of onset varies, but incidence rises dramatically after age 50 and is highest among blacks and men.

Interrupting blood flow

In TIA, microemboli released from a thrombus may temporarily interrupt blood flow, especially in the small distal branches of the brain's arterial tree. Small spasms in those arterioles may precede TIA and also impair blood flow.

A transient experience

The most distinctive characteristics of TIAs are the transient duration of neurologic deficits and the complete return of normal function. The signs and symptoms of TIA correlate with the location of the affected artery. They include double vision, unilateral blindness, staggering or uncoordinated gait, unilateral weakness or numbness, falling because of weakness in the legs, dizziness, and speech deficits, such as slurring and thickness.

Preventing a stroke

During an active TIA, treatment aims to prevent a stroke and consists of aspirin or anticoagulants to minimize the risk of thrombosis. After or between attacks, preventive treatment includes carotid endarterectomy or cerebral microvascular bypass.

What causes it

Factors that increase the risk of stroke include:
- arrhythmias (especially atrial fibrillation)
- atherosclerosis
- cardiac enlargement
- diabetes mellitus
- drug abuse
- ECG changes
- family history of cerebrovascular disease
- gout
- high serum triglyceride levels
- history of TIA
- hormonal contraceptive use
- hypertension
- lack of exercise
- orthostatic hypotension
- rheumatic heart disease
- sickle cell disease
- smoking.
    Major causes of stroke include:
- embolism
- hemorrhage
- thrombosis.

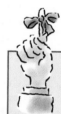

Memory jogger

Here are some key points to remember about TIA:

T: Temporary episode that clears within 12 to 24 hours.

I: It's usually considered a warning sign of Impending stroke.

A: Aspirin and Anticoagulants given during a TIA may minimize the risk of thrombosis.

What to look for

When taking the patient's history, you may uncover risk factors for stroke. You may observe loss of consciousness, dizziness, or seizures. Obtain information from a family member or friend if necessary. Neurologic examination provides most of the information about the physical effects of stroke.

Physical findings depend on:
• the artery affected and the portion of the brain it supplies (see *Neurologic deficits in stroke*, page 576)
• the severity of the damage
• the extent of collateral circulation that develops to help the brain compensate for a decreased blood supply.

Reflecting on reflexes

Assessment of motor function and muscle strength commonly shows a loss of voluntary muscle control and hemiparesis or hemiplegia on one side of the body. In the initial phase, flaccid paralysis with decreased deep tendon reflexes may occur. These reflexes return to normal after the initial phase, accompanied by an increase in muscle tone and, in some cases, muscle spasticity on the affected side.

Sensory impairment: Slight to severe

Vision testing usually reveals reduced vision or blindness on the affected side of the body and, in patients with left-sided hemiplegia, problems with visual-spatial relations. Sensory assessment may reveal sensory losses, ranging from slight impairment of touch to the inability to perceive the position and motion of body parts. The patient may also have difficulty interpreting visual, tactile, and auditory stimuli.

Whose side are you on, anyway?

If the stroke occurs in the brain's left hemisphere, it produces signs and symptoms on the right side of the body. If it occurs in the right hemisphere, signs and symptoms appear on the left side. However, a stroke that damages cranial nerves produces signs on the same side as the damage.

What tests tell you

These tests are used to diagnose stroke:
• Cerebral angiography details disruption or displacement of the cerebral circulation by occlusion or hemorrhage. It's the test of choice for examining the entire cerebral circulation.

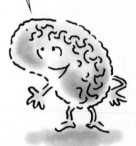

Remember that my right hemisphere controls the left side of the body and my left hemisphere controls the right side of the body.

Neurologic deficits in stroke

In stroke, functional loss reflects damage to the brain area normally perfused by the occluded or ruptured artery. Whereas one patient may experience only mild hand weakness, another may develop unilateral paralysis. Hypoxia and ischemia may produce edema that affects distal parts of the brain, causing further neurologic deficits. The signs and symptoms that accompany stroke at different sites are described below.

Site	Signs and symptoms	Site	Signs and symptoms
Middle cerebral artery	• Aphasia • Dysphasia • Dyslexia (reading problems) • Dysgraphia (inability to write) • Visual field cuts • Hemiparesis on the affected side, which is more severe in the face and arm than in the leg	Anterior cerebral artery	• Confusion • Weakness • Numbness on the affected side (especially in the arm) • Paralysis of the contralateral foot and leg with accompanying footdrop • Incontinence • Poor coordination • Impaired motor and sensory functions • Personality changes, such as flat affect and distractibility
Internal carotid artery	• Headaches • Weakness • Paralysis • Numbness • Sensory changes • Vision disturbances such as blurring on the affected side • Altered level of consciousness • Bruits over the carotid artery • Aphasia • Dysphasia • Ptosis	Vertebral or basilar artery	• Mouth and lip numbness • Dizziness • Weakness on the affected side • Vision deficits, such as color blindness, lack of depth perception, and diplopia • Poor coordination • Dysphagia • Slurred speech • Amnesia • Ataxia
		Posterior cerebral artery	• Visual field cuts • Sensory impairment • Dyslexia • Coma • Blindness from ischemia in the occipital area

• Digital subtraction angiography evaluates the patency of the cerebral vessels and identifies their position in the head and neck. It also detects and evaluates lesions and vascular abnormalities.
• CT scan detects structural abnormalities, edema, and lesions, such as nonhemorrhagic infarction and aneurysms. It differentiates stroke from other disorders, such as primary metastatic tumor and subdural, intracerebral, or epidural hematoma. Patients with TIA commonly have a normal CT scan.

• PET scan provides data on cerebral metabolism and cerebral blood flow changes, especially in ischemic stroke.
• Single-photon emission CT identifies cerebral blood flow and helps diagnose cerebral infarction.
• MRI and magnetic resonance angiography evaluate the lesion's location and size. MRI doesn't distinguish hemorrhage, tumor, or infarction as well as a CT scan, but it provides superior images of the cerebellum and brain stem.
• Transcranial Doppler studies evaluate the velocity of blood flow through major intracranial vessels, which can indicate the vessels' diameter.
• Cerebral blood flow studies measure blood flow to the brain and help detect abnormalities.
• Ophthalmoscopy may show signs of hypertension and athero-sclerotic changes in the retinal arteries.
• EEG may detect reduced electrical activity in an area of cortical infarction and is especially useful when CT scan results are inconclusive. It can also differentiate seizure activity from stroke.
• Oculoplethysmography indirectly measures ophthalmic blood flow and carotid artery blood flow.

How it's treated

Medical treatment for stroke commonly includes physical rehabilitation, dietary and drug regimens to help decrease risk factors, and measures to help the patient adapt to specific deficits, such as speech impairment and paralysis.

Drugs commonly used for stroke therapy include:
• thrombolytic therapy, such as recombinant tPA, given within the first 3 hours of an ischemic stroke to restore circulation to the affected brain tissue and limit the extent of brain injury
• anticonvulsants, such as phenytoin, to treat or prevent seizures
• stool softeners, such as docusate, to avoid straining, which increases intracranial pressure
• corticosteroids, such as dexamethasone, to minimize cerebral edema
• anticoagulants, such as heparin, warfarin, and ticlopidine, to reduce the risk of thrombotic stroke
• analgesics, such as codeine, to relieve headache that may follow hemorrhagic stroke.

Surgery

Depending on the stroke's cause and extent, the patient may also undergo surgery. A craniotomy may be done to remove a hematoma, an endarterectomy to remove atherosclerotic plaque from the inner arterial wall, or extracranial-intracranial bypass to circumvent an artery that's blocked by occlusion or stenosis. Ventricular shunts may be necessary to drain CSF if hydrocephalus occurs.

Tuberculosis

Tuberculosis is an infectious disease that primarily affects the lungs but can invade other body systems as well. In tuberculosis, pulmonary infiltrates accumulate, cavities develop, and masses of granulated tissue form within the lungs. Tuberculosis may occur as an acute or a chronic infection.

Incidence is highest in people who live in crowded, poorly ventilated, unsanitary conditions, such as prisons, tenement houses, and homeless shelters. Others at high risk for tuberculosis include alcoholics, I.V. drug abusers, elderly people, and those who are immunocompromised.

What causes it

Tuberculosis results from exposure to *Mycobacterium tuberculosis* and, sometimes, other strains of mycobacteria. Here's what happens:
• Transmission — An infected person coughs or sneezes, spreading infected droplets. When someone without immunity inhales these droplets, the bacilli are deposited in the lungs.
• Immune response — The immune system responds by sending leukocytes, and inflammation results. After a few days, leukocytes are replaced by macrophages. Bacilli are then ingested by the macrophages and carried off by the lymphatics to the lymph nodes.
• Tubercle formation — Macrophages that ingest the bacilli fuse to form epithelioid cell tubercles, tiny nodules surrounded by lymphocytes. Within the lesion, caseous necrosis develops and scar tissue encapsulates the tubercle. The organism may be killed in the process.
• Dissemination — If the tubercles and inflamed nodes rupture, the infection contaminates the surrounding tissue and may spread through the blood and lymphatic circulation to distant sites. This process is called *hematogenous dissemination*.

What to look for

After exposure to *M. tuberculosis*, roughly 5% of infected people develop active tuberculosis within 1 year. They may complain of a low-grade fever at night, a productive cough that lasts longer than

3 weeks, and symptoms of airway obstruction from lymph node involvement.

In other infected people, microorganisms cause a latent infection. The host's immunologic defense system may destroy the bacillus. Alternatively, the encapsulated bacilli may live within the tubercle. It may lie dormant for years, reactivating later to cause active infection.

Adding insult to injury

Tuberculosis can cause massive pulmonary tissue damage, with inflammation and tissue necrosis eventually leading to respiratory failure. Bronchopleural fistulas can develop from lung tissue damage, resulting in pneumothorax. The disease can also lead to hemorrhage, pleural effusion, and pneumonia. Small mycobacterial foci can infect other body organs, including the kidneys, skeleton, and CNS.

With proper treatment, the prognosis for a patient with tuberculosis is usually excellent.

What tests tell you

These tests are used to diagnose tuberculosis:
• Chest X-rays show nodular lesions, patchy infiltrates (mainly in upper lobes), cavity formation, scar tissue, and calcium deposits.
• A tuberculin skin test reveals infection at some point but doesn't indicate active disease.
• Stains and cultures of sputum, CSF, urine, drainage from abscesses, or pleural fluid show heat-sensitive, nonmotile, aerobic, acid-fast bacilli.
• CT scanning and MRI allow the evaluation of lung damage and may confirm a difficult diagnosis.
• Bronchoscopy shows inflammation and altered lung tissue. It may also be performed to obtain sputum if the patient can't produce an adequate sputum specimen.

How it's treated

The usual treatment for tuberculosis is daily oral doses of isoniazid or rifampin, with ethambutol added in some cases, for at least 9 months. After 2 to 4 weeks, the disease is no longer infectious, and the patient can resume normal activities while continuing to take medication.

The patient with atypical mycobacterial disease or drug-resistant tuberculosis may require second-line drugs, such as capreomycin, streptomycin, para-aminosalicylic acid, pyrazinamide, and cycloserine. However, he may find it difficult to follow this lengthy treatment regimen. Therefore, the incidence of noncompliance is high. This noncompliance has led to the development of resistant strains of tuberculosis in recent years.

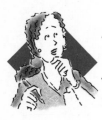

Quick quiz

1. A diagnostic test that can confirm metabolic acidosis is:
A. ABG analysis.
B urinalysis.
C. anion gap.
D. electrolyte level.

Answer: A. Arterial pH below 7.35 confirms metabolic acidosis. With severe acidotic states, pH may fall to 7.10 and $Paco_2$ may be normal or less than 34 mm Hg as compensatory mechanisms take hold.

2. A characteristic sign in respiratory alkalosis is:
A. hypoventilation.
B. deep, rapid breathing.
C. positive Homans' sign.
D. vomiting.

Answer: B. The cardinal sign of respiratory alkalosis is deep, rapid breathing, possibly exceeding 40 breaths/minute and much like the Kussmaul's respirations that characterize diabetic acidosis. Such hyperventilation usually leads to CNS and neuromuscular disturbances.

3. In a patient with arterial occlusive disease, treatment involves:
A. exercise.
B. low-cholesterol diet.
C. pain medication.
D. surgery.

Answer: D. Acute arterial occlusive disease usually requires surgery to restore circulation to the affected area.

4. Perioral paresthesia, twitching, tetany, and seizures are signs and symptoms of:
A. hypercalcemia.
B. hypocalcemia.
C. hypernatremia.
D. hyponatremia.

Answer: B. Characteristic signs and symptoms of hypocalcemia include perioral paresthesia, twitching, carpopedal spasm, tetany, seizures and, possibly, cardiac arrhythmias. Although Chvostek's and Trousseau's signs are reliable indicators of hypocalcemia, they aren't specific.

5. For a patient with hyperglycemia, a rapid acting insulin that may be administered is:
  A. Humalog.
  B. regular.
  C. NPH.
  D. lente.

Answer: A. Insulin may be rapid-acting (Humalog), fast-acting (regular), intermediate-acting (NPH and lente), or a premixed combination of fast-acting and intermediate-acting. Purified human insulin is commonly used today.

Scoring

☆☆☆ If you answered all five questions correctly, amazing! Your knowledge of disorders is proliferating with remarkable speed and efficiency.

☆☆ If you answered four questions correctly, good work! Your learning skill is a remarkable combination of environmental, genetic, dietary, and other unspecified factors.

☆ If you answered fewer than four questions correctly, no worries! Review the chapter and your understanding will achieve an admirable level of homeostasis.

Appendices and index

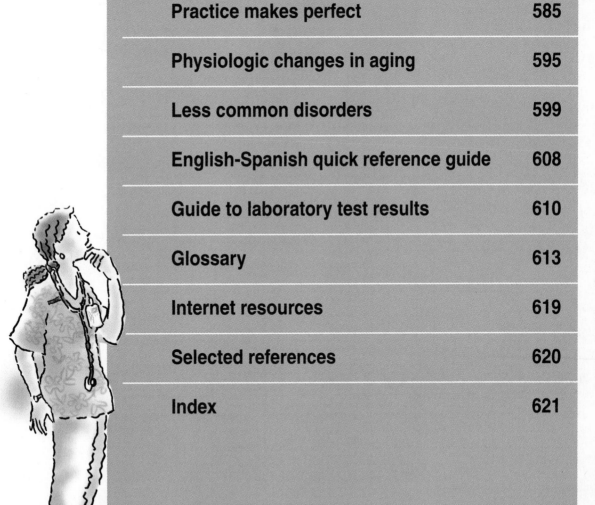

Practice makes perfect

Chapter 1

1. During a respiratory assessment of a patient, you percuss a resonant sound. This sound is indicative of:

    A.   air collection.
    B.   hyperinflated lung.
    C.   normal lung tissue.
    D.   consolidation.

Answer: C. Resonant sounds are heard over normal lung tissue. In most cases, they can be percussed over nearly all of the chest.

2. While counting a patient's pulse rate, you identify an irregular rhythm. To determine an accurate rate, you should count the beats for:

    A.   30 seconds and then multiply by 2.
    B.   15 seconds and then multiply by 4.
    C.   60 seconds.
    D.   10 seconds and then multiply by 6.

Answer: C. If the rhythm is irregular, count the beats for 60 seconds to obtain an accurate pulse rate.

3. During a patient's musculoskeletal assessment, you notice that he can't move his left arm away from his side. This should be documented as impaired:

    A.   supination.
    B.   abduction.
    C.   extension.
    D.   adduction.

Answer: B. Abduction is the ability to move the limb away from the midline.

4. To assess stereognosis, you should ask the patient to close his eyes and then you should:

    A.   grasp his index finger and move it back and forth.
    B.   draw a large number on his palm and ask him to identify the number.
    C.   place a common object in his hand and ask him to identify it.
    D.   touch one of his limbs and ask him to identify the location that you touched.

Answer: C. The ability to discriminate the size, shape, weight, texture, and form of an object is known as *stereognosis*. To test stereognosis, ask the patient to close his eyes, place a common object in his hand, and then ask him to identify the object.

5. During a patient interview, the nurse helps the patient redirect attention to a question about a specific issue. This communication technique is known as:

    A.   rephrasing.
    B.   clarification.
    C.   collaboration.
    D.   focusing.

Answer: D. Focusing is a technique that helps the patient redirect his attention back to a specific issue. It fosters patient self-control and helps the patient avoid vague generalizations so that he can accept responsibility for facing problems.

Chapter 2

6. What percentage of blood does atrial kick provide to the ventricles?

    A.   10%
    B.   20%
    C.   25%
    D.   30%

Answer: D. Contraction of the atria normally provides the ventricles with about 30% of their blood.

7. The immediate treatment of choice for asystole is:

    A.   epinephrine.
    B.   cardiopulmonary resuscitation (CPR).
    C.   atropine.
    D.   transcutaneous pacing.

Answer: B. The immediate treatment of choice for asystole is CPR. Start CPR as soon as you determine that a patient has no pulse. Subsequent treatment focuses on identifying and either treating or removing the underlying cause.

8. The condition in which a premature ventricle contraction (PVC) strikes on the downslope of the preceding T wave can be described as:

    A.   unifocal.
    B.   compensatory pause.
    C.   R-on-T phenomenon.
    D.   bigeminy.

Answer: C. When a PVC strikes on the downslope of the preceding normal T wave, it's known as the *R-on-T phenomenon.* This event can trigger more serious rhythm disturbances.

9. In accelerated junctional rhythm, heart rate is usually:

    A.   between 60 and 100 beats/minute.
    B.   between 100 and 200 beats/minute.
    C.   between 150 and 250 beats/minute.
    D.   greater than 300 beats/minute.

Answer: A. Accelerated junctional rhythm results when an irritable focus in the atrioventricular junction speeds up and takes over as the heart's pacemaker. The accelerated rate is usually between 60 and 100 beats/minute.

10. If a patient with atrial fibrillation is symptomatic, the treatment of choice is:
- A. defibrillation.
- B. synchronized cardioversion.
- C. digoxin.
- D. beta-adrenergic blockers.

Answer: B. For a symptomatic patient with atrial fibrillation, immediate synchronized cardioversion is necessary. Cardioversion is most successful if used within the first 3 days of treatment and is less successful if the rhythm has existed for a long time.

Chapter 3

11. Which of the following conditions can increase a patient's international normalized ratio (INR)?
- A. Hypovolemia
- B. Respiratory failure
- C. Heart failure
- D. Cirrhosis

Answer: D. Elevated INR values may indicate cirrhosis, disseminated intravascular coagulation, hepatitis, vitamin K deficiency, salicylate intoxication, uncontrolled oral anticoagulation, or massive blood transfusion.

12. The presence of which factor may result in an elevated platelet count?
- A. Cold temperature
- B. Low altitude
- C. Sedentary lifestyle
- D. Furosemide

Answer: A. High altitudes, persistent cold temperatures, strenuous exercise, and excitement increase platelet count.

13. Which condition may result in hypokalemia?
- A. Myocardial infarction
- B. Burns
- C. Crush injuries
- D. Vomiting

Answer: D. Depletion of total body potassium occurs with vomiting, diarrhea, GI and renal disorders, gastric suctioning, diabetic ketoacidosis and insulin administration without potassium supplements, diuretic use, excessive aldosterone secretion, and excessive licorice ingestion.

14. Which factor might influence the results of a prostate-specific antigen (PSA) test?
  A. Placing the specimen on ice
  B. Collecting the specimen in the morning
  C. Performing the test in conjunction with a digital rectal examination
  D. Failing to fast prior to the test
Answer: C. Collect a PSA specimen either before or at least 48 hours after a digital rectal examination to avoid falsely elevated PSA levels.

15. Coinciding high levels of triglycerides and cholesterol may occur in which condition?
  A. Coronary artery disease (CAD)
  B. Nephrotic syndrome
  C. Diabetes mellitus
  D. Cirrhosis
Answer: A. High levels of triglycerides and cholesterol reflect an increased risk of CAD.

Chapter 4

16. To determine the proper length of a feeding tube prior to insertion, the nurse should measure:
  A. from the mouth to the upper curvature of the stomach.
  B. from the mouth to the xiphoid process.
  C. from the tip of the nose to the upper curvature of the stomach.
  D. from the tip of the nose to the earlobe and then to the xiphoid process.
Answer: D. To determine the tube length needed to reach the stomach, first extend the distal end of the tube from the tip of the patient's nose to his earlobe. Coil this portion of the tube around your fingers so the end remains curved until you insert it. Then extend the uncoiled portion from the earlobe to the xiphoid process.

17. You are about to use a handheld resuscitation bag on a patient and see secretions in his mouth. You should first:
  A. insert an oral airway.
  B. suction the airway.
  C. turn the patient on his side.
  D. use the handheld resuscitation bag on the patient.
Answer: B. Before using the handheld resuscitation bag, check the patient's upper airway for foreign objects or secretions. If present, remove them. Suction the patient to remove secretions that may obstruct the airway. If necessary, insert an oropharyngeal or nasopharyngeal airway to maintain airway patency.

18. A patient is on bedrest and prone to pressure ulcers. In the supine position, common pressure ulcer sites include:
    A.   sacrum.
    B.   xiphoid process.
    C.   knees.
    D.   groin.
Answer: A. Common pressure ulcer sites for patients confined to the supine position include the sacrum, coccyx, ischial tuberosities, and greater trochanters. Other common sites include the skin over the vertebrae, scapulae, elbows, knees, and heels in bed-bound and relatively immobile patients.

19. How long should a patient who has undergone a lumbar puncture remain on bed rest?
    A.   2 hours
    B.   4 hours
    C.   6 hours
    D.   8 hours
Answer: D. The patient may be ordered to lie flat for 8 to 12 hours after the procedure. If necessary, place a patient-care reminder on his bed to alert other staff members of this requirement.

20. A patient with a chest tube has fluctuations in the water-seal chamber when he breathes. You should:
    A.   check for air leaks.
    B.   check the drainage.
    C.   monitor the fluctuations.
    D.   clamp the chest tube.
Answer: C. If a patient with a chest tube has fluctuations in the water-seal chamber when he breathes, you should monitor the fluctuations. Normal fluctuations of 2″ to 4″ (5 to 10 cm) reflect pressure changes in the pleural spaces during respiration. To check for fluctuation when a suction system is being used, momentarily disconnect the suction system so that the air vent is opened and observe for fluctuations.

Chapter 5

21. The most common complication among patients receiving I.V. therapy is:
    A.   infiltration.
    B.   phlebitis.
    C.   fluid overload.
    D.   sepsis.
Answer: A. Infiltration (infused fluid leaking into the surrounding tissues) is a serious risk associated with I.V. therapy. It occurs when a venous access device punctures the vein wall or migrates out of the vein.

22. A commonly used central venous insertion site is the:
   A.   femoral vein.
   B.   brachial vein.
   C.   vena cava.
   D.   subclavian vein.
Answer: D. Commonly used central venous insertion sites include the subclavian, internal and external jugular, and brachiocephalic veins. Rarely, the femoral and brachial veins may be used.

23. Which nursing action can be used to help prevent air embolism when changing central venous I.V. tubing?
   A.   Place the patient in Trendelenburg's position.
   B.   Place the patient in the supine position.
   C.   Ask the patient to perform Valsalva's maneuver.
   D.   Avoid clamping the central venous catheter.
Answer: C. To help prevent air embolism when changing central venous I.V. tubing, teach the patient Valsalva's maneuver and ask him to demonstrate it to you at least twice. The patient may also need to perform Valsalva's maneuver when the catheter is open to the air.

24. During central venous catheter insertion, a patient complains of chest pain and shortness of breath and becomes cyanotic. He's most likely experiencing:
   A.   air embolism.
   B.   thrombosis.
   C.   local infection.
   D.   pneumothorax.
Answer: D. Signs of pneumothorax include chest pain, dyspnea, cyanosis, decreased breath sounds on affected side, and abnormal chest X-ray.

25. If a nurse suspects air embolism, she should:
   A.   set up for and assist with chest tube insertion.
   B.   have the patient perform Valsalva's maneuver.
   C.   clamp the catheter and turn the patient on his left side.
   D.   clamp the catheter and turn the patient on his right side.
Answer: C. The nurse should clamp the catheter and turn the patient on his left side, head down, so air can enter the right atrium and be dispersed via the pulmonary artery. This position should be maintained for 20 to 30 minutes.

Chapter 6

26. Pain rating scales are used to quantify pain:

    A.   quality.

    B.   onset.

    C.   intensity.

    D.   duration.

Answer: C. Pain rating scales are used to quantify pain intensity—one of pain's most subjective characteristics.

27. An anticonvulsant drug that may be used to treat neuropathic pain is:

    A.   gabapentin.

    B.   bupivacaine.

    C.   chlorzoxazone.

    D.   ropivacaine.

Answer: A. Anticonvulsant drugs may be used to treat neuropathic pain (pain generated by peripheral nerves). These agents include carbamazepine, clonazepam, divalproex sodium, gabapentin, lamotrigine, oxcarbazepine, phenytoin, tiagabine, topiramate, valproic acid, and zonisamide.

28. A physical therapy measure that involves the use of dry or moist heat to decrease pain is:

    A.   hydrotherapy.

    B.   thermotherapy.

    C.   cryotherapy.

    D.   transcutaneous electrical nerve stimulation.

Answer: B. Thermotherapy refers to the application of dry or moist heat to decrease pain, relieve stiff joints, ease muscle aches and spasms, improve circulation, and increase the pain threshold.

29. A patient is undergoing range-of-motion (ROM) exercises as part of a physical therapy routine. The nurse moves each of the patient's joints through its entire range. This type of ROM is known as:

    A.   passive ROM.

    B.   active ROM.

    C.   active-assistive ROM.

    D.   exercise.

Answer: A. Passive ROM refers to movement of a joint through its entire range without active muscle contraction. In this form of ROM, another person moves the patient's limb (or other body part) for him.

30. Which alternative and complementary therapy involves the concept of vital energy flowing in balance?

    A.   Yoga
    B.   Meditation
    C.   Therapeutic Touch
    D.   Biofeedback

Answer: C. Central to Therapeutic Touch is the concept of a universal life force, which is thought to permeate space and sustain all living organisms. Practitioners believe that, in healthy people, this vital energy flows freely in and through the body in a balanced way that nourishes all body organs; they also believe that illness is a result of disequilibrium in the energy field.

Chapter 7

31. Which color indicates a healthy wound and normal healing?

    A.   Black
    B.   Blue
    C.   Yellow
    D.   Red

Answer: D. If a wound bed is red (the color of healthy granulation tissue), the wound is healthy and normal healing is underway. When a wound begins to heal, a layer of pale pink granulation tissue covers the wound bed. As this layer thickens, it becomes beefy red.

32. The debridement technique that involves moisture-retentive dressings is:

    A.   sharp.
    B.   autolytic.
    C.   chemical.
    D.   mechanical.

Answer: B. Autolytic debridement involves the use of moisture-retentive dressings to cover the wound bed. Necrotic tissue is dissolved through self-digestion of enzymes in the wound fluid.

33. The type of wound that occurs when a mechanical force, such as shearing, scrapes the skin causing a partial-thickness wound is:

    A.   laceration.
    B.   skin tear.
    C.   bite.
    D.   abrasion.

Answer: D. An abrasion occurs when a mechanical force, such as friction or shearing, scrapes away a partial thickness of skin. Unless an unusually large amount of skin is involved or an infection develops, an abrasion is one of the least complicated traumatic wounds.

34. The type of dressing that's impermeable to oxygen and water and turns to a gel over time is:

A. hydrocolloid.
B. foam.
C. contact.
D. composite.

Answer: A. Hydrocolloid dressings are adhesive, moldable wafers made of a carbohydrate-based material. Most have a waterproof backing. They're impermeable to oxygen, water, and water vapor, and most hydrocolloid dressings provide some degree of absorption. These dressings turn to gel as they absorb moisture.

35. Growth factors are an example of which therapeutic modality?

A. Hydrotherapy
B. Laser therapy
C. Biotherapy
D. Hyperbaric oxygen therapy

Answer: C. Two biotherapy methods used in wound treatment include growth factors and living skin equivalents.

Chapter 8

36. Zamivir and oseltamivir are treatments for influenza:

A. types A and B.
B. types B and C.
C. types A and C.
D. type C only.

Answer: A. The neuramidase inhibitors zamivir and oseltamivir are indicated for influenza types A and B.

37. A patient with intermittent, crampy, abdominal pain that intensifies with stress or after meals and is accompanied by constipation alternating with diarrhea is experiencing:

A. gastroenteritis.
B. gastroesophageal reflux disease.
C. irritable bowel syndrome.
D. peptic ulcers.

Answer: C. The most commonly reported symptom of irritable bowel syndrome is intermittent, crampy, lower abdominal pain, which is usually relieved by defecation or passage of flatus. It typically occurs during the day and intensifies with stress or 1 to 2 hours after meals. The patient may experience constipation alternating with diarrhea, with one being the dominant problem. Mucus is usually passed through the rectum. Abdominal distention and bloating are common.

38. *Borrelia burgdorferi* is the causative organism of:
   A.   hepatitis.
   B.   tuberculosis.
   C.   Lyme disease.
   D.   multiple sclerosis.

Answer: C. Lyme disease is caused by the spirochete *Borrelia burgdorferi*, which is carried by deer ticks.

39. Dressler's syndrome may occur as a complication of:
   A.   myocardial infarction (MI).
   B.   multiple sclerosis.
   C.   pulmonary embolism.
   D.   stroke.

Answer: A. Dressler's syndrome, also known as *post-MI pericarditis*, can occur days to weeks after an MI. It causes residual pain, malaise, and fever.

40. A patient's X-rays show narrowing of joint spaces and cyst-like bony deposits. These findings may indicate:
   A.   osteoporosis.
   B.   osteoarthritis.
   C.   otitis media.
   D.   rheumatoid arthritis.

Answer: B. X-rays of a patient with osteoarthritis typically show narrowing of the joint space or margins and cystlike bony deposits in joint space and margins. Sclerosis of the subchondral space, joint deformity due to degeneration or articular damage, bony growths at weight-bearing areas, and fusion of joints may also occur.

Physiologic changes in aging

Aging is characterized by the loss of some body cells and reduced metabolism in other cells. These processes cause a decline in body function and changes in body composition. This chart will help you recognize the gradual changes in body function that normally accompany aging so you can adjust your assessment techniques accordingly.

Area of assessment	Age-related changes
Nutrition	• Protein, vitamin, and mineral requirements usually unchanged • Energy requirements possibly decreased by about 200 calories per day because of diminished activity • Loss of calcium and nitrogen (in patients who aren't ambulatory) • Diminished absorption of calcium and vitamins B_1 and B_2 due to reduced pepsin and hydrochloric acid secretion • Decreased salivary flow and decreased sense of taste (may reduce appetite) • Diminished intestinal motility and peristalsis of the large intestine • Brittle teeth due to thinning of tooth enamel • Decreased biting force • Diminished gag reflex • Limited mobility (may affect ability to obtain or prepare food)
Skin	• Facial lines resulting from subcutaneous fat loss, dermal thinning, decreasing collagen and elastin, and 50% decline in cell replacement • Delayed wound healing due to decreased rate of cell replacement • Decreased skin elasticity (may seem almost transparent) • Brown spots on skin due to localized melanocyte proliferation • Dry mucous membranes and decreased sweat gland output (as the number of active sweat glands declines) • Difficulty regulating body temperature because of decrease in size, number, and function of sweat glands and loss of subcutaneous fat
Hair	• Decreased pigment, causing gray or white hair • Thinning as the number of melanocytes declines • Pubic hair loss resulting from hormonal changes • Facial hair increase in postmenopausal women and decrease in men
Eyes and vision	• Baggy and wrinkled eyelids due to decreased elasticity, with eyes sitting deeper in sockets • Thinner and yellow conjunctivae; possible pingueculae (fat pads) • Decreased tear production due to loss of fatty tissue in lacrimal apparatus • Corneal flattening and loss of luster • Fading or irregular pigmentation of iris

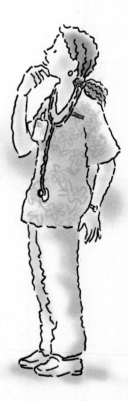

Area of assessment	Age-related changes
Eyes and vision *(continued)*	• Smaller pupil, requiring three times more light to see clearly; diminished night vision and depth perception • Scleral thickening and rigidity; yellowing due to fat deposits • Vitreous degeneration, revealing opacities and floating debris • Lens enlargement; loss of transparency and elasticity, decreasing accommodation • Impaired color vision due to deterioration of retinal cones • Decreased reabsorption of intraocular fluid, predisposing to glaucoma
Ears and hearing	• Atrophy of the organ of Corti and the auditory nerve (sensory presbycusis) • Inability to distinguish high-pitched consonants • Degenerative structural changes in the entire auditory system
Respiratory system	• Nose enlargement from continued cartilage growth • General atrophy of tonsils • Tracheal deviation due to changes in the aging spine • Increased anteroposterior chest diameter as a result of altered calcium metabolism and calcification of costal cartilage • Lung rigidity; decreased number and size of alveoli • Kyphosis • Respiratory muscle degeneration or atrophy • Declining diffusing capacity • Decreased inspiratory and expiratory muscle strength; diminished vital capacity • Lung tissue degeneration, causing decrease in lungs' elastic recoil capability and increase in residual capacity • Poor ventilation of the basal areas (from closing of some airways), resulting in decreased surface area for gas exchange and reduced partial pressure of oxygen • Oxygen saturation decreased by 5% • 30% reduction in respiratory fluids, heightening risk of pulmonary infection and mucus plugs • Lower tolerance for oxygen debt
Cardiovascular system	• Slightly smaller heart size • Loss of cardiac contractile strength and efficiency • 30% to 35% diminished cardiac output by age 70 • Heart valve thickening, causing incomplete closure (systolic murmur) • 25% increase in left ventricular wall thickness between ages 30 and 80 • Fibrous tissue infiltration of the sinoatrial node and internodal atrial tracts, causing atrial fibrillation and flutter • Vein dilation and stretching • 35% decrease in coronary artery blood flow between ages 20 and 60 • Increased aortic rigidity, causing increased systolic blood pressure disproportionate to diastolic, resulting in widened pulse pressure

Area of assessment	Age-related changes
Cardiovascular system *(continued)*	• Electrocardiogram changes: increased PR interval, QRS complex, and QT interval; decreased amplitude of QRS complex; shift of QRS axis to the left • Heart rate takes longer to return to normal after exercise • Decreased strength and elasticity of blood vessels, contributing to arterial and venous insufficiency • Decreased ability to respond to physical and emotional stress
GI system	• Diminished mucosal elasticity • Reduced GI secretions, affecting digestion and absorption • Decreased motility, bowel wall and anal sphincter tone, and abdominal wall strength • Liver changes: decreases in weight, regenerative capacity, and blood flow • Decline in hepatic enzymes involved in oxidation and reduction, causing less efficient metabolism of drugs and detoxification of substances
Renal system	• Decline in glomerular filtration rate • 53% decrease in renal blood flow secondary to reduced cardiac output and atherosclerotic changes • Decrease in size and number of functioning nephrons • Reduction in bladder size and capacity • Weakening of bladder muscles, causing incomplete emptying and chronic urine retention • Diminished kidney size • Impaired clearance of drugs • Decreased ability to respond to variations in sodium intake
Male reproductive system	• Reduced testosterone production, resulting in decreased libido as well as atrophy and softening of testes • 48% to 69% decrease in sperm production between ages 60 and 80 • Prostate gland enlargement, with decreasing secretions • Decreased volume and viscosity of seminal fluid • Slower and weaker physiologic reaction during intercourse, with lengthened refractory period
Female reproductive system	• Declining estrogen and progesterone levels (about age 50) cause: -cessation of ovulation; atrophy, thickening, and decreased size of ovaries -loss of pubic hair and flattening of labia majora -shrinking of vulval tissue, constricted introitus, and loss of tissue elasticity -vaginal atrophy; thin and dry mucus lining; more alkaline pH of vaginal environment -shrinking uterus -cervical atrophy, failure to produce mucus for lubrication, thinner endometrium and myometrium -pendulous breasts; atrophy of glandular, supporting, and fatty tissue -nipple flattening and decreased size -more pronounced inframammary ridges.

Area of assessment	Age-related changes
Neurologic system	• Degenerative changes in neurons of central and peripheral nervous system • Slower nerve transmission • Decrease in number of brain cells by about 1% per year after age 50 • Hypothalamus less effective at regulating body temperature • 20% neuron loss in cerebral cortex • Slower corneal reflex • Increased pain threshold • Decrease in stage III and IV of sleep, causing frequent awakenings; rapid eye movement sleep also decreased
Immune system	• Decline beginning at sexual maturity and continuing with age • Loss of ability to distinguish between self and nonself • Loss of ability to recognize and destroy mutant cells, increasing incidence of cancer • Decreased antibody response, resulting in greater susceptibility to infection • Tonsillar atrophy and lymphadenopathy • Lymph node and spleen size slightly decreased • Some active blood-forming marrow replaced by fatty bone marrow, resulting in inability to increase erythrocyte production as readily as before in response to such stimuli as hormones, anoxia, hemorrhage, and hemolysis • Diminished vitamin B_{12} absorption, resulting in reduced erythrocyte mass and decreased hemoglobin level and hematocrit
Musculoskeletal system	• Increased adipose tissue • Diminished lean body mass and bone mineral contents • Decreased height from exaggerated spinal curvature and narrowing intervertebral spaces • Decreased collagen formation and muscle mass • Increased viscosity of synovial fluid, more fibrotic synovial membranes
Endocrine system	• Decreased ability to tolerate stress • Blood glucose concentration increases and remains elevated longer than in a younger adult • Diminished levels of estrogen and increasing levels of follicle-stimulating hormone during menopause, causing coronary thrombosis and osteoporosis • Reduced progesterone production • 50% decline in serum aldosterone levels • 25% decrease in cortisol secretion rate

Less common disorders

Disease and causes	Pathophysiology	Signs and symptoms
Amyloidosis • Pressure caused by accumulation and infiltration of amyloid that leads to atrophy of nearby cells; abnormal immunoglobulin synthesis and reticuloendothelial cell dysfunction may occur • Familial inheritance in persons with Portuguese ancestry • May occur with tuberculosis, chronic infection, rheumatoid arthritis, multiple myeloma, Hodgkin's disease, paraplegia, brucellosis, and Alzheimer's disease	A rare, chronic disease of abnormal fibrillar scleroprotein accumulation that infiltrates body organs and soft tissues. Perireticular type affects the inner coats of blood vessels whereas pericollagen type affects the outer coats. Amyloidosis can result in permanent, even life-threatening, organ damage.	• Proteinuria, leading to nephrotic syndrome and eventually to renal failure • Heart failure caused by cardiomegaly, arrhythmias, and amyloid deposits in subendocardium, endocardium, and myocardium • Stiffness and enlargement of tongue, decreased intestinal motility, malabsorption, bleeding, abdominal pain, constipation, and diarrhea • Appearance of peripheral neuropathy • Liver enlargement, usually with azotemia, anemia, albuminuria and, rarely, jaundice
Ankylosing spondylitis • No known cause; strongly associated with presence of human leukocyte antigen-B27 • Familial inheritance	Fibrous tissue of the joint capsule is infiltrated by inflammatory cells that erode the bone and fibrocartilage. Repair of the cartilaginous structures begins with the proliferation of fibroblasts, which synthesize and secrete collagen. The collagen forms fibrous scar tissue that eventually undergoes calcification and ossification, causing the joint to fuse or lose flexibility.	• Intermittent lower back pain that's most severe after inactivity or in the morning • Stiffness, limited lumbar spine motion • Pain and limited expansion of chest • Peripheral arthritis in shoulders, hips, and knees • Kyphosis in advanced stages • Hip deformity and limited range of motion • Mild fatigue, fever, and anorexia or weight loss

Anthrax
• Infection of the skin, lungs, or GI tract that results from contact with *Bacillus anthracis* spores
	After infection, bacterium produces toxins that enter susceptible cells, leading to cell death; mechanism unknown.	Incubation is 12 hours to 5 days.
		• Red-brown bump on skin enlarges and swells around edges; a black scab forms after the bump blisters and hardens
		• Swollen lymph nodes
		• Muscle ache and headache
		• Nausea, vomiting, fever
		   Pulmonary anthrax
		• Respiratory problems that may progress to respiratory failure
		• Shock and coma
		   GI anthrax (rare)
		• Extensive bleeding; tissue death
		• Fatal if enters the bloodstream

Disease and causes	Pathophysiology	Signs and symptoms
Aspergillosis • Fungal infection caused by *Aspergillus* species; transmitted by inhalation of fungal spores or invasion of spores through wounds or injured tissue	*Aspergillus* species produce extracellular enzymes, such as proteases and peptidases that contribute to tissue invasion, leading to hemorrhage and necrosis.	Incubation is a few days to weeks. • May produce no symptoms or mimic tuberculosis, causing a productive cough and purulent or blood-tinged sputum, dyspnea, empyema, and lung abscesses *Allergic aspergillosis* • Wheezing, dyspnea, pleural pain, and fever *Aspergillosis endophthalmitis* • Appears 2 to 3 weeks after eye surgery • Cloudy vision, eye pain, and reddened conjunctiva • Purulent exudate on exposure to anterior and posterior chambers of the eye
Bell's palsy • Considered an idiopathic facial paralysis; infectious cause suggested	Blockage of the seventh cranial nerve due to inflammation around the nerve where it leaves bony tissue leads to unilateral or bilateral facial weakness or paralysis. The blockage may result from hemorrhage, tumor, meningitis, or local trauma.	• Unilateral facial weakness or paralysis, with aching at the jaw angle • Drooping mouth, causing salivation • Distorted taste • Impaired ability to fully close the eye on the affected side • Loss of taste and tinnitus
Botulism • Paralytic illness caused by an endotoxin produced by *Clostridium botulinum;* commonly caused by consumption of inadequately cooked, contaminated foods	The endotoxin acts at the neuromuscular junction of skeletal muscle, preventing acetylcholine release and blocking neural transmission, eventually resulting in paralysis.	Appears 12 to 36 hours after digesting food; severity depends on amount consumed *Initial signs* • Dry mouth, sore throat, weakness, dizziness, vomiting, and diarrhea *Cardinal signs* • Acute symmetrical cranial nerve impairment, followed by weakness and muscle paralysis • Mental or sensory processes not typically affected; if they are affected, they're usually associated with fever
Bronchiectasis • Conditions associated with continued damage to bronchial walls and abnormal mucociliary clearance cause tissue breakdown to adjacent airways; such conditions include cystic fibrosis, immunologic disorders, and recurrent bacterial respiratory tract infections	Inflammation and destruction of the structural components of the bronchial wall lead to chronic abnormal dilatation.	*In early stages* • Asymptomatic with complaints of frequent pneumonia or hemoptysis • Chronic cough producing foul-smelling, mucopurulent secretions • Coarse crackles during inspiration • Wheezing, dyspnea, sinusitis, fever, and chills

Disease and causes	Pathophysiology	Signs and symptoms
Bronchiectasis *(continued)*		*In advanced stage* • Chronic malnutrition and right-sided heart failure caused by hypoxic pulmonary vasoconstriction
Bronchiolitis • No known cause; may be associated with specific diseases or conditions, such as bone marrow, heart, or lung transplantation; rheumatoid arthritis; lupus erythematosus; and Crohn's disease	Infection or other unknown factors cause necrosis of the bronchial epithelium and destruction of ciliated epithelial cells. As the submucosa becomes edematous, cellular debris and fibrin form plugs in the bronchioles.	*Subacute symptoms* • Fever, persistent nonproductive cough, dyspnea, malaise, and anorexia • Physical assessment reveals dry crackles *Less common* • Productive cough, hemoptysis, chest pain, general aches, and night sweats
Celiac disease • Results from a complex interaction involving dietary, genetic, and immunologic factors	Ingestion of gluten causes injury to the villi in the upper small intestine, leading to a decreased surface area and malabsorption of most nutrients. Inflammatory enteritis also results, leading to osmotic diarrhea and secretory diarrhea.	• Recurrent diarrhea, abdominal distention, stomach cramps, weakness, or increased appetite without weight gain • Normochromic, hypochromic, or macrocytic anemia • Osteomalacia, osteoporosis, tetany, and bone pain in lower back, rib cage, and pelvis • Peripheral neuropathy, paresthesia, or seizures • Dry skin, eczema, psoriasis, dermatitis herpetiformis, and acne rosacea • Amenorrhea, hypometabolism, and adrenocortical insufficiency • Mood changes and irritability
Cholera • Acute enterotoxin-mediated GI infection caused by gram-negative bacillus, which is transmitted through water and food that's contaminated with fecal material from carriers or people with active infections	After ingestion of a significant inoculum, colonization of the small intestine occurs. The secretion of a potent enterotoxin results in a massive outpouring of isotonic fluid from the mucosal surface of the small intestine. Profuse diarrhea, vomiting, fluid and electrolyte loss occurs and may lead to hypovolemic shock, metabolic acidosis, and death.	Incubation period is several hours to 5 days • Acute, painless, profuse watery diarrhea, and vomiting • Intense thirst, weakness, and loss of skin tone • Muscle cramps • Cyanosis • Oliguria • Tachycardia • Falling blood pressure, fever, and hypoactive bowel sounds

Disease and causes	Pathophysiology	Signs and symptoms
Creutzfeldt-Jakob disease • Rare form of dementia • Prion infection	Organism infects the central nervous system, leading to myelin destruction and neuronal loss.	• Myoclonic jerking, ataxia, aphasia, vision disturbances, paralysis, and early abnormal EEG
Endocarditis • Infection of the endocardium of the heart caused by bacteria, viruses, fungi, rickettsiae, and parasites	Endothelial damage allows microorganisms to adhere to the surface, where they proliferate and promote the propagation of endocardial vegetation.	• Weakness and fatigue • Weight loss, fever, night sweats, and anorexia • Arthralgia, splenomegaly, and new systolic murmur
Esophageal varices • Portal hypertension	Shunting of blood to the venae cavae caused by portal hypertension, leading to dilation of esophageal veins.	• Hemorrhage and subsequent hypotension • Compromised oxygen supply • Altered level of consciousness
Fanconi's syndrome • Inherited renal tubular transport disorder	Changes in the proximal renal tubules caused by atrophy of epithelial cells and loss of proximal tube volume result in a shortened connection to glomeruli by an unusually narrow segment. Malfunction of the proximal renal tubules leads to hyperkalemia, hypernatremia, glycosuria, phosphaturia, aminoaciduria, uricosuria, retarded growth, and rickets.	Mostly normal appearance at birth with slightly lower birth weights • After 6 months: weakness, failure to thrive, dehydration, cystine crystals in the corners of the eye, and retinal pigment degeneration • Yellow skin with little pigmentation • Slow linear growth
Hypersplenism • Increased activity of the spleen, where all types of blood cells are removed from circulation due to chronic myelogenous leukemia, lymphomas, Gaucher's disease, hairy cell leukemia, and sarcoidosis	Spleen growth may be stimulated by an increase in its workload, such as the trapping and destroying of abnormal red blood cells.	• Enlarged spleen • Cytopenia
Idiopathic pulmonary fibrosis • Chronic progressive lung disease associated with inflammation and fibrosis • No known cause	Interstitial inflammation made up of an alveolar septal infiltrate of lymphocytes, plasma cells, and histiocytes. Fibrotic areas are composed of dense acellular collagen. Areas of honeycombing that form are composed of cystic fibrotic air spaces, commonly lined with bronchiolar epithelium and filled with mucus. Smooth muscle hyperplasia may occur in areas of fibrosis and honeycombing.	• Dyspnea • Nonproductive cough • Chest heaviness • Wheezing • Anorexia • Weight loss

Disease and causes	Pathophysiology	Signs and symptoms
Kaposi's sarcoma • Acquired immunodeficiency syndrome-related cancer	A malignant cancer arising from vascular endothelial cells, Kaposi's sarcoma affects endothelial tissue, which compromises all blood vessels.	• Red-purple circular lesions, slightly raised on the face, arms, neck, and legs • Internal lesions, especially in GI tract and brain, identified by biopsy
Keratitis • Inflammation of cornea caused by microorganisms, trauma, or autoimmune disorders	Bacterial infection leading to ulceration of the cornea.	• Decreased visual acuity • Pain • Photophobia
Kyphosis • An excessive anteroposterior curving of the spine caused by a congenital anomaly, tuberculosis, syphilis, malignant or compression fracture, arthritis, or rickets	Pathophysiology is related to causative factor.	• Abnormally rounded thoracic curve
Latex allergy • Hypersensitivity to products containing natural latex	Latex protein allergens trigger release of histamine and other mediators of the systemic allergic cascade in sensitized persons.	• Local dermatitis to anaphylactic reaction
Legionnaires' disease • Infection caused by gram-negative bacillus, *Legionella pneumophila*	Transmission of disease occurs with inhalation of organism carried in aerosols produced by air-conditioning units, water faucets, shower heads, humidifiers, and contaminated respiratory equipment.	• Dry cough • Myalgia • GI distress • Pneumonia • Cardiovascular collapse
Leprosy • Infection caused by *Mycobacterium leprae*	Chronic, systemic infection with progressive cutaneous lesions that attacks the peripheral nervous system.	• Skin lesions • Anesthesia • Muscle weakness • Paralysis
Medullary sponge kidney • Genetic disorder	Collecting ducts in the renal pyramids dilate, forming cavities, clefts, and cysts that produce such complications as calcium oxylate calculi and infections.	• Renal calculi • Hematuria • Infection (fever, chills, and malaise)

Disease and causes	Pathophysiology	Signs and symptoms
Myocarditis • Inflammation of the myocardium caused by bacterial, fungal, viral, or protozoal infections; heat stroke; ionizing radiation; rheumatic fever; and diphtheria	Initial infection triggers an autoimmune, cellular and, possibly, humoral response resulting in myocardial inflammation and necrosis.	• Rapid, irregular, and weak pulse • Chest tenderness • First heart sound resembles second heart sound • Fatigue
Neurofibromatosis • Inherited disorder	Group of developmental disorders of the nervous system, muscles, bones, and skin that affects the cell growth of neural tissue.	• Café-au-lait spots • Multiple, pediculated, soft tumors • Hearing loss
Osgood-Schlatter disease • No known cause	Osteochondrosis of the tibia; disease of the growth or ossification centers in children.	• Frequent fractures • Pain at inferior aspect of patella
Pediculosis • Infestation by the lice parasite	Ectoparasite that attaches itself to the hair shaft with claws, and feeds on blood several times daily; resides close to the scalp to maintain its body temperature. Itching may be caused by an allergic reaction to louse saliva or irritability.	• Itching • Eczematous dermatitis • Inflammation • Tiredness • Irritability • Weakness • Lice present in hair (head, axillary, and pubic)
Pheochromocytoma • Polyglandular multiple endocrine neoplasia	Tumor of the chromaffin cells of the adrenal medulla that causes an increased production of catecholamines.	• Hypertension • High blood glucose • High lipid levels • Headache • Palpitations • Sweating • Dizziness • Constipation • Anxiety
Pleurisy • Several causes, including lupus, rheumatoid arthritis, and tuberculosis	Inflammation of the pleura with exudation into the thoracic cavity and lung surface.	• Chilliness • Stabbing chest pain • Fever • Suppressed cough • Pallor • Dyspnea

Disease and causes	Pathophysiology	Signs and symptoms
Polycythemia vera • No known cause; possibly caused by a multipotential stem cell defect	Increased production of red blood cells, neutrophils, and platelets inhibits blood flow to microcirculation, resulting in intravascular thrombosis.	Usually no symptoms in early stages In later stages, related to expanded blood volume and system affected • Weakness, light-headedness, headache, vision disturbances, and fatigue • Hepatomegaly and splenomegaly
Pyloric stenosis • Congenital; no known cause	Pyloric sphincter muscle fibers thicken and become inelastic, leading to a narrowed opening. The extra peristaltic effort that's necessary leads to hypertrophied muscle layers of the stomach.	• Progressive nonbilious vomiting, leading to projectile vomiting at ages 2 to 4 weeks
Retinal detachment • Caused by trauma; can also occur after cataract surgery, severe uveitis, and primary or metastatic choroidal tumors	The neural retina separates from the underlying retinal pigment epithelium.	• Floaters, flashing lights, scotoma in peripheral visual field (painless) and, eventually, a curtain or veil occurs in the field of vision
Retinitis pigmentosa • Autosomal recessive disorder in 80% of affected children • Less commonly transmitted as an X-linked trait	Slow, degenerative changes in the rods cause the retina and pigment epithelium to atrophy. Irregular black deposits of clumped pigment are in equatorial region of retina and eventually in the macular and peripheral areas.	• Progressive night blindness, visual field constriction with ring scotoma, and loss of acuity progressing to blindness
Reye's syndrome • No known cause • Viral agents and drugs (especially salicylates) have been implicated	Mitochondrial dysfunction and fatty vacuolization of the liver and renal tubules leading to hepatic injury and central nervous system damage.	• Vomiting • Change in mental status progressing from lethargy to disorientation to coma
Rocky Mountain spotted fever • Infection caused by *Rickettsia rickettsii* carried by several tick species	*R. rickettsii* multiply within endothelial cells and spread through the bloodstream. Focal areas of infiltration lead to thrombosis and leakage of red blood cells into surrounding tissue.	• Fever, headache, mental confusion, and myalgia • Rash develops as small macules progress to maculopapules and petechiae (Initially, rash starts on wrists and ankles and spreads to trunk. A rash noted on palms and soles is especially diagnostic.)

Disease and causes	Pathophysiology	Signs and symptoms
Sarcoidosis • No known cause • Evidence suggests that the disease is the result of exaggerated cellular immune response to a limited class of antigens	Organ dysfunction results from an accumulation of T lymphocytes, mononuclear phagocytes, and nonsecreting epithelial granulomas, which distort normal tissue architecture.	• Mainly generalized, most commonly involving the lung, with resulting respiratory symptoms • Fever, fatigue, and malaise
Scabies • Human itch mite (*Sarcoptes scabiei* var. *hominis*)	Mite burrows superficially beneath stratum corneum, depositing eggs that hatch, mature, and reinvade the skin.	Occur from sensitization reaction against excreta that mites deposit • Intense itching, worsens at night; threadlike lesions on wrists, between fingers, and on elbows, axillae, belt line, buttocks, and male genitalia
Sjögren's syndrome • Autoimmune rheumatic disorder with no known cause; genetic and environmental factors may be involved	Lymphocytic infiltration of exocrine glands causes tissue damage that results in xerostomia and dry eyes.	*In xerostomia* • Dry mouth; difficulty swallowing and speaking; ulcers on the tongue, buccal mucosa and lips; severe dental caries *In ocular involvement* • Dry eyes; gritty, sandy feeling; decreased tearing; burning, itching, redness; and photosensitivity *Extraglandular* • Arthralgias, Raynaud's phenomenon, lymphadenopathy, and lung involvement
Strabismus • Eye malalignment that's frequently inherited; controversy exists whether amblyopia is caused by or results from strabismus	In paralytic (nonconcomitant) strabismus, paralysis of one or more ocular muscles may be caused by an oculomotor nerve lesion. In nonparalytic (concomitant) strabismus, unequal ocular muscle tone is caused by supranuclear abnormality within the central nervous system.	• Eye malalignment noticeable by external eye examination, ophthalmoscopic observation of the corneal light reflex in center of pupils, diplopia, and other vision disturbances
Thrombocythemia • *Primary:* no known cause • *Secondary:* caused by chronic inflammatory disorders, iron deficiency, acute infection, neoplasm, hemorrhage, or postsplenectomy	A clonal abnormality of a multipotent hematopoietic stem cell results in increased platelet production, although platelet survival is usually normal. If combined with degenerative vascular disease, may lead to serious bleeding or thrombosis.	• Weakness, hemorrhage, nonspecific headache, paresthesia, dizziness, and easy bruising

Disease and causes	Pathophysiology	Signs and symptoms
Thrombophlebitis • Caused by endothelial damage, accelerated blood clotting, and reduced blood flow	Alteration in epithelial lining causes platelet aggregation and fibrin entrapment of red blood cells, white blood cells, and additional platelets; the thrombus initiates a chemical inflammatory process in the vessel epithelium that leads to fibrosis, which may occlude the vessel lumen or embolize.	• Varies with site and length of affected vein • Affected area usually extremely tender, swollen, red, and warm to the touch
Trigeminal neuralgia • No known cause; possibly a compression neuropathy • At surgery or autopsy, the intracranial arterial and venous loops are found to compress the trigeminal nerve root at the brain stem	Painful disorder along the distribution of one or more of the trigeminal nerve's sensory divisions, most commonly the maxillary.	• Searing or burning pain lasting seconds to 2 minutes at the trigeminal nerve distribution • Touching a trigger point typically elicits pain
Vitiligo • No known cause; usually acquired but may be familial (autosomal dominant) • Possible immunologic and neurochemical basis suggested	Destruction of melanocytes (humoral or cellular) and circulating antibodies against melanocytes results in hypopigmented areas.	• Progressive, symmetrical areas of complete pigment loss with sharp borders, generally appearing in periorificial areas, flexor wrists, and extensor distal extremities
Wilson's disease • Inherited copper toxicosis	Defective mobilization of copper from hepatocellular lysosomes for excretion by way of bile allows excessive copper retention in the liver, brain, kidneys, and corneas, leading to tissue necrosis and subsequent hepatic and neurologic disorders.	• Kayser-Fleischer ring (rusty brown ring of pigment at periphery of corneas) • Signs of hepatitis leading to cirrhosis • Tremors, unsteady gait, muscular rigidity, inappropriate behavior, and psychosis • Hematuria, proteinuria, and uricosuria

English-Spanish quick reference guide

Use this list to help you communicate with your Spanish-speaking patients.

anemia	la anemia	heartbeat	el latido
angina	la angina	– irregular	– irregular
appendicitis	la apendicitis	– rhythmical	– riftmico
arteriosclerosis	la arteriosclerosis	– slow	– lento
arthritis	la artritis	– fast (tachycardia)	– taquicardia
asthma	el asma	heartburn	las agruras (el ardor), acedía
backache	el dolor de espalda	heart disease	la enfermedad del corazón
blindness	la ceguera	heart failure	el fallo cardíaco
bronchitis	la bronquitis	heart murmur	el soplo del corazón
burn (first,	la quemadura (de primer,	hemorrhage	la hemorragia
second, or third degree)	segundo o tercer grado)	hemorrhoids	las almorranas, las hemorroides
bursitis	la bursitis	hepatitis	la hepatitis
cancer	el cáncer	hernia	la hernia
chickenpox	la varicela, las viruelas locas	herpes	el herpes
chills	los escalofrios	high blood pressure	la presión alta
cold	el catarro, el resfriado	hives	la urticaria
cold sores	lasúlceras de la boca	hoarseness	la ronquera
constipation	el estreñimiento	ill	enfermo(a)
convulsion	la convulsión	illness	la enfermedad
cough	la tos	immunization	la inmunización
cramps	los calambres	infarct	el infarto
deafness	la sordera	infection	la infección
diabetes	la diabetes	inflammation	la inflamación
diarrhea	la diarrea	injury	el daño la lastimadura, la herida
discharge	el flujo	itch	la picazón, la comezón
dizziness	el vértigo, el mareo	jaundice	la piel amarilla, la ictericia
eczema	el eccema	kidney stone	el cálculo en el riñón,
emphysema	el enfisema		la piedra en el riñón
epilepsy	la epilepsia	laryngitis	la laringitis
fainting spell	el desmayo	lesion	la lesión, el daño
fatigue	la fatiga	leukemia	la leucemia
fever	la fiebre	lice	los piojos
flu	la influenza, la gripe	lump	el bulto
food poisoning	el envenenamiento por	malignancy	el tumor, la malignidad
	comestibles	malignant	maligno(a)
fracture	la fractura	measles	el sarampión
gallbladder attack	el ataque de la vesícula biliar	meningitis	la meningitis
gallstone	el cálculo biliar	menopause	la menopausia
gastric ulcer	la úlcera gástrica	metastasis	la metástasis
glaucoma	el glaucoma	migraine	la migrañia, la jaqueca
gonorrhea	la gonorrea	multiple sclerosis	la esclerosis múltiple
headache	el dolor de cabeza	mumps	las paperas
heart attack	el ataque al corazón	muscular dystrophy	la distrofia muscular
		mute	mudo(a)

English	Spanish
obese	obeso(a)
overdose	la sobredosis
overweight	el sobrepeso
pain	el dolor
– growing pain	– el dolor de crecimiento
– labor pain	– el dolor de parto
– phantom limb pain	– el dolor de miembro fantasma
– referred pain	– el dolor referido
– sharp pain	– el dolor agudo
– shooting pain	– el dolor punzante
– burning pain	– el dolor que arde
– intense pain	– el dolor intenso
– severe pain	– el dolor severo
– intermittent pain	– el dolor intermitente
– throbbing pain	– el dolor palpitante
palpitation	la palpitación
paralysis	la parálisis
Parkinson's disease	la enfermedad de Parkinson
pneumonia	la pulmonía
psoriasis	la psoriasis
pus	el pus
rash	la roncha, el salpullido, la erupción
relapse	la recaída
renal	renal
rheumatic fever	la fiebre reumitáca
roseola	la roséola
rubella	la rubéola
rupture	la ruptura
scab	la costra
scar	la cicatriz
scratch	el rasguño
senile	senil
shock	el choque
sore	la llaga
spasm	el espasmo
sprain	la torcedura
stomachache	el dolor del estómago
stomach ulcer	la úlcera del estómago
suicide	el suicidio
swelling	la hinchazón
syphilis	la sífilis
tachycardia	la taquicardia
toothache	el dolor de muela
toxemia	la toxemia
trauma	el trauma
tuberculosis	la tuberculosis
tumor	el tumor
ulcer	la úlcera
unconsciousness	la pérdida del conocimiento
virus	el virus
vomit	el vómito, los vómitos
wart	la verruga
weakness	la debilidad
wheeze	el jadeo, la silba
wound	la herida
yellow fever	la fiebre amarilla

Guide to laboratory test results

This chart provides normal values for common laboratory tests, including chemistry, hematology, and coagulation tests. Where indicated, conventional and SI units are given.

Comprehensive metabolic panel

Laboratory test	Conventional	SI Units
Albumin	3.5-5 g/dl	35-50 g/L
Alkaline phosphatase	45-115 U/L	45-115 U/L
ALT	Male: 10-40 U/L	0.17-0.68 µkat/L
	Female: 7-35 U/L	0.12-0.60 µkat/L
AST	12-31 U/L	0.21-0.53 µkat/L
Bilirubin, total	0.2-1 mg/dl	3.5-17 µmol/L
BUN	8-20 mg/dl	2.9-7.5 mmol/L
Calcium	8.2-10.2 mg/dl	2.05-2.54 mmol/L
Carbon dioxide	22-26 mEq/L	22-26 mmol/L
Chloride	100-108 mEq/L	100-108 mmol/L
Creatinine	Male: 0.8-1.2 mg/dl	62-115 µmol/L
	Female: 0.6-0.9 mg/dl	53-97 µmol/L
Glucose	70-100 mg/dl	3.9-6.1 mmol/L
Potassium	3.5-5 mEq/L	3.5-5 mmol/L
Protein, total	6.3-8.3 g/dl	64-83 g/L
Sodium	135-145 mEq/L	135-145 mmol/L

Lipid panel

Laboratory test	Conventional	SI Units
Total cholesterol	< 200 mg/dl	< 5.18 mmol/L
HDL cholesterol	$\geq$ 60mg/dl	$\geq$ 1.55 mmol/L
LDL cholesterol	< 130 mg/dl	< 3.36 mmol/L
VLDL cholesterol	< 130 mg/dl	< 3.4 mmol/L
Triglycerides	< 150 mg/dl	< 1.7 mmol/L

Thyroid panel

Laboratory test	Conventional	SI Units
T_3	80-200 ng/dl	1.2-3 nmol/L
T_4, free	0.9-2.3 ng/dl	10-30 nmol/L
T_4, total	5-13.5 mcg/dl	60-165 mmol/L
TSH	0.4-4.2 mIU/L	0.4-4.2 mIU/L

Other chemistry tests

Laboratory test	Conventional	SI Units
A/G ratio	3.4-4.8 g/dl	34-38 g/dl
Ammonia	< 50 ng/dl	< 36 µmol/L
Amylase	26-102 U/L	0.4-1.74 µkat/L
Anion gap	8-14 mEq/L	8-14 mmol/L
Bilirubin, direct	< 0.5 mg/dl	< 6.8 µmol/L
Calcitonin	Male: < 16 pg/ml	< 16 ng/L
	Female: < 8 pg/ml	< 8 ng/L
Calcium, ionized	4.65-5.28 mg/dl	1.1-1.25 mmol/L
Cortisol	a.m.: 7-25 mcg/dl	0.2-0.7 µmol/L
	p.m.: 2-14 mcg/dl	0.06-0.39 µmol/L
C-reactive protein	< 0.8 mg/dl	< 8 mg/L
Ferritin	Male: 20-300 ng/ml	20-300 mcg/L
	Female: 20-120 ng/ml	20-120 mcg/L
Folate	1.8-20 ng/ml	4.45-3 nmol/L
GGT	Male: 7-47 U/L	0.12-1.80 µkat/L
	Female: 5-25 U/L	0.08-0.42 µkat/L
Hb_{A1c}	4%-7%	0.04-0.07
Homocysteine	< 12 µmol/L	< 12 µmol/L
Iron	Male: 65-175 mcg/dl	11.6-31.3 µmol/L
	Female: 50-170 mcg/dl	9-30.4 µmol/L
Iron-binding capacity	250-400 mcg/dl	45-72 µmol/L
Lactic acid	0.5-2.2 mEq/L	0.5-2.2 mmol/L
Lipase	10-73 U/L	0.17-1.24 µkat/L
Magnesium	1.3-2.2 mg/dl	0.65-1.05 mmol/L
Osmolality	275-295 mOsm/kg	275-295 mOsm/kg
Phosphate	2.7-4.5 mg/dl	0.87-1.45 mmol/L
Prealbumin	19-38 mg/dl	190-380 mg/L
Uric acid	Male: 3.4-7 mg/dl	202-416 µmol/L
	Female: 2.3-6 mg/dl	143-357 µmol/L

Hematology tests

Laboratory test	Conventional	SI Units
Hemoglobin	Male: 14-17.4 g/dl	140-174 g/L
	Female: 12-16 g/dl	120-160 g/L
Hematocrit	Male: 42%-52%	0.42-0.52
	Female: 36%-48%	0.36-0.48
Red blood cell	Male: 4.5-5.5 million/mm³	$4.5\text{-}5.5 \times 10^{12}$/L
	Female: 4-5 million/mm³	$4\text{-}5 \times 10^{12}$/L

(continued)

Hematology tests
(continued)

Laboratory test	Conventional	SI Units
Leukocytes	4,000-10,000/mm^3	4-10 × 10^9/L
• Bands	0%-5%	0.03-0.08
• Basophils	0%-1%	0-0.01
• Eosinophils	1%-4%	0.01-0.04
• Lymphocytes	25%-40%	0.25-0.40
– B-Lymphocytes	270-640/mm^3	—
– T-Lymphocytes	1,400-2,700/mm^3	—
• Monocytes	2%-8%	0.02-0.08
• Neutrophils	54%-75%	0.54-0.75
Platelets	140,000-400,00/mm^3	140-400 × 10^9/L

Coagulation tests

Laboratory test	Conventional	SI Units
Activated clotting time	107 sec ± 13 sec	107 sec ± 13 sec
Bleeding time	3-6 min	3-6 min
D-dimer	< 250 mcg/L	< 1.37nmol/L
Fibrinogen	200-400 mg/dl	2-4 g/L
INR (therapeutic target)	2.0-3.0	2.0-3.0
Partial thromboplastin time	21-35 sec	21-35 sec
Prothrombin time	10-14 sec	10-14 sec

Glossary

aberrant conduction: abnormal pathway of an impulse traveling through the heart's conduction system

ablation: removal of a body part or the destruction of its function; surgical or radiofrequency removal of an irritable focus in the heart is used to prevent tachyarrhythmias

acidosis: condition in which excess acid or reduced bicarbonate in the blood drops the arterial pH below 7.35

action potential: electrical impulse across nerve or muscle fibers that have been stimulated

active transport: movement of solutes from an area of lower concentration to one of higher concentration (the solutes are said to move against the concentration gradient)

addiction: physical or psychological dependence on a substance or activity, characterized by a craving beyond the individual's voluntary control

adrenergic agonist: drug that mimics the effects of the sympathetic nervous system

adrenergic blocking drug: drug that interferes with transmission of nerve impulses to adrenergic receptors, allowing a parasympathetic response

afterload: resistance that the left ventricle must work against to pump blood through the aorta

agonist: drug that enhances or stimulates a receptor

air embolism: systemic complication of I.V. therapy that occurs when air is introduced into the venous system and includes such signs and symptoms as respiratory distress, unequal breath sounds, weak pulse, increased central venous pressure, decreased blood pressure, and loss of consciousness

albumin: protein that can't pass through capillary walls and that draws water into the capillaries by osmosis during reabsorption

alopecia: baldness that's partial or complete, local or general; in chemotherapy, caused by the destruction of rapidly dividing cells in the hair shaft or root

amplitude: height of a waveform

anaphylactic reaction (anaphylaxis): severe allergic reaction that may include flushing, chills, anxiety, agitation, generalized itching, palpitations, paresthesia, throbbing in the ears, wheezing, coughing, seizures, and cardiac arrest

angioedema: life-threatening reaction causing sudden swelling of tissues around the face, neck, lips, tongue, throat, hands, feet, genitals, or intestines

antagonist: drug that nullifies the action of an agonist drug at a receptor site

antibody: immunoglobulin molecule synthesized in response to a specific antigen

antidiuretic hormone (ADH): hormone produced in the hypothalamus and stored in the posterior pituitary gland that responds to osmolarity and blood pressure changes and also promotes water reabsorption by the kidneys

antigen: major component of blood that exists on the surface of blood cells and can initiate an immune response (a particular antigen can also induce the formation of a corresponding antibody when given to a person who doesn't normally have the antigen)

arrhythmia: disturbance of the normal cardiac rhythm from the abnormal origin, discharge, or conduction of electrical impulses

atrial kick: amount of blood pumped into the ventricles as a result of atrial contraction; contributes approximately 30% of total cardiac output

automaticity: ability of a cardiac cell to initiate an impulse on its own

bacterial phlebitis: painful inflammation of a vein that can occur with peripherally inserted central catheters; usually occurs after a long period of I.V. therapy

bactericidal: causing death of bacteria

bioavailability: rate and extent to which a drug enters the circulation, thereby gaining access to target tissue

biological response modifiers: agents used in biological therapy that alter the body's response to cancer

biphasic electrocardiogram complex: complex containing both an upward and a downward deflection; usually seen when the electrical current is perpendicular to the observed lead

blood-brain barrier: barrier separating the parenchyma of the central nervous system from the circulating blood, preventing certain substances from reaching the brain or cerebrospinal fluid

body surface area (BSA): area covered by a person's external skin that's calculated in square meters (m^2) according to height and weight; used to calculate safe pediatric dosages for all drugs and safe dosages for adult patients receiving extremely potent drugs or drugs requiring great precision, such as antineoplastic and chemotherapeutic agents

bundle-branch block: cardiac conduction abnormality in which an impulse is slowed or blocked as it travels through one of the bundle branches

capture: successful pacing of the heart, represented on the ECG tracing by a pacemaker spike followed by a P wave or QRS complex

cardiac output: amount of blood ejected from the left ventricle per minute; normal value is 4 to 8 L/minute

carotid sinus massage: manual pressure applied to the carotid sinus to slow the heart rate

central venous (CV) therapy: treatment in which drugs or fluids are infused directly into a major vein; used in emergencies, when a patient's peripheral veins are inaccessible, or when a patient needs infusion of a large volume of fluid, multiple infusion therapies, or long-term venous access (in CV therapy, a catheter is inserted with its tip in the superior vena cava, inferior vena cava, or right atrium of the heart)

central venous pressure (CVP): important indicator of circulatory function and the pumping ability of the right side of the heart; measured with a catheter placed in or near the right atrium

compensatory pause: period following a premature contraction during which the heart regulates itself, allowing the sinoatrial node to resume normal conduction

conduction: transmission of certain forms of energy, such as electrical impulses through the myocardium

conductivity: ability of one cardiac cell to transmit an electrical impulse to another cell

cross-sensitivity: hypersensitivity to similar I.V. drugs (if a patient is hypersensitive to a particular drug, he may be hypersensitive to other chemically similar drugs)

cytokines: type of biological response modifier— includes interferon, interleukins, tumor necrosis factor, and colony-stimulating factors

cytotoxic: destructive to cells

depolarization: response of a cell to an electrical impulse that causes movement of ions across the cell membrane, which triggers contraction

diastole: phase of the cardiac cycle when both atria (atrial diastole) or both ventricles (ventricular diastole) are at rest and filling with blood

diffusion: movement of solutes from an area of higher concentration to one of lower concentration by passive transport (a fluid movement process that requires no energy)

diluent: liquid used to reconstitute I.V. drugs that are supplied in powder form; for example, normal saline solution, sterile water for injection, dextrose 5% in water (some drugs should be reconstituted with diluents that contain preservatives)

drip factor: number of drops to be delivered per milliliter of solution in an I.V. administration set; measured in gtt/ml (drops per milliliter); listed on the package containing the I.V. tubing administration set

drip rate: number of drops of I.V. solution to be infused per minute; based on the drip factor and calibrated for the selected I.V. tubing

extracellular fluid (ECF): any fluid in the body that isn't contained inside the cells, including interstitial fluid, plasma, and transcellular fluid

extravasation: infiltration of irritating fluids, resulting in damage to surrounding tissues; a medical emergency

flow rate: number of milliliters of I.V. fluid to administer over 1 hour; based on the total volume to be infused in milliliters and the amount of time for the infusion

gluconeogenesis: conversion of protein to carbohydrates for energy; essential visceral proteins (serum albumin and transferrin) and somatic body proteins (skeletal, smooth muscle, and tissue proteins) are converted to energy in starvation or severe nutrient deficiencies; when essential body proteins break down, a negative nitrogen balance results (more protein is used by the body than is taken in)

glycogenolysis: in metabolism, the mobilization and conversion of glycogen to glucose in the body

hematoma: localized mass of extravasated blood that's confined within an organ or tissue

hemolytic reaction: life-threatening reaction to transfusions that occurs as a result of incompatible ABO or Rh blood or improper blood storage

hemothorax: bleeding into the pleural cavity; treated with the insertion of a chest tube for draining blood

hepatotoxicity: quality of being toxic to or capable of destroying liver cells

hirsutism: excessive growth of dark, coarse body hair in a masculine distribution

histamine-2 receptors: cells in the gastric mucosa that respond to histamine release by increasing gastric acid secretion

human leukocyte antigen (HLA): antigen that's essential to immunity; part of the histocompatibility system, which controls compatibility between transplant or transfusion recipients and donors

(generally, the closer the HLA match between donor and recipient, the less likely the tissue or organ will be rejected)

hydrothorax: infusion of a solution into the chest

hyperglycemia: high blood glucose seen especially in patients with diabetes mellitus; signs and symptoms include increased thirst, blurred vision, frequent urination, and fatigue

hyperosmolar hyperglycemic nonketotic syndrome (HHNS): metabolic syndrome that occurs primarily in patients with diabetes that's characterized by hyperglycemia, hyperosmolarity, and an absence of significant ketosis

hypertonic solution: solution with higher osmolarity (concentration) than the normal range of serum (275 to 295 mOsm/L), such as dextrose 5% in half-normal saline solution, dextrose 5% in normal saline solution, and dextrose 5% in lactated Ringer's solution

hypocalcemia: calcium deficiency; signs and symptoms include tingling in the fingers, muscle cramps, nausea, vomiting, hypotension, cardiac arrhythmias, and seizures

hypoglycemia: low blood glucose; signs and symptoms include sweating, shaking, and irritability

hypokalemia: low blood potassium; signs and symptoms include muscle weakness, paralysis, paresthesia, and arrhythmias

hypomagnesemia: low blood magnesium; patient may complain of tingling around the mouth or paresthesia in the fingers and may show signs of mental changes, hyperreflexia, tetany, and arrhythmias

hypophosphatemia: low blood phosphates; patient may be irritable or weak and may have paresthesia; in extreme cases, coma and cardiac arrest can occur

hypotonic solution: solution with lower osmolarity (concentration) than the normal range of serum (275 to 295 mOsm/L)—such as half-normal saline solution, 0.33% saline solution, or dextrose 2.5% in water—which hydrates cells while reducing fluid in the circulatory system

hypovolemic shock: shock due to loss of systemic volume; caused by internal bleeding, hemorrhage, or sepsis; signs and symptoms include increased heart rate, decreased blood pressure, mental confusion, and cool, clammy skin

idiosyncratic reaction: an inherent inability to tolerate certain therapeutic chemicals (for example, a tranquilizer may cause excitation rather than sedation in a particular patient)

incompatibility: an adverse reaction to I.V. therapy that results when I.V. solutions, drugs, or blood products are mixed together (in I.V. medication therapy, the more complex the solution, the greater the risk of incompatibility; in transfusion therapy, incompatibility of donor and recipient blood can cause serious adverse effects)

induration: tissue firmness that may occur around a wound margin following blanchable erythema or chronic venous congestion

infiltration: infusion of I.V. solution into surrounding tissues rather than the blood vessel; symptoms include discomfort, decreased skin temperature around the site, blanching, absent backflow of blood, and slower flow rate

insulin lipodystrophy: thickening of tissues and accumulation of fat at an injection site; results from too-frequent injection of insulin in the same site

interstitial fluid (ISF): extracellular fluid that bathes all cells in the body; accounts for about 75% of extracellular fluid

intracellular fluid (ICF): fluid that's contained inside the cells of the body

intrathecal: within the spinal canal

irritant: agent that, when used locally, produces a local inflammatory reaction

isotonic solution: solution with osmolarity that's within the normal range for serum (275 to 295 mOsm/L), such as lactated Ringer's solution and normal saline solution

micronutrients: essential dietary elements required only in small quantities; also called trace elements or trace minerals; examples include zinc, copper, chromium, iodide, selenium, and manganese

myelosuppression: interference with and suppression of the blood-forming stem cells in the bone marrow; a possible complication of chemotherapy

nadir: lowest point in some series of measurements, such as white blood cell, hemoglobin, or platelet levels

necrotic: pertaining to localized tissue death

nephrotoxicity: quality of being toxic to or capable of destroying kidney cells

neutropenia: abnormal decrease in circulating neutrophils

nociceptor: sensory receptor that conveys nociceptive information about a noxious stimulus

nomogram: table for estimating body surface area when a patient's weight and height are known

nonvesicant: agent that doesn't cause blisters

opioid: natural, semisynthetic, or synthetic drug that relieves pain by binding to opioid receptors in the nervous system

osmolarity: concentration of a solution expressed in milliosmols of solute per liter of solution

osmosis: passive transport of fluid across a membrane from an area of lower concentration to one of higher concentration that stops when the solute concentrations are equal

ototoxicity: potentially irreversible damage to the auditory and vestibular branches of the eighth cranial nerve; may cause hearing or balance loss

oxygen-hemoglobin affinity: tendency of hemoglobin to hold oxygen (When oxygen's hemoglobin affinity increases, oxygen stays in the patient's bloodstream and isn't released into other tissues. Oxygen's hemoglobin affinity can increase during blood storage, causing oxygen to stay in a patient's bloodstream rather than being released into other tissues. Signs of this reaction include a depressed respiratory rate, especially in patients with chronic lung disease.)

parasympatholytic drug: drug that blocks the effects of the parasympathetic nervous system, allowing a sympathetic response

parasympathomimetic drug: drug that mimics the effects of the parasympathetic nervous system

parenteral: any route other than the GI tract by which drugs, nutrients, or other solutions may enter the body (for example, I.V., I.M., or subcutaneously)

parenteral nutrition: therapy that provides calories from dextrose and one or more nutrients that keep the body functioning; ordered when a nutritional assessment reveals a nonfunctional GI tract, increased metabolic need, or a combination of both; administered through either a peripheral or central venous infusion device; solutions may contain one or more of the following: dextrose, proteins, lipids, electrolytes, vitamins, and trace elements

passive transport: fluid movement that requires no energy and in which solutes move from an area of higher concentration to one of lower concentration (this change is called moving down the concentration gradient and results in an equal distribution of solutes)

peripheral parenteral nutrition (PPN): delivery of nutrients through a short cannula inserted into a peripheral vein; generally provides fewer nonprotein calories than total parenteral nutrition because lower dextrose concentrations are used

peripherally inserted central catheter (PICC): central venous access device that's inserted through a peripheral vein with the tip ending in the superior or inferior vena cava; generally used when patients need frequent blood transfusions or infusions of caustic drugs or solutions; especially useful if the patient doesn't have reliable routes for short-term I.V. therapy

phlebitis: inflammation of a vein

photosensitivity reaction: increased reaction of the skin to sunlight; may result in edema, papules, urticaria, or acute burns

physiologic pump: mechanism that's involved in the active transport of solutes; for example, the sodium-potassium pump, which moves sodium ions out of cells to the extracellular fluid and potassium ions into cells from the extracellular fluid

pneumothorax: air in the thorax; signs and symptoms include chest pain, dyspnea, cyanosis, or decreased or absent breath sounds on the affected side (a thoracotomy should be performed and a chest tube inserted if pneumothorax is severe enough for intervention)

polymorphic ventricular tachycardia: type of ventricular tachycardia in which the QRS complexes change from beat to beat

pressure ulcer: wound that's the clinical manifestation of localized tissue death due to lack of blood flow in areas under pressure

pruritus: itching

reentry mechanism: failure of a cardiac impulse to follow the normal conduction pathway; instead, it follows a circular path

refractory period: brief period during which excitability in a myocardial cell is depressed

repolarization: recovery of the myocardial cells after depolarization during which the cell membrane returns to its resting potential

retrograde depolarization: depolarization that occurs backward toward the atrium instead of downward toward the ventricles; results in an inverted P wave

rhesus (Rh) system: in blood physiology, a major blood antigen system that consists of Rh-positive and Rh-negative groups (Rh-positive blood has a variant of the Rh antigen called a D antigen or D factor; Rh-negative blood doesn't have this antigen. A person with Rh-positive blood doesn't carry anti-Rh antibodies because they would destroy his red blood cells.)

saline lock: an intermittent infusion device that's flushed with saline

sepsis: infection of tissues with disease-causing microorganisms or their toxins; signs and symptoms include elevated temperature, glucose in the urine (glycosuria), chills, malaise, increased white blood cells (leukocytosis), and altered level of consciousness

stomatitis: inflammation of the mouth; in chemotherapy, painful mouth ulcers apparent 3 to 7 days after treatment begins, with symptoms ranging from mild to severe (accompanying pain can lead to malnutrition and fluid and electrolyte imbalance if the patient can't chew and swallow adequate food and fluid; treatment includes scrupulous oral hygiene and topical anesthetic mixtures)

tardive dyskinesia: disorder characterized by involuntary repetitious movements of the muscles of the face, limbs, and trunk; most commonly results from extended periods of treatment with phenothiazine drugs

tension pneumothorax: type of pneumothorax in which air leaks into the lungs but can't escape, causing pressure in the lungs and eventually leading to lung collapse; a medical emergency in which the patient exhibits signs of acute respiratory distress, asymmetrical chest wall movement and, possibly, a tracheal shift away from the midline (a chest tube must be inserted immediately, before respiratory and cardiac decompensation occur)

teratogenic: pertaining to the production of physical defects in an embryo or a fetus

thrombocytopenia: blood platelet depletion

thrombogenic: device or process that may cause or lead to thrombosis formation

thrombophlebitis: inflammation of the vein due to the formation of a blood clot

thrombosis: development of a thrombus (blood clot)

titration: gradual addition of a component to a solution that ends when no more of the component can be consumed by reaction in the solution (with I.V. therapy, you can accurately titrate medication doses by adjusting the concentration of the infusate and the administration rate)

total parenteral nutrition (TPN): delivery of nutrients through a central line and usually through the subclavian vein with the tip of the catheter in the superior vena cava; usually indicated when parenteral nutrition is needed for more than 5 days

transcellular fluids: form of extracellular fluid that includes cerebrospinal fluid, lymph, and fluids in such spaces as the pleural and abdominal cavities

transfusion reaction: adverse reaction to transfusion therapy, the most severe of which is a hemolytic reaction, which destroys red blood cells and may become life-threatening; signs include fever, chills, rigors, headache, and nausea

universal donor: person with group O blood, which lacks both A and B antigens and can be transfused in limited amounts in an emergency to any patient — regardless of the recipient's blood type — with little risk of adverse reaction

universal recipient: person with AB blood type, which has neither anti-A nor anti-B antibodies; may receive A, B, AB, or O blood

urticaria: vascular reaction of the skin characterized by the eruption of hives and severe itching

Valsalva's maneuver: maneuver involving forced exhalation against a closed glottis that increases pressure within the thoracic cavity, thereby impeding venous return of blood to the heart

vasoconstriction: narrowing of the lumen of a blood vessel

vasopressor: drug that stimulates contraction of the muscular tissue of the capillaries and arteries

vesicant: agent that causes or forms blisters

Internet resources

AIDS
CDC National Prevention Information
    Network
www.cdcnpin.org
Association of Nurses in AIDS Care
www.anacnet.org

Alzheimer's disease
The Alzheimer's Association
www.alz.org

Arthritis
Arthritis Foundation
www.arthritis.org
National Institute of Arthritis and
    Musculoskeletal and Skin Diseases
www.nih.gov/niams

Asthma
Asthma & Allergy Foundation of America
www.aafa.org
American Academy of Allergy, Asthma &
    Immunology
www.aaaai.org
American Lung Association
www.lungusa.org

Cancer
American Cancer Society
www.cancer.org
Skin Cancer Foundation
www.skincancer.org
Cancer Information Service
http://cis.nci.nih.gov

Dermatology
American Academy of Dermatology
www.aad.org

Diabetes
American Diabetes Association
www.diabetes.org
Juvenile Diabetes Research Foundation
    International
www.jdf.org

Gastrointestinal disorders
Crohn's and Colitis Foundation of America
www.ccfa.org
National Institute of Diabetes & Digestive &
    Kidney Diseases
www.niddk.nih.gov

Heart disease
American Heart Association
www.americanheart.org

Hemophilia
National Hemophilia Foundation
www.hemophilia.org

Hepatitis
American Liver Foundation
www.liverfoundation.org

Infectious diseases
Centers for Disease Control and Prevention
www.cdc.gov

Lyme disease
Lyme Disease Foundation
www.lyme.org

Miscellaneous
National Library of Medicine
www.nlm.nih.gov
American Academy of Family Physicians
www.aafp.org
National Heart, Lung, and Blood Institute
www.nhlbi.nih.gov
United Ostomy Association
www.uoa.org
Wound, Ostomy & Continence Nurse
    Society
www.wocn.org

Multiple sclerosis
National Multiple Sclerosis Society
www.nmss.org

Orthopedics
National Osteoporosis Foundation
www.nof.org

Pain
American Chronic Pain Association
www.theacpa.org
America Pain Society
www.ampainsoc.org

Parkinson's disease
National Parkinson Foundation
www.parkinson.org
American Parkinson Disease Foundation
www.apdaparkinson.com

Pediatrics
American Academy of Pediatrics
www.aap.org

Psychiatric and mental illness
National Mental Health Association
www.nmha.org

Renal
National Kidney Foundation
www.kidney.org

Sickle cell anemia
Sickle Cell Disease Association of America
www.sicklecelldisease.org

Stroke
National Stroke Association
www.stroke.org
National Institute of Neurological Disorders
    and Stroke
www.ninds.nih.gov

Thyroid
Thyroid Foundation of America
www.tsh.org

Selected references

ACLS Provider Manual, Dallas: American Heart Association, 2004.

"ASPAN Pain and Comfort Clinical Guideline," *Journal of Perianesthia Nursing* 18(4):232-36, August 2003.

Assessment Made Incredibly Easy, 3rd ed. Philadelphia: Lippincott Williams & Wilkins, 2005.

Bickley, L. *Bates' Guide to Physical Examination and History Taking,* 8th ed., Philadelphia: Lippincott Williams & Wilkins, 2005.

Cardiovascular Care Made Incredibly Easy. Philadelphia: Lippincott Williams & Wilkins, 2005.

Comprehensive Accreditation Manual for Hospitals: The Official Handbook, Oakbrook Terrace, Ill.: Joint Commission on Accreditation of Healthcare Organizations, 2005.

ECG Interpretation Made Incredibly Easy, 3rd ed. Philadelphia: Lippincott Williams & Wilkins, 2005.

English and Spanish Medical Words & Phrases, 3rd ed. Philadelphia: Lippincott Williams & Wilkins, 2004.

Fischbach, F.T. *A Manual of Laboratory and Diagnostic Tests,* 7th ed. Philadelphia: Lippincott Williams & Wilkins, 2004.

Guideline for the Management of Cancer Pain in Adults and Children, Glenview Ill.: American Pain Society, 2005.

Handbook of Geriatric Nursing Care, 2nd ed. Philadelphia: Lippincott Williams & Wilkins, 2003.

Hess, C. *Clinical Guide to Wound Care,* 5th ed. Philadelphia: Lippincott Williams & Wilkins, 2005.

Infusion Nurses Society. "Infusion Nursing Standards of Practice," *Journal of Intravenous Nursing* 23(6S): S1-S85. November/December 2000.

Masoorli, S., and Angeles, T. "Getting a Line on Central Venous Access Devices," *Nursing2002* 32(4):36-47. April 2002.

Medication Administration Made Incredibly Easy. Philadelphia: Lippincott Williams & Wilkins, 2003.

Nursing2006 Drug Handbook, 26th ed. Philadelphia: Lippincott Williams & Wilkins, 2006.

Nursing Diagnoses: Definitions and Classification 2005-2006. Philadelphia: North American Nursing Diagnosis Association, 2005.

Nursing Procedures, 4th ed. Philadelphia: Lippincott Williams & Wilkins, 2004.

Pain Management Made Incredibly Easy. Philadelphia: Lippincott Williams & Wilkins, 2003.

Pathophysiology Made Incredibly Easy, 3rd ed. Philadelphia: Lippincott Williams & Wilkins, 2006.

Perry, A., and Potter, P. *Clinical Nursing Skills and Techniques,* 5th ed. St. Louis: Mosby–Year Book, Inc., 2002.

"Pressure Ulcers in Adults: Prediction and Prevention." *Clinical Practice Guideline Number 3 AHCPR Pub. No 92-0047, May 1992.*

Psychiatric Nursing Made Incredibly Easy. Philadelphia: Lippincott Williams & Wilkins, 2004.

"Treatment of Pressure Ulcers." *Clinical Guideline Number 15 AHCPR Publication No. 95-0652: December 1994.*

Wound Care Made Incredibly Easy. Philadelphia: Lippincott Williams & Wilkins, 2003.

Index

i refers to an illustration; t refers to a table; **boldface** indicates color pages.

i refers to an illustration; t refers to a table; **boldface** indicates color pages.

i refers to an illustration; t refers to a table; **boldface** indicates color pages.

i refers to an illustration; t refers to a table; **boldface** indicates color pages.

i refers to an illustration; t refers to a table; **boldface** indicates color pages.

i refers to an illustration; t refers to a table; **boldface** indicates color pages.